THE KETOGENIC BIBLE

The Authoritative Guide to Ketosis

Dr. Jacob Wilson & Ryan Lowery, PhD (c)

Victory Belt Publishing

Las Vegas

First Published in 2017 by Victory Belt Publishing Inc.

ISBN-13: 978-1-628601-04-6

Interior Design by Yordan Terziev and Boryana Yordanova

Printed in Canada

TC 0117

Acknowledgments

> If I have seen further, it is by standing upon the shoulders of giants.
> —Sir Isaac Newton

This book is truly the result of work by a conglomeration of amazing people who have inspired us to be better and to dive deeper, and who have supported us each and every step of the way. Without them, this book would not have been possible and the research along with the passion we share for this very topic would not exist.

To begin, we want to thank our friends and colleagues who helped inspire this book and have supported us throughout its writing: Victoria Adelus, Dr. Peter Attia, Tom Bilyeu, Luciano Bruno, Dr. Stephen Cunnane, Dr. Dom D'Agostino, David Diamond, Brunno Falcao, Bella Falconi, Josh Field, Glen Finkel, Dr. Ken Ford, Andy and Sal Frisella, Dr. Jason Fung, Ben Greenfield, Chris Harding, Dr. Maleah Holland, Jordan Joy, the communities at Ketogains, Ketogenic.com, and Ketovangelist, Dr. Eric Kossoff, Emily Maguire, Drew Manning, Yemeni Mesa, Jimmy Moore, Dr. Mary Newport, Tim Noakes, Daniel Orrego, Ben Pakulsi, Ron and Shannon Penna, Dr. David Perlmutter, Dr. Stephen Phinney, Craig Preisendorf, Dr. Angela Poff, Dr. Mike Roberts and the entire Auburn crew, Dr. Adrienne Scheck, Dr. Thomas Seyfried, Tim Skwiat, Karen Thompson, Brian Underwood, the Victory Belt team, Leanne Vogel, Dr. Jeff Volek, Shawn Wells, Dr. Eric Westman, Todd White, Robb Wolfe, and many more.

We are blessed to be surrounded by "giants" who have been extremely successful and fulfilled, and who continue to share our mission to help change people's lives and make this world a better place. Thank you all for being mentors and leaders for us every day.

> Teamwork is the ability to work together toward a common vision. The ability to direct individual accomplishments toward organizational objectives. It is the fuel that allows common people to attain uncommon results.
> —Andrew Carnegie

You are only as good as your team. Fortunately, our team at ASPI is much more than that—we truly constitute a family. Every single person there had a hand in making this book become a reality, and without each and every one of them it would not have been possible: Andres Ayesta, Andrew Barninger, Sam Beeler, Alex Burton, Jalissa Harris, Paul Hauser, Dr. Ashley Holly, Chris Irvin, Matthew Sharp, Matt Stefan, William Wallace, Acadia Webber, and our entire training staff. All of you continue to impress us with your unwavering commitment to change lives through science and innovation. That commitment comes through in this work of art we all put together, and for that, we are forever grateful.

> When everything goes to hell, the people who stand by you without flinching—they are your family.
> —Jim Butcher

From the bottom of our hearts, we would like to dedicate this book to our family and friends in thanks for their unwavering support, especially over the last several years. In order to write this book, we sacrificed birthdays, holidays, weekends, and even vacations, yet every step of the way our family and friends were there to support us. To our immediate family (Anita, Floyd, Stephanie, Gabriel, and Raudel, and Joan, Galen, and Steven), thank you for always being there for us during late-night calls and whenever we needed it the most. Everyone's love and guidance helped us conquer the unimaginable, and we hope to inspire and help people to the same degree you have helped us over the years. We love every one of you tremendously and hope this book serves as a symbol of our determination to change the world for the best.

CONTENTS

INTRODUCTION

They say that a lifetime flashes by in what seems like the blink of an eye. That minute can either come and go or create a revelation heard 'round the world. We were raised to help inspire people to do the latter. We believe that this is our calling and that the ketogenic diet is a medium to inspire others and change the world as we know it.

Where It All Started: Jacob's Story

My story begins in Richmond, California. I was born to Floyd and Anita Wilson, the two best parents a kid could hope for. My parents grew up in San Francisco and had very little as kids. Working sometimes three or four jobs to take care of us, my dad realized that his children needed a strong education. I remember my parents making a huge deal anytime I brought home a drawing, poem, or paper. They made me feel as if the scribbled portrait I'd made was a work that Picasso himself would have been proud of! On the first Halloween that I dressed up for—I must have been about five years old—my parents bought me a scientist's kit. It had a lab coat, funny glasses, and a chemistry set. The instant I put on the lab coat, I realized my calling: I would be a scientist. This was no fleeting moment.

I was the second of two boys. As you can imagine, my mom had to be a saint to deal with that much testosterone! My dad was obsessed with sports, and this drove us to take up hockey. I loved hockey and memorized every key athlete in NHL history. After graduating from high school in two and a half years, I knew that I wanted to take a shot at the big time. My dad encouraged me to go to the mecca of hockey: Canada.

Canadian Junior Hockey is the equivalent of college football in the United States. It is literally a national pastime; the entire country takes great pride in the sport. Up there, the competition is fierce. I was only five-foot-eight and weighed 150 pounds soaking wet. This predicament caused me to study the impact of nutrition, psychology, and training on human performance and body composition in an effort to gain weight to maximize my performance. Soon I became fascinated with these topics and decided to dedicate my life to them. After several years of hockey, I threw myself into school full-time. This passion carried me all the way through my PhD, where I studied a substance called beta-hydroxy-beta-methylbutyrate (HMB), which is very similar to the ketone body beta-hydroxybutyrate (BHB). We found that when HMB was given to humans, it sped recovery, blunted age-related declines in muscle mass, and elevated protein synthesis, an important process for building muscle.

In 2008, near the end of my doctoral program, I met Dominic D'Agostino at an experimental biology conference. I noticed that Dr. D'Agostino didn't consume many carbohydrates. In fact, his diet consisted primarily of sardines and coconut oil! I grew fascinated and found out that he was studying BHB. His strict ketogenic diet allowed him to eat only twice a day without crashing. The diet fascinated me. After graduating from Florida State University in 2010 with my doctorate in skeletal muscle physiology, I started a research laboratory dedicated to nutrition and human performance at University of Tampa.

In Tampa, I kept in touch with Dr. D'Agostino and developed a great relationship with his lab. I also was fortunate to cross paths with the brightest young star and scientist I have come across to date. His name is Ryan Lowery. It's rare to meet a true genius, but Ryan is one such person. Soon after we met in 2010, we attended the national conference of the National Strength and Conditioning Association (NSCA), which opened us up to a whole new world of research. Since then, we have published more than 100 papers, book chapters, and abstracts together.

Beginnings:
The Lowery Perspective

They say that the people who are crazy enough to think they can change the world are the ones who actually do. Fortunately for me, I'm surrounded by Jacob and an entire crazy team, all of whom share the same vision: to inspire and change lives through science and innovation. I never would have dreamed of getting to this point, but very early on in my life, I knew that I had a bigger mission, and when the stars align, anything is possible.

For me, it all started in Butler, New Jersey, a small suburb about an hour outside of New York City. Butler has that *Friday Night Lights* feel, where football takes precedence and you know every person in your high school graduating class. Growing up, I was fortunate to have a tight-knit group of friends who shared my passion for sports. These friends, along with my teachers and coaches, pushed me to work hard both in the classroom and on the field. Fortunately, my relentless work ethic combined with incredible support and guidance allowed me achieve some great feats that set me on my current path. I attribute that work ethic to the principles my parents instilled in my brother, Steven, and me from an early age. My dad, Galen, and my mom, Joan—my biggest supporters and greatest mentors—taught us three core values:

1) Respect

2) Passion

3) Optimism

They instilled within us a commitment to excellence and a sense of humility. Like most teenagers, we thought it was overkill at the time, but as I sit here writing this, I am so grateful for what they taught me. Above all, my parents stressed the importance of education, personal development, and helping others along the way.

The summer before I entered junior high school, I fractured my elbow in a freak accident while playing outside. After seeing a physical therapist regularly for over a year, I decided I wanted to pursue physical therapy as a career. I always knew I wanted to help people and be in and around sports, but I could never wrap my head around what to do. The vision was being painted; I could see it now: Dr. Lowery, DPT. I had that vision prior to becoming a teenager and still strive to get there, one day, via a slightly different path. Sometimes in life things happen that just don't make sense and can take the wind out of our sails. For me, that crushing blow came in junior high, when I experienced the first big loss of my life.

Septicemia, adult respiratory distress syndrome, severe coronary heart disease, multi-organ failure, diabetes, and obesity: It pains me to type these diagnoses from the official autopsy report of Marlayne Makovec, my 62-year-old grandmother, whose life ended far too early and abruptly. The autopsy read, "She was an obese woman in moderate to severe respiratory distress, lethargic." That doesn't define my grandmother. It doesn't mention that she was the most caring, considerate, and passionate person I had ever known. It doesn't mention that she was the glue holding our entire family together. It doesn't mention that she left behind a loving husband, beautiful children, and numerous grandchildren, all of whom loved her more than you can imagine. All that was written were the reasons she was no longer here. My grandmother was gone, and it was the first real loss I saw my family endure. How did it happen? Could it have been prevented?

The experience of losing my grandmother and the questions her death raised stayed with me through the next several years of my life. I was your typical high school student-athlete, ranking at the top of my class while also serving as captain of the baseball and football teams. Though it was hundreds of miles away from my family and friends, I ended up committing to the University of Tampa to play baseball and pursue my undergraduate degree. I was determined to figure out a way to use my past experiences for good and to help change people's lives for the better so that they didn't have to have experiences similar to my grandmother's.

Upon entering my first health science class freshman year, I realized that God had a much larger vision for me and that Tampa was exactly where I needed to be to live out that vision. Much to my surprise, I encountered a professor lecturing with much excitement on the same topics I was interested in. I'd found a guy who shared my vision and passion to impact the world. That professor was

Jacob Wilson. Fortunately for me, he saw the same enthusiasm in me early on. Jacob took me under his wing and introduced me to the world of research. He's been a mentor to me ever since, and we have never looked back. Along the way, Jacob and I, along with Shawn Wells, another incredible mentor and friend, attended a national conference that ultimately would play a vital role in why we are writing this book today.

The Turning Point

At the 2011 National Strength and Conditioning Association conference, we attended a lecture by our now good friends and colleagues, Dr. Jeff Volek and Dr. Steve Phinney, true pioneers in the ketogenic dieting field. These scientists gave a phenomenal presentation on ketogenic dieting and performance. At the end, an audience member stood up and asked, "What data is there on ketogenic dieting and resistance training in athletes?" In response, Dr. Volek said, "We currently do not have any controlled studies on this topic." Almost simultaneously, we looked at each other and said the exact same thing: "We have a lot of work to do!"

From that point forward, we jumped headfirst into researching ketogenic dieting, exogenous ketones, and their impact on body composition, molecular signaling, and performance. We have conducted extensive research not only on the ketogenic diet and resistance training but also on the impact of both the diet and exogenous ketones on aging, mitochondrial health, and cognitive function. More recently, we stepped out of traditional academia and created the most advanced laboratory in the world for the study of human performance: the Applied Science and Performance Institute (ASPI), located in Tampa, Florida. Our mission is to help people see the world not as it is but as it could be by redefining the limits of science—to truly change lives through science and innovation and #makepositivitylouder. Every day we strive to help improve lives, educate people, and create a lasting impact that will live long beyond us.

About This Book

This book is the culmination of decades of research broken down in a simple, relatable manner. *The Ketogenic Bible* is targeted toward people who are just being introduced to ketosis, yet it also appeals to those looking for more scientific information on how ketosis can be applied in specific situations. Whether you have no idea what ketosis is or you are a leading researcher in this field, this book is intended to serve as a resource for you.

Because we are scientists, we have included hundreds, if not thousands, of citations throughout this book. Don't let these citations intimidate you; rather, view them as affirmation that the information presented here is more than just opinion.

We created this book so that if you are interested in understanding more about ketosis, you can equip yourself with the tools necessary to answer any question that you have or that someone else throws your way. *The Ketogenic Bible* features:

- a detailed history of the ketogenic diet
- a general guide to what ketosis and the ketogenic diet are
- areas in which the ketogenic diet can be advantageous
- advanced as well as quick and easy ketogenic recipes
- the first material ever published in a book on exogenous ketones and their role in ketosis

Feel free to skip around the book, especially if you are interested in a certain aspect of the ketogenic diet or exogenous ketone supplementation. Use this book as a guide to further your exploration and understanding of ketosis as a whole.

The Ketogenic Bible is the result of countless hours spent both in the lab and interacting with the greatest minds in the world on this topic. From the bottom of our hearts, we hope that you enjoy reading this book as much as we have enjoyed the journey we took to construct it.

Chapter 1:

KETOSIS: THE BASICS

Because you've picked up this book, you likely are interested in learning more about the ketogenic lifestyle and what it means to be in a state of ketosis.

For our entire lives, we've been told that the primary source of energy for our bodies is carbohydrates, or glucose. However, there is an alternative fuel source that our bodies can use under various conditions—a fuel source that is more efficient and often underutilized. That source is ketones.

Ketone bodies are produced when the body metabolizes, or breaks down, fat. The cells in the body are able to utilize these ketones as fuel to help power everyday functions. There are three kinds of ketone bodies:

- acetoacetate (AcAc)

- beta-hydroxybutyrate (BHB)

- acetone (Acetone is actually produced by breaking down acetoacetate, making it more of a by-product, but for our purposes, it can be considered a ketone body.)

Each type of ketone body serves unique functions and can be tested for. For example, BHB in the blood can be tested using a finger prick, AcAc in the urine can be measured using a urine strip, and acetone in the breath can be measured using a breath meter.

All of us, at some point in our lives and routinely throughout the day, have some amount of ketones in our blood, yet we often don't realize it. For example, if you ate dinner at 5 p.m. and didn't eat again until 10 a.m. the next day, you likely would be in a minor state of ketosis since you hadn't eaten food and had been fasting for seventeen hours. Our bodies naturally make ketones under these circumstances; however, most people never achieve a consistent state of ketosis due to the constant supply of carbohydrates in their diet. Therefore, instead of breaking down and metabolizing fat, our bodies metabolize carbohydrates—or, rather, glucose. In other words, when glucose is available in the blood, the body will use that to make energy instead of dietary fat or stored body fat. However, when glucose isn't as readily available (glucose is still around but isn't as high), the body turns to breaking down fat, and ketones become its primary fuel source.

Ketosis is, essentially, the state of having elevated ketone levels, typically above 0.5 millimole per liter, or mmol/L. How a state of ketosis is induced, how high a person's blood ketones are, and what benefits are achieved from that degree of ketosis vary widely from individual to individual.

Normal Carbohydrate Diet
Ketone levels of 0–0.4 mmol/L, blood glucose levels of 80–120, and no change in blood pH.

Prolonged Fasting / Ketogenic Diet
Ketone levels of 0.5–7 mmol/L, blood glucose levels of 60–120, and no change in blood pH. Results in improvements in health.

Diabetic Ketoacidosis
Ketone levels of >15–25 mmol/L, blood glucose levels of >200, and very low blood pH. Can be fatal!

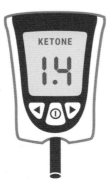

Figure 1.1. *Differences in degrees of ketosis.*

The Other Fuel

For centuries, scientists have known that body cells are fueled by glucose; however, it wasn't until the 1950s that scientists found out our bodies can function on an entirely unique energy source: ketones. Over a hundred years ago, in 1915, Dr. Francis Benedict published a landmark paper on fasting and fuel utilization. He discovered that the body can hold only a small amount of glycogen, the stored form of glucose—about 2,000 calories' worth. At that time it was believed that after glycogen runs out, the only way to fuel the body would be to break down muscle and organs (bodily tissue) at an accelerated rate in order to provide glucose (Cahill, 2006). (The liver can turn protein into glucose through a process called gluconeogenesis; more on that on page 18.) The result would be sustained glucose for the brain at the expense of the body's other vital tissues—certainly not an ideal process.

For a long time, ketones were even believed to be toxic. This misunderstanding dates back to the 1920s and the discovery of insulin. As doctors started to use it to treat diabetes, they found that too much insulin caused blood glucose to drop dangerously low, a condition known as hypoglycemia, which could result in unconsciousness, coma, and even death. When patients with hypoglycemia were given carbohydrates, the symptoms were reversed. (We've all experienced some form of hypoglycemia. Some people refer to this as being "hangry.") This led scientists to believe that the brain and central nervous system were fueled entirely by glucose (Owen, 2005). Since individuals with uncontrolled diabetes had ketones in their blood, researchers believed that ketones were toxic by-products of the disease. It wasn't until George Cahill started challenging this theory in the 1960s that people started to realize that glucose isn't the only fuel for the brain and that the previously thought "toxic by-product" might be an alternative fuel source for our bodies (Cahill et al., 1966).

Around the mid-1950s, researchers began to consider using fasting to treat obesity (Cahill et al., 1966) and started investigating the impact of fasting on fuel utilization in the brain and other tissues. Dr. Cahill and his colleagues, profound scientists, began to question the idea that the brain depends solely on glucose for energy, especially in a fasted state. Cahill reasoned that since the body can hold only a limited amount of glycogen, if glucose were the body's only fuel (with protein as a costly emergency backup that would damage body tissues), then fasting would result in death in eight to eighteen days. Believing that there had to be an alternative explanation for how the body is fueled, Cahill rolled the dice and had six students fast for eight days. (A study like this would never be approved today, but it provided incredible findings.) One of two things could happen: either the students would die, or they would live and Cahill would have discovered that there is an alternative source of energy for the brain. Since George Cahill is a legend in history books and not a prisoner in the state penitentiary, you can guess the outcome. He found that the students' glucose levels fell from around 80 mg/dL on day 1 to 65 mg/dL on day 3 and stayed at that level for the five remaining days of the study. On day 3, their blood ketone levels had risen from 0 to 1.6 mmol/L, and on day 8, those levels had risen to 4.2 mmol/L—without negatively affecting the pH, or acidity, of their blood. Additionally, their fasting insulin levels were cut in half. Cahill's research provided the first proof that the brain can use a fuel source other than glucose: ketones.

Diet-Induced Ketosis and the Ketogenic Diet Defined

Fortunately, scientists soon discovered that the absence of carbohydrates, even in the presence of food consumption (i.e., the origins of a ketogenic diet), could mimic this fasted state and that ketosis could be induced by altering the diet instead. Soon thereafter, researchers began to focus on the kind of diet that induces ketosis—one that triggers the production of ketones—the ketogenic diet.

Ms. B's Forty-Day Fast

Ms. B., a very intelligent nurse who happened to be overweight (approximately 280 pounds), wanted to change her body composition and improve her health. Fearing heart failure, she entered a six-week starvation study conducted by a researcher in Dr. Cahill's lab named Dr. Owen. When Dr. Owen was asked why he would undertake such an extreme experiment, he answered, "Jesus fasted forty days and forty nights; and afterward he hungered" (Matthew 4:2). What his team found was astonishing! Results showed that Ms. B. derived two-thirds of the fuel for her brain from ketones, while her blood ketone levels did not exceed 7 mmol/L even after forty-plus days of fasting. From here, the scientists were confident that ketones could provide an additional source of energy during times of decreased fuel availability and that our bodies knew how to properly regulate this fuel.

Non-starvation, diet-induced ketosis (nutritional ketosis) differs from starvation-induced ketosis in that the production of ketones is typically lower due to the fact that food is being consumed. Although it's different for everyone, a well-formulated ketogenic diet is typically high in fat (more than 65 percent) and extremely low in carbohydrate (5 to 10 percent) (Veech et al., 2004). Research shows that ketone levels tend not to rise above 7 mmol/L during diet-induced ketosis and usually remain far below this level. For example, Dr. Jeff Volek's lab found that following three and six weeks of ketogenic dieting, normal-weight men had an average concentration of BHB in the blood close to 0.5 mmol (Sharman et al., 2002). These results were confirmed by a study of individuals with cardiovascular risk factors, which found that after six weeks of a calorie-restricted ketogenic diet, BHB levels had risen only to, on average, 0.5 mmol (Ballard et al., 2013). Moreover, our lab found that even in highly trained, physically active, healthy men, ketone levels generally do not rise above 1.5 mmol after eight weeks on a strict ketogenic diet combined with resistance exercise.

So what exactly comprises a ketogenic diet? There are many different explanations, but they all share one essential feature: significantly reduced carbohydrates. Here are some definitions from published studies:

- Less than 50 grams of carbohydrates per day (or 5 to 10 percent of total daily caloric intake) and dietary fat as high as 90 percent of total daily caloric intake (Paoli et al., 2013).

- Less than 50 grams of carbohydrates per day, regardless of fat, protein, or caloric intake (Westman et al., 2003).

- Four times as much fat as carbohydrates, with protein regulated so that 90 percent of calories are derived from fat (Swink et al., 1977).

- Less than 50 grams of carbohydrates per day, or approximately 10 percent of total daily calories from carbohydrates (i.e., 200 calories on a 2,000-calorie-per-day diet) (Accurso et al., 2008).

- High fat, low protein, low carbohydrates (Freeman, 1998).

- An ad libitum ("free-feeding") diet consisting of less than 50 grams of carbohydrates per day (Gregory et al., 2017).

All these definitions focus on the intake of fat, protein, and carbohydrates, known as macronutrients. This makes sense because consuming carbohydrates, too much protein, and too little fat can prevent the production of ketones. (We'll look closer at optimal macronutrient ratios in Chapter 3.) However, we want to use a more general definition that doesn't mandate specific amounts of macronutrients but instead focuses on the overall goal of a ketogenic diet. For our purposes, a ketogenic diet is one in which glucogenic (glucose-producing) substrates (non-fiber carbohydrates and glucogenic amino acids) are low enough to force the body to rely primarily on fat as fuel and increase the production of ketone bodies.

Why not specify macronutrient ratios? You may have heard people recommend a ketogenic diet that is 80 percent fat, 15 percent protein, and 5 percent carbohydrate. However, it is difficult to tell whether someone will get into ketosis from macronutrient ratios alone without knowing other individualized variables, such as physical activity level, total caloric intake, and health conditions. For instance, a friend of ours was trying to bulk up and wanted to do it via a ketogenic diet. His daily caloric intake was around 4,500 calories. If he were following the recommendation that 5 to 10 percent of his calories should come from carbohydrates, he would have been consuming anywhere from 56 to 113 grams of carbohydrates and 225 to 282 grams of protein a day—likely enough to prevent ketosis, especially if he wasn't exercising. Setting macronutrient goals can be helpful for someone who is just starting out on a ketogenic diet (we offer some suggestions on page 182), but keep in mind that it must be taken in context and factor in individual goals (e.g., therapeutic use versus enhancement of athletic performance versus weight loss). There is no one-size-fits-all approach for a ketogenic diet, and thus the ratios and, in particular, the actual amount of each macronutrient may vary slightly from person to person depending on goals and health parameters such as insulin sensitivity, body composition, gender, and activity level.

> A ketogenic diet is one in which glucogenic (glucose-producing) substrates (non-fiber carbohydrates and glucogenic amino acids) are low enough to force the body to rely primarily on fat as fuel and increase the production of ketone bodies.

The Physiology of Diet-Induced Ketosis

Why is lowering carbohydrates so important for ketosis? Because it helps create two necessary conditions. First, blood glucose levels need to drop—and reducing carbohydrates via a ketogenic diet has been shown to lower fasting blood glucose (Brehm et al., 2003; Samaha et al., 2003). Second, the body's glycogen stores need to be depleted. On a ketogenic diet, the glycogen stored in the liver can be depleted in approximately forty-eight hours (Adam-Perrott et al., 2006).

Both lower blood glucose and depleted glycogen stores are crucial for ketosis because they force the body to use a fuel other than glucose. The body naturally utilizes glucose whenever it's available, whether in the bloodstream (from the food we eat) or from the breakdown of stored glycogen. Thus, by lowering both the amount of glucose taken in from food and the amount of glucose stored as glycogen, the body is able start burning fat/ketones as its primary fuel source.

THE PHYSIOLOGY OF DIET-INDUCED KETOSIS

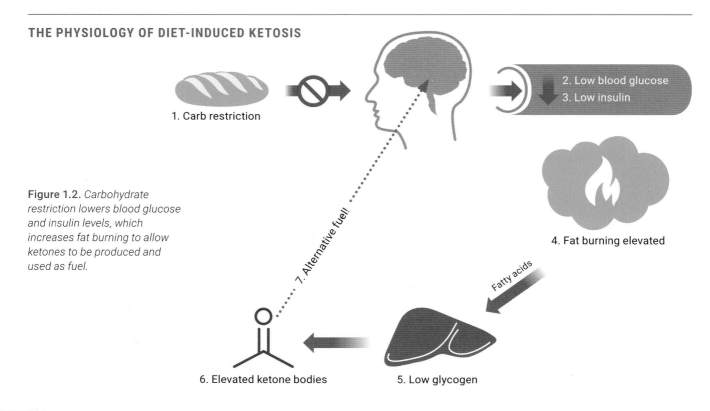

1. Carb restriction

2. Low blood glucose
3. Low insulin

4. Fat burning elevated

Fatty acids

5. Low glycogen

6. Elevated ketone bodies

7. Alternative fuel!

Figure 1.2. *Carbohydrate restriction lowers blood glucose and insulin levels, which increases fat burning to allow ketones to be produced and used as fuel.*

There's a second reason that lowered blood glucose helps induce ketosis. Carbohydrates are the primary trigger for the release of the hormone insulin, which triggers the uptake of glucose from the bloodstream into the cells. Insulin also halts the utilization of fat as fuel and promotes its storage—so when insulin is high, fat isn't burned. However, when insulin is low, the body can break down triglycerides (the stored form of fat) to be used as fuel. Burning fat is, of course, what produces ketone bodies.

To summarize, the physiology of diet-induced ketosis involves the lowering of blood glucose, stored glycogen, and insulin levels. The result is an enhanced release and reliance on fat as fuel. Finally, these fats are converted to ketone bodies, which can provide an alternative and more effective fuel source for the body.

Doesn't Eating Fat Make You Fat?

"You are what you eat" is a common, overly simplistic phrase that nutritionists use to convey that if you eat "bad" food, your health will suffer. Most people take this phrase out of context to mean, "If I don't eat fat, I can't get fat." If that were the case, then someone could drink fifteen sodas a day and eat cereal for every meal and still be a lean machine. Could it happen? Maybe for someone who's extremely insulin sensitive. Is it likely? Absolutely not.

Let us start out by saying that fat is not the culprit. If we were in court, a not-guilty verdict would bound to be issued once the evidence was presented. As mentioned earlier, if you drastically reduce your carbohydrate intake, you need to make up for that energy deficit through one or both of the other macronutrients: fat and protein. Often people err on the side of caution and adopt the old Atkins approach of going low-carb but eating super high amounts of protein and only moderate amounts of fat. Unfortunately, this approach likely wouldn't result in an ability to adapt to using fat as fuel (known

as becoming keto-adapted) because the liver can create glucose from certain amino acids/proteins through the process of gluconeogenesis. Therefore, rather than consume just "low carb" and high protein, individuals on a ketogenic diet eat very low carb and increase their fat intake while maintaining or slightly increasing their protein intake. The body then adjusts to utilizing fat as its primary fuel source.

Our entire lives we've been told that high amounts of dietary fat are what lead to heart disease, diabetes, high cholesterol, and even obesity. Understandably, people are often hesitant to embrace a lifestyle in which bacon and butter aren't so bad after all. It's fat that makes us fat, right? Wrong. If we look at the historic rates of obesity in the United States, we see a phenomenon worth pointing out.

During the 1980s, nutritional guidelines and strategic food marketing convinced people that consuming fat led to serious complications, including obesity. (We will touch on why this was the case more in Chapter 2.) Everywhere we turned, low-fat food options were popping up, almost as if fat were a plague and we needed to avoid it as such. Yet, at the same time, the prevalence of obesity began to increase dramatically (see Figure 1.3). By following the low-fat recommendations and consuming more fast and packaged foods labeled "low-fat" (which nearly always has added sugar to make up for the taste lost by reducing fat) while exercising less, our society actually got *fatter*. How could this be?

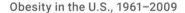

Obesity in the U.S., 1961–2009

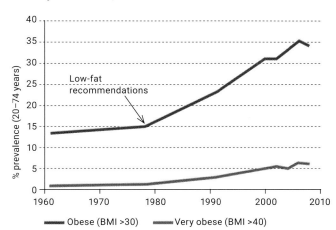

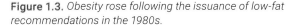

Figure 1.3. *Obesity rose following the issuance of low-fat recommendations in the 1980s.*

Scientists have been scratching their heads over this phenomenon for decades. Is it the fat, the carbohydrates, or possibly the combination of the two that is leading to obesity and other metabolic issues? A landmark experiment may hold the answer.

Dr. Robert Wolfe is one of the foremost authorities on metabolism. His laboratory conducted a study in which fat was infused into subjects' blood; it showed that when fat was infused by itself, it was used as fuel, and none of the early indicators of obesity, like elevated insulin and glucose levels, were seen (Klein et al., 1992). In the next phase of the study, the researchers infused fat and carbohydrate together into subjects' blood. This time, fat was not utilized as fuel; instead, both fat and carbohydrate utilization was impaired. The experiment clearly indicated that fat by itself isn't what is making us fat. Rather, it is the combination of high amounts of fat *and* high amounts of carbohydrates. (No surprise that this is what makes up 95 percent of fast-food meals!) As we will discuss throughout this book, when carbohydrates (and thus insulin) are low and fat consumption is high, the general results are loss of body fat; improvements in insulin, glucose, and cholesterol levels; and an overall improvement in health.

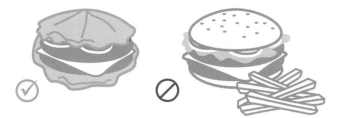

Figure 1.4. *A lettuce wrap is an easy way to avoid the combination of high-fat and high-carb found in foods like cheeseburgers.*

Keto Adaptation

Most of us have been consuming a carbohydrate-rich diet for our entire lives. While fasting or following a ketogenic diet can help you start producing ketones, it takes time for your body to switch to burning fat as its primary fuel source. Imagine getting a call today and finding out that you had to move to a different country tomorrow and stay for six months. It would take you time to learn the language and adapt to the culture. You could get by, but the longer you were there, the more you would adapt to the culture and the easier life would become. Similarly, when adopting a ketogenic lifestyle, it takes time to truly adapt, but keep in mind that the implications for health, from improvements in conditions like obesity and diabetes to enhanced athletic performance and longevity, can be profound.

Take a moment and imagine a friend of yours who is thin. This individual, like most of us, is probably storing 1,600 to 2,000 calories in the form of glycogen. How much fat do you think this individual is storing? It may astound you to learn that even a thin person may be storing 30,000 to 60,000 calories in the form of fat! In an average-sized individual, this number can go to 100,000, and someone who's obese may be storing 200,000 calories' worth of fat. Thus we are in no short supply of energy—all of us have body fat. However, we often lack the ability to tap into and utilize that body fat.

Research shows that babies and children have a significant ability to tap into these fat stores (Coggan et al., 2000; Martinez et al., 1992), but as we age, we become more reliant on our much smaller carbohydrate stores (Martinez et al., 1992).

In fact, babies are born in a state of ketosis and are able to utilize ketone bodies at a rate that is five to forty times greater than adults (Platt and Deshpande, 2005). We would venture to say that the diminished ability to use fat as fuel is an impact of our dietary choices, with an emphasis on grains and other carbohydrates. Research shows that high-carbohydrate diets begin to "fix" our metabolisms to prefer carbohydrates as fuel (Volek et al., 2015). You often hear people say that glucose is the body's preferred energy source; however, an alternative explanation may be that our natural state is to be in ketosis, but our dietary habits interrupt this process and program our bodies to develop a carbohydrate-dependent metabolism.

Is there a way to get back to tapping into our larger energy reserve? Yes, and it involves a process called keto adaptation.

Keto adaptation is the body's response to carbohydrate restriction. When we're keto-adapted, we've shifted from relying primarily on carbohydrates for our energy needs to relying primarily on fat (and therefore ketones) (Volek et al., 2015). Research tends to show significant declines in physical performance after one week of following a ketogenic diet; however, performance levels are restored after about six weeks, although it sometimes takes longer (Phinney et al., 1983; Volek et al., 2015). From this, it is generally surmised that keto adaptation can take anywhere from several weeks to a couple of months. However, based on long-term data collected from elite athletes who have adopted a very low carbohydrate diet, we contend that keto adaptations are still occurring even a year after initiation of the diet (Volek et al.,

2016). (We'll explore this topic in more depth in Chapter 5.) The series of adaptations that occur following a ketogenic diet is extensive. There is no clear-cut point at which someone is completely adapted and all of these changes have been made. Several factors are involved, including previous diet, exercise habits, insulin sensitivity, and much more. Research shows that these keto adaptations include, but are not limited to, increasing the number of mitochondria (fat-burning machinery) in a cell, elevating blood ketone levels, and enhancing the body's ability to take in and use ketones at the cellular level (Volek et al., 2015; Volek et al., 2016).

Diabetic Ketoacidosis

Mention the word *ketosis* to someone, and almost inevitably this question will come up: "Shouldn't you be worried about going into a state of ketoacidosis?" It is important to understand the difference between the physiological effects of a ketogenic diet (in other words, ketosis) and ketoacidosis.

Ketoacidosis occurs when there is uncontrolled ketone production, which is typically accompanied

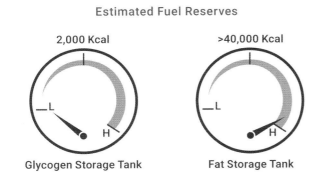

Estimated Fuel Reserves

2,000 Kcal   >40,000 Kcal

Glycogen Storage Tank   Fat Storage Tank

Figure 1.5. *Our bodies have a limited glycogen storage capacity; meanwhile, we have nearly unlimited fat stores to tap into.*

by high concentrations of blood glucose (i.e., diabetes). In ketoacidosis, blood ketone levels reach 15 to 25 mmol/L, and the acidity of the blood also increases (Cartwright et al., 2012). The potential cause for harm comes from the alarming rise in acidity or lowering of the pH of the blood.

A healthy human body tightly regulates blood acid concentrations. If your blood has a pH of less than 7, it's acidic; if the pH is higher than 7, it's basic, or alkaline (the opposite of acidic). Human blood is usually slightly alkaline, with a pH ranging from 7.35 to 7.45. Any deviation from this norm, even by the most modest of margins, can prove fatal (see Figure 1.6).

The most common form of ketoacidosis is diabetic ketoacidosis. This usually occurs in type 1 diabetics but also can occur in type 2 diabetics. What's the difference? In type 1 diabetics, the pancreas does not produce insulin. In type 2 diabetics, the cells of the body are resistant to insulin and/or the pancreas produces inadequate amounts of insulin. (We discuss these issues in more detail in Chapter 5.)

It is clear that insulin is a key player in both types of diabetes, but what is its role? Insulin's main jobs are to:

1) take glucose into the cells to be used for energy, and

2) keep fat metabolism in check

During fasting or on a low-carbohydrate diet, insulin levels drop and insulin sensitivity—insulin's ability to interact efficiently with the cells—improves. In a person who is insulin sensitive, less insulin is required to move a greater amount of glucose into the cells.

However, when insulin is absent (as it is in people with type 1 diabetes) or the cells are resistant to its effects (as in people with type 2 diabetes), glucose is not taken up into cells efficiently and therefore cannot be utilized for energy. Under these conditions, carbohydrate consumption causes blood glucose levels to skyrocket from a normal level of 80 to 100 mg/dL (during fasting) to levels greater than 300 mg/dL! Many scientists have referred to this phenomenon as "starvation in the face of plenty" (Figure 1.7). The energy (glucose) is there, knocking on the door to the cell, but it can't get in, so it floats around in the blood, potentially causing harm.

When cells sense that both glucose and insulin are low (or cells simply aren't responding to insulin), the liver increases the process known as gluconeogenesis, literally "making glucose from new." It is the formation of glucose from non-carbohydrate substrates. To make this glucose, the body uses either amino acids (whether from the diet or from muscle tissues), the glycerol backbone of fat molecules, or lactate produced by the muscles. At the same time, since cells perceive that they are starving because no energy is getting in, fatty acid breakdown is increased in order to produce ketone bodies.

However, in situations involving ketoacidosis, there is plenty of glucose in the blood; the cells just aren't able to absorb it (i.e., they are resistant to it). When blood glucose gets too high, the kidneys are unable to filter and reabsorb it properly, leading to glucose being excreted in the urine. Because glucose isn't properly filtrated, it brings with it the fluid portion of the blood, which also is excreted in the urine. This results in a lower blood volume with a high concentration of ketone bodies. In this case, these extremely elevated levels of ketone bodies, which are slightly acidic in nature, increase blood acidity and must be treated immediately. This is ketoacidosis.

It is important to remember that ketoacidosis is typically not seen in healthy individuals implementing a ketogenic diet or even supplementing with exogenous ketones, since both of those are controlled processes that raise blood ketone levels to, at most, 5 to 7 mmol/L. Ketoacidosis, on the other hand, is uncontrolled, with blood ketone levels starting at 15 to 25 mmol/L.

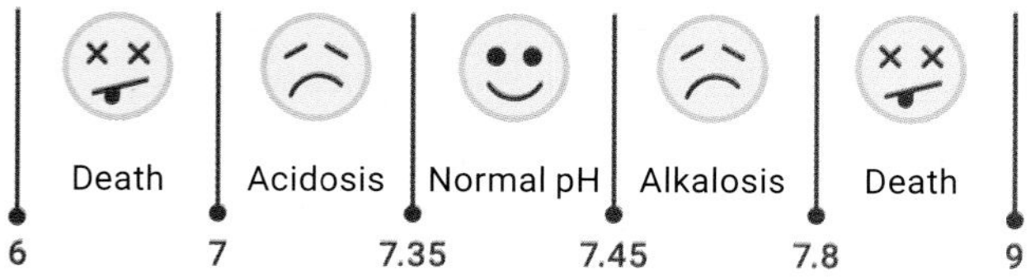

| Death | Acidosis | Normal pH | Alkalosis | Death |
| 6 | 7 | 7.35 | 7.45 | 7.8 | 9 |

Figure 1.6. *Range of blood pH levels.*

Insulin Resistance: "Starvation in the Face of Plenty"

The best way we've found to explain insulin resistance and "starvation in the face of plenty" is with a silly yet simple depiction of a little town called Resistance. In Resistance, when it rains (i.e., someone eats carbohydrates), green sludge (i.e., glucose) rises from the ground and floods the streets (i.e., the bloodstream). The city calls in its cleaning crew (i.e., insulin) to clean up the streets, and the crew does so by sweeping the sludge into people's houses (i.e., cells). The cleaners knock on people's doors, the people open their doors, the cleaners brush the sludge in, and then they're on their way. The people don't really mind—it's not a lot of sludge, and they know that getting it off the streets benefits the town. But if it begins to rain all the time (i.e., frequent carbohydrate consumption constantly raises blood glucose), the

people of Resistance get tired of all this sludge in their houses. Eventually, when the cleaners come to push the sludge into houses, fewer and fewer people answer the door. This is insulin resistance: when cells stop responding to insulin's signals. There's so much sludge on the street that the town calls in more cleaners (more insulin) to force the sludge into the houses. But then the sludge begins pouring out the windows. The houses (cells) already have too much sludge and can't take on any more, so no matter how hard the cleaners try, they can't push the sludge into the houses, and the sludge stays on the street (in the blood). With all this readily available glucose/sludge sitting around in the blood, our bodies shut off a process known as lipolysis, or fat breakdown, and instead of burning fat, we end up storing it.

Figure 1.7. *Insulin resistance explained.*

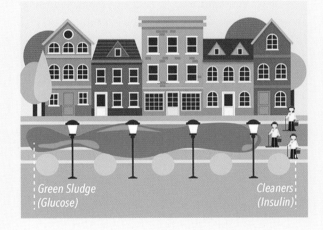

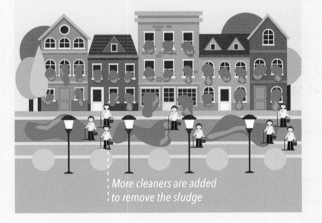

Is the Ketogenic Diet Just Another Low-Carb Diet?

Unfortunately, the definition of a low-carbohydrate diet is confounded by the fact that there is no minimum recommended daily allowance for carbohydrates. However, a commonly accepted definition is that a low-carb diet is one that supplies less than 50 percent of its calories from carbohydrates (Feinman et al., 2003). This is in

stark contrast to the less-than-50-grams-per-day recommendation for very-low-carbohydrate ketogenic diets. (If the friend we mentioned earlier in the chapter who was eating around 4,500 calories per day used the 50 percent definition, he'd be "low-carb" if he ate 550 grams of carbs a day! We all know that this is anything but low-carb.)

As previously discussed, a ketogenic diet is one in which glucogenic substrates are low enough to force the body to transition from metabolizing glucose to burning fat and subsequently producing ketones. So while a ketogenic diet is low in carbohydrates, a low-carb diet isn't necessarily ketogenic.

A classic study (Young et al., 1971) demonstrated a clear difference between low-carb and ketogenic diets. Scientists took overweight young men and placed them on "low-carbohydrate" diets consisting of 30, 60, or 100 grams of carbohydrates per day. They found that after nine weeks, the 100-gram group was not in ketosis at all, while the 30-gram group had achieved high levels of ketosis. Moreover, the 30-gram group lost more fat than both the 60-gram group and the 100-gram group despite there being no differences in total calories or protein consumed. This study clearly demonstrates that not all low-carbohydrate diets are the same, and certainly not all are ketogenic. You must understand this concept to derive optimal benefits from this book.

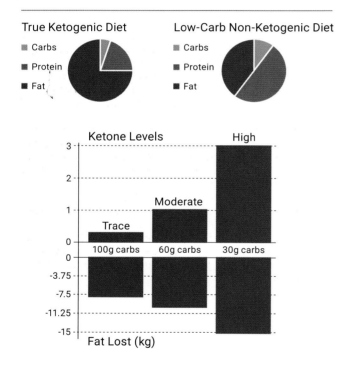

Figure 1.8. *Differences in body fat lost between a low-carb diet and a ketogenic diet.*

Source: Adapted from Young et al., 1971.

CHAPTER SUMMARY

This chapter provided a strong foundation for understanding ketosis that will be needed throughout the remainder of the book. We explained that ketosis is characterized by blood ketone levels above 0.3 mmol/L. In general, a ketogenic diet is one in which glucogenic substrates (non-fiber carbohydrates and glucogenic amino acids) are low enough to force the body to rely primarily on fat for energy and increase the production of ketone bodies. This type of dietary strategy allows individuals to enter a state of keto adaptation, in which their fuel source switches from primarily carbohydrates to primarily fat and ketones. The process of keto adaptation varies in duration and continues to provide benefits the longer you eat ketogenic. Fat in and of itself does not make you fat; rather, copious amounts of dietary fat in the presence of substantial carbohydrates (a hallmark of the standard Western diet) can make you both fat and insulin resistant.

Early research on diabetics found that when the disease state was left untreated, blood ketone levels would rise to levels greater than 15 mmol/L. The result was ketoacidosis, a lowering of blood pH due to an uncontrollable rise in ketones even in the presence of high amounts of glucose. This led researchers to believe that ketones were a toxic by-product of metabolic dysfunction and disease. However, research from starvation studies and ketogenic dieting has taught us that ketones are a high-powered energy source that can replace glucose and serve as the body's dominant fuel source.

References

Adam-Perrot, A., P. Clifton, and F. Brouns. "Low-carbohydrate diets: nutritional and physiological aspects." *Obesity Reviews* 7, no. 1 (2006): 49–58. doi: 10.1111/j.1467-789X.2006.00222.x

Ballard, K. D., E. E. Quann, B. R. Kupchak, B. M. Volk, D. M. Kawiecki, M. L. Fernandez, ... and J. S. Volek. "Dietary carbohydrate restriction improves insulin sensitivity, blood pressure, microvascular function, and cellular adhesion markers in individuals taking statins." *Nutrition Research* 33, no. 11 (2013): 905–12. doi: 10.1016/j.nutres.2013.07.022

Bliss, M. *The Discovery of Insulin.* Chicago: University of Chicago Press: 1982.

Brehm B. J., R. J. Seeley, S. R. Daniels, and D. A. D'Alessio. "A randomized trial comparing a very low carbohydrate diet and a calorie restricted low fat diet on body weight and cardiovascular risk factors in healthy women." *Journal of Clinical Endocrinology & Metabolism* 88 (2003): 1617–23. doi: 10.1210/jc.2002-021480

Cahill Jr., G. F. "Fuel metabolism in starvation." *Annual Review of Nutrition* 26 (2006): 1–22. doi: 10.1146/annurev.nutr.26.061505.111258

Cahill Jr., G. F., M. G. Herrera, A. Morgan, J. S. Soeldner, J. Steinke, P. L. Levy, ... and D. M. Kipnis. "Hormone-fuel interrelationships during fasting." *Journal of Clinical Investigation* 45, no. 11 (1966): 1751. doi: 10.1172/JCI105481

Cartwright, M. M., W. Hajja, S. Al-Khatib, M. Hazeghazam, D. Sreedhar, R. N. Li, ... and R. W. Carlson. "Toxigenic and metabolic causes of ketosis and ketoacidotic syndromes." *Critical Care Clinics* 28, no. 4 (2012): 601–31. doi: 10.1016/j.ccc.2012.07.001

Coggan A. R., C. A. Raguso, A. Gastaldelli, L. S. Sidossis, and C. W. Yeckel. "Fat metabolism during high-intensity exercise in endurance-trained and untrained men." *Metabolism* 49, no. 1 (2000): 122–28.

Feinman, R. D., and E. J. Fine. "Thermodynamics and metabolic advantage of weight loss diets." *Metabolic Syndrome and Related Disorders* 1, no. 3 (2003): 209–19. doi: 10.1089/154041903322716688

Gregory, R. M., H. Hamdan, D. M. Torisky, and J. D. Akers. "A low-carbohydrate ketogenic diet combined with 6-weeks of CrossFit training improves body composition and performance." *International Journal of Sports and Exercise Medicine* 3, no. 2 (2017). In press. doi: 10.23937/2469-5718/1510054

Hatori, M., C. Vollmers, A. Zarrinpar, L. DiTacchio, E. A. Bushong, S. Gill, ... and M. H. Ellisman. "Time-restricted feeding without reducing caloric intake prevents metabolic diseases in mice fed a high-fat diet." *Cell Metabolism* 15, no. 6 (2012): 848–60. doi: 10.1016/j.cmet.2012.04.019

Klein, S., and R. R. Wolfe. "Carbohydrate restriction regulates the adaptive response to fasting." *American Journal of Physiology-Endocrinology and Metabolism* 262, no. 5 (1992): E631–36.

Lin, S., T. C. Thomas, L. H. Storlien, and X. F. Huang. "Development of high fat diet-induced obesity and leptin resistance in C57Bl/6J mice." *International Journal of Obesity* 24, no. 5 (2000): 639–46.

Martinez L. R., and E. M. Haymes. "Substrate utilization during treadmill running in prepubertal girls and women." *Medicine and Science in Sports and Exercise* 24 (1992): 975–83.

Owen, O. E. "Ketone bodies as a fuel for the brain during starvation." *Biochemistry and Molecular Biology Education* 33, no. 4 (2005): 246–51.

Paoli, A., A. Rubini, J. S. Volek, and K. A. Grimaldi. "Beyond weight loss: a review of the therapeutic uses of very-low-carbohydrate (ketogenic) diets." *European Journal of Clinical Nutrition* 67, no. 8 (2013): 789–96. doi: 10.1038/ejcn.2013.116

Phinney, S. D., E. S. Horton, E. A. H. Sims, J. S. Hanson, and E. Danforth, Jr. "Capacity for moderate exercise in obese subjects after adaptation to a hypocaloric, ketogenic diet." *Journal of Clinical Investigation* 66 (1980): 1152–61. doi: 10.1172/JCI109945

Platt, M. W., and S. Deshpande. "Metabolic adaptation at birth." *Seminars in Fetal and Neonatal Medicine* 10, no. 4 (2005): 341–50. doi: 10.1016/j.siny.2005.04.001

Samaha, F. F., N. Iqbal, P. Seshadri, K. L. Chicano, D. A. Daily, J. McGrory, T. Williams, M. Williams, E. J. Gracely, and L. Stern. "A low-carbohydrate as compared with a low-fat diet in severe obesity." *New England Journal of Medicine* 348 (2003): 2074–81. doi: 10.1056/NEJMoa022637

Sharman, M. J., W. J. Kraemer, D. M. Love, N. G. Avery, A. L. Gómez, T. P. Scheett, and J. S. Volek. "A ketogenic diet favorably affects serum biomarkers for cardiovascular disease in normal-weight men." *Journal of Nutrition* 132, no. 7 (2002): 1879–85.

Veech, R. L. "The therapeutic implications of ketone bodies: the effects of ketone bodies in pathological conditions: ketosis, ketogenic diet, redox states, insulin resistance, and mitochondrial metabolism." *Prostaglandins, Leukotrienes and Essential Fatty Acids* 70, no. 3 (2004): 309–19. doi: 10.1016/j.plefa.2003.09.007

Volek, J. S., T. Noakes, and S. D. Phinney. "Rethinking fat as a fuel for endurance exercise." *European Journal of Sport Science* 15, no. 1 (2015): 13–20. doi: 10.1080/17461391.2014.959564

Young, C. M., S. S. Scanlan, H. S. Im, and L. Lutwak. "Effect on body composition and other parameters in obese young men of carbohydrate level of reduction diet." *American Journal of Clinical Nutrition* 24, no. 3 (1971): 290–96.

Chapter 2

THE PAST, PRESENT, AND FUTURE OF KETOGENIC DIETING

> Everyone has a doctor in him; we
> just have to help him in his work.
> The natural healing force within
> each one of us is the greatest force in
> getting well. . . . To eat when you are
> sick is to feed your sickness.
>
> —**Hippocrates**

Imagine if Alexander Fleming hadn't left his dirty petri dish in a lab sink when he left for vacation in the summer of 1928; we might not have penicillin. Imagine if Perry Spencer hadn't had a chocolate bar in his pocket that melted when he stood next to a magnetron (a system that generates microwaves for radar systems); we might not have the microwave oven. Imagine if John Pemberton hadn't mixed his "headache and addiction cure" of coca leaves, sugar syrup, and kola nuts with carbonated water; we might not have Coca-Cola.

You may not know their names, but these people have affected your life in some way. Similarly, several other key players whose names may be unknown to you have had a significant impact on the development of the ketogenic diet. Throughout this chapter, we will take a journey back in time and highlight significant individuals and events in the history of the ketogenic diet, including the first low-carb advocates, the emergence of the ketogenic diet, its fall from favor and resurgence, the introduction of low-fat recommendations, and the development of exogenous ketones.

Where It All Started

The concept of restricting carbohydrates to lose weight and improve health dates back to the mid-1800s. Jean Anthelme Brillat-Savarin, a French lawyer, politician, and "father of low-carbohydrate diets," was the first to connect obesity and carbohydrates. In his 1825 book *The Physiology of Taste,* he states that a major cause of obesity "is the floury and starchy substances which man makes the prime ingredients of his daily nourishment. . . . All animals that live on farinaceous food grow fat willy-nilly; and man is no exception to the universal law."

Not long after, English undertaker William Banting began following a low-carbohydrate diet on the advice of Dr. William Harvey. Numerous medical treatments, starvation diets, and extreme exercise hadn't worked for this five-foot-five, 202-pound sixty-five-year-old, but by limiting carbohydrates—his diet cut out bread, sugar, potatoes, milk, and beer—he experienced an incredible transformation. Banting was so ecstatic with his weight loss that in 1863 he published *A Letter on Corpulence,* which sold thousands of copies. By 1866, London and much of Europe were experiencing full Banting mania. Though not entirely the same as a ketogenic diet, the Banting diet paved the way for later carbohydrate-restriction strategies and is still extremely popular in South Africa, with advocates like Dr. Tim Noakes, coauthor of the book *The Real Meal Revolution.*

Despite the Banting diet trend, in order to fully understand the origins of the ketogenic diet, we must begin with fasting, whose health benefits eventually led researchers and doctors to the ketogenic diet as we know it today.

KETO TIMELINE

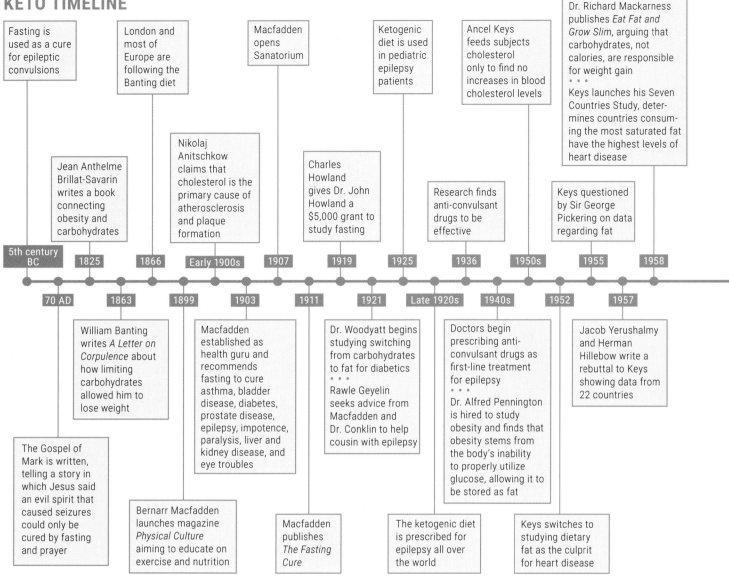

Fasting is used as a cure for epileptic convulsions — 5th century BC

Jean Anthelme Brillat-Savarin writes a book connecting obesity and carbohydrates — 1825

London and most of Europe are following the Banting diet — 1825

Nikolaj Anitschkow claims that cholesterol is the primary cause of atherosclerosis and plaque formation — 1866

Macfadden opens Sanatorium — 1907

Charles Howland gives Dr. John Howland a $5,000 grant to study fasting — 1919

Ketogenic diet is used in pediatric epilepsy patients — 1925

Ancel Keys feeds subjects cholesterol only to find no increases in blood cholesterol levels — 1925

Research finds anti-convulsant drugs to be effective — 1936

Dr. Richard Mackarness publishes *Eat Fat and Grow Slim*, arguing that carbohydrates, not calories, are responsible for weight gain
• • •
Keys launches his Seven Countries Study, determines countries consuming the most saturated fat have the highest levels of heart disease — 1958

Keys questioned by Sir George Pickering on data regarding fat — 1955

The Gospel of Mark is written, telling a story in which Jesus said an evil spirit that caused seizures could only be cured by fasting and prayer — 70 AD

William Banting writes *A Letter on Corpulence* about how limiting carbohydrates allowed him to lose weight — 1863

Macfadden established as health guru and recommends fasting to cure asthma, bladder disease, diabetes, prostate disease, epilepsy, impotence, paralysis, liver and kidney disease, and eye troubles — 1899

Bernarr Macfadden launches magazine *Physical Culture* aiming to educate on exercise and nutrition — 1899

Macfadden publishes *The Fasting Cure* — 1903

Dr. Woodyatt begins studying switching from carbohydrates to fat for diabetics
• • •
Rawle Geyelin seeks advice from Macfadden and Dr. Conklin to help cousin with epilepsy — 1911

The ketogenic diet is prescribed for epilepsy all over the world — 1921

Doctors begin prescribing anti-convulsant drugs as first-line treatment for epilepsy
• • •
Dr. Alfred Pennington is hired to study obesity and finds that obesity stems from the body's inability to properly utilize glucose, allowing it to be stored as fat — Late 1920s

Keys switches to studying dietary fat as the culprit for heart disease — 1940s

Jacob Yerushalmy and Herman Hillebow write a rebuttal to Keys showing data from 22 countries — 1957

Timeline markers: 5th century BC · 70 AD · 1825 · 1863 · 1866 · 1899 · Early 1900s · 1903 · 1907 · 1911 · 1919 · 1921 · 1925 · Late 1920s · 1936 · 1940s · 1950s · 1952 · 1955 · 1957 · 1958

In ancient times, fasting was used as a sacred and nutritional therapy for various conditions, including epilepsy. Plenty of accounts dating as far back as the fifth century BC describe abstinence from food as an effective cure for epileptic convulsions (Temkin, 1994). In the King James Version of the Bible, Mark describes Jesus curing a boy who experienced seizures, saying, "This kind [of evil spirit] can come forth by nothing, but by prayer and fasting" (Mark 9:17–29). In the modern era, doctors and scientists recognized that fasting is beneficial for a variety of health conditions and therefore attempted to dig deeper and discover exactly why it has these effects. The ultimate question became: is it possible to receive the benefits of fasting while still consuming calories?

The story begins with an unlikely hero: Bernarr Macfadden. In today's social media era, fitness enthusiasts can be found on every platform, from Instagram to Facebook to Snapchat. Everywhere you turn, familiar faces fill our screens with their incredible physiques, showing off the phenomenal work they have done in the gym, in the kitchen, and sometimes in Photoshop. However, in the early twentieth century, Macfadden was the health and fitness guru for both the fitness and the medical communities. Nicknamed "Body Love" by *Time* magazine, he paved the way for our current understanding of fasting and ketosis (Hunt, 1989).

Growing up, Macfadden faced a lot of hardship at home. His father was an abusive alcoholic, and his mother suffered from depression. By the

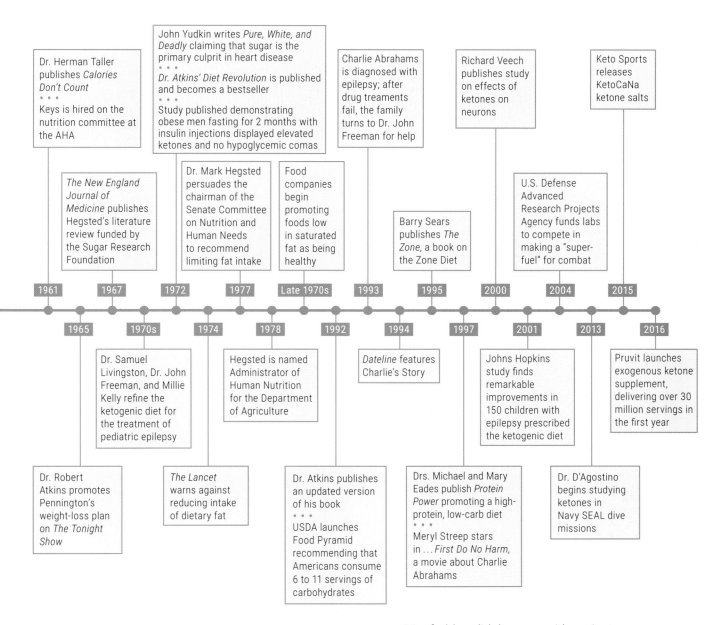

Dr. Herman Taller publishes *Calories Don't Count*
• • •
Keys is hired on the nutrition committee at the AHA

John Yudkin writes *Pure, White, and Deadly* claiming that sugar is the primary culprit in heart disease
• • •
Dr. Atkins' Diet Revolution is published and becomes a bestseller
• • •
Study published demonstrating obese men fasting for 2 months with insulin injections displayed elevated ketones and no hypoglycemic comas

Charlie Abrahams is diagnosed with epilepsy; after drug treatments fail, the family turns to Dr. John Freeman for help

Richard Veech publishes study on effects of ketones on neurons

Keto Sports releases KetoCaNa ketone salts

The New England Journal of Medicine publishes Hegsted's literature review funded by the Sugar Research Foundation

Dr. Mark Hegsted persuades the chairman of the Senate Committee on Nutrition and Human Needs to recommend limiting fat intake

Food companies begin promoting foods low in saturated fat as being healthy

Barry Sears publishes *The Zone*, a book on the Zone Diet

U.S. Defense Advanced Research Projects Agency funds labs to compete in making a "super-fuel" for combat

| 1961 | 1967 | 1972 | 1977 | Late 1970s | 1993 | 1995 | 2000 | 2004 | 2015 |

| 1965 | 1970s | 1974 | 1978 | 1992 | 1994 | 1997 | 2001 | 2013 | 2016 |

Dr. Samuel Livingston, Dr. John Freeman, and Millie Kelly refine the ketogenic diet for the treatment of pediatric epilepsy

Hegsted is named Administrator of Human Nutrition for the Department of Agriculture

Dateline features Charlie's Story

Johns Hopkins study finds remarkable improvements in 150 children with epilepsy prescribed the ketogenic diet

Pruvit launches exogenous ketone supplement, delivering over 30 million servings in the first year

Dr. Robert Atkins promotes Pennington's weight-loss plan on *The Tonight Show*

The Lancet warns against reducing intake of dietary fat

Dr. Atkins publishes an updated version of his book
• • •
USDA launches Food Pyramid recommending that Americans consume 6 to 11 servings of carbohydrates

Drs. Michael and Mary Eades publish *Protein Power* promoting a high-protein, low-carb diet
• • •
Meryl Streep stars in *...First Do No Harm*, a movie about Charlie Abrahams

Dr. D'Agostino begins studying ketones in Navy SEAL dive missions

time he was eleven years old, both of his parents had died. Macfadden had no real family left, so he spent a year in an orphanage, where he was vaccinated using a medically unsound method and nearly perished, leading to a lifelong distrust of the mainstream medical community. Macfadden was a weak and sickly child, yet in his late teens he began experimenting with dumbbells, walking three to six miles per day, and using natural remedies to heal his body. Against all odds, he ended up making a name for himself in what was the start of a huge fitness industry (Hunt, 1989).

> "Weakness is a crime!
> Don't be a criminal."
> —Bernarr Macfadden

Macfadden didn't agree with mainstream medical practices and objected to doctors' lack of understanding of naturopathic treatments such as fasting. This, along with his infatuation with bodybuilding and fitness, led Macfadden in 1899 to launch his own magazine, *Physical Culture*, which set out to educate readers on the importance of being physically active, eating healthy, and limiting tobacco, alcohol, and even white bread (Macfadden called it the "staff of death"). By 1903, the magazine's circulation had reached over 100,000 copies a month, and it ultimately established Macfadden as America's first health guru.

Soon after achieving wide acclaim, Macfadden began making incredible promises that his tactics could cure any disease and allow people to live to over 100 years old. His formula was simple: exercise, get sunlight, avoid alcohol and tobacco, monitor diet, and regularly fast for a period ranging from three days to three weeks. Following these rules, he believed, could alleviate and cure nearly any disease, including asthma, bladder disease, diabetes, prostate disease, epilepsy, impotence, paralysis, liver and kidney disease, and even eye troubles (Hunt, 1989).

Feeling overwhelmingly confident in his abilities, Macfadden opened the Bernarr Macfadden Sanatorium in Battle Creek, Michigan, in 1907. (It was later moved to Chicago and renamed the Bernarr Macfadden Healthatorium.) It operated for several decades and served more than 300,000 individuals actively seeking to improve their health. (Interestingly, Macfadden's sanitarium competed with Harvey Kellogg's famous sanitarium, also in Battle Creek. It was eventually bought by Kellogg. Not surprisingly, Kellogg's sanitarium encouraged a low-fat, low-protein diet with an emphasis on whole grains.) This sanctuary was unlike any other, containing reading rooms, state-of-the-art fitness equipment, and even a sixty-foot swimming pool.

Macfadden and his leading osteopathic doctor, Hugh Conklin, were known for calling out mainstream medical doctors with their slogan, "We will take those you have given up on and cure them." Though he received a lot of negative press for his bold claims about his ability to cure people (he was even arrested on obscenity charges for discussing sexually transmitted infections and premarital sex in *Physical Culture*), Macfadden's popularity rose thanks to clients such as Upton Sinclair, who advocated ferociously for Macfadden and published the book *The Fasting Cure* in 1911. Most importantly, Macfadden brought attention to the need for research to improve our understanding of the effects of fasting, sex, and physical activity on overall health (Bennett, 2013).

Fast-forward a decade to 1921 and meet Rawle Geyelin, a prominent physician from New York who had a personal interest in fasting. His young cousin had been dealing with epilepsy for four years, and he'd watched as every treatment recommended by the leading doctors in the field, such as bromide and phenobarbital (Luminal, a brand of phenobarbital, was one of the most popular epilepsy drugs), failed to work. Dr. Geyelin and his cousin's family sought advice from two individuals who claimed to have all the answers: Bernarr Macfadden and Dr. Hugh Conklin in Battle Creek, Michigan.

"When the importance of physical culture is recognized it will enter into every phase of human life. . . . There is hardly a question in life [of] which physical culture should not be a part."
—Bernarr Macfadden

Dr. Conklin took Dr. Geyelin's young cousin under his care and had him fast for multiple days over the next several months. Just when the family thought that a solution would never be found, the boy's seizures stopped the second day after he started fasting, and he remained seizure-free for more than two years without drugs, just periodic fasting (Geyelin, 1921). Blown away by the results, Geyelin started using the same fasting treatment with a group of his patients with epilepsy to see if he could confirm the results his cousin had seen. After putting thirty patients on a twenty-day fast, he found that 87 percent became seizure-free. Geyelin went on to state, "When one wanted to turn a clouded mentality to a clear one it could almost always be done with fasting" (Geyelin, 1929).

Due to the sheer novelty of and excitement over his findings, Dr. Geyelin shared his results with an audience at an American Medical Association convention. You can imagine the gasps from the doctors in the auditorium who saw scientific data supporting this ridiculed, self-proclaimed healer, Bernarr Macfadden. Prior to Geyelin's data, numerous absurd and even barbaric therapeutic modalities—such as bloodletting, trephining (boring a hole into the skull), removing the ovaries and adrenal glands—and countless herbs and drugs had been

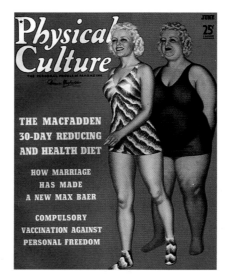

Figure 2.1. *A cover of* Physical Culture *magazine making claims about health and beauty.*

used in an attempt to cure what seemed at the time to be an incurable condition. The idea that a simple treatment like restricting food could cure epilepsy was met with skepticism and frustration (Wheless, 2008), even though fasting had eliminated seizures in 87 percent of Geyelin's patients and Dr. Conklin reported that his "water diet"—fasting—had cured epilepsy in 90 percent of the children he treated who were younger than ten. (And in 80 percent of adolescents ten to fifteen years old, 65 percent of patients fifteen to twenty-five, and 50 percent of patients between twenty-five and forty. Above age forty, the percentage was very low.)

Despite Conklin's and Geyelin's successes, their explanation for why fasting worked as a treatment for epilepsy—that it cleared the body of harmful toxins—was unsubstantiated. Astonished by the fact that some of the best doctors in the world had overlooked this form of treatment, in 1919 Charles Howland, the father of Geyelin's cousin, gave his brother, Dr. John Howland, a professor of pediatrics at Johns Hopkins, a $5,000 grant to determine whether there was a scientific rationale for the success of the "starvation" treatment that had helped heal his son (Wheless, 2004). With these start-up funds, Howland set up his laboratory and—because, as any respectable researcher can tell you, you are only as good as the team around you—recruited Dr. James Gamble, a clinical chemist, to help look at the metabolic and biochemical responses to fasting.

Gamble set up a series of studies to examine various blood and tissue markers in response to short-term fasting. He noted that patients undergoing fasting had differences in electrolyte balance and acid/base balance, but he failed to come up with a direct explanation for why fasting had beneficial results for epilepsy. The door was starting to open. Yet nobody could determine exactly what was going on that could be the key answer that would pave the way for decades to come (Wheless, 2004).

In 1921, Dr. Rollin Woodyatt, an endocrinologist in Chicago, was fascinated by the fact that fasting clears glucose from the bloodstream, even in diabetics. He sought to determine the effects of shifting the bulk of a diabetic's nutrition from carbohydrates to fat. His theory was that this (like fasting) would allow the body to "rest" the pancreas (since the pancreas produces insulin to manage glucose from carbohydrates) and use fat as fuel. In doing so, he discovered that even in non-diabetic, healthy subjects, ketone bodies such as beta-hydroxybutyrate (BHB) and acetone were present.

At the same time, over 300 miles north, Dr. Russel Wilder of the Mayo Clinic also was looking to fat as the key to receiving the benefits of fasting while still consuming calories. When the body metabolizes fat, particles called ketone bodies are produced, and it is these ketones that the body utilizes as fuel. Wilder proposed that the benefits Conklin saw with his patients were likely due to ketonemia, or high levels of ketones in the blood. With that in mind, Wilder suggested that this state (which would eventually become known as ketosis) could be achieved by means other than fasting, such as minimizing carbohydrate intake and having a high fat intake. Wilder immediately began putting his epileptic patients on a ketone-producing diet and coined the term by which we know it today: "ketogenic diet."

While the scientific community eagerly waited to see data on the results of Wilder's ketogenic diet, Dr. Mynie Peterman, a Mayo Clinic pediatrician, put the diet to the test in several of his pediatric epileptic patients in 1925. To say that the results were incredible is an understatement. Children on the diet experienced a significant drop in number of seizures and in some cases became free of seizures altogether. Even more striking was the fact that they seemed to sleep better, were less irritable, and displayed increased alertness (Peterman, 1925). News of Peterman's results spread quickly, and by the late 1920s doctors all over the country were prescribing the ketogenic diet for the treatment of epilepsy. For families and doctors, the choice was simple: implement a ketogenic diet or give patients sedatives, which came with brutal side effects.

With the 1930s came the Great Depression and ultimately the crash of scientific funding. Research money was scarce, so animal studies became more prevalent because they were much easier to control and therefore allowed researchers more flexibility to examine complex conditions such as those that occur with epilepsy. The ketogenic diet was still the treatment of choice for epilepsy until the brilliant team of neurosurgeon Tracy Putnam and neurologist Houston Merritt began seeking alternatives to phenobarbital, the sedative discussed earlier. One such alternative, a phenobarbital derivative called phenytoin, appeared mildly sedative but held huge promise for treating seizures. Branded Dilantin, it became the first truly anti-convulsant drug, and by 1940, doctors were prescribing it as a first-line treatment for epilepsy. This scientific discovery may go down in history as one of the best/worst breakthroughs: while it prompted researchers to find new, beneficial anti-convulsant drugs, it also led to a reduction in the use of the ketogenic diet (Wheless, 2004).

Over the next decade, dozens of anti-convulsive compounds were discovered, and pharmaceutical companies competed to develop the best "cure in a pill." However, Putnam and Merritt soon came to realize that their discovery, as important as it was, created a major hurdle for the scientific research into the root cause of epilepsy and why the ketogenic diet was an effective therapy for it. (Doctors felt that they had a strong cure and thus were less proactive in trying to identify and address the root cause instead of just masking it with pharmaceutical agents.) Over the years, fewer and fewer children were placed on a ketogenic diet; instead, they were given combinations of various drugs. Soon thereafter, few doctors, nutritionists, or researchers gave the ketogenic diet any attention—especially after they learned of the research done by a man who would change our food industry for years to come. His name was Ancel Keys.

The Study Heard 'Round the World

If you're familiar with the name Ancel Keys, it's probably due to the "Great Man" theory of history—the idea that history is changed by "strong personalities steer[ing] events using their own personal charisma, intelligence, wisdom, or wits" (Teicholz, 2014). In the history of nutrition, Ancel Keys was, by far, the Greatest Man.

Keys, an influential nutrition scientist, had an interesting career: he started out studying fish physiology and went on to develop the famous Seven Countries Study. Little did he know the impact that his work would have for decades to come.

Until Keys's work in the early 1950s, the reigning theory on the cause of arterial plaque—a key risk factor for heart disease—was based on studies done in the early 1900s by Russian pathologist Nikolaj Anitschkow. These studies pointed to the notion that consuming large amounts of cholesterol could induce atherosclerosis and plaque formation in the arteries (Bailey, 1916). Despite several limitations in the study design, they paved the way for years of research that led to a negative perception of dietary cholesterol. But in the early 1950s, Keys discredited this theory: he fed subjects up to 3,000 milligrams of cholesterol per day (the equivalent of about sixteen eggs) and found that it had no significant effect on blood cholesterol levels (Keys, 1950). Many other studies had similar results showing that high dietary cholesterol (cholesterol consumed in the diet) didn't necessarily lead to high blood cholesterol levels, and the focus on dietary cholesterol began to fade.

However, heart disease was on the rise, and scientists were scrambling to find a solution to stop the epidemic. They were looking for a scapegoat, and it just so happened that they closed their eyes in a crowded room, picked at random, and called out an innocent individual known as fat as the culprit. Keys led the charge: in 1952, he switched his focus from dietary cholesterol to dietary fat and thus began the development of his "diet-heart hypothesis," which eventually linked dietary fat and heart disease in the minds of millions and led to a low-fat craze that persisted for decades.

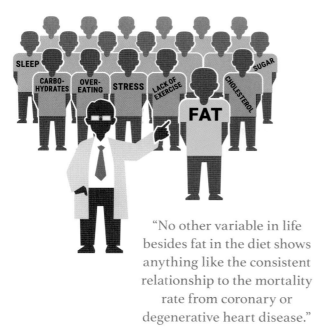

"No other variable in life besides fat in the diet shows anything like the consistent relationship to the mortality rate from coronary or degenerative heart disease."

—Ancel Keys, 1954

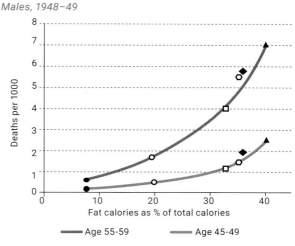

Figure 2.2. *Ancel Keys's Correlative Study showing that higher fat consumption was associated with higher death rates.*

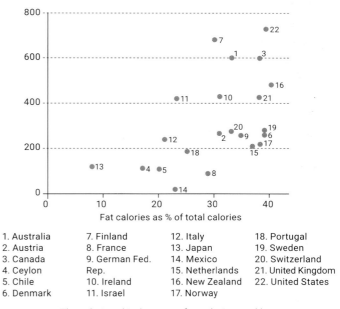

Figure 2.3. *The relationship between fat calories and heart disease in twenty-two countries.*

It was time for Ancel Keys to take his stand. In 1953, he published a paper called "Atherosclerosis: A Problem in Newer Public Health" in which he began to associate fat consumption with heart disease mortality. In 1955, at the World Health Organization, Keys was questioned by British physician Sir George Pickering. Pickering asked Keys to provide evidence for his hypothesis that the consumption of dietary fat was associated with heart disease. Keys referred to a graph from his paper on atherosclerosis in which he compared fat intake and heart disease mortality in six countries: the United States, Canada, Australia, England, Italy, and Japan (Keys, 1953). The results, he believed, were straightforward: Americans consumed the greatest amount of dietary fat and had the most deaths from heart disease. The Japanese ate the least fat and had the fewest deaths from heart disease. Therefore, dietary fat caused heart disease. After much questioning about this correlation, Keys left the conference feeling defeated and set out on a quest to prove his point to his colleagues. If only he could do a larger study, he thought, maybe that would "show them."

Around this same time, President Dwight Eisenhower suffered his first heart attack, and interest in nutrition and its impact on heart health grew exponentially. More researchers jumped into the fold, looking to find the magic bullet to help our president, our country, and ultimately our own hearts. In 1957, Jacob Yerushalmy and Herman Hilleboe, two attendees of the WHO meeting, wrote a rebuttal to Keys titled "Fat in the Diet and Mortality from Heart Disease: A Methodological Note." This paper included data from twenty-two countries rather than just the six that Keys had looked at. Yerushalmy and Hilleboe still found a positive correlation between calories from fat and incidence of heart disease, but their takeaways were very different from Keys's. For example, the death rate from heart disease in Finland was more than twenty times that in Mexico, even though fat consumption rates in the two nations were similar. When the researchers looked at deaths from all causes rather than isolating heart disease, they found that mortality had a *negative* correlation with fat intake: people in countries with higher fat intakes were actually living longer. When all the data were presented, the only positive correlation with deaths from all causes was consumption of *carbohydrates* (Yerushalmy and Hilleboe, 1957).

> It is well known that the indirect method merely suggests that there is an association between the characteristics studied and mortality rates and . . . is not in itself proof of a cause-effect relationship.
> —Yerushalmy and Hilleboe, 1957

But perhaps the most important thing to remember about these studies is that *correlation doesn't equal causation*. One example we like to use is that the murder rate is highly correlated with a rise in ice cream sales. In this case, someone could make the same argument as Keys and state that eating ice cream causes people to become murderers. Obviously, this isn't the case, but this example demonstrates the importance of knowing

the difference between correlation and causation. Ice cream sales tend to rise in the summer months; crime rates also increase during this time for numerous reasons. However, a chocolate chip cookie dough sundae won't make someone a murderer (unless it doesn't have sprinkles, of course).

> "The collector walks with blinders on; he sees nothing but the prize."
> —Anne Morrow Lindbergh

In 1958, Keys and several of his colleagues around the world initiated the Seven Countries Study, which examined the association between diet (particularly saturated fat intake) and cardiovascular disease, comparing the health and diets of nearly 13,000 middle-aged men in the United States, Japan, and Europe. Keys determined that countries in which people consumed large amounts of saturated fat in meat and dairy saw higher levels of heart disease than those in which people ate more grains, fish, nuts, and vegetables (Keys, 1980). This led to what became known as the diet-heart hypothesis: that eating saturated fat raises blood cholesterol and therefore increases the risk of heart disease. In Keys's eyes, it was as if (in an anachronistic analogy)

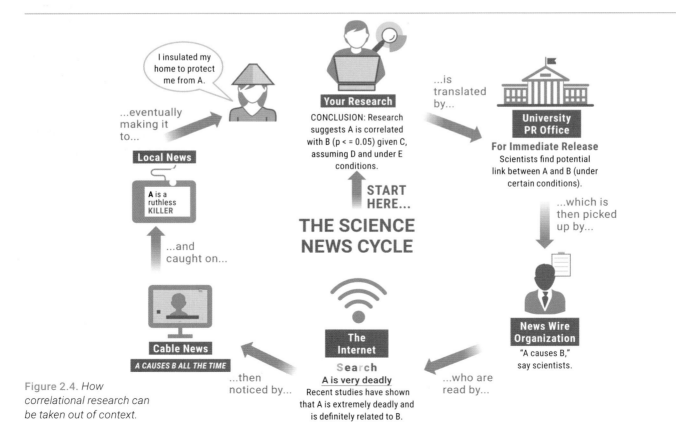

Figure 2.4. How correlational research can be taken out of context.

he was the hero of *Rocky II*, knocked to the canvas by his colleagues but persevering to become the last man standing at the end of the fight.

Except there was one big problem: Rocky beat Apollo fair and square, but in this instance, Keys rigged the fight. A strategic fighter, Keys found advantages in the form of what researchers term "selection bias." Instead of selecting countries randomly, Keys chose to report on and discuss only those likely to support his hypothesis, including Yugoslavia, Finland, and Italy. He excluded countries like France, Switzerland, Sweden, and West Germany, where people consumed a lot of fat yet didn't suffer from high rates of heart disease. Regardless, keep in mind that the Seven Countries Study focused on *correlation, not causation.* At no point has it ever been determined that eating fat *causes* heart disease; the study simply looked for a correlation between rates of heart disease and consumption of saturated fat.

These major problems notwithstanding, the damage was done. Based on the Seven Countries Study, Americans began to believe that eating fat increased the risk of heart disease. Ancel Keys may not have predicted the impact his work would have on nutrition, but it was tremendous: his results led the U.S. government to institute dietary guidelines, policies, and food-labeling procedures that demonized fat, particularly saturated fat, and are still around today . . . at least for now.

The year 1961 turned out to be one of the most important in the history of nutrition. Keys sealed saturated fat's fate by landing a position on the nutrition committee of the American Heart Association and instituting the country's first-ever nutrition guidelines advising a limited intake of

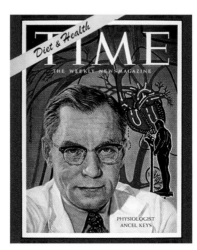

Figure 2.5. *Dr. Ancel Keys on the cover of* Time *magazine.*

saturated fat. He appeared on the cover of *Time* magazine for his philosophies and findings on solving the health crisis, and the idea that eating fat was linked to poor health spread rapidly. In 1977, Dr. Mark Hegsted, a nutrition researcher and huge advocate for Keys's conclusions, helped persuade Senator George McGovern, chairman of the Senate Committee on Nutrition and Human Needs, to include a recommendation for limiting fat intake in that year's *Dietary Goals for the United States.* These guidelines, which were based on observational studies, "partial" scientists, and questionable methodologies, had severe limitations. Hegsted, who was named Administrator of Human Nutrition for the Department of Agriculture in 1978, claimed, "Important benefits could be expected from following the low-fat recommendations. And for the risks? None can be identified." If only he could have looked into the future, I'm sure he would have taken those words back.

Hello from the Other Side

Not all scientists agreed that fat is the major culprit in heart disease. One British scientist in particular was screaming at the top of his lungs that another macronutrient was the real driving force, yet no one wanted to listen. In 1972, John Yudkin claimed in his book *Pure, White, and Deadly,* "If only a small fraction of what we know about the effects of sugar were to be revealed in relation to any other material used as a food additive, that material would promptly be banned" (Yudkin, 1972). Yudkin kept trying to wrap his head around how everyone was overlooking the health implications of sugar, a pure carbohydrate lacking fiber and nutrition that had been a part of the Western diet for only a couple hundred years.

While most health authorities labeled saturated fat as the scapegoat, Yudkin postulated that it likely was the recent introduction of sugar that was making people sick. Not only were the low-fat recommendations misguided, but they could actually be dangerous if they encouraged people to consume more sugar. In 1974, *The Lancet,* a British medical journal, warned against significantly reducing dietary fat, reinforcing the idea that the cure should not be worse than the disease. These scientists knew that

if dietary fat were drastically reduced, there would be an equally drastic increase in one of the other two macronutrients, and it wasn't going to be protein. First, protein is significantly more expensive, and second, sugar can make even the worst of the worst carbohydrates taste sweet. But Yudkin was shot down by both Keys and various government bodies anytime he attempted to present new evidence pointing to sugar, not fat, as the culprit in heart disease (Yudkin, 1964).

It was David versus Goliath, except in this case, there were ten Goliaths and only one David; Yudkin and his colleagues were vastly outnumbered by the disciples of Keys's work. During the 1960s and '70s, researchers and individuals who opposed Keys's work tended to lose support and funding, which had a detrimental impact on their ability to continue to conduct research. It was almost as if anyone who opposed Keys's work was committing scientific funding suicide.

In the mid-1900s, a plethora of data was gathered that could and should have freed us from the perception that saturated fat was the culprit. Unfortunately, the ideology with the louder voice won, and that voice belonged to Ancel Keys.

KETO CONCEPT

The Sugargate Scandal

In the 1950s and '60s, nutrition debates were peaking. In one corner was Ancel Keys, who targeted fat as the cause of heart disease, and in the other were Yudkin and others, who claimed that sugar was the problem. Prominent Harvard nutritionist Mark Hegsted sided with Keys. In addition to urging the government to advocate for reducing fat intake in its official recommendations, Hegsted was paid the equivalent of $48,000 by a trade group called the Sugar Research Foundation to write a literature review (an analysis of multiple studies done on a single topic) aimed at countering early research linking sucrose (table sugar) to coronary heart disease.

As every criminal defense attorney knows, the key to a good defense is providing an alternative theory of the crime—a narrative with some coherence and probability that lays the blame at the feet of someone other than the accused. Hegsted certainly understood this. To counter the claim that sugar was linked to heart disease, he shifted the focus to dietary fat and cholesterol intake. His study was published in 1967 in the *New England Journal of Medicine* (McGandy et al., 1967). At the time, researchers did not have to disclose conflicts of interest, so no one knew about Hegsted's big payday. His pay-for-play agreement with the sugar industry is a classic example of how an ethically irresponsible decision can have an effect for generations to come.

The Resurgence of the Ketogenic Diet

"It is no measure of health to be well-adjusted to a profoundly sick society."
—Jiddu Krishnamurti

Despite the development of anti-convulsant drugs and the demonization of fat, some rare places never let the ketogenic diet die. The Johns Hopkins Hospital headed the ketogenic charge in the 1970s under the leadership of neurologists Dr. Samuel Livingston and Dr. John Freeman and dietitian Millie Kelly, who together refined the ketogenic diet specifically to treat epilepsy in children. New studies were surfacing on the effects of fasting, ketogenic dieting, and elevations in ketone levels on various markers of health.

One such study (Drenick et al., 1972) took a group of obese men with insignificant blood ketone levels and injected them with insulin to observe the clinical signs of hypoglycemia. The subjects then fasted for two months straight, losing an average of 33 kilograms (72.6 pounds). Their blood ketone levels were elevated to around 8 mmol/L, and finally the researchers repeated the insulin injections expecting to see similar results, with signs of hypoglycemia and potentially even reaching the point of a coma. Surprisingly, there were no adverse responses in the men, even when the insulin caused their blood glucose levels to drop "dangerously low." This study pointed to the fact that when ketones are elevated to a significant degree, they may be able to offer protection from hypoglycemia by providing an alternative fuel source for the brain. Scientists were becoming more fascinated with ketones, the therapeutic benefits of fasting, and the potential benefits of elevating ketones through nutritional means. It's the latter that would ultimately lead to the resurgence of the ketogenic diet.

Ask someone if they've ever tried a low-carbohydrate diet and you'll often hear them say, "Yeah, I've done Atkins before." Robert C. Atkins was an American physician and cardiologist who struggled with obesity and decided to try the diet advocated by Dr. Alfred Pennington. In the years following World War II, Pennington had been hired by DuPont, a large American chemical company, to uncover the reasons behind a rapidly growing obesity problem among

its staff. He concluded that obesity was not due merely to overeating but also to the body's inability to properly utilize glucose. Basically, he recommended that instead of seeing it as an energy balance issue, we should focus on what our bodies do with the food we eat—burn it or store it as fat. Pennington's diet became popularly known as the DuPont Diet and was published by *Holiday* magazine in the 1950s. Pennington published an editorial in the *New England Journal of Medicine* in 1953 discussing the role of carbohydrates in obesity.

Atkins found immediate and lasting weight loss on Pennington's diet and began prescribing a similar approach for his patients who struggled to lose weight. In 1965, he promoted his weight-loss plan on *The Tonight Show,* and in 1972 he published *Dr. Atkins' Diet Revolution,* which became an instant bestseller. The diet wasn't necessarily ketogenic (though the two often overlap)—Atkins's approach was centered around high protein, inclusion of fats, and lower carbohydrates. The low-carb craze took the world by storm, and the idea of losing weight without severely restricting calories became extremely popular. Atkins certainly wasn't the first person to recommend this kind of diet, but he made a big impression on the nutrition industry that lasted for years and paved the way for scientists and researchers to investigate the effects of a low-carb, and eventually a ketogenic, diet.

Though Atkins was making waves by advocating a high-fat, high-protein diet, his voice was soon drowned out by the voices of Hegsted and McGovern,

---

Was There a Pre-Atkins Revolution?

Pennington wasn't the only doctor to advocate a low-carb diet in the 1950s. In 1958, Dr. Richard Mackarness, a physician at an obesity and food allergy clinic in Britain, published *Eat Fat and Grow Slim,* which argues that carbohydrates, rather than calories, are the real offenders responsible for weight gain. A couple years later, Dr. Herman Taller published his book *Calories Don't Count.* Taller was one of the first to say that diets need to be individualized, as not everyone responds to food in the same way. Rather, he stated, "The crux of the matter is not how many calories we take in, but what our bodies do with those calories." Not everyone can tolerate carbohydrates to the same degree; instead, we need to personalize nutrition.

These two books were popular, but they made nowhere near the headlines that Robert Atkins would make with his book a decade later.

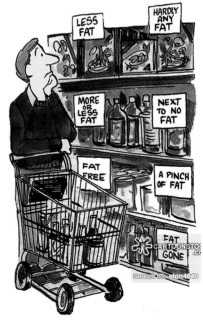

Figure 2.6. *Grocery store shelves lined with "low-fat" marketing phrases in order to entice customers with the "health" benefits of products.*

who issued the new dietary guidelines with low-fat recommendations just a couple years after Atkins published his book. With the government placing the blame for cardiovascular disease squarely on fat consumption, several large food corporations jumped at the chance to claim that their products were healthy by changing their formulations so they could advertise that they were "low-fat" (Wartella et al., 2010). Beginning in the late 1970s and continuing to this day, food companies have attempted to catch consumers' eyes with bold claims on product labels suggesting that the products promote good health because they are "low in saturated fat."

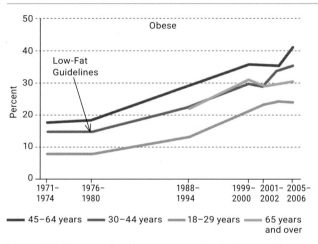

Figure 2.7. *Obesity rates have continued to climb since the introduction of these low-fat recommendations.*

Source: National Center for Health Statistics (US). Health, United States, 2008: With Special Feature on the Health of Young Adults. Hyattsville (MD): National Center for Health Statistics (US); 2009 Mar. Chartbook.

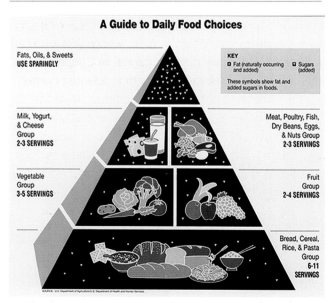

Figure 2.8. *The USDA Food Pyramid.*

Over the next twenty years, research into the ketogenic diet exploded because of the popularity of Atkins and a renewed interest in epilepsy. At the same time, the government's dietary recommendations didn't seem to be panning out; obesity continued to rise at a steady rate. In 1992, Atkins published *Dr. Atkins' New Diet Revolution,* an update to the 1972 bestseller. Shortly thereafter, Barry Sears released *The Zone,* a hugely popular diet book that distinguished between good and bad carbohydrates, and Drs. Michael and Mary Dan Eades published *Protein Power,* which advocated a high-protein, low-carb diet. Both books alluded to the fact that the advice to eat low-fat wasn't ideal and that processed carbohydrates were causing a lot of the health issues plaguing society. But in 1992, the USDA launched its Food Pyramid recommending that Americans consume six to eleven daily servings of bread, cereal, rice, pasta, and other grains while using fats and oils "sparingly." What we really needed was to flip that pyramid upside down.

One Last Chance

In 1993, Charlie Abrahams, the son of Hollywood movie producer Jim Abrahams and his wife, Nancy, was facing an incredible challenge. At just one year old, Charlie had been diagnosed with epilepsy. As time passed, his situation worsened—so much so that at twenty months old, he was having up to 100 seizures per day. Charlie was put on one medication after another, to no avail. Jim Abrahams said later in a *Dateline* interview, "You pour the drugs down your child's throat despite the fact that something inside you says, 'Wait a minute, this can't be right.'" The Abrahamses were relentless in their pursuit of a solution, yet they met dead end after dead end. Charlie's health was deteriorating rapidly, but giving up was never an option.

After scouring through hundreds of books on epilepsy searching for a solution, Abrahams stumbled upon *Seizures and Epilepsy in Childhood: A Guide for Parents,* by Dr. John Freeman, one of the pediatric neurologists at Johns Hopkins who had been using a ketogenic diet to treat epilepsy. Deep within this book,

Dr. Freeman briefly mentions a dietary protocol he had used to treat the condition. Charlie had traveled thousands of miles to see some of the best doctors in the world, taken some of the most powerful drugs, undergone surgery, and even seen faith healers and herbalists, without effect. With no other options left, the Abrahamses packed their bags and flew to Baltimore to see Dr. Freeman and learn about his diet that had been successful in treating epilepsy: the ketogenic diet.

Charlie was immediately put on a strict ketogenic diet. Within forty-eight hours, his seizures had completely stopped. As the days, weeks, and even months passed, Charlie remained seizure-free, and his growth and development rapidly improved (Wheless, 2004). The ketogenic diet was the answer the Abrahamses had been looking for. To spread the word to other families struggling with epilepsy, Jim Abrahams created the Charlie Foundation, an organization that has put out videos and other content to increase awareness of the ketogenic diet as a treatment for epilepsy and has funded research into the use of ketogenic therapies for a wide variety of conditions.

The ketogenic diet got a huge boost in October 1994, when an episode of the popular TV show *Dateline* featured Charlie's incredible story, raising awareness and invigorating the research community to explore the ketogenic diet further. Then, in 1997, Abrahams produced a TV movie starring Meryl Streep called …*First Do No Harm,* which showcases Charlie Abrahams's experience with the ketogenic diet. More than eight million viewers watched the movie on the night it aired. Parents and kids from all over the world began flocking to Johns Hopkins to try the ketogenic diet, and in 2001 a study from there concluded that more than 150 kids with epilepsy had seen remarkable improvements on the ketogenic diet.

The Abrahamses' advocacy was exactly what scientists and researchers in the ketogenic realm needed. It was a sign of hope and highlighted the significant impact that the ketogenic diet can have on health. In the 1990s and early 2000s, thousands of studies on the ketogenic diet investigated its effect on everything from epilepsy to cancer to Alzheimer's to body composition and performance. Throughout this book, we will delve into each of these areas in more detail and discuss new research and emerging support for the ketogenic diet.

Exogenous Ketones: An Emerging Area of Research

Over the course of the history of the ketogenic diet, scientists have discovered that elevations in ketone production cause some unique physiological responses that may offer health benefits (which we'll explore more in the rest of this book). It's not always easy to increase our level of ketones by altering our diet. But what if we could achieve elevated ketones by taking exogenous ketones—those that are consumed orally rather than produced by the body—in a food or supplement? To find the first example of research into this practice, we have to go back more than seventy years to a study on the motility of bull sperm. (Yes, you read that correctly: bull sperm.) Lardy and Phillips (1945) discovered that beta-hydroxybutyrate (BHB) and acetoacetate (AcAc), two ketone bodies, increased bull sperm motility while simultaneously decreasing cellular oxygen consumption. This interesting finding would go unexplained until legendary German physician and biochemist Hans Krebs decided to mentor a student to investigate further how ketones could increase the metabolic efficiency of cells.

Krebs is credited with the discovery of the key sequences of metabolic reactions that produce energy inside our cells, now called the Krebs cycle, for which he earned a Nobel Prize in 1953. Krebs was also a colleague of Otto Warburg, whom you will read a lot about when we discuss cancer in Chapter 5. In the late 1950s, Krebs worked with a scientist named Richard Veech to determine the redox state of the cell: how much energy is being used and wasted and whether the cell is efficient at what it's supposed to do. This research laid the foundation for how taking ketones could impact human health by improving the efficiency of cells. In the early 1990s, Veech and his colleagues began publishing more of their studies showing that ketone bodies were having positive effects on cardiac efficiency and improving the energy production in mitochondria (the powerhouse of a cell) (Kashiwaya et al., 1997). At around the same time, other studies were showing that BHB not only reduced food consumption and body weight (we will discuss this more in the body composition and appetite section) but also improved insulin sensitivity (Arase et al., 1988; Amiel et al., 1991). Could it be possible for people to receive the health benefits of ketones even if they weren't sticking to a strict ketogenic diet?

In 2000, Veech and his colleagues published a study on the effects of one kind of ketone on neurons that are representative of Alzheimer's and Parkinson's disease (Kashiwaya et al., 2000). Soon after, in 2004, the U.S. Defense Advanced Research Projects Agency (DARPA) gave several groups—including Dr. Veech and his lab—$2 million each per year as part of a competition to find a "superfuel" for the U.S. Special Forces to use in combat. Veech and his research partner, Kieran Clarke, soared to the top of the competition and received further funding from DARPA to dig deeper into the effects of the use of ketones on performance. This eventually led to the development of an FDA-approved food: ketone esters (discussed more in Chapter 4).

A couple years later, Dr. Dominic D'Agostino began investigating the impact of ketogenic dieting on simulated Navy SEAL dive missions. These divers tend to develop oxygen rebreather–related seizures because they dive to significant depths and constantly rebreathe excess oxygen from their tanks. Dr. D'Agostino was looking for ways to prevent these seizures from occurring. One possible solution was to develop a method to help stabilize the brain during deep dives. D'Agostino looked at the effects of different ketone esters in animal studies that simulated what Navy SEAL divers do in a deep dive with an oxygen rebreather (D'Agostino et al., 2013). Just one dose of the ketone ester delayed the onset of seizure activity *significantly.*

There are very few "aha" moments in a scientist's lifetime, and this surely was one for Dr. D'Agostino and his team. It was clear that there was something very interesting going on with brain energy metabolism and exogenous ketones. D'Agostino and several other researchers have since conducted numerous studies investigating the effects of exogenous ketones on various conditions. (In Chapters 4 and 5, we dig deeper into those studies, the different forms of exogenous ketones [esters, salts, etc.], and emerging data on dosage, timing, and applications.)

Unfortunately, there are two downsides to ketone esters: one, they are currently very expensive, and two, they taste like jet fuel. To sell exogenous ketones to the public, something needed to change. Chemist Patrick Arnold brought to market a more palatable ketone mineral salt solution (BHB-sodium, BHB-calcium, BHB-magnesium, and BHB-potassium). Though it was available, many people still didn't understand what ketones were, what they could be used for, and what the long-term implications of utilizing them were. However, shortly thereafter, a network marketing company called Pruvit set out to bring ketones to the masses. Fast-forward to today, and Pruvit has delivered over 30 million servings of exogenous ketones to people with incredible results and has begun running research trials to take an even deeper look at its product.

Other network marketing companies, along with traditional brick-and-mortar stores, are now carrying products containing exogenous ketones. It is only a matter of time before exogenous ketones become mainstream; we would be surprised if you don't see them at your local health food store or even in grocery stores in the very near future. More studies investigating the impact of ketone mineral salts, ketone esters, and other ketogenic agents on health and human performance are rapidly emerging (which we will discuss later in this book), and we promise you that this is just the beginning.

CHAPTER SUMMARY

In this chapter, we took a journey back over a century to look at the origin of fasting, how it was used in the early 1900s, and why fat was demonized. We discussed the resurrection of the ketogenic diet and even presented an overview of the hot new topic of exogenous ketones. We hope you now have a better understanding of why we are in this situation and why the current dietary guidelines read the way they do. Read on for a scientific overview of ketosis, the ketogenic diet, its implications, and delicious keto-friendly recipes.

References

Amiel, S. A., H. R. Archibald, G. Chusney, A. J. Williams, and E. A. Gale. "Ketone infusion lowers hormonal responses to hypoglycaemia: evidence for acute cerebral utilization of a non-glucose fuel." *Clinical Science* 81, no. 2 (1991): 189–94.

Arase, K., J. S. Fisler, N. S. Shargill, D. A. York, and G. A. Bray. "Intracerebroventricular infusions of 3-OHB and insulin in a rat model of dietary obesity." *American Journal of Physiology-Regulatory, Integrative and Comparative Physiology* 255, no. 6 (1988): R974–81.

Atkins, R. C. *Dr. Atkins' Diet Revolution: The High Calorie Way to Stay Thin Forever.* D. McKay Co., 1972.

Bailey, C. H. "Atheroma and other lesions produced in rabbits by cholesterol feeding." *Journal of Experimental Medicine* 23, no. 1 (1916): 69–84.

Banting, W. *Letter on Corpulence,* addressed to the public...with addenda. (1869). Harrison.

Bennett, J. *Muscles, Sex, Money, & Fame.* Lulu.com, 2013.

Brillat-Savarin, J. A. (MFK Fisher, trans.). "The physiology of taste: Or, meditations on transcendental gastronomy." Washington, D.C.: Counterpoint, 1999. (Original work published 1825.)

Conklin, H. W. "Cause and treatment of epilepsy." *Journal of the American Osteopathic Association* 22, no. 1 (1922): 11–14.

D'Agostino, D. P., R. Pilla, H. E. Held, C. S. Landon, M. Puchowicz, H. Brunengraber, ... and J. B. Dean. "Therapeutic ketosis with ketone ester delays central nervous system oxygen toxicity seizures in rats." *American Journal of Physiology-Regulatory, Integrative and Comparative Physiology* 304, no. 10 (2013): R829–36.

Drenick, E. J., L. C. Alvarez, G. C. Tamasi, and A. S. Brickman. "Resistance to symptomatic insulin reactions after fasting." *Journal of Clinical Investigation* 51, no. 10 (1972): 2757.

Freeman, J. M. *Seizures and Epilepsy in Childhood: A Guide for Parents.* Baltimore: Johns Hopkins University Press, 1997.

Geyelin, H. R. "Fasting as a method for treating epilepsy." *Med Rec* 99 (1921): 1037–9.

Geyelin, H. R. "The relation of chemical influences, including diet and endocrine disturbances, to epilepsy." *Annals of Internal Medicine* 1929 (2): 678–81.

Hendricks, M. "High fat and seizure free." *Johns Hopkins Magazine,* April 1995: 14–20.

Hunt, W. R. *Body Love: The Amazing Career of Bernarr Macfadden.* Chicago: Popular Press, 1989.

Kashiwaya, Y., T. Takeshima, N. Mori, K. Nakashima, K. Clarke, and R. L. Veech. "d-β-Hydroxybutyrate protects neurons in models of Alzheimer's and Parkinson's disease." *Proceedings of the National Academy of Sciences* 97, no. 10 (2000): 5440–4.

Kashiwaya, Y., M. T. King, and R. L. Veech. "Substrate signaling by insulin: a ketone bodies ratio mimics insulin action in heart." *American Journal of Cardiology* 80, no. 3A (1997): 50A–64A.

Kearns, C. E., L. A. Schmidt, and S. A. Glantz. "Sugar industry and coronary heart disease research: a historical analysis of internal industry documents." *JAMA Internal Medicine* 176, no. 11 (2016): 1680–5. doi: 10.1001/jamainternmed.2016.5394.

Keys, A. "Atherosclerosis: A Problem in Newer Public Health." *Atherosclerosis* 1 (1953): 19.

Keys, A. "Epidemiological studies related to coronary heart disease: characteristics of men aged 40–59 in seven countries." *Acta Medica Scandinavica* 180, no. 460 (1966): 4–5.

Keys, A. "Seven countries. A multivariate analysis of death and coronary heart disease." Cambridge, MA: Harvard University Press, 1980.

Keys, A., O. Mickelsen, E. V. O. Miller, and C. B. Chapman. "The relation in man between cholesterol levels in the diet and in the blood." American Association for the Advancement of Science. *Science* 112 (1950): 79–81.

Lardy, H. A., and P. H. Phillips. "Studies of fat and carbohydrate oxidation in mammalian spermatozoa." *Archives of Biochemistry* 6, no. 1 (1945): 53–61.

Lennox, W. G., and S. Cobb. "Studies in epilepsy. VIII: The clinical effect of fasting." *Archives of Neurology & Psychiatry* 20 (1928): 771–9.

Lozano, R., C. J. Murray, A. D. Lopez, and T. Satoh. "Miscoding and misclassification of ischaemic heart disease mortality." *Global Program on Evidence for Health Policy Discussion Paper* (2001): 12.

Mackarness, R. *Eat Fat and Grow Slim.* London: Harvill Press, 1958.

McGandy, R. B., D. M. Hegsted, and F. J. Stare. "Dietary fats, carbohydrates and atherosclerotic vascular disease." *New England Journal of Medicine* 277, no. 4 (1967): 186–92.

McGovern, G. "Dietary goals for the United States." *Report of the Select Committee on Nutrition and Human Needs of the United States Senate.* Washington, D.C.: U.S. Government Printing Office, 1977.

Milton, K. "Hunter-gatherer diets—a different perspective." *American Journal of Clinical Nutrition* 71, no. 3 (2000): 665–7.

Noakes, T., J. Proudfoot, and S. A. Creed. *The Real Meal Revolution: The Radical, Sustainable Approach to Healthy Eating.* London: Hachette UK, 2015.

Pennington, A. W. "A reorientation on obesity." *New England Journal of Medicine* 248, no. 23 (1953): 959–64.

Peterman, M. G. "The ketogenic diet in epilepsy." *Journal of the American Medical Association* 84, no. 26 (1925): 1979–83.

Swink T. D., E. P. G. Vining, and J. M. Freeman. "The ketogenic diet: 1997." *Advances in Pediatrics* 44 (1997): 297–329.

Taller, H. *Calories Don't Count.* New York: Simon & Schuster, 1961.

Teicholz, N. *The Big Fat Surprise: Why Butter, Meat and Cheese Belong in a Healthy Diet.* New York: Simon & Schuster, 2014.

Temkin, O. *The Falling Sickness: A History of Epilepsy from the Greeks to the Beginnings of Modern Neurology.* Baltimore: Johns Hopkins University Press, 1994.

Wartella, E. A., A. H. Lichtenstein, and C. S. Boon, eds. "History of Nutrition Labeling." In *Institute of Medicine Committee on Examination of Front-of-Package Nutrition Rating Systems and Symbols.* Washington, D.C.: National Academies Press, 2010.

Welch, H. W., F. J. Goodnow, S. Flexner, et al. "Memorial meeting for Dr. John Howland." Bull. 000 Johns Hopkins Hospital 41 (1927): 311–21.

Westman, E. C., J. S. Volek, and S. D. Phinney. *New Atkins for a New You: The Ultimate Diet for Shedding Weight and Feeling Great.* New York: Fireside, 2010.

Wheless, J. W. "History and origin of the ketogenic diet." In *Epilepsy and the Ketogenic Diet* (31–50). Humana Press, 2004.

Yerushalmy, J., and H. E. Hilleboe. "Fat in the diet and mortality from heart disease; a methodologic note." *New York State Journal of Medicine* 57, no. 14 (1957): 2343–54.

Yudkin, J. "Patterns and trends in carbohydrate consumption and their relation to disease." *Proceedings of the Nutrition Society* 23 (1964): 149–62.

Yudkin, J. *Pure, White, and Deadly: The New Facts About the Sugar You Eat as a Cause of Heart Disease, Diabetes, and Other Killers.* London: Davis-Poynter Limited, 1972.

Chapter 3:

CONSTRUCTING A WELL-FORMULATED KETOGENIC DIET

It is comical to watch people gawk and stare as they walk by a table of individuals who are eating a keto-friendly meal. It's even more hilarious when those individuals pull out their ketone meters and test their ketone levels after eating. Upon beginning this diet, it's almost as if people treat their ketones like a game of Pokemon Go. Register a 0.3 mmol and it's like catching a Pidgey (very easy); register over 2.0 mmol and it's as if you caught a Dragonite (very difficult). The biggest challenge, however, comes in the individuality of the results. For instance, we were recently having lunch with two of our colleagues: one of them ate just bacon and cream cheese, while the other ate salmon, a large green salad, and broccoli cooked in coconut oil and butter. Almost as if the restaurant had turned into a Poke-Gym, the ketone meters came out and the battle was on.

After a brief period, the results were in. Both of them had played a Pikachu (moderately difficult) and ended up at around 0.8 mmol. How could this be? The composition of their meals differed drastically, yet they ended up with the same levels of ketones. Does that mean both meals were well-formulated? This chapter addresses that very question.

There are numerous ways to induce nutritional ketosis. You could refrain from eating entirely (i.e., fast) or, at the opposite end of the spectrum, you could consume 70 to 100 percent of your calories in the form of fat. A ketogenic diet is by nature a low-carbohydrate diet; however, a low-carbohydrate diet is not always a ketogenic diet. Further questions arise as to how many and which types of carbohydrates you should consume. What about protein, which the body can convert to glucose? And what about macronutrient ratios? Ketogenic and non-ketogenic nutrients? It all boils down to these essential questions:

What is the role of each macronutrient, and how do they function as part of a well-formulated ketogenic diet that will place you in a state of nutritional ketosis and simultaneously optimize your health, satiety, and long-term success?

Let's dive in and discuss what it means to develop a well-formulated ketogenic diet.

Ketogenicity and the Ketogenic Ratio

A diet's *ketogenicity* is its ability to induce ketogenesis (the production of ketones) in the body and therefore elevate blood ketone levels. To understand ketogenicity, scientists have developed an equation known as the Ketogenic Ratio (Cohen et al., 2009):

$$\text{Ketogenic Ratio} = \frac{\text{ketogenic factors}}{\text{anti-ketogenic factors}}$$

Ketogenic factors are foods that contribute to the body's ability to induce ketosis, while anti-ketogenic factors oppose it. An example of a ketogenic factor is MCT oil, which is digested rapidly, contributing to the production of ketones (see page 56 for more on MCT oil). Bread would be an anti-ketogenic factor, since it is primarily carbohydrates, which raise blood glucose and insulin and thus prevent the production of ketones. Fats tend to be ketogenic, while carbohydrates serve as anti-ketogenic factors. Protein gets a bit tricky since it is both ketogenic and anti-ketogenic. (Some amino acids found in protein, such as leucine and lysine, can be ketogenic, while others, like alanine, are anti-ketogenic.) For the sake of the Ketogenic Ratio, protein and carbohydrates are classified as anti-ketogenic factors, and fat is the ketogenic factor.

Therefore, we can say that the Ketogenic Ratio = grams of fat / (grams of protein + grams of carbohydrate).

A 3:1 ratio means that there are 3 grams of fat for every 1 gram of protein and carbohydrates. So if a snack contains 21 grams of fat and 7 grams of carbohydrates and protein combined, it would have a 3:1 ratio. As another example, say you took an egg (which has 6 grams of protein and 5 grams of fat) and cooked it in 7 grams of coconut oil. You would be consuming roughly 12 grams of fat, 6 grams of protein, and 0 grams of carbohydrates, or a 2:1 ratio.

Most people tend to eat a more modified ratio of around 2:1, with 2 grams of fat (ketogenic) for every 1 gram of protein and carbohydrates (anti-ketogenic). This ratio falls more in line with a 75 to 80 percent fat, 15 to 20 percent protein, and 5 percent carbohydrate based diet. When it comes to therapeutic modalities such as epilepsy, a 4:1 ratio is commonly prescribed. In this case, nearly 90 percent of the diet is fat and 10 percent is a combination of protein and carbs.

This equation has a basic clinical application because it provides a foundation to start with and build from. However, this method has limitations because:

1) it assumes that protein is completely anti-ketogenic, and

2) it takes only macronutrient percentages into consideration rather than total calories.

Research shows that this method truly predicts ketogenicity only when an individual is in calorie balance, meaning that calories consumed equal calories expended (Cohen et al., 2009). As discussed earlier, being keto-adapted increases fat utilization; therefore, this equation doesn't take into account the stored body fat being burned. This is why a person may be at a 2:1 or even a 1:1 ratio, yet still be in a state of ketosis (Heilbronn et al., 2005).

Finally, the Ketogenic Ratio doesn't take into account that not all carbohydrates affect the body in the same way. As we will discuss later in this book, green vegetables (fibrous carbohydrates) may be ketogenic, while pasta (a non-fibrous carbohydrate) is not. Because fibrous carbohydrates don't have a glucose or insulin response and are not completely digested, they don't inhibit ketogenesis like sugar or sugary foods do. Therefore, while the Ketogenic Ratio is nice as a basic guideline, you still must account for other factors—such as total calories consumed; sources of fat, carbohydrate, and protein; activity level; and meal frequency—when designing the best approach for *you*.

Carbohydrates

Carbohydrates are basically carbon-based (*carbo*) substances that contain water (*hydrates*). Carbohydrates can be classified as monosaccharides, disaccharides, or polysaccharides:

- **Monosaccharides,** or simple carbohydrates, are the basic structures of carbohydrates. Examples of monosaccharides include glucose (the simplest form of sugar), fructose (fruit sugar), and galactose (a sugar found in milk).

- Two monosaccharides bound together are known as a **disaccharide**. Examples of disaccharides include sucrose (table sugar), which is glucose bound to fructose, and lactose (another sugar found in milk), which is glucose bound to galactose.

- More than ten units of monosaccharides bound together are known as **polysaccharides**. Polysaccharides include starches (breads and cereals), cellulose (roughage), dextrin (baked potatoes), and pectin (jam).

On a ketogenic diet, carbohydrate levels are kept low to prevent spikes in blood glucose and, consequently, insulin.

Glycemic Index and Glycemic Load

Until the last two decades, people divided carbohydrates into simple and complex carbs to describe how fast they were digested and subsequently how rapidly they raised blood glucose. *Simple* was the term used to describe mono- and disaccharides, which make blood sugar rise rapidly, while *complex* was used to describe polysaccharides, which elicit a slower increase in blood glucose. This classification makes sense because the simpler the molecule, the easier it is to break down. The more chains (i.e., polysaccharides) to be broken, the longer it takes to absorb. However, we now realize that nutrition is much more complex. Scientists have developed two new scales that go into a little more detail: the glycemic index and glycemic load.

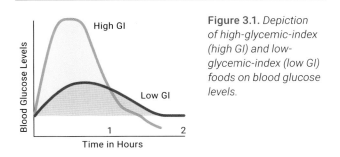

Figure 3.1. *Depiction of high-glycemic-index (high GI) and low-glycemic-index (low GI) foods on blood glucose levels.*

KETO CONCEPT

Blood Sugar

Our bodies use glucose to fuel cells—so when we refer to blood sugar, we're talking about the amount of glucose that's in the bloodstream. For the average person on a carbohydrate-based diet, blood glucose fluctuates from 80 to 120 mg/dL when fasting. When a person's blood glucose ranges from 125 mg/dL when fasting to more than 200 mg/dL after eating, that individual is said to be either pre-diabetic or diabetic. One way to track blood glucose is with a glucometer. Upon waking in the morning, use the glucometer to check your fasted glucose level to see where you are. If you really want to take it to the next level, check your blood glucose before certain meals or snacks and then 30, 60, and 90 minutes after eating those meals or snacks and see how they affect you. Within two hours after a meal, your blood glucose should return to the normal range (80 to 120 mg/dL); however, in individuals who are insulin resistant/pre-diabetic, these numbers can remain elevated for several hours after a carbohydrate-rich meal. Blood glucose varies from person to person, so it's important to be your own scientist here. Your blood glucose should be lower on a ketogenic diet than on a carbohydrate-based diet. Don't be alarmed if your fasting blood glucose level drops below 80 mg/dL on a ketogenic diet, as this is common. Just make sure to monitor it.

The glycemic index is a scale from 1 to 100 that describes how fast a food raises blood glucose after it is consumed. Pure glucose is set at 100, and everything else is compared to that. For example, a slice of white bread is given a GI of about 75; meanwhile, peanuts have a GI of 14.

Glycemic load is also a measure of how carbohydrates impact blood sugar, but it takes into account an extra variable: the total amount of carbohydrates in a food and how those carbohydrates affect blood sugar levels. To determine glycemic load, you take the amount of carbohydrates per serving of the food, multiply by its glycemic index, and then divide by 100.

$$\text{Glycemic Load} = \left(\frac{\text{total carbohydrates}}{\text{per serving}} \times \text{GI} \right) / 100$$

So the glycemic load in that slice of white bread is calculated as follows:

(15 x 75) / 100 = 11.25

The amount of carbohydrates a food contains doesn't show up in its glycemic index, but it has a big effect on the food's glycemic load. For example, carrots have a glycemic index of 47—on the high end of low—and contain 5 grams of carbohydrates per serving. However, when you calculate their glycemic load, they are a 2.4—on the low end of low. In contrast, whole-wheat pasta has a glycemic index of 48 (on the high end of low) but contains 40 grams of carbohydrates, so its glycemic load is fairly high at 19.2.

GLYCEMIC INDEX (GI)		GLYCEMIC LOAD (GL)	
Low	0–55	Low	0–10
Intermediate	56–69	Intermediate	11–19
High	≥70	High	≥20

The takeaway here is that using only the glycemic index to evaluate carbohydrate sources may limit our ability to develop a well-formulated ketogenic diet that includes carbohydrate sources that have a low glycemic load. While numerous factors affect the absorption of a carbohydrate (both how fast it's absorbed and how much of it is absorbed), the two factors that are often overlooked are fiber and water content.

Fiber and Total Carbohydrates versus Net Carbohydrates

Many people attempt to avoid carbohydrates altogether on a ketogenic diet. However, that also means avoiding fiber, which has important health benefits, especially for the gut. Dietary fibers are carbohydrates that are not broken down in the small intestine and instead make it to the large intestine, where they are broken down by bacteria. The great thing about fiber is that it has been shown to lower body fat, assist in managing diabetes, improve insulin sensitivity, decrease the risk of heart disease, elevate satiety, and foster beneficial bacteria in our guts (Slavin, 2013; see Figure 3.2). Moreover, the fermentation of fiber in the gut produces short-chain fatty acids (SCFA), such as acetate, butyrate, and propionate, which are also ketogenic.

Research demonstrates that most individuals switching from a normal carbohydrate-based diet to a ketogenic diet drastically lower their fiber intake. In fact, one study found that decreasing carbohydrates from 400 to 23 grams daily also decreased fiber intake from 28 to 6 grams (Duncan et al., 2007). As a result, subjects decreased both their healthy bacteria as well as the production of healthy short-chain fatty acids. We believe it is paramount to maintain fiber intake on a ketogenic diet (by consuming green leafy vegetables and fibrous foods) and focus on reducing net carbohydrates: total carbohydrates minus fiber (see the table, opposite).

Resistant Starch and Butyrate

Resistant starches do exactly what their name implies: resist digestion. These types of starches have been shown to improve insulin sensitivity and reduce appetite. However, too much resistant starch can lead to bloating or GI discomfort due to the fact that it doesn't get digested. Once it's fermented by the bacteria in the gut, a short-chain fatty acid known as butyrate is produced. Butyrate is actually the preferred fuel of the cells that line the colon, and there is a host of data showing its beneficial effects on human health and function. Finding ways to increase butyrate levels while lowering carbohydrates on a ketogenic diet can significantly improve gut bacteria and long-term success with the diet.

Several lines of evidence support focusing on net carbs instead of total carbs, but we will focus on just two of them. The first is that fiber, even though it is counted as a carbohydrate, should be resistant to digestion, so it does not increase blood glucose or insulin levels—and often lowers them (Slavin et al., 2013). Second, research shows that foods high in fiber could allow carbohydrates in the diet to be increased from 4 to 10 percent without hindering seizure control in epileptic patients (Pfeifer et al., 2005). Thus we suggest counting net carbs and including high-fiber foods in your diet. Green and cruciferous vegetables are great ways to add fiber and volume.

The total amount of net carbohydrates in a diet will vary from person to person. However, a classic study found that in overweight but healthy college-age people, blood ketone levels were highest when the subjects ate 30 grams of net carbohydrates a day, were moderate when they ate 60 grams, and were near zero when they ate 100 grams (Young et al., 1971). It is still not clear whether someone on a long-term ketogenic diet needs fiber; ketones (beta-hydroxybutyrate) and fatty acids could help maintain gut health and function by increasing butyrate without the need for dietary fiber. However, upon starting the diet, we recommend that you include fibrous vegetables to help improve short-chain fatty acid production and keep satiety high and hunger at bay.

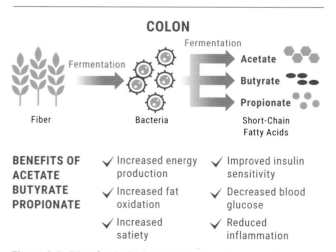

COLON

Fermentation → Fiber → Bacteria → Fermentation → Short-Chain Fatty Acids: Acetate, Butyrate, Propionate

BENEFITS OF ACETATE BUTYRATE PROPIONATE
- ✓ Increased energy production
- ✓ Increased fat oxidation
- ✓ Increased satiety
- ✓ Improved insulin sensitivity
- ✓ Decreased blood glucose
- ✓ Reduced inflammation

Figure 3.2. Fiber feeds the bacteria in the gut, which ultimately produces short-chain fatty acids like butyrate. These short-chain fatty acids have a wide range of potential benefits.

VEGETABLE	FAT	CARBS	FIBER	NET CARBS	PROTEIN	CALORIES	SERVING
Asparagus	0.4 g	7 g	4 g	3 g	4 g	40	1 cup raw
Beets	0.2 g	13 g	4 g	9 g	2 g	58	1 cup raw
Bell peppers, green	0.3 g	7 g	3 g	4 g	1 g	30	1 cup raw
Bell peppers, red	0.4 g	9 g	3 g	6 g	1 g	39	1 cup raw
Broccoli	0.6 g	11 g	5 g	6 g	4 g	55	1 cup raw
Brussels sprouts	0.8 g	11 g	4 g	7 g	4 g	56	1 cup raw
Red cabbage	0.11 g	5.16 g	1.5 g	3.66 g	1 g	22	1 cup raw
Napa cabbage	0.1 g	7 g	2 g	5 g	1 g	28	1 cup raw
Carrots	0.3 g	12 g	4 g	8 g	1 g	52	1 cup raw
Cauliflower	0.1 g	5 g	2 g	3 g	2 g	25	1 cup raw
Celery	0.1 g	5 g	2 g	3 g	2 g	25	1 cup raw
Collard greens	0.2 g	2 g	1 g	1 g	1 g	11	1 cup raw
Corn, yellow	1.38 g	19.07 g	2 g	17.07 g	3.34 g	88	1 ear raw
Cucumber	0.2 g	3 g	1 g	2 g	1 g	14	1 cup raw
Eggplant	0.2 g	5 g	3 g	2 g	1 g	20	1 cup raw
Fennel	0.1 g	6.3 g	2.7 g	3.6 g	1 g	27	1 cup raw
Green beans	0.1 g	8 g	4 g	4 g	2 g	34	1 cup raw
Green peas	0.6 g	21 g	7 g	14 g	8 g	117	1 cup raw
Kale	0.5 g	7.3 g	2.6 g	4.7 g	2.5 g	36	1 cup raw
Leeks	0.3 g	13 g	2 g	11 g	1 g	54	1 cup raw
Mushrooms, white	0.2 g	2 g	1 g	1 g	2 g	15	1 cup raw
Mushrooms, cremini	0.07 g	3.1 g	1.4 g	1.7 g	1.8 g	16	1 cup raw
Mushrooms, portobello	0.29 g	3.3 g	0.29 g	3.01 g	2 g	18	1 mushroom
Mushrooms, shiitake	0.49 g	6.8 g	2.5 g	4.3 g	2 g	34	1 cup
Olives, black	1.9 g	1 g	1 g	0 g	0 g	21	5 medium olives
Olives, green	2.6 g	1 g	1 g	0 g	0 g	25	5 medium olives
Onions	0.1 g	16 g	2 g	14 g	1 g	67	1 cup raw
Lettuce, romaine	0.1 g	1 g	1 g	0 g	0 g	6	1 cup raw
Lettuce, iceberg	0.08 g	1.69 g	0.7 g	0.99 g	0.51 g	8	1 cup raw
Spinach	0.1 g	1 g	1 g	0 g	1 g	7	1 cup raw
Squash, summer	0.2 g	4 g	1 g	3 g	1 g	18	1 cup raw
Squash, butternut	0.07 g	8.18 g	1.4 g	6.78 g	0.7 g	32	½ cup
Tomato	0.4 g	7 g	2 g	5 g	2 g	32	1 cup raw
Turnip greens	0.17 g	3.92 g	1.8 g	2.12 g	0.82 g	18	1 cup raw
Zucchini	0.2 g	4 g	1 g	3 g	1 g	18	1 cup raw

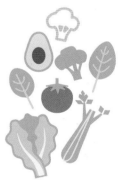

KETO CONCEPT

Volume of Foods

One complaint that people have when ketogenic dieting with low-fiber foods is that the volume of food is not enough to make them feel full. Think about the last time you ate cereal or fruit snacks. Personally, we both could easily eat four bowls of cereal and an entire bag of gummy worms without feeling full. However, when was the last time you "overate" broccoli or Brussels sprouts? When following a ketogenic diet, it's easy to make low-fiber meals or snacks that aren't very satiating. For example, when we first tried a ketogenic diet several years ago, we were hooked on something called keto mousse, a delicious combination of heavy cream, coconut butter, protein, and macadamia nuts. A serving is only about a cup, but it is calorically dense (nearly 750 calories). You can imagine how easy it would be to overindulge in a food like that.

One possible solution to this satiety problem is to include low-calorie, high-fiber foods, such as green and cruciferous vegetables. For example, instead of keto mousse, you could have a large salad with bacon and blue cheese and pork rind "croutons," and then have some ground beef with broccoli. The increased volume of food along with the increased fiber would likely make you feel way fuller and wouldn't have you snacking soon thereafter. So make sure to incorporate low-calorie, high-fiber veggies (such as those in the table above), especially while you are adapting to the ketogenic diet, so that you feel satiated.

Does Net Really Mean Net?

Pick up a protein bar or "sugar-free" snack and the label might say "low net carbs" or even "0 net carbs." Unfortunately, because of how nutrition labeling works, that figure doesn't always mean that the bar is a good choice on a ketogenic diet. First, some of the "fibers" that are used in these items actually do increase blood glucose and insulin levels, thus they technically aren't fibers. The FDA is currently looking deeper into these false fibers to require companies to adjust their product labels accordingly.

Second, instead of fibers, companies sometimes use sugar alcohols to sweeten their treats. Given the current nutritional labeling regulations, these sugar alcohols can be subtracted from the overall carbohydrate count; even if an item has 20 grams of carbohydrates and 15 grams of sugar alcohols, it can be labeled as having "5 net carbohydrates." Similar to the mislabeled "fibers," some of these sugar alcohols (for example, the maltitol found in sugar-free gummy bears) can have an effect on blood glucose and, worse, tear up your stomach if consumed in high amounts. Be cautious about consuming these types of foods, especially at the onset of a ketogenic diet. Beware of marketing gimmicks such as net carbs, and research the fiber or sugar alcohol being used to ensure that it won't raise your blood glucose or leave you running for the bathroom. If you feel like being your own scientist, sample various foods or snacks and use your glucometer to measure how they affect your glucose levels. For more information, go to www.ketogenic.com/nutrition/guidetofiber to see what makes up a "true" fiber.

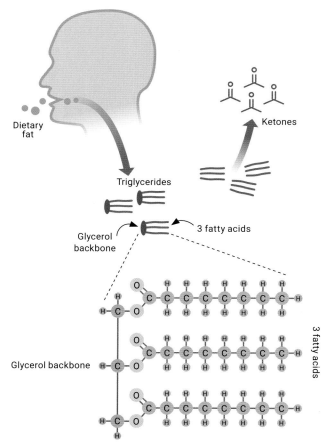

Figure 3.3. *The process of dietary fat getting broken down into triglycerides and eventually fatty acids and ketones.*

level. Fats come in the form of triglycerides in our diet and also are stored as triglycerides, molecules that consist of a glycerol backbone connected to three fatty acids. The liver can use the glycerol backbone to create glucose during gluconeogenesis, but the remainder of the fat molecule is nearly all ketogenic—breaking it down produces ketones. For this reason, fat should comprise the majority of your diet, representing 60 to 90 percent of total calories.

Fats

Let's face it: fat has been vilified for decades. The fact that we have written a book in which we recommend eating large amounts of fat is really a disruptive concept to the nutrition industry. What we want to do is give you a Fat 101 tutorial.

First, though, a quick explanation of why fat is the preferred macronutrient for ketosis on a molecular

Saturated and Unsaturated Fats

To explain what saturated and unsaturated fats are, we first have to look at the molecular structure of fat. A molecule of a carbohydrate, such as glucose, contains six carbon atoms. But a fat molecule can have from two to eighty carbon atoms! Each carbon atom can form a bond with four other atoms. Two of these bonds will always be used to connect it to the next carbon in the chain. If the remaining two bonds are connected to hydrogens, the fat is said to be *saturated* with hydrogen atoms; if they don't bond with hydrogen atoms, the fat is considered *unsaturated.*

Imagine a line of people standing with their arms and legs outstretched. Each limb represents a potential bond. Everyone joins hands with the people on either side of them, so there are two bonds left to be made (with their legs). Those individuals who have people grabbing onto their legs would be considered saturated since all four limbs are connected to others; meanwhile, those who don't have anyone clinging to their legs would be considered unsaturated.

Unsaturated fats can be further divided into monounsaturated and polyunsaturated fats. Monounsaturated fats have a single double bond (i.e., one person clinging to one leg), while polyunsaturated fats have more than one double bond (no one grabbing onto either leg).

Most people can easily identify saturated fats. They are solid at room temperature and include animal-based fats such as lard, dairy-based fats such as butter, and coconut-based fats such as coconut oil. Conversely, unsaturated fats are liquid at room temperature and are typically vegetable-based; monounsaturated fats include olive oil, nut oils, and avocado oil, while polyunsaturated fats include canola oil and fish oil. Increased consumption of monounsaturated and polyunsaturated fatty acids has been shown to increase blood ketones (Fuehrlein et al., 2004) and lower blood triglycerides (Volek et al., 2000), which are a risk factor for heart

disease. Saturated fats often are feared due to the correlational research discussed earlier in the book. However, saturated fats convey many health benefits, including elevating HDL cholesterol and increasing LDL cholesterol size (which is a good thing; we want large LDL, not little particles that can get stuck and lead to plaque formation and buildup). In the presence of a low-carbohydrate diet, saturated fats are easily metabolized and broken down (Mensink et al., 2003; Forsythe et al., 2010).

Finally, there are trans fats, which are produced when a manufacturer turns unsaturated fat into saturated fat by adding hydrogens to vegetable oil to make it solid at room temperature. Products like margarine are high in trans fats—stay away from these! Trans fats are the one type of fat we recommend steering clear of due to their negative effects on health, such as raising total LDL cholesterol and lowering HDL cholesterol. Trans fats are commonly used by fast-food chains because they can be used repeatedly for frying. However, the FDA recently stepped in to state that trans fats are no longer "generally recognized as safe" and is requiring companies to remove them from manufacturing and food-making processes in the near future.

We recommend that you consume fat from a variety of sources. Trying to avoid particular fats can have repercussions in other areas of health. For example, research shows that avoiding eggs in an effort to reduce saturated fat intake is less beneficial for raising good cholesterol than consuming a diet higher in eggs (Mutungi et al., 2008).

Essential Fatty Acids

Essential fatty acids are those fatty acids that aren't synthesized in the body and therefore must be obtained from food. They are classified as polyunsaturated omega-3, omega-6, and omega-9 fatty acids based on the position of the first double bond (on the third, sixth, or ninth carbon). Omega-3 essential fatty acids include alpha-linolenic acid (ALA), found in plants, and eicosapentaenoic acid (EPA) and docosahexaenoic acid (DHA), found in animal foods, especially fish (Swanson et al., 2012).

ALA has potential ketogenic properties. Recent research has shown that consuming 2 grams of

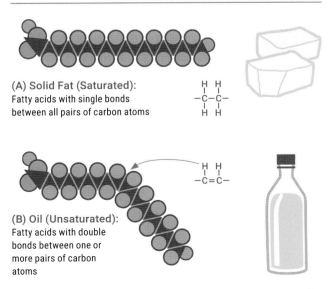

(A) Solid Fat (Saturated): Fatty acids with single bonds between all pairs of carbon atoms

$$-\overset{\displaystyle H}{\underset{\displaystyle H}{C}}-\overset{\displaystyle H}{\underset{\displaystyle H}{C}}-$$

(B) Oil (Unsaturated): Fatty acids with double bonds between one or more pairs of carbon atoms

$$-\overset{\displaystyle H}{C}=\overset{\displaystyle H}{C}-$$

Figure 3.4. *The difference between saturated and unsaturated fatty acids.*

ALA daily in the form of flax seed raised post-meal ketone production by 26 percent (Hennebelle et al., 2016) and that supplementing with 2.5 grams per day of omega-3 fatty acids from fish oil (1.8 grams of EPA and 0.7 grams of DHA) had positive effects on subjects' blood lipid profiles (Volek et al., 2000). Blood lipid profiles (cholesterol, triglycerides, fatty acids, etc.) are important because they can be predictors of cardiovascular disease risk. Omega-6 fatty acid needs appear to be met readily through a normal ketogenic diet without the need to supplement.

Based on all this data, we recommend consuming salmon, mackerel, or even Dr. D'Agostino's favorite, sardines, frequently since these fish are high in omega-3 fatty acids and ALA. In addition, we suggest adding foods like flax seed to keto-friendly milkshakes or other recipes and selecting a daily fish oil supplement with at least 2 grams of EPA and DHA combined. For more recommendations, see Chapter 6.

Short- and Medium-Chain Fatty Acids

In a fat molecule, each carbon atom is bound to multiple hydrogen atoms, making it a hydrocarbon. Since the carbon atoms are linked to each other, we can think of a fat molecule as a chain of hydrocarbons. Short-chain fatty acids are comprised of fewer than six carbon atoms; medium-chain fatty acids (MCFA) are comprised of six to ten carbon atoms; and long-chain fatty acids are comprised of more than ten carbon atoms.

Our lab has found that of these fats, short-chain fatty acids are the most ketogenic and that, in general, a shorter carbon chain is more ketogenic. While short-chain fatty acids are abundant in dairy-based fats such as butter and cream, supplements containing SCFAs tend to taste and smell rancid. However, theoretically, if someone could mask the smell and taste of butyrate (an SCFA), it could be the most ketogenic fatty acid of all. For this reason, most people prefer to supplement with MCT oil or powder, which contains medium-chain fatty acids plus a glycerol backbone (making it a triglyceride). We will discuss MCTs since they are a common staple in the ketogenic diet.

MCTs are less likely than long-chain triglycerides (LCTs) to be stored as fat because their shorter carbon chain length enables them to be digested rapidly. (LCTs are commonly found in most foods and oils.) The shorter chain length allows MCTs to be broken down into medium-chain fatty acids (breaking off the glycerol backbone and leaving the three fatty acids) by enzymes in saliva and stomach juices. Following this breakdown, medium-chain fatty acids move from the digestive tract to the liver for immediate energy production. Long-chain fatty acids, on the other hand, can be broken down only by pancreatic enzymes (bile acids and lipases). Once broken down, they are transported from the small intestine on chylomicrons (little "boats") through the lymphatic system before entering the bloodstream, giving them a greater chance of being taken up by adipose (fat) tissue for storage. Compared to short- and medium-chain fatty acids, which can go directly to the liver without chylomicrons, long-chain fatty acids require more transport to break down.

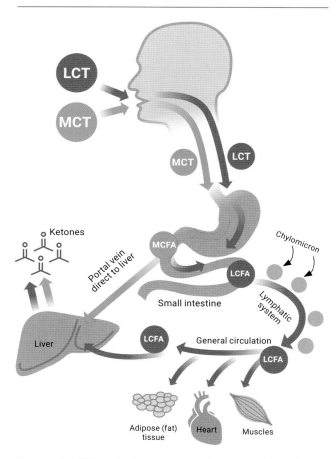

Figure 3.5. *MCTs are broken down rapidly compared to LCTs, which need transportation and enzymes to be broken down, thereby making the process lengthier.*

The unique aspect of MCTs is that they have been found to be much more ketogenic than normal long-chain fatty acids. Moreover, MCT supplementation has been shown to increase metabolism in the short term (St-Onge et al., 2003), raise blood ketones (Van Wymelbeke et al., 1998), and enhance fat loss (Tsuji et al., 2001). (We discuss MCT supplementation in more detail in Chapter 4.) Foods high in MCTs are coconut oil (50 percent) and butter and heavy cream (from 4 to 12 percent). You can also take MCT supplements in oil or powder form. Unfortunately, for many people, MCT supplementation may cause an upset stomach. Therefore, we recommend starting low (2 to 5 grams) and working your way up to 5 to 10 grams per serving to test your tolerance and help reduce upset stomach.

In summary, fats form the cornerstone of a ketogenic diet. We recommend that roughly 60 to 80 percent of your diet come from this energy source, depending on your ultimate goal (e.g., weight loss versus overall health). Fats should come from a variety of animal sources—red meat (ground beef and steak), poultry (chicken thighs), fish, and dairy (butter and cream)—as well as from plant sources, such as coconut oil, olive oil, nuts, and avocados, and from pure MCTs.

Protein

The third macronutrient is protein. Unlike carbohydrates and fats, proteins are thought to be used primarily to build hair, nails, enzymes, and various organ systems like skeletal muscle, the heart, and the brain. In addition to serving as building blocks for body tissues, proteins signal several reactions in the body, including the release of hormones such as glucagon and insulin and the stimulation of muscle building via increased protein synthesis. While proteins can be used as an energy source, this is not their primary function. However, research shows that dietary protein is essential for muscle repair and optimizing muscle mass. There are a number of factors to consider when it comes to dietary protein on a ketogenic diet, particularly the amount and quality of protein that needs to be consumed for general health.

Research demonstrates that consuming protein improves exercise performance and protects against muscle loss when consumption is between 1.2 and 1.5 grams of protein per kilogram of body weight while in a ketogenic state (Phinney et al., 2004). So a person who weighs 100 kilograms (220 pounds) would want to consume 120 to 150 grams of protein per day in order to reap the most benefits from protein. As part of an average 2,000-calorie diet, this would mean 20 to 30 percent of the diet coming from protein. It has been proposed that protein intake should not exceed 20 to 25 percent of a person's diet, as a higher intake might make it difficult to get into ketosis because protein contains glucogenic amino acids (e.g., alanine) that theoretically could be utilized to make glucose when needed. However, research in epilepsy patients showed that a modified Atkins diet consisting of approximately 64 percent fat and 31 percent protein (a 2:1 ratio) was as effective as a traditional 4:1 ratio ketogenic diet at reducing seizure risk (Kossoff et al., 2008). One thing that does appear certain is that consuming less than 1.0 to 1.2 grams of protein per kilogram of body weight results in declines in both lean mass and endurance performance (Phinney et al., 2004).

In summary, protein is a critical nutrient for tissue repair, functionality, and skeletal muscle health, as well as immune support. We recommend that individuals on a ketogenic diet consume a minimum of 1.0 to 1.2 grams of protein per kilogram of body weight, but no more than 1.7 grams per kilogram of body weight. This typically works out to 20 to 30 percent of total calories. Those who are sedentary or not training may want to stay on the lower end of that range, while individuals who train frequently may fare better on the upper end.

To calculate this recommendation for yourself, do the following:

1) Divide your weight in pounds by 2.2; this is your weight in kilograms.

2) Multiple your weight in kilograms by a number between 1.2 and 1.7 to arrive at your recommended protein intake.

Micronutrient and Electrolyte Considerations

Micronutrients are nutrients that we need in small quantities to survive. They include vitamins and minerals, such as calcium, iron, zinc, magnesium, and sodium. Research suggests that when people start a ketogenic diet, their micronutrient intake often declines. This is because, in focusing on selecting fatty foods, they eliminate nearly all carbohydrates, including vegetables, which are a great source of micronutrients. For example, broccoli, cauliflower, spinach, and even avocados and eggs (with the yolks) are packed with essential vitamins and minerals. This is why we preach about consuming whole foods in order to meet these micronutrient requirements.

Electrolytes are perhaps the greatest concern for ketogenic dieters. Electrolytes, which include sodium and potassium, are charged substances that are required for normal bodily functions, such as nervous system regulation and muscle activity. Drops in electrolytes seem to occur primarily in the first week after beginning a ketogenic diet.

Sodium

Sodium helps the body regulate water levels, blood pressure, and pH balance. On a ketogenic diet, insulin levels drop in the absence of carbohydrates, causing the body to start excreting excess sodium and water. Insulin increases sodium retention by boosting sodium reabsorption; therefore, low insulin levels lead to increased fluid and sodium excretion (DeFronzo, 1981). The typical person gets sufficient sodium through the traditional Western diet, but ketogenic dieters often suffer from low sodium levels due to excessive excretion at the onset of the diet; this leads to a need for increased sodium intake. In a twenty-eight-day study, obese individuals consumed either a low-carbohydrate or a high-carbohydrate diet. Compared to the high-carbohydrate group, the low-carbohydrate group demonstrated greater urinary sodium excretion in the first week, but this disappeared over the twenty-eight-day period,

demonstrating that adaptations occurred as they became keto-adapted (Rabast et al., 1981). Keep in mind that a sodium intake that is too low can be just as dangerous as an intake that is too high. As with all essential nutrients, the graph for risk association with sodium and health problems is U-shaped, such that both low and high intakes of sodium are associated with an increased risk of cardiovascular disease and all-cause mortality (Alderman, 1998).

Potassium

Potassium is an important mineral that helps the body maintain pH balance, build proteins, sustain normal growth, and control the electrical activity of the heart. Like sodium levels, potassium levels can drop on a ketogenic diet due to water excretion (Phinney et al., 1983). One study comparing low-carb and high-carb diets found that potassium excretion was greater in the low-carbohydrate group for the first two weeks, but after four weeks, potassium excretion on a low-carbohydrate diet did not differ from a high-carbohydrate diet (Rabast et al., 1981).

Magnesium and Calcium

Magnesium plays many roles, including helping to maintain normal nerve and muscle function and heart rate, supporting a healthy immune system, regulating blood glucose levels, and aiding in energy production (Guerrera et al., 2009). Magnesium deficiencies are common; however, due to the excretion of key minerals that occurs due to low insulin levels on a ketogenic diet, magnesium also should be supplemented or eaten in the form of foods such as avocados or nuts.

Calcium is essential for cardiovascular health. Calcium deficiencies aren't as apparent on a ketogenic diet due to common food choices containing adequate amounts, such as fish, cheese, and greens, but some people find themselves lacking in dietary calcium. The Western diet has succumbed to the calcium-fortified craze by fortifying milk and even cereal with calcium to ensure that our levels are sufficient. However, many of these fortified foods contain too many carbs for someone on a ketogenic diet. Still, it is recommended that calcium come from food first and supplements second, as data strongly suggests a greater benefit from calcium derived from food (Napoli et al., 2007).

Electrolyte Supplementation

Overall, electrolyte levels appear to drop at the beginning of a ketogenic diet before returning to normal levels once a person is keto-adapted. In addition to the studies cited above, a study of obese adolescents demonstrated normal electrolyte levels after consuming a ketogenic diet for eight weeks (Willi et al., 1998). However, a large six-month study demonstrated a decrease in blood sodium in obese individuals combined with an increase in urinary calcium excretion over that period (Westman et al., 2002). Similarly, a six-week low-carbohydrate, high-protein diet also showed an increase in calcium excretion (Reddy et al., 2002).

Therefore, sodium, potassium, calcium, and even magnesium may need to be supplemented on a ketogenic diet, especially at the onset. In fact, Dr. Stephen Phinney recommends 3 to 5 grams of sodium and 2 to 3 grams of potassium daily for individuals who are exercising regularly. Deciding whether you need to supplement will likely depend on the types of foods you are eating. You could get sufficient amounts of these electrolytes from food, but individuals who exercise regularly need to be liberal with sodium intake because they lose it rapidly during exercise through both urine and sweat. Many people who have headaches or feel lethargic in the early stage of the diet see quick improvements when they add an electrolyte supplement that boosts sodium, potassium, magnesium, and/or calcium levels. Depending on your diet (for example, whether you eat mineral-rich foods or add salt to your meat), these ketogenic aids can be stopped or continued for as long as needed.

Meal Frequency and Intermittent Eating

The general trend over the last few decades has been to eat small, frequent meals. Bodybuilders, who are trying to turn on that switch known as muscle protein synthesis as much as possible, have popularized this approach. With the goal of maximizing that response, some individuals tend to consume five to seven meals per day, eating every few hours. The theory is that small, frequent meals may stoke our metabolism and lead to greater increases in fat loss. However, multiple studies have shown that increasing meal frequency does not appear to significantly affect body composition, nor does it boost metabolism (La Bounty et al., 2011; Schoenfeld et al., 2015).

However, *restricting* the number of times you eat while maintaining a ketogenic lifestyle appears to have several advantages. First, research shows that fasting elevates blood ketone levels due to the absence of carbohydrates and a reliance on fat as a fuel source (Varady et al., 2013). (We will discuss this more later in the book.) While strict, long-term fasting is likely not the lifestyle that most individuals will choose, intermittent eating (periodic fasting) protocols are an alternative.

There are two basic structures for intermittent eating: alternate-day eating and time-restricted feeding. (You may know these instead as "alternate-day fasting" and "intermittent fasting," but for some people the word *fasting* is scary. These are the same concepts, just reworded for a different perspective.)

In alternate-day eating, you switch between days of normal eating and days of restricting calories to 25 percent of normal intake (Varady et al., 2013). For example, if you normally eat 2,000 calories, you might eat that amount on Monday but consume only 500 calories on Tuesday and continue to rotate.

In time-restricted feeding, you eat during a certain window every day. This window can last anywhere from four to twelve hours.

Both protocols have resulted in fat loss and a sparing of muscle mass (Hatori et al., 2012). Moreover, individuals experience hunger on fasting

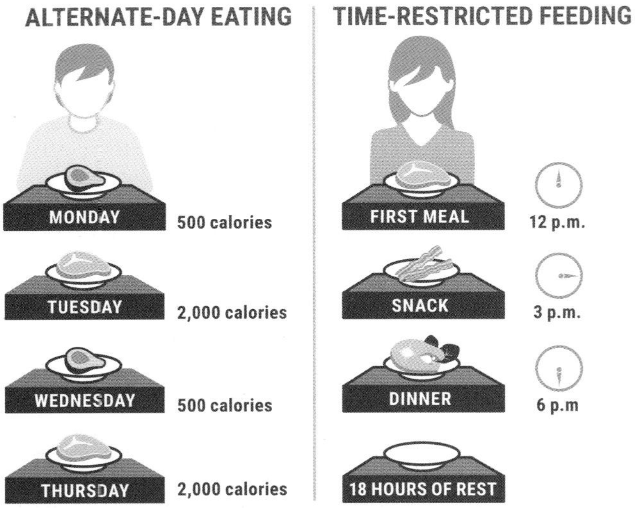

ALTERNATE-DAY EATING

MONDAY	500 calories
TUESDAY	2,000 calories
WEDNESDAY	500 calories
THURSDAY	2,000 calories

TIME-RESTRICTED FEEDING

FIRST MEAL	12 p.m.
SNACK	3 p.m.
DINNER	6 p.m
18 HOURS OF REST	

Figure 3.6. *Alternate-day eating and time-restricted feeding are the two basic forms of intermittent eating.*

days during the first two weeks, but after that they tend to adapt (Varady et al., 2013). Why? It's possible that because intermittent eating raises ketone levels, after an adjustment period the body is able to switch easily between getting fuel from food and getting fuel from ketones (Johnson et al., 2007).

Thus we suggest that you use one of the following meal-frequency plans for ketogenic dieting:

- Consume a normal breakfast and dinner, but have coffee or another noncaloric beverage instead of a meal at lunchtime (time-restricted feeding of ten to twelve hours).

- Fast in the morning and eat only in the afternoon and evening (time-restricted feeding). For example, you might eat between 1:00 p.m. and 8:00 p.m. Perhaps once or twice a week, shorten the eating window (say, from 4 p.m. to 9 p.m.). This would allow you to see how you respond to intermittent eating and discover what works best with your lifestyle.

- Every other day, reduce your normal caloric intake (breakfast, moderate lunch, and dinner) to 500 to 1,000 calories (alternate-day eating).

- Have coffee with heavy cream or MCTs for breakfast and lunch and eat a normal dinner (time-restricted feeding). This is a type of "fat fast" that mimics the normal fasting response, yet you consume calories in the form of straight fat.

As we will discuss in later chapters, the meal frequency you select will ultimately depend on whether your goal is muscle gain, fat loss, weight maintenance, or health outcome, and most importantly on your lifestyle. By fine-tuning the eating window, intermittent eating can help further the benefits of the ketogenic diet.

CHAPTER SUMMARY

For relatively healthy individuals, we recommend following a ketogenic diet that emphasizes a variety of healthy saturated and unsaturated fats, vegetables, and protein sources. In general, you should aim to keep net carbohydrates to less than 10 percent of your diet and eat at least 15 grams of fiber each day. Fats should make up between 60 and 80 percent of your daily calories. We suggest keeping protein in the range of 1.2 to 1.7 grams per kilogram of body weight daily, or around 20 to 30 percent of your diet.

Micronutrients such as sodium, potassium, magnesium, and calcium tend to be depleted on a ketogenic diet, particularly at the beginning of the keto adaptation phase. We recommend taking an electrolyte supplement that contains sodium and potassium and eating magnesium- and calcium-rich foods daily.

Finally, meal frequency should be dictated by your personal goal. Because intermittent eating increases ketone levels, it can be useful in conjunction with a ketogenic diet. The spacing and frequency of meals can be adjusted according to your preference, but we recommend eating no more than three meals a day. In the "Keto for You" section of Chapter 6, we go into more detail about how to design and follow a ketogenic diet that is tailored to your unique needs and goals.

References

Alderman M. H., H. Cohen, and S. Madhavan. "Dietary sodium intake and mortality: the National Health and Nutrition Examination Survey (NHANES I)." *The Lancet* 351, no. 9105 (1998): 781–5.

Cohen, I. A. "A model for determining total ketogenic ratio (TKR) for evaluating the ketogenic property of a weight-reduction diet." *Medical Hypotheses* 73, no. 3 (2009): 377–81.

DeFronzo, R. A. "The effect of insulin on renal sodium metabolism." *Diabetologia* 21, no. 3 (1981): 165–71.

Duncan, S. H., et al. "Reduced dietary intake of carbohydrates by obese subjects results in decreased concentrations of butyrate and butyrate-producing bacteria in feces." *Applied and Environmental Microbiology* 73.4 (2007): 1073–8.

Forsythe, C. E., S. D. Phinney, R. D. Feinman, B. M. Volk, D. Freidenreich, E. Quann, ... and D. M. Bibus. "Limited effect of dietary saturated fat on plasma saturated fat in the context of a low carbohydrate diet." *Lipids* 45, no. 10 (2010): 947–62.

Fuehrlein, B. S., M. S. Rutenberg, J. N. Silver, M. W. Warren, D. W. Theriaque, G. E. Duncan, ... and M. L. Brantly. "Differential metabolic effects of saturated versus polyunsaturated fats in ketogenic diets." *Journal of Clinical Endocrinology & Metabolism* 89, no. 4 (2004): 1641–5.

Guerrera, M. P., S. L. Volpe, and J. J. Mao. "Therapeutic uses of magnesium." *American Family Physician* 80, no. 2 (2009): 157–62.

Hatori, M., C. Vollmers, A. Zarrinpar, L. DiTacchio, E. A. Bushong, S. Gill, ... and M. H. Ellisman. "Time-restricted feeding without reducing caloric intake prevents metabolic diseases in mice fed a high-fat diet." *Cell Metabolism* 15, no. 6 (2012): 848–60.

Heilbronn, L. K., S. R. Smith, C. K. Martin, S. D. Anton, and E. Ravussin. "Alternate-day fasting in nonobese subjects: effects on body weight, body composition, and energy metabolism." *American Journal of Clinical Nutrition* 81, no. 1 (2005): 69–73.

Hennebelle, M., A. Courchesne-Loyer, V. St-Pierre, C. Vandenberghe, C. A. Castellano, M. Fortier, ... and S. C. Cunnane. "Preliminary evaluation of a differential effect of an α-linolenate-rich supplement on ketogenesis and plasma ω-3 fatty acids in young and older adults." *Nutrition* 32, nos. 11–12 (2016): 1211–6.

Johnson, J. B., W. Summer, R. G. Cutler, B. Martin, D. H. Hyun, V. D. Dixit, ... and O. Carlson. "Alternate day calorie restriction improves clinical findings and reduces markers of oxidative stress and inflammation in overweight adults with moderate asthma." *Free Radical Biology and Medicine* 42, no. 5 (2007): 665–74.

Kossoff, E. H., H. Rowley, S. R. Sinha, and E. P. Vining. "A prospective study of the modified Atkins diet for intractable epilepsy in adults." *Epilepsia* 49, no. 2 (2008): 316–9.

La Bounty, P. M., B. I. Campbell, J. Wilson, E. Galvan, J. Berardi, S. M. Kleiner, ... and A. Smith. "International Society of Sports Nutrition position stand: meal frequency." *Journal of the International Society of Sports Nutrition* 8, no. 1 (2011): 1.

Mensink, R. P., P. L. Zock, A. D. Kester, and M. B. Katan. "Effects of dietary fatty acids and carbohydrates on the ratio of serum total to HDL cholesterol and on serum lipids and apolipoproteins: a meta-analysis of 60 controlled trials." *American Journal of Clinical Nutrition* 77, no. 5 (2003): 1146–55.

Mutungi, G., J. Ratliff, M. Puglisi, M. Torres-Gonzalez, U. Vaishnav, J. O. Leite, ... and M. L. Fernandez. "Dietary cholesterol from eggs increases plasma HDL cholesterol in overweight men consuming a carbohydrate-restricted diet." *Journal of Nutrition* 138, no. 2 (2008): 272–6.

Napoli, N., J. Thompson, R. Civitelli, and R. C. Armamento-Villareal. "Effects of dietary calcium compared with calcium supplements on estrogen metabolism and bone mineral density." *American Journal of Clinical Nutrition* 85, no. 5 (2007): 1428–33.

Pfeifer, H. H., and E. A. Thiele. "Low-glycemic-index treatment: a liberalized ketogenic diet for treatment of intractable epilepsy." *Neurology* 65, no. 11 (2005): 1810–2.

Pfeifer, H. H., D. A. Lyczkowski, and E. A. Thiele. "Low glycemic index treatment: implementation and new insights into efficacy." *Epilepsia* 49, suppl 8 (2008): 42–45.

Phinney, S. D. "Ketogenic diets and physical performance." *Nutrition & Metabolism* 1, no. 1 (2004): 1.

Phinney, S. D., B. R. Bistrian, W. J. Evans, E. Gervino, and G. L. Blackburn. "The human metabolic response to chronic ketosis without caloric restriction: preservation of submaximal exercise capability with reduced carbohydrate oxidation." *Metabolism* 32, no. 8 (1983): 769–76.

Rabast, U., K. H. Vornberger, and M. Ehl. "Loss of weight, sodium and water in obese persons consuming a high-or low-carbohydrate diet." *Annals of Nutrition and Metabolism* 25, no. 6 (1981): 341–9.

Reddy, S. T., C. Y. Wang, K. Sakhaee, L. Brinkley, and C. Y. Pak. "Effect of low-carbohydrate high-protein diets on acid-base balance, stone-forming propensity, and calcium metabolism." *American Journal of Kidney Diseases* 40, no. 2 (2002): 265–74.

Schoenfeld, B. J., A. A. Aragon, and J. W. Krieger. "Effects of meal frequency on weight loss and body composition: a meta-analysis." *Nutrition Reviews* 73, no. 2 (2015): 69–82.

St-Onge, M. P., et al. "Medium-versus long-chain triglycerides for 27 days increases fat oxidation and energy expenditure without resulting in changes in body composition in overweight women." *International Journal of Obesity* 27, no. 1 (2003): 95–102.

Swanson, D., R. Block, and S. A. Mousa. "Omega-3 fatty acids EPA and DHA: health benefits throughout life." *Advances in Nutrition: An International Review Journal* 3, no. 1 (2012): 1–7.

Tsuji, H., et al. "Dietary medium-chain triacylglycerols suppress accumulation of body fat in a double-blind, controlled trial in healthy men and women." *Journal of Nutrition* 131.11 (2001): 2853–9.

Van Wymelbeke, V., A. Himaya, J. Louis-Sylvestre, and M. Fantino. "Influence of medium-chain and long-chain triacylglycerols on the control of food intake in men." *American Journal of Clinical Nutrition* 68, no. 2 (1998): 226–34.

Varady, K. A., S. Bhutani, M. C. Klempel, C. M. Kroeger, J. F. Trepanowski, J. M. Haus, ... and Y. Calvo. "Alternate day fasting for weight loss in normal weight and overweight subjects: a randomized controlled trial." *Nutrition Journal* 12, no. 1 (2013): 1.

Volek, J. S., A. L. Gómez, and W. J. Kraemer. "Fasting lipoprotein and postprandial triacylglycerol responses to a low-carbohydrate diet supplemented with n-3 fatty acids." *Journal of the American College of Nutrition* 19, no. 3 (2000): 383–91.

Westman, E. C., W. S. Yancy, J. S. Edman, K. F. Tomlin, and C. E. Perkins. "Effect of 6-month adherence to a very low carbohydrate diet program." *American Journal of Medicine* 113, no. 1 (2002): 30–36.

Willi, S. M., M. J. Oexmann, N. M. Wright, N. A. Collop, and L. L. Key. "The effects of a high-protein, low-fat, ketogenic diet on adolescents with morbid obesity: body composition, blood chemistries, and sleep abnormalities." *Pediatrics* 101, no. 1 (1998): 61–67.

Chapter 4:

SUPPLEMENTING WITH KETONES

Typically, the liver produces ketones only under certain physiological conditions, such as fasting, extreme caloric restriction, or consuming a ketogenic diet. Because some individuals find these methodologies too radical or restrictive, scientists have attempted to isolate ketone bodies and provide them in supplement form so that people can reap the benefits of ketones without necessarily fasting or following a ketogenic diet. These supplements are known as *exogenous* ketones because they are produced outside the body, as opposed to the *endogenous* ketones that are made inside the body, as explained in the first section of this chapter.

Let us be clear that supplementing with exogenous ketones is *not* the same thing as following a ketogenic diet; however, there are overlapping features in which an elevation in ketones generates many of the same effects on health. In this chapter, we will discuss the research behind exogenous ketones, the data involving their use, various types and bioavailability, and potential therapeutic and practical applications.

Ketones: The Fourth Macronutrient

Walk into most medical facilities and tell a doctor that you are trying to increase the number of ketones in your body, and you might find yourself sent to the psych ward for further screening. Rather than throw you into a padded room, we want to help you understand the context and applications in which individuals might want to elevate their ketone levels by supplementing with exogenous ketones.

If we go back in time to the discovery of ketones, it was well established that *extreme* overproduction of ketone bodies was a by-product of diabetes, thus it was given the name *diabetic ketoacidosis*. This is why many physicians associate high levels of ketones with danger (VanItalie and Nufert, 2003). However, as discussed earlier in this book, the levels of ketones seen with ketoacidosis are far higher than those seen in individuals following a ketogenic diet. Similar to the diet, taking exogenous ketones can raise ketone levels significantly, but safely. Although ketones developed a bad rap for their association with ketoacidosis, more and more studies are identifying other potential applications and physiological functions of ketone bodies at reasonable levels.

Figure 4.1. *The typical range of blood ketone levels when individuals are dieting, taking exogenous ketones, or experiencing the potentially fatal state of ketoacidosis. As you can see, the diet or supplementation do not approach the levels of blood ketones seen in ketoacidosis.*

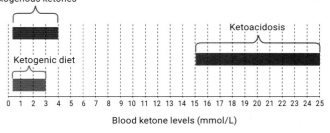

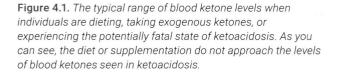

Blood ketone levels (mmol/L)

When fatty acids are broken down in the liver, a molecule called acetyl-CoA is produced. The acetyl-CoA then enters the mitochondria—the energy-creating part of a cell—where it is used to produce energy in the form of ATP. However, when there is an abundance of acetyl-CoA (a result of increased fat oxidation), the excess not used by the mitochondria can be diverted for the formation of ketone bodies through a metabolic process called *ketogenesis*.

How does this happen? Why is there a buildup of acetyl-CoA that eventually leads to the production of endogenous ketones?

During periods of low glucose availability, our bodies increase lipolysis (the process of breaking down fat). In a process known as the Krebs cycle, intermediates like oxaloacetate (OAA) (an important last step in the Krebs cycle; see Figure 4.2) are sent to the brain to help produce glucose via gluconeogenesis. Think of the Krebs cycle as an assembly line for the production of cars. The first step in that assembly line is the frame of a car (which represents acetyl-CoA entering the Krebs cycle). Following that are several stages in which various parts are added to the car: the tires might be added next, then the interior components, etc. The final step in the assembly line is putting the engine in the car. (The engine is similar to OAA.) Now, imagine that the production manager of the assembly line gets a call from his boss saying the engines that are not already placed in cars are needed in another building (OAA getting shuttled toward the brain). As a result, there are fewer engines available to keep the assembly line moving forward (i.e., less OAA to keep the Krebs cycle going). Because there are not enough engines available for the number of car frames (amount of acetyl-CoA) being produced, a backup occurs in the assembly line. The backup goes all the way back to the first step—the frame of the car—to a point where no more frames can enter the assembly line. This backup of frames (like the buildup of acetyl-CoA) leads the production manager to send the extra frames off to be used elsewhere. In the Krebs cycle, these "frames" (i.e., acetyl-CoA) are shuttled toward ketogenesis to form the ketone bodies acetoacetate (AcAc) and beta-hydroxybutyrate (BHB).

Ketone Body Metabolism and Uptake

Ketone bodies are small lipid-derived molecules that may serve as a circulating energy source for tissues in times of fasting or prolonged exercise (Newman and Verdin, 2014). Early studies have looked at variations in ketone bodies in normal men over the course of a typical day and have found a wide variation in ketone concentrations. However, one thing that is certain is that most people have some sort of elevation in ketones at some point in the day (Johnson et al., 1958). This brings up the question: Are we meant to have slightly elevated ketone concentrations throughout the day, but our consumption of carbohydrate-rich foods repeatedly blunts this response? Could it be that a state of ketosis is naturally occurring in all of us at different times throughout a typical day? Something to think about.

It is well established that the cells' uptake of ketones is proportional to the amount of ketones present in the blood (Courchesne-Loyer et al., 2016). However, to take up ketones into tissues, we need the help of monocarboxylic acid transporters (MCTs; to avoid confusion with medium-chain triglycerides, also known as MCTs, we will refer to these as MCT transporters). The rate at which ketones are taken into the cells depends on how available MCT transporters are. The number of MCT transporters varies from individual to individual, which can affect how much

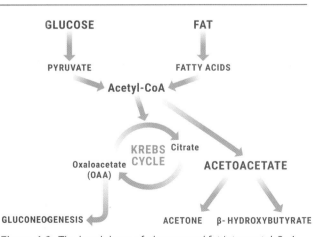

Figure 4.2. *The breakdown of glucose and fat into acetyl-CoA. Fat breakdown can overwhelm acetyl-CoA, causing a buildup of extra acetyl-CoA that is shuttled toward ketone production. OAA can be shuttled toward gluconeogenesis, leading to a further backup in the Krebs cycle.*

and how rapidly ketones are taken up (Newman and Verdin, 2014). For instance, if Person A and Person B are following the same ketogenic protocol, Person A might have a baseline fasting ketone level of 0.7 mmol/L, while Person B might be at 1.6 mmol/L. Similarly, when supplementing with ketones, Person B might see a sharp rise in ketone levels that persists for an extended period, while Person A sees a sharp rise in ketone levels that drops rapidly. Why? One possible explanation is that Person A has more MCT transporters than Person B and therefore is a better "ketone user" whose body tissues take them up fast.

Imagine that you are driving your car through the Lincoln Tunnel into New York City (see Figure 4.3). All the cars in the tunnel represent ketone bodies, and the tunnel itself represents an MCT transporter facilitating their uptake into the cell (i.e., the city). There is a limit to the number of cars that can be in the tunnel at one time. If you are trying to travel through that tunnel on a weekday morning, hundreds of cars could be backed up. One logical fix would be to build a second tunnel right next to it, doubling the number of cars that can get into the city at a time.

Similarly, our bodies can increase MCT transporters in order to allow more ketones to be taken up into the cells. One way to do so is to increase exercise. Exercise boosts the body's capacity to utilize ketones and take them up into skeletal muscle due to the fact that lactate, which is produced during exercise, and ketones both use MCT transporters. When exercising, the lactic acid that is built up in your muscles is also cleared by MCT transporters. Thus, exercise itself may cause the amount of MCT transporters to increase. Therefore,

the more physically active you are, the more MCT transporters you are likely to have. This is why individuals who are fit, lean, or exercising tend to see lower plasma levels of ketones than obese and/or sedentary individuals: their ketones are more efficiently transported from the bloodstream into the cells. Thus it is important to keep in mind that blood ketone levels may not be the most accurate indication of your level of ketosis.

KETO CONCEPT

Chasing Ketones

The concept of "chasing ketones" is prevalent among ketogenic dieters. Often, people tend to "chase" higher ketone levels, leaving them frustrated when they dip below expectations. However, think about what we discussed above. What if that dip in ketone levels just means that you are taking them up into your tissues better and they are being utilized rather than just hanging around in your blood? The point is that you shouldn't get discouraged about small fluctuations or changes in blood ketone levels, and you shouldn't go battling your friends and family over whose ketone levels are higher. Over time, whether you are on a ketogenic diet or supplementing with exogenous ketones, you will likely begin to see lower blood ketone levels as your number of MCT transporters increases and the uptake of ketones into your tissues improves.

Medium-Chain Triglycerides (MCTs)

An important distinction needs to be made between medium-chain triglycerides (MCTs) and exogenous ketones. People often use the two terms interchangeably; however, their makeup, delivery, and function differ significantly. For example, MCTs are broken down in the liver, with ketones being the by-products of that breakdown process. Exogenous ketones, on the other hand, don't need to be broken down because they are ketones already.

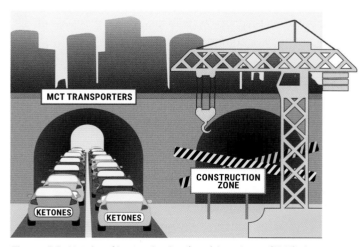

Figure 4.3. *Uptake of ketone bodies (cars) into tissue (NYC) via MCT transporters (tunnel).*

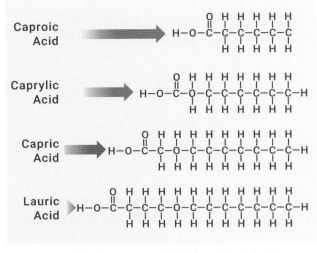

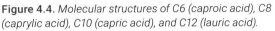

Figure 4.4. *Molecular structures of C6 (caproic acid), C8 (caprylic acid), C10 (capric acid), and C12 (lauric acid).*

MCTs are bound to glycerol and contain three fatty acids with carbon side chain lengths ranging from six to twelve carbons (C6, C8, etc.). These medium-chain fatty acids (MCFAs) include:

- Caproic acid (C6: hexanoic)
- Caprylic acid (C8: octanoic)
- Capric acid (C10: decanoic)
- Lauric acid (C12: dodecanoic)*

Due to their smaller molecular size, MCFAs are less calorically dense than long-chain fatty acids (8.3 calories versus 9.2 calories per gram) and therefore are labeled as a more "efficient" source of dietary fat; that is, MCFAs are more easily digested and produce ketones at a faster rate (Karen and Welma, 2015; Koji and Truyoshi, 2010). In addition, the metabolism of MCTs differs from that of long-chain triglycerides (LCTs) in that MCTs can be absorbed directly into the blood without the need for pancreatic enzymes or transportation through the gastrointestinal tract, making them faster-absorbing. MCTs go straight to the liver, where they can be used as a source of instant energy or turned into ketones. (See page 56 for more on the metabolism of MCTs.)

Several versions of pure MCT oil (which usually contains a combination of C8 and C10) and MCT powder are available today. While both forms can be advantageous, several of the MCT powders on the market are mixed with maltodextrin (derived from starch and absorbed like glucose) and therefore could have some effects on glucose, so

be cautious. Also keep in mind that many people experience gastrointestinal distress when using MCT oil, especially initially. MCTs do not require enzymes to break them down, so they are rapidly absorbed and delivered. This rapid introduction of fat can overwhelm our bodies and leave our stomachs in distress, which might result in a sprint to the restroom. Over time, the body can adapt and eventually build up a tolerance; however, we suggest that if you want to try MCT oil, you build up your intake slowly.

As discussed earlier, acetyl-CoA is produced during fat oxidation and then either is used by the mitochondria to produce energy or, if there is excess acetyl-CoA, is converted to ketone bodies through a metabolic process called ketogenesis.

MCTs are rapidly digested and broken down to acetyl-CoA, which can lead to a buildup of acetyl-CoA and a subsequent increase in ketone bodies (Dias, 1990). That said, there is much dispute about which of the MCTs is most important for enhancing ketogenesis. For example, caprylic acid (C8) is thought to be the most ketogenic MCT (McGarry, 1971; Wang et al., 2015). It makes the most sense on paper: one C8 molecule is broken down into two C4 ketones. However, other, earlier studies showed that caproic acid (C6) may be more ketogenic than caprylic acid (Schultz et al., 1949). Many people have questioned the benefits, if any, of lauric acid (C12) with respect to its effects on ketogenesis. Recently, a group out of Tokyo found that coconut oil (which is about 50 percent C12) has a negligible effect on blood ketones. But wait: when the C12 MCT was isolated, these researchers found that it activated ketogenesis in cells within the central nervous system, indicating that lauric acid may be advantageous for providing fuel for neurons and thus may benefit cognition and brain-related disorders (Nonaka et al., 2016).

There is also much debate about the effective dose of MCTs needed to enhance ketone production. To elevate ketone levels from zero to around 0.3 mmol/L using MCTs only, research indicates that you would need to consume 20 to 100 grams or more, which could be challenging due to the gastric distress you might experience if you consumed such a large amount (Van Wymelbeke et al., 1998; Freund and Weinsier, 1966; Courchesne-Loyer et al., 2013; Bergen et al., 1966). In fact, one study (Misell et al.,

2001) found no significant elevation in blood ketone levels in endurance athletes who consumed upwards of 60 grams of MCT oil per day. As you can imagine, all the subjects in this study experienced gastric distress, and as a result, no performance benefit was seen with MCT oil supplementation.

MCT supplements and foods that are high in MCTs are great to incorporate into a ketogenic diet; however, you should not rely on MCTs alone to elevate your blood ketone levels. Look for an MCT powder that is bound to soluble corn fiber rather than maltodextrin to get the best effects and to incorporate a combination of C8, C6, C10, and even C12 into your diet. If you're looking to boost your ketone levels to higher, therapeutic levels, exogenous ketone supplementation is more effective at rapidly increasing plasma ketone levels.

The Effects of Exogenous Ketones: A Unique "Superfuel"

Our bodies typically can create three different types of ketone bodies: beta-hydroxybutyrate (BHB), acetoacetate (AcAc), and acetone. Two of these, beta-hydroxybutyrate and acetoacetate, have been found to have unique metabolic properties in studies looking at their application outside the context of a ketogenic diet. Research dating back to the 1940s showed that both BHB and AcAc improved oxygen efficiency and increased sperm motility in animals (Lardy and Phillips, 1945). Researchers also began looking at the effects of infusing BHB or AcAc and the impact on insulin and glucose (Nath and Brahmachari, 1944; Tidwell and Axelrod, 1948). These studies had mixed results: some indicated that infusing ketones caused hyperglycemia (a rise in blood glucose), while others saw hypoglycemia (a drop in blood glucose). Thus, in the 1940s, scientists came to understand that ketone bodies improve oxygen efficiency and increase sperm motility, and the data was mixed when it came to whether ketones themselves had any effect on the pancreas or insulin secretion.

Two critical pieces of the puzzle that were determined early on were that ketone bodies are utilized in proportion to their presence in the blood—if a lot of ketones are present, cells tend to use a lot of ketones—and that even in the presence of glucose, ketones are used *preferentially*. Yes, you read that right: dating back over seventy years, we had information showing that ketones are the brain's preferred energy source, even when given the choice between glucose and ketones. This being the case, more researchers became interested in supplementing with various ketones to look at elevating blood levels and the impact it would have on various metabolic functions. Is it possible that even individuals who are not keto-adapted and aren't eating a ketogenic diet can still receive some of the benefits of ketosis?

The 1950s and '60s saw an explosion of research investigating the effects of infusing various doses and types of ketone bodies in animals and humans. One early study showed that following a rapid intravenous infusion of BHB, blood ketones rose significantly, and there was a consistent drop in blood glucose (Neptune, 1956). Other studies during this time (such as Madison et al., 1964) showed that infusions of ketones resulted in:

- Decreases in blood glucose
- A 50 percent drop in liver glucose output

It is not clear what caused the consistent drop in glucose. However, the reason for the differing results among these early ketone infusion studies may be that ketone levels as high as 3.5 mmol triggered the pancreas to secrete more insulin (i.e., the higher the level over 3.5 mmol/L, the more insulin was secreted) to prevent further endogenous ketone production. This increase in insulin would cause a decrease in blood glucose levels. However, other studies have shown that in a fasted state, concentrations of BHB below 5 mmol/L were unable to trigger insulin to be released (Biden and Taylor, 1983). More studies need to be done looking at a dose-dependent response on blood ketone levels and any insulin release associated with too-high levels of blood BHB. Currently, it seems that under well-controlled conditions (i.e., on a ketogenic diet or with ketone supplementation), we would normally see elevations in ketones of about 0.3 to 3.5 mmol/L; therefore, insulin wouldn't be released to a degree that would impair the breakdown of fat.

The Ketone-Insulin Conundrum

On paper, the theory sounds simple: increased production or elevation in ketones ➡ stimulation of insulin ➡ lowered blood glucose and the release of free fatty acids from adipose (fat) tissue ➡ the prevention of fatal ketoacidosis. However, in human trials, this theory doesn't pan out. In fact, one study found that AcAc lowered blood glucose but had no effect on insulin release (Fajans et al., 1964). Another study found that a BHB infusion had no significant effect on insulin levels (Senior and Loridan, 1968). Interestingly enough, the biggest instigators of insulin secretion in these two studies were amino acids, which are responsible for stimulating muscle growth—and certain amino acids have been shown to reduce diet-induced obesity and improve insulin sensitivity (Zhang et al., 2007). Lastly, a third study investigated a low-carbohydrate ketogenic diet with supplemental ketones over twenty-four months in an infant with glycogen storage disease (inability to break down

glycogen for use as fuel). Free fatty acids (indicative of lipolysis) were not correlated with ketone levels, even when those levels were well over 3 mmol/L (Valayannopoulos et al., 2011). Thus it is important to understand that any short-term effects of exogenous ketones (for example, on insulin secretion, free fatty acids, and lipolysis) don't always lead to long-term effects, especially when it comes to body composition and optimal health. And even if exogenous ketones do have an effect on insulin, that effect would likely be comparable to what's seen after drinking a protein shake, which means that it is likely negligible and wouldn't have long-term negative effects on fat storage or breakdown.

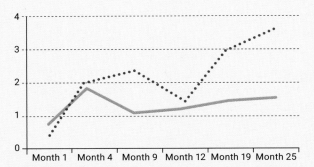

Change in levels of total ketone bodies (in mmol/L, gray dotted line) and free fatty acids (in g/L, yellow line) during the study.

Figure 4.6. *Elevating ketones to a normal physiological range (up to 3 mmol/L) does not significantly increase insulin levels in humans.*

Source: Senior and Loridan, 1968.

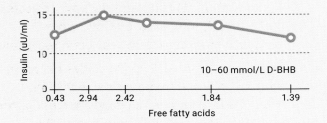

Figure 4.5. *Changes in ketone bodies and their relationship to free fatty acids in the blood.*

Source: Valayannopoulos et al., 2011.

Ketone Salts versus Ketone Esters

Currently, the number of ketone supplements on the market is exploding, primarily in the form of ketone salts, which are cheaper to produce and more palatable than the "jet fuel" esters. Since launching its supplement, Keto OS, in 2015, a company called Pruvit has delivered nearly 30 million servings. Now, numerous other companies are launching ketone-based supplements, riding on Pruvit's coattails and attempting to capitalize on the "ketone conversation." Let's break down what these supplements actually are.

Ketone Salts

Ketone salts are white powdered substances that are becoming more available. They consist of a BHB molecule bound to a mineral salt, such as sodium, calcium, magnesium, or potassium (though potassium BHB is very hydroscopic and nearly impossible to make in powdered form). In addition, it is now possible to bind BHB to amino acids, such as lysine, arginine, creatine, citrulline, agmatine, and leucine; however, these products are not technically ketone salts, are less popular, and are just starting to emerge in the market (e.g., Keto Aminos).

People tend to be wary of the mineral/salt load of ketone supplements. As a society, we have demonized sodium (as we did fat several decades ago), and most ketone supplements use a BHB bound to sodium as a main source of ketones. In general, the mineral content of the ketone salt varies depending on the molecule to which it is bound.

Ketone Salt	Average BHB	Average Mineral Load	Per Gram of Supplement
BHB sodium	81.8%	18.2%	818 mg BHB, 182 mg sodium
BHB calcium	83.8%	16.2%	838 mg BHB, 162 mg calcium
BHB magnesium	89.5%	10.5%	895 mg BHB, 105 mg magnesium
BHB potassium	72.5%	27.5%	725 mg BHB, 275 mg potassium

It is important to be aware of the mineral loads of these supplements and factor them into your daily intake. Some people who are being treated for various conditions need to pay particular attention to this to avoid excess consumption of certain minerals.

For more information about ketone salts, go to Ketogenic.com and check out the article "To Ketone or Not to Ketone: Mineral Salts."

Ketone Esters

To avoid potential issues with the mineral loads of ketone salts, various ketone esters have been developed. Ketone esters are salt-free liquids that exist in monoester (one), diester (two), and even triester (three) form. This means that instead of the ketone molecule being bound to a mineral, as is the case with ketone salts, the ketone molecule is bound to a different substance via an ester bond.

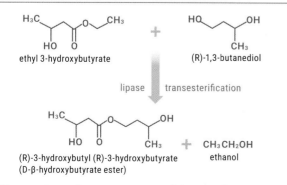

Figure 4.7. *A schematic overview of the manufacturing of the D-β-hydroxybutyrate ester.*

Retrieved from the FDA GRAS filing by Drs. Veech and Clarke.

Do Ketones Have Calories?

One aspect of ketones that is often overlooked is that they are a fuel source and therefore do have calories. In the GRAS (Generally Recognized as Safe) Notice for the D-BHB ester developed by Dr. Veech and Kieran Clarke, the caloric value is listed at 4.7 kcal/gram. It is estimated that the true caloric value falls somewhere between 4.7 kcal/gram and 5.4 kcal/gram for beta-hydroxybutyrate. So watch out for ketone supplements that claim to have zero calories—that claim is an easy way to spot those companies that either use improper labeling or are "fairy dusting" their products with BHB.

As you can see, during the synthesis of the D-β-hydroxybutyrate ester, ethanol is produced as a by-product. However, when properly developed and made, most of the ethanol is removed via vacuum.

Most of the esters have been studied for their safety and efficacy in animals (Desrochers et al., 1995; Kesl et al., 2016) and in healthy adult subjects (Clark et al., 2012) with no adverse outcomes.

The biggest limitations of these esters, however, are:

- **Cost:** The R/D form of BHB (the body's biological form) is significantly more expensive than the DL-BHB or RS-BHB form, which is used in most ketone salts. (We will discuss this more below.) The process of making pure R/D BHB is challenging, yet several researchers and companies are making significant strides.

- **Taste:** In an article he wrote after testing with the ketone ester, our colleague, Dr. Peter Attia, described the taste as "jet fuel." To say that ketone esters have a sharp, bitter taste is an understatement. We've sampled many different esters, and we like to describe it as being like drinking a bottle of gin or vodka passed down from your grandfather's grandfather, mixed with a bit of rubbing alcohol. Part of the issue with the taste may stem from impurities within the ester, thus a better distillation process may aid in the flavor profile (similar to distilled vodkas).

We are confident that these esters will soon come to market in a palatable form; the only remaining hurdle will be the cost.

The History of Ketone Esters

The first esters were developed and studied by Dr. Ronald Birkhahn and Dr. Henri Brunengraber, both leading authorities and researchers in the field of ketones. The first acceptable form for administering large amounts of ketone bodies was used by Birkhahn et al. (1979), who described the synthesis of the monoesterglycerol and acetoacetate (AcAc), often referred to as monoacetoacetin. The breakdown of monoacetoacetin yields AcAc, a physiologic fuel. Birkhahn's early studies of monoacetoacetin showed that it could be safely infused in normal and injured rats and exerted a protein-sparing effect. Birkhahn wasn't satisfied, though, so he set out to make his ester better. He sought to create an ester of DL-3-hydroxybutyrate (BHB) and glycerol, known as monoglyceride (Birkhahn et al., 1997). The researchers concluded that animals continuously infused with glyceryl mono-DL-BHB did not exhibit symptoms of toxicity but did show indications that this compound was utilized for *energy*.

Around the same time, another group (Desrochers et al., 1995) began working on synthesizing the monoester and diester of a compound called 1-3-butanediol (1,3 BD) and either AcAc or DL-BHB. (1,3 BD is an alcohol that, when broken down, can be converted to BHB.) This set the stage for various combinations of D,L (or R, S)

DIFFERENT TYPES OF KETONE ESTERS	
BASE	BOUND TO
Acetoacetate	Monoester glycerol
Acetoacetate	Triesterglycerol
DL-BHB	Monoester glycerol
DL-BHB	Triesterglycerol
Acetoacetate	Monoester 1,3-butanediol
Acetoacetate	Diester 1,3-butanediol
DL-BHB	Monoester 1,3-butanediol
DL-BHB	Diester 1,3-butanediol
D-BHB	Monoester 1,3-butanediol

1,3 BD and either BHB or AcAc. (The D,L nomenclature is synonymous with R,S and simply refers to the isomer being used.)

More recently, Dr. Dom D'Agostino's lab began working with the D,L-1,3-butanediol acetoacetate diester (BD-AcAc2) for studies looking at CNS oxygen toxicity and seizures (D'Agostino et al., 2013). Dr. Richard Veech has been a strong advocate of using only the D isomer (not the mixed D,L) in his ester. His lab, along with others, has conducted several bioavailability studies on the impact of this ester on blood BHB and performance, both with remarkable results. Both of these esters show tremendous promise and need more research to establish what benefits and limitations they may have.

In summary, exogenous ketones come in many forms—salts, monoesters, diesters, and a combination of different isomers (e.g., D/R-BHB, L/S-BHB, or a combination of the two, such as DL-BHB, aka RS-BHB). Ketone salts are cheaper and more palatable than ketone esters. They can raise blood ketone levels quickly and sustain that elevation for a short time. Ketone esters typically combine 1,3-BD with either AcAc or BHB to make non-ionized sodium-free precursors of ketone bodies. Doing so eliminates any concerns that one may have with mineral/salt load and can potentially elevate plasma ketone levels for a longer period due to a processed conversion of 1,3-BD in the liver to ketone bodies. To date, ketone esters are not commercially available and have been used only in research settings due to their high cost and harsh taste; however, companies are working on both of these aspects in an attempt to bring them to market.

Ketone Isomers: Is There a Difference?

An *isomer* is a compound that has the same type and number of atoms as another compound, but arranged in a different sequence. The two main ketone isomers are D-BHB (also known as R-BHB) and L-BHB (also known as S-BHB). These isomers are classified as *enantiomers,* meaning that they are mirror images of each other, but are not identical. Hold up both hands in front of you. What you see is that they are nearly identical, but if you place your left hand over your right, they don't match up perfectly. Similarly, isomers like D-BHB and L-BHB are mirror images. In most cases, there is a biological form that our bodies can use and/or produce, with the other form being either less effective or not effective at all.

Are Exogenous Ketones Safe?

To date, both ketone esters and ketone salts have GRAS (Generally Recognized as Safe) approval at various doses. The biggest safety concerns with ketone salts are the mineral load and possible impurities. However, the mineral load needs to be taken in the context of a well-formulated diet, your degree of physical activity, etc. DL-BHB has been administered orally for several months without adverse effects, even at high doses (32 grams per day), in two 6-month-old infants with chronic low levels of glucose (Plecko et al., 2002).

In addition, sodium BHB supplementation in infants who have multiple acyl-CoA dehydrogenase deficiency (MADD)—a disorder involving dysregulated fatty acid oxidation and usually treated with a low-fat, low-protein, high-carbohydrate diet plus avoiding long fasting periods, has shown no adverse effects over several years (Van Hove et al., 2003). Rather, neurological function improved, with progressive improvement of brain MRI following supplementation.

Kesl et al. (2016) recently did a safety study of ketone salts in animals. After several weeks at a high dosage, they found no adverse effects.

All that being said, with ketone salts becoming more and more popular in the U.S., it is important to be wary of impurities from ketone salt production, such as crotonic acid and other impurities that can reside in the raw materials. Products from manufacturers trying to take shortcuts often have high elevations of these impurities that, when consumed in large amounts, may have contraindications over time. Therefore, look for products that are third-party-tested and research-backed and that use the highest-quality natural forms of BHB.

The body produces D-BHB, so it's naturally biologically active—it slots into place easily. Think of it like a game of Tetris. A biologically active substance fits perfectly into its spot in the body, while its non-biologically active counterpart doesn't fit exactly right and leaves you with too much open space in your game.

As previously discussed, most ketone supplements utilize the mixed isomer, or racemic, form of ketones (DL-BHB). Why? First, the mixed isomer is significantly cheaper to produce. However, if the biologically active form (D-BHB) makes up 50 percent or less of the racemic form, what is the other portion (the L-BHB) doing? Is it even necessary? Unlike D-BHB, L-BHB is not biologically active. So how do our bodies handle L-BHB? Well, it is not completely wasted: L-BHB is metabolized via S-BHB CoA, which eventually gets converted to D-BHB and other by-products (Desrochers et al., 1992).

One study showed that the degree of ketogenesis and uptake was significantly higher in rats given D 1,3 BD (the biologically active form) compared to L 1,3 BD. The degree of ketogenesis was ninefold in the D-BHB condition and three-and-a-half-fold in the L-BHB condition, while uptake was 80 to 102 percent in the D-BHB condition and 29 to 38 percent in the L-BHB condition. Other studies have seen similar results. In fact, Gueldry and Bralet (1995) looked at the difference of D versus L versus DL-BD and also DL-BHB on various markers. They found the following:

	Increase in Plasma BHB	Increase in Plasma AcAc
D-BD	1183%	1043%
L-BD	183%	271%
DL-BD	742%	414%
DL-BHB	667%	600%

Clearly, the D isomer generates the larger increase in plasma BHB and AcAc, while the L isomer generates little increase in either. It is also interesting to note that animals fed L 1,3 BD displayed increased fatty acid synthesis (the formation of fatty acids—which we don't want); therefore, the L isomer appears to be more readily stored as fat than the D isomer (Robinson and Williamson, 1980; Desrochers et al., 1992; Tsai et al., 1996). If you remember what we talked about earlier in regard to lipolysis and ketones impacting the breakdown and storage of fat, it appears that the L isomer increases fatty acid synthesis more than the D isomer.

The D-BHB isomer seems to be the one that is primarily responsible for the beneficial effects of ketone supplementation. One possibility is that L-BHB has some blood glucose–lowering effects in animals (Meenakshi et al., 1995), but this hasn't been confirmed (McKenzie, 1902). Even though the brain takes up D-BHB significantly better than L-BHB (Robinson and Williamson, 1980), Dr. D'Agostino's lab has seen positive results with the racemic (D,L) form of 1,3 BD in a variety of therapeutic applications (such as seizures, oxygen toxicity, and cancer). However, it is uncertain how these same studies would have turned out if the active D isomer had been given alone.

The type of ketone isomer may play a unique role in the attenuation of seizures. Some studies indicate that the decrease in seizures that occurs as a result of lack of oxygen to the brain may be unrelated to the degree of ketosis, meaning that even though D-BHB initiates a greater degree of ketosis, something else may be driving the attenuation of seizures (Chavko et al., 1999). One study found that L-BHB was more effective than D-BHB for seizures; the authors indicated that the anticonvulsant properties may be related to acetone and AcAc levels. However, previous studies showed that when properly metabolized, D-BHB increased AcAc more than L-BHB. Additionally, preliminary research from our lab showed that L-BHB had no effect on blood ketone levels, even at a moderately high dose (10 grams). In fact, some researchers suggest that L-BHB might actually get in the way and block the binding sites for D-BHB, which could be counterproductive for the effects that we want ketones to have.

It is plausible that individuals would need less than half of the amount of a ketone supplement that contained only D-BHB to get the same effects as the mixed-isomer ketone supplement (DL-BHB). This relates to efficacy and the elevation of plasma BHB levels in the body, which could have huge implications when discussing dosing strategies, especially with ketone salts.

Finally, our lab has found that D-BHB has a greater effect on performance than DL-BHB; however, more research comparing the direct effects of D-BHB and L-BHB on performance, brain uptake and metabolism, and therapeutic potential is needed. The current evidence favors supplementing with D-BHB alone rather than with the mixed isomer.

CHAPTER SUMMARY

Take a deep breath. That was a ton of information about exogenous (supplemental) ketones and their potential applications. It is a lot to take in, but we hope you continue to utilize this as a resource for years to come.

To summarize this chapter, ketone supplementation has been around for decades and has finally been brought to the mainstream by companies like Pruvit. MCT transporters act as tunnels to help take up ketones into the cells and can be increased with exercise. Medium-chain triglycerides are not the same as exogenous ketones; you would likely need 20-plus grams of MCTs to get even a small bump (0.3 mmol/L) in blood ketone levels. Ketone salts are typically bound to mineral salts, such as sodium, calcium, and magnesium, while ketone esters (which are mostly liquid) are bound to either glycerol or 1,3 BD. Ketone salts are cheaper and more palatable than ketone esters, and there is ongoing research investigating their effects on multiple variables. The different isomers of ketones include D-BHB and L-BHB. Most ketones on the market are a mixed-isomer (racemic) form of the two (i.e., DL-BHB); however, our lab and others have shown that the D isomer is more bioavailable than the L isomer.

The area of exogenous ketones is constantly evolving, and over the years we are sure to see new data and technologies emerge to improve delivery, bioavailability, and more. In our lab, we're continuing to test new applications for these supplements and discover possible limitations for their use. Nonetheless, the potential of exogenous ketones is very promising, and we are excited to see more research and reports on this topic. In later chapters, we will look more at potential therapeutic applications for supplemental ketones and how you might implement them into your lifestyle with or even without a ketogenic diet.

References

Abou-Hamdan, M., E. Cornille, M. Khrestchatisky, M. de Reggi, and B. Gharib. "The energy crisis in Parkinson's disease: a therapeutic target." In *Etiology and Pathophysiology of Parkinson's Disease,* A. Q. Rana, ed. (2011). INTECH Open Access Publisher. doi: 10.5772/17369.

Abraham, R. "Ketones: controversial new energy drink could be next big thing in cycling." *Cycling Weekly,* last modified January 9, 2015. www.cyclingweekly.co.uk/news/latest-news/ketones-controversial-new-energy-drink-next-big-thing-cycling-151877

Alzheimer's Association. "2015 Alzheimer's disease facts and figures." *Alzheimer's & Dementia: Journal of the Alzheimer's Association* 11, no. 3 (2015): 332–84.

Amiel, S. A., H. R. Archibald, G. Chusney, A. J. Williams, and E. A. Gale. "Ketone infusion lowers hormonal responses to hypoglycaemia: evidence for acute cerebral utilization of a non-glucose fuel." *Clinical Science* 81, no. 2 (1991): 189–94.

Arase, K., J. S. Fisler, N. S. Shargill, D. A. York, and G. A. Bray. "Intracerebroventricular infusions of 3-OHB and insulin in a rat model of dietary obesity." *American Journal of Physiology-Regulatory, Integrative and Comparative Physiology* 255, no. 6 (1988): R974–81.

Belanger, H. G., R. D. Vanderploeg, and T. McAllister. "Subconcussive blows to the head: a formative review of short-term clinical outcomes." *Journal of Head Trauma Rehabilitation* 31, no. 3 (2016): 159–66.

Bergen, S. S., S. A. Hashim, and T. B. Van Itallie. "Hyperketonemia induced in man by medium-chain triglyceride." *Diabetes* 15, no. 10 (1966): 723–5.

Bergsneider, M., D. A. Hovda, E. Shalmon, D. F. Kelly, P. M. Vespa, N. A. Martin, ... and D. P. Becker. "Cerebral hyperglycolysis following severe traumatic brain injury in humans: a positron emission tomography study." *Journal of Neurosurgery* 86, no. 2 (1997): 241–51.

Biden, T. J., and K. W. Taylor. "Effects of ketone bodies on insulin release and islet-cell metabolism in the rat." *Biochemical Journal* 212, no. 2 (1983): 371–7.

Biros, M. H., and R. Nordness. "Effects of chemical pretreatment on posttraumatic cortical edema in the rat." *American Journal of Emergency Medicine* 14, no. 1 (1996): 27–32.

Bonuccelli, G., A. Tsirigos, D. Whitaker-Menezes, S. Pavlides, R. G. Pestell, B. Chiavarina, ... and F. Sotgia. "Ketones and lactate 'fuel' tumor growth and metastasis: evidence that epithelial cancer cells use oxidative mitochondrial metabolism." *Cell Cycle* 9, no. 17 (2010): 3506–14.

Boumezbeur, F., G. F. Mason, R. A. de Graaf, K. L. Behar, G. W. Cline, G. I. Shulman, ... and K. F. Petersen. "Altered brain mitochondrial metabolism in healthy aging as assessed by in vivo magnetic resonance spectroscopy." *Journal of Cerebral Blood Flow & Metabolism* 30, no. 1 (2010): 211–21.

Cahill Jr., G. F. "Starvation in man." *New England Journal of Medicine* 282, no. 12 (1970): 668–75.

Chavko, M., J. C. Braisted, and A. L. Harabin. "Attenuation of brain hyperbaric oxygen toxicity by fasting is not related to ketosis." *Undersea & Hyperbaric Medicine* 26, no. 2 (1999): 99.

Chini, C. C., M. G. Tarragó, and E. N. Chini. "NAD and the aging process: role in life, death and everything in between." *Molecular and Cellular Endocrinology* (2016). doi: 10.1016/j.mce.2016.11.003.

Ciarlone, S. L., J. C. Grieco, D. P. D'Agostino, and E. J. Weeber. "Ketone ester supplementation attenuates seizure activity, and improves behavior and hippocampal synaptic plasticity in an Angelman syndrome mouse model." *Neurobiology of Disease* 96 (2016): 38–46.

Clarke, K., K. Tchabanenko, R. Pawlosky, E. Carter, M. T. King, K. Musa-Veloso, ... and R. L. Veech. "Kinetics, safety and tolerability of (R)-3-hydroxybutyl (R)-3-hydroxybutyrate in healthy adult subjects." *Regulatory Toxicology and Pharmacology* 63, no. 3 (2012): 401–8.

Clarke, K., and P. Cox. (2013). U.S. Patent Application No. 14/390,495.

Costantini, L. C., L. J. Barr, J. L. Vogel, and S. T. Henderson. "Hypometabolism as a therapeutic target in Alzheimer's disease." *BMC Neuroscience* 9, no. 2 (2008): 1.

Courchesne-Loyer, A., M. Fortier, J. Tremblay-Mercier, R. Chouinard-Watkins, M. Roy, S. Nugent, ... and S. C. Cunnane. "Stimulation of mild, sustained ketonemia by medium-chain triacylglycerols in healthy humans: estimated potential contribution to brain energy metabolism." *Nutrition* 29, no. 4 (2013): 635–40.

Courchesne-Loyer, A., E. Croteau, C. A. Castellano, V. St-Pierre, M. Hennebelle, and S. C. Cunnane. "Inverse relationship between brain glucose and ketone metabolism in adults during short-term moderate dietary ketosis: A dual tracer quantitative positron emission tomography study." *Journal of Cerebral Blood Flow & Metabolism* (2016). doi: 10.1177/0271678X16669366.

Cox, P. J., T. Kirk, T. Ashmore, K. Willerton, R. Evans, A. Smith, ... and M. T. King. "Nutritional ketosis alters fuel preference and thereby endurance performance in athletes." *Cell Metabolism* 24, no. 2 (2016): 256–68.

Cunnane, S., S. Nugent, M. Roy, A. Courchesne-Loyer, E. Croteau, S. Tremblay, ... and H. Begdouri. "Brain fuel metabolism, aging, and Alzheimer's disease." *Nutrition* 27, no. 1 (2011): 3–20.

Cunnane, S. C., A. Courchesne-Loyer, C. Vandenberghe, V. St-Pierre, M. Fortier, M. Hennebelle, ... and C. A. Castellano. "Can ketones help rescue brain fuel supply in later life? Implications for cognitive health during aging and the treatment of Alzheimer's disease." *Frontiers in Molecular Neuroscience* 9 (2016): 53.

D'Agostino, D. P., R. Pilla, H. E. Held, C. S. Landon, M. Puchowicz, H. Brunengraber, ... and J. B. Dean. "Therapeutic ketosis with ketone ester delays central nervous system oxygen toxicity seizures in rats." *American Journal of Physiology-Regulatory, Integrative and Comparative Physiology* 304, no. 10 (2013): R829–36.

Dahlhamer, J. M. "Prevalence of inflammatory bowel disease among adults aged ≥ 18 years—United States, 2015." *Morbidity and Mortality Weekly Report* 65 (2016).

Desrochers, S., F. David, M. Garneau, M. Jetté, and H. Brunengraber. "Metabolism of R-and S-1, 3-butanediol in perfused livers from meal-fed and starved rats." *Biochemical Journal* 285, no. 2 (1992): 647–53.

Desrochers, S., P. Dubreuil, J. Brunet, M. Jette, F. David, B. R. Landau, and H. Brunengraber. "Metabolism of (R, S)-1, 3-butanediol acetoacetate esters, potential parenteral and enteral nutrients in conscious pigs." *American Journal of Physiology-Endocrinology and Metabolism* 268, no. 4 (1995): E660–7.

Egan, B., and D. P. D'Agostino. "Fueling performance: ketones enter the mix." *Cell Metabolism* 24, no. 3 (2016): 373–5.

Felts, P. W., O. B. Crofford, and C. R. Park. "Effect of infused ketone bodies on glucose utilization in the dog." *Journal of Clinical Investigation* 43, no. 4 (1964): 638.

Fine, E. J., C. J. Segal-Isaacson, R. D. Feinman, S. Herszkopf, M. C. Romano, N. Tomuta, ... and J. A. Sparano. "Targeting insulin inhibition as a metabolic therapy in advanced cancer: a pilot safety and feasibility dietary trial in 10 patients." *Nutrition* 28, no. 10 (2012): 1028–35.

Freund, G., and R. L. Weinsier. "Standardized ketosis in man following medium chain triglyceride ingestion." *Metabolism* 15, no. 11 (1966): 980–91.

Frey, S., G. Geffroy, V. Desquiret-Dumas, N. Gueguen, C. Bris, S. Belal, ... and G. Lenaers. "The addition of ketone bodies alleviates mitochondrial dysfunction by restoring complex I assembly in a MELAS cellular model." *Biochimica et Biophysica Acta* 1863, no. 1 (2017): 284–91.

Gasior, M., A. French, M. T. Joy, R. S. Tang, A. L. Hartman, and M. A. Rogawski. "The anticonvulsant activity of acetone, the major ketone body in the ketogenic diet, is not dependent on its metabolites acetol, 1, 2-propanediol, methylglyoxal, or pyruvic acid." *Epilepsia* 48, no. 4 (2007): 793–800.

Goldstein, J. L., and B. Cryer. "Gastrointestinal injury associated with NSAID use: a case study and review of risk factors and preventative strategies." *Drug, Healthcare and Patient Safety* 7 (2015): 31.

Gueldry, S., and J. Bralet. "Effect of D- and L-1, 3-butanediol isomers on glycolytic and citric acid cycle intermediates in the rat brain." *Metabolic Brain Disease* 10, no. 4 (1995): 293–301.

Hashim, S. A., and T. B. VanItallie. "Ketone body therapy: from the ketogenic diet to the oral administration of ketone ester." *Journal of Lipid Research* 55, no. 9 (2014): 1818–26.

Hoge, C. W., D. McGurk, J. L. Thomas, A. L. Cox, C. C. Engel, and C. A. Castro. "Mild traumatic brain injury in US soldiers returning from Iraq." *New England Journal of Medicine* 358, no. 5 (2008): 453–63.

Hootman, J. M., R. Dick, and J. Agel. "Epidemiology of collegiate injuries for 15 sports: summary and recommendations for injury prevention initiatives." *Journal of Athletic Training* 42, no. 2 (2007): 311.

Hu, Z. G., H. D. Wang, W. Jin, and H. X. Yin. "Ketogenic diet reduces cytochrome c release and cellular apoptosis following traumatic brain injury in juvenile rats." *Annals of Clinical & Laboratory Science* 39, no. 1 (2009): 76–83.

Izumi, Y., K. Ishii, H. Katsuki, A. M. Benz, and C. F. Zorumski. "Beta-hydroxybutyrate fuels synaptic function during development. Histological and physiological evidence in rat hippocampal slices." *Journal of Clinical Investigation* 101, no. 5 (1998): 1121.

Johnson, R. E., F. Sargent, and R. Passmore. "Normal variations in total ketone bodies in serum and urine of healthy young men." *Quarterly Journal of Experimental Physiology and Cognate Medical Sciences* 43, no. 4 (1958): 339–44.

Kashiwaya, Y., C. Bergman, J. H. Lee, R. Wan, M. T. King, M. R. Mughal, ... and R. L. Veech. "A ketone ester diet exhibits anxiolytic and cognition-sparing properties, and lessens amyloid and tau pathologies in a mouse model of Alzheimer's disease." *Neurobiology of Aging* 34, no. 6 (2013): 1530–9.

Kashiwaya, Y., K. Sato, N. Tsuchiya, S. Thomas, D. A. Fell, R. L. Veech, and J. V. Passonneau. "Control of glucose utilization in working perfused rat heart." *Journal of Biological Chemistry* 269, no. 41 (1994): 25502–14.

Kashiwaya, Y., T. Takeshima, N. Mori, K. Nakashima, K. Clarke, and R. L. Veech. "d-β-hydroxybutyrate protects neurons in models of Alzheimer's and Parkinson's disease." *Proceedings of the National Academy of Sciences* 97, no. 10 (2000): 5440–4.

Kashiwaya, Y., R. Pawlosky, W. Markis, M. T. King, C. Bergman, S. Srivastava, ... and R. L. Veech. "A ketone ester diet increases brain malonyl-CoA and uncoupling proteins 4 and 5 while decreasing food intake in the normal Wistar rat." *Journal of Biological Chemistry* 285, no. 34 (2010): 25950–6.

Katayama, Y., D. P. Becker, T. Tamura, and D. A. Hovda. "Massive increases in extracellular potassium and the indiscriminate release of glutamate following concussive brain injury." *Journal of Neurosurgery* 73, no. 6 (1990): 889–900.

Keith, H. M. "Factors influencing experimentally produced convulsions." *Archives of Neurology & Psychiatry* 29, no. 1 (1933): 148–54.

Keith, H. M. G. W. Stavraky, C. H. Rogerson, D. H. Hardcastle, and K. Duguid. "Experimental convulsions induced by administration of thujone." *Journal of Nervous and Mental Disease* 84, no. 1 (1936): 84.

Kemper, M. F., A. Miller, R. J. Pawlosky, and R. L. Veech. "Administration of a novel β-hydroxybutyrate ester after radiation exposure suppresses in vitro lethality and chromosome damage, attenuates bone marrow suppression in vivo." *FASEB Journal* 30, suppl 1 (2016): 627.3.

Kephart, W., M. Holland, P. Mumford, B. Mobley, R. Lowery, M. Roberts, and J. Wilson. "The effects of intermittent ketogenic dieting as well as ketone salt supplementation on body composition and circulating health biomarkers in exercising rodents." *FASEB Journal* 30, suppl 1 (2016): lb383.

Kesl, S. L., A. M. Poff, N. P. Ward, T. N. Fiorelli, C. Ari, A. J. Van Putten, ... and D. P. D'Agostino. "Effects of exogenous ketone supplementation on blood ketone, glucose, triglyceride, and lipoprotein levels in Sprague–Dawley rats." *Nutrition & Metabolism* 13 (2016): 9.

Kesl, S. L., M. Wu, L. J. Gould, and D. P. D'Agostino. "Potential mechanisms of action for exogenous ketone enhancement of ischemic wound healing in young and aged Fischer rats." *FASEB Journal* 30, suppl 1 (2016): 1036.9.

Laffel, L. "Ketone bodies: a review of physiology, pathophysiology and application of monitoring to diabetes." *Diabetes/Metabolism Research and Reviews* 15, no. 6 (1999): 412–26.

Lardy, H. A. and P. H. Phillips. "Studies of fat and carbohydrate oxidation in mammal an spermatozoa." *Archives of Biochemistry* 6, no. 1 (1945): 53–61.

Lee, Y. S., W. S. Kim, K. H. Kim, M. J. Yoon, H. J. Cho, Y. Shen, ... and C. Hohnen-Behrens. "Berberine, a natural plant product, activates AMP-activated protein kinase with beneficial metabolic effects in diabetic and insulin-resistant states." *Diabetes* 55, no. 8 (2006): 2256–64.

Likhodii, S. S., I. Serbanescu, M. A. Cortez, P. Murphy, O. C. Snead, and W. M. Burnham. "Anticonvulsant properties of acetone, a brain ketone elevated by the ketogenic diet." *Annals of Neurology* 54, no. 2 (2003): 219–26.

Liu, Y., F. Liu, K. Iqbal, I. Grundke-Iqbal, and C. X. Gong. "Decreased glucose transporters correlate to abnormal hyperphosphorylation of tau in Alzheimer disease." *FEBS Letters* 582, no. 2 (2008): 359–64.

Loridan, L., and B. Senior. "Effects of infusion of ketones in children with ketotic hypoglycemia." *Journal of Pediatrics* 76, no. 1 (1970): 69–74.

Maalouf, M. P. G. Sullivan, L. Davis, D. Y. Kim, and J. M. Rho. "Ketones inhibit mitochondrial production of reactive oxygen species production following glutamate excitotoxicity by increasing NADH oxidation." *Neuroscience* 145, no. 1 (2007): 256–64.

Madison, L. L., D. Mebane, R. H. Unger, and A. Lochner. "The hypoglycemic action of ketones. II. Evidence for a stimulatory feedback of ketones on the pancreatic beta cells." *Journal of Clinical Investigation* 43, no. 3 (1964): 408–15.

Magee, B. A., N. Potezny, A. M. Rofe, and R. A. Conyers. "The inhibition of malignant cell growth by ketone bodies." *Australian Journal of Experimental Biology and Medical Science* 57, no. 5 (1979): 529–39.

McKenzie, A. "CXL.—The resolution of β-hydroxybutyric acid into its optically active components." *Journal of the Chemical Society, Transactions* 81 (1902): 1402–12.

McNally, M. A., and A. L. Hartman. "Ketone bodies in epilepsy." *Journal of Neurochemistry* 121, no. 1 (2012): 28–35.

Meenakshi, C., K. Latha Kumari, and C. S. Shyamala Devi. "Biochemical studies on the effects of S-1, 3-butanediol of diabetes induced rats." *Indian Journal of Physiology and Pharmacology* 39 (1995): 145–8.

Mejía-Toiber, J., T. Montiel, and L. Massieu. "D-β-hydroxybutyrate prevents glutamate-mediated lipoperoxidation and neuronal damage elicited during glycolysis inhibition in vivo." *Neurochemical Research* 31, no. 12 (2006): 1399–408.

Misell, L. M., N. D. Lagomarcino, V. Schuster, and M. Kern. "Chronic medium-chain triacylglycerol consumption and endurance performance in trained runners." *Journal of Sports Medicine and Physical Fitness* 41, no. 2 (2001): 210.

Murray, A. J., N. S. Knight, M. A. Cole, L. E. Cochlin, E. Carter, K. Tchabanenko, ... and R. M. Deacon. "Novel ketone diet enhances physical and cognitive performance." *FASEB Journal* fj-201600773R (2016).

Nair, K. S., S. L. Welle, D. Halliday, and R. G. Campbell. "Effect of beta-hydroxybutyrate on whole-body leucine kinetics and fractional mixed skeletal muscle protein synthesis in humans." *Journal of Clinical Investigation* 82, no. 1 (1988): 198.

Nath, M. C., and H. D. Brahmachari. "Experimental hyperglycaemia by injection of intermediary fat metabolism products in rabbits." *Nature* 154 (1944): 487.

Neptune, E. M. "Changes in blood glucose during metabolism of ß-hydroxybutyrate." *American Journal of Physiology–Legacy Content* 187, no. 3 (1956): 451–3.

Newman, J. C., and E. Verdin. "β-hydroxybutyrate: much more than a metabolite." *Diabetes Research and Clinical Practice* 106, no. 2 (2014): 173–81.

Newport, M. T. "Alzheimer's disease: what if there was a cure?" *ReadHowYouWant* (2013).

Newport, M. T., T. B. VanItallie, Y. Kashiwaya, M. T. King, and R. L. Veech. "A new way to produce hyperketonemia: use of ketone ester in a case of Alzheimer's disease." *Alzheimer's & Dementia* 11, no. 1 (2015): 99–103.

Nonaka, Y., T. Takagi, M. Inai, S. Nishimura, S. Urashima, K. Honda, ... and S. Terada. "Lauric acid stimulates ketone body production in the KT-5 astrocyte cell line." *Journal of Oleo Science* 65, no. 8 (2016): 693–9.

Paoli, A., G. Bosco, E. M. Camporesi, and D. Mangar. "Ketosis, ketogenic diet and food intake control: a complex relationship." *Frontiers in Psychology* 6 (2015): 27.

Papandreou, D., E. Pavlou, E. Kalimeri, and I. Mavromichalis. "The ketogenic diet in children with epilepsy." *British Journal of Nutrition* 95, no. 01 (2006): 5–13.

Plecko, B., S. Stoeckler-Ipsiroglu, E. Schober, G. Harrer, V. Mlynarik, S. Gruber, ... and O. Ipsiroglu. "Oral β-hydroxybutyrate supplementation in two patients with hyperinsulinemic hypoglycemia: monitoring of β-hydroxybutyrate levels in blood and cerebrospinal fluid, and in the brain by in vivo magnetic resonance spectroscopy." *Pediatric Research* 52, no. 2 (2002): 301–6.

Poff, A. M., C. Ari, P. Arnold, T. N. Seyfried, and D. P. D'Agostino. "Ketone supplementation decreases tumor cell viability and prolongs survival of mice with metastatic cancer." *International Journal of Cancer* 135, no. 7 (2014): 1711–20.

Poff, A., N. Ward, T. Seyfried, and D. D'Agostino. "Combination ketogenic diet, ketone supplementation, and hyperbaric oxygen therapy inhibits metastatic spread, slows tumor growth, and increases survival time in mice with metastatic cancer (123.7)." *FASEB Journal* 28, suppl 1 (2014): 123.7.

Poff, A., S. Kesl, N. Ward, and D. D'Agostino. "Metabolic effects of exogenous ketone supplementation–an alternative or adjuvant to the ketogenic diet as a cancer therapy?" *FASEB Journal* 30, suppl 1 (2016): 1167.2.

Prins, M. L., and C. C. Giza. "Induction of monocarboxylate transporter 2 expression and ketone transport following traumatic brain injury in juvenile and adult rats." *Developmental Neuroscience* 28, nos. 4–5 (2006): 447–56.

Prins, M. L., S. M. Lee, L. S. Fujima, and D. A. Hovda. "Increased cerebral uptake and oxidation of exogenous βHB improves ATP following traumatic brain injury in adult rats." *Journal of Neurochemistry* 90, no. 3 (2004): 666–72.

Prins, M. L., L. S. Fujima, and D. A. Hovda. "Age-dependent reduction of cortical contusion volume by ketones after traumatic brain injury." *Journal of Neuroscience Research* 82, no. 3 (2005): 413–20.

Reger, M. A., S. T. Henderson, C. Hale, B. Cholerton, L. D. Baker, G. S. Watson, ... and S. Craft. "Effects of β-hydroxybutyrate on cognition in memory-impaired adults." *Neurobiology of Aging* 25, no. 3 (2004): 311–4.

Rho, J. M., G. D. Anderson, S. D. Donevan, and H. S. White. "Acetoacetate, acetone, and dibenzylamine (a contaminant in l-(+)-β-hydroxybutyrate) exhibit direct anticonvulsant actions in vivo." *Epilepsia* 43, no. 4 (2002): 358–61.

Ritter, A. M., C. S. Robertson, J. C. Goodman, C. F. Contant, and R. G. Grossman. "Evaluation of a carbohydrate-free diet for patients with severe head injury." *Journal of Neurotrauma* 13, no. 8 (1996): 473–85.

Robinson, A. M., and D. H. Williamson. "Physiological roles of ketone bodies as substrates and signals in mammalian tissues." *Physiological Reviews* 60, no. 1 (1980): 143–87.

Rodger, S. "Oral ketone supplementation: effect on cognitive function, physiology and exercise performance." Master's Thesis (2015).

Rossi, R., S. D. Örig, E. Del Prete, and E. Scharrer. "Suppression of feed intake after parenteral administration of D-β-hydroxybutyrate in pygmy goats." *Journal of Veterinary Medicine Series* A 47, no. 1 (2000): 9–16.

Rothwell, N. J., and M. J. Stock. "A role for brown adipose tissue in diet-induced thermogenesis." *Nature* 281, no. 5726 (1979): 31.

Sato, K., Y. Kashiwaya, C. A. Keon, N. Tsuchiya, M. T. King, G. K. Radda, ... and R. L. Veech. "Insulin, ketone bodies, and mitochondrial energy transduction." *FASEB Journal* 9, no. 8 (1995): 651–8.

Schultz, L. H., V. R. Smith, and H. A. Lardy. "The effect of the administration of various fatty acids on the blood ketone levels of ruminants." *Journal of Dairy Science* 32, no. 9 (1949): 817–22.

Seale, P., and M. A. Lazar. "Brown fat in humans: turning up the heat on obesity." *Diabetes* 58, no. 7 (2009): 1482–4.

Senior, B., and L. Loridan. "Direct regulatory effect of ketones on lipolysis and on glucose concentrations in man." *Nature* 219, no. 5149 (1968): 83–4.

Sherwin, R. S., R. G. Hendler, and P. Felig. "Effect of ketone infusions on amino acid and nitrogen metabolism in man." *Journal of Clinical Investigation* 55, no. 6 (1975): 1382.

Simpson, I. A., K. R. Chundu, T. Davies-Hill, W. G. Honer, and P. Davies. "Decreased concentrations of GLUT1 and GLUT3 glucose transporters in the brains of patients with Alzheimer's disease." *Annals of Neurology* 35, no. 5 (1994): 546–51.

Skinner, R., A. Trujillo, X. Ma, and E. A. Beierle. "Ketone bodies inhibit the viability of human neuroblastoma cells." *Journal of Pediatric Surgery* 44, no. 1 (2009): 212–6.

Smith, S. L., D. J. Heal, and K. F. Martin. "KTX 0101: a potential metabolic approach to cytoprotection in major surgery and neurological disorders." *CNS Drug Reviews* 11, no. 2 (2005): 113–40.

Srivastava, S., Y. Kashiwaya, M. T. King, U. Baxa, J. Tam, G. Niu, ... and R. L. Veech. "Mitochondrial biogenesis and increased uncoupling protein 1 in brown adipose tissue of mice fed a ketone ester diet." *FASEB Journal* 26, no. 6 (2012): 2351–62.

Suzuki, M., M. Suzuki, Y. Kitamura, S. Mori, K. Sato, S. Dohi, ... and A. Hiraide. "Beta-hydroxybutyrate, a cerebral function improving agent, protects rat brain against ischemic damage caused by permanent and transient focal cerebral ischemia." *Japanese Journal of Pharmacology* 89, no. 1 (2002): 36–43.

Thio, L. L., M. Wong, and K. A. Yamada. "Ketone bodies do not directly alter excitatory or inhibitory hippocampal synaptic transmission." *Neurology* 54, no. 2 (2000): 325–31.

Thomas, G. N. W. "Sugar and migraine." *British Medical Journal* 2, no. 3326 (1924): 598.

Tidwell, H. C., and H. E. Axelrod. "Blood sugar after injection of acetoacetate." *Journal of Biological Chemistry* 172, no. 1 (1948): 179–84.

Tieu, K., C. Perier, C. Caspersen, P. Teismann, D. C. Wu, S. D. Yan, ... and S. Przedborski. "D-β-hydroxybutyrate rescues mitochondrial respiration and mitigates features of Parkinson disease." *Journal of Clinical Investigation* 112, no. 6 (2003): 892–901.

Tsai, Y. C., Y. C. Chou, A. B. Wu, C. M. Hu, C. Y. Chen, F. A. Chen, and J. A. Lee. "Stereoselective effects of 3-hydroxybutyrate on glucose utilization of rat cardiomyocytes." *Life Sciences* 78, no. 12 (2006): 1385–91.

Valayannopoulos, V., F. Bajolle, J. B. Arnoux, S. Dubois, N. Sannier, C. Baussan, ... and A. Vassault. "Successful treatment of severe cardiomyopathy in glycogen storage disease type III With D, L-3-hydroxybutyrate, ketogenic and high-protein diet." *Pediatric Research* 70, no. 6 (2011): 638–41.

Van Hove, J. L., S. Grünewald, J. Jaeken, P. Demaerel, P. E. Declercq, P. Bourdoux, ... and J. V. Leonard. "D, L-3-hydroxybutyrate treatment of multiple acyl-CoA dehydrogenase deficiency (MADD)." *The Lancet* 361, no. 9367 (2003): 1433–5.

VanItallie, T. B., and T. H. Nufert. "Ketones: metabolism's ugly duckling." *Nutrition Reviews* 61, no. 10 (2003): 327–41.

Van Wymelbeke, V., A. Himaya, J. Louis-Sylvestre, and M. Fantino. "Influence of medium-chain and long-chain triacylglycerols on the control of food intake in men." *American Journal of Clinical Nutrition* 68, no. 2 (1998): 226–34.

Veech, R. L., B. Chance, Y. Kashiwaya, H. A. Lardy, and G. F. Cahill. "Ketone bodies, potential therapeutic uses." *IUBMB Life* 51, no. 4 (2001): 241–7.

Veech, R. L. "The therapeutic implications of ketone bodies: the effects of ketone bodies in pathological conditions: ketosis, ketogenic diet, redox states, insulin resistance, and mitochondrial metabolism." *Prostaglandins, Leukotrienes and Essential Fatty Acids* 70, no. 3 (2004): 309–19.

Wang, D., A. Pannerec, J. Feige, N. Christinat, M. Masoodi, and E. Mitchell. "Cognition and synaptic-plasticity related changes in aged rats supplemented with 8-and 10 carbon medium chain triglycerides." *FASEB Journal* 29, suppl 1 (2015): LB291.

Wang, Y., N. Liu, W. Zhu, K. Zhang, J. Si, M. Bi, ... and J. Wang. "Protective effect of β-hydroxybutyrate on glutamate induced cell death in HT22 cells." *International Journal of Clinical Experimental Medicine* 9, no. 12 (2016): 23433–9.

West, A. C., and R. W. Johnstone. "New and emerging HDAC inhibitors for cancer treatment." *Journal of Clinical Investigation* 124, no. 1 (2014): 30–39.

White, H., and B. Venkatesh. "Clinical review: ketones and brain injury." *Critical Care* 15, no. 2 (2011): 1.

Williams, S., C. Basualdo-Hammond, R. Curtis, and R. Schuller. "Growth retardation in children with epilepsy on the ketogenic diet: a retrospective chart review." *Journal of the Academy of Nutrition and Dietetics* 102, no. 3 (2002): 405.

Yin, J. X., M. Maalouf, P. Han, M. Zhao, M. Gao, T. Dharshaun, ... and E. M. Reiman. "Ketones block amyloid entry and improve cognition in an Alzheimer's model." *Neurobiology of Aging* 39 (2016): 25–37.

Youm, Y. H., K. Y. Nguyen, R. W. Grant, E. L. Goldberg, M. Bodogai, D. Kim ... and S. Kang. "The ketone metabolite [beta]-hydroxybutyrate blocks NLRP3 inflammasome-mediated inflammatory disease." *Nature Medicine* 21, no. 3 (2015): 263–269.

Young, C. M., S. S. Scanlan, H. S. Im, and L. Lutwak. "Effect on body composition and other parameters in obese young men of carbohydrate level of reduction diet." *American Journal of Clinical Nutrition* 24, no. 3 (1971): 290–6.

Zhang, Y., K. Guo, R. E. LeBlanc, D. Loh, G. J. Schwartz, and Y. H. Yu. "Increasing dietary leucine intake reduces diet-induced obesity and improves glucose and cholesterol metabolism in mice via multimechanisms." *Diabetes* 56, no. 6 (2007): 1647–54.

Zhao, W., M. Varghese, P. Vempati, A. Dzhun, A. Cheng, J. Wang, ... and G. M. Pasinetti. "Caprylic triglyceride as a novel therapeutic approach to effectively improve the performance and attenuate the symptoms due to the motor neuron loss in ALS disease." *PLOS ONE* 7, no. 11 (2012): e49191.

Zilberter, M., A. Ivanov, S. Ziyatdinova, M. Mukhtarov, A. Malkov, A. Alpár, ... and A. Pitkänen. "Dietary energy substrates reverse early neuronal hyperactivity in a mouse model of Alzheimer's disease." *Journal of Neurochemistry* 125, no. 1 (2013): 157–71.

"GRAS Exemption Claim for (R)-3-hydroxybutyl (R)-3-hydroxybutyrate." www.fda.gov/downloads/Food/IngredientsPackagingLabeling/GRAS/NoticeInventory/UCM403846

"Sports Concussion Statistics." Head Case. 2016. www.headcasecompany.com/concussion_info/stats_on_concussions_sports

Chapter 5

POTENTIAL APPLICATIONS

Section 1:
Appetite Control and Weight Loss

In 2015, we spoke at a conference about some of our newest research on how a well-formulated ketogenic diet can aid in fat loss. Fast-forward one year, and we were speaking at an educational event centered around ketogenic dieting. A gentleman came up to us and gave us both a big hug. With tears in his eyes, he said, "Thank you for saving my life." In 2015, he explained, he heard our talk about the ketogenic diet and fat loss. The week before that presentation, he'd been rushed to the hospital after feeling faint; he was severely obese, his liver enzymes were through the roof, his blood lipid profile was highly atherosclerotic (exhibiting high LDL and low HDL cholesterol levels), and his fasting blood glucose level was well over 500 mg/dL (a normal level is under 100 mg/dL). Just walking from his car to his office had become difficult. His doctor told him that if he didn't reduce his weight, change his eating habits, and start exercising, he wouldn't live much longer. After attending our seminar, the man decided to implement a ketogenic diet along with exercise and even periodic exogenous ketones (discussed in Chapter 4) to see if it was the change he needed to lose weight. A year later, he'd lost more than 100 pounds, his fasting blood glucose had dropped to 97 mg/dL, and he felt like a new man.

We've heard thousands of similar testimonials. Can the ketogenic diet be an effective tool for weight loss? We certainly believe it can.

It is no surprise that we are facing a global obesity epidemic. According to the National Health and Nutrition Examination Surveys (NHANES), 35 percent of adult men and 40 percent of adult women in the United States today are obese (Malik et al., 2013). The obesity epidemic seems to be driven primarily by environments that encourage overconsumption of food, consumption of high-sugar foods, and a lack of physical activity (Swinburn et al., 2011). We are constantly bombarded with strategic advertising for cheap, readily available snacks, such as king-sized candy bars, chips, cake, and cereal. We've spoken with some of the top companies that sell these sugar-laden food items, and there is an entire strategy around their marketing to appeal to your senses. Every commercial, whether it is targeted toward you or, worse, your children, is meant to drive a desire to buy. There is a reason behind every one of those animated bunnies, tigers, and leprechauns featured in food commercials aimed at kids. Inevitably, we all fall victim to these marketing ploys and end up buying in, whether we like to admit it or not.

The U.S. government's current recommendations for weight loss center around low-fat, calorie-restricted diets; however, these diets tend to fail over the long term (Liu et al., 2014; Sumithran et al., 2013). In fact, studies have revealed that the majority of weight lost on a low-fat diet is gained back within three to five years (MacLean et al., 2011). There are two possible reasons for this: increased hunger and a slower metabolism. First, studies show that low-calorie, low-fat diets can result in elevated desire to eat, hunger, and food consumption in just a couple weeks' time (Sumithran et al., 2011; Doucet et al., 2000). Second, after following a calorie-restricted diet, our metabolism adapts: when we cut back on calories our bodies adjust to expend fewer calories for basic functions, like keeping our bodily systems running. That slowing of the metabolism can remain in place for as much as six years after we stop dieting; the more extreme the diet, the higher the likelihood of this effect persisting for a longer time (Fothergill et al., 2016)! Low-fat, low-calorie diets force us to battle both an elevation in hunger and a slower, adapted metabolism—setting us up for the ultimate disaster of weight regain. For a diet to be effective and sustainable, it needs to prevent weight regain and place hunger within the dieter's control.

The Hunger Problem

Many people assume that the solution to the obesity epidemic is simple: eat less and move more. Certainly we are eating more and moving less than we did before the epidemic began. Data from the USDA Economic Research Service states that we are eating over 350 more calories per day now than Americans did fifty years ago (Cecil et al., 2008). It's difficult to say what's behind that increase, but inarguably as a society we are not only eating more, but also moving less. According to the Centers for Disease Control and Prevention, only 21 percent of adults in the United States meet the 2008 Physical Activity Guidelines for Americans, which consist of 150 minutes per week of moderate-intensity aerobic activity (or 75 minutes of vigorous aerobic activity) and strength training at least two days per week. We

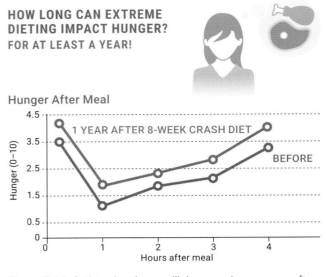

HOW LONG CAN EXTREME DIETING IMPACT HUNGER? FOR AT LEAST A YEAR!

Hunger After Meal

Figure 5.1.1. Satiety signals are still depressed even a year after an extreme crash diet.

Source: Adapted from Sumithran, 2011.

are sitting more than ever, and our desk jobs leave us with bad posture as well as a lack of movement throughout the day.

While eating less and moving more could work, the reality is that weight loss is much more complex. Studies have found more than thirty gene variants that may explain differences in body weight between lean and obese individuals. The first gene to be linked to obesity was the fat mass and obesity-associated (FTO) gene (Cecil et al., 2008). In obese individuals, variations in this gene result in reduced feelings of fullness after a meal and an impaired ability to regulate appetite (Llewellyn et al., 2014). Thus it's possible that these individuals have a more difficult time feeling full than their leaner counterparts. While one person may feel full after eating a small lunch, another might perceive that meal as just a snack and still be hungry for more.

Hunger is a physiological need to eat, but there is a difference between hunger and appetite. For example, say you wake up late in the morning and don't get a chance to even drink some coffee before heading to work. As soon as you get to the office, you are bombarded with phone calls and meetings, and before you realize it, it is afternoon and your stomach is growling. That's hunger. You decide to take your lunch break and go with a colleague to get a big Cobb salad with blue cheese, bacon, eggs, and steak. The fullness you experience afterward is known as satiety; the suppressed hunger following a meal is known as satiation. Then you head back to the office and find that someone brought in freshly baked chocolate chip cookies and brownies. Though you are still full from lunch, you may be tempted to have a treat. That's appetite. However, because you're so full, you're able to resist the desire to eat the cookie or brownie (at least we hope you are!).

Three main processes regulate food intake, all of which are controlled in an area of the brain known as the hypothalamus. First, similar to how a thermostat regulates the temperature in a house, our bodies have an internal "nutrient stat." When the nutrient stat detects that levels of nutrients like glucose, fatty acids, and ketones are high, the brain sends out signals for hunger to be low (Obici et al., 2002). Second, our bodies have a mechanical response to food. When the volume of food we eat expands and distends our guts (Martin et al., 2007), our brains receive a mechanical signal that we are full. Imagine a balloon that expands when you blow it up. When we consume a large quantity of food (e.g., overindulging on turkey and stuffing at Thanksgiving), our stomachs literally expand and fill up (sometimes causing us to undo a button or loosen up a notch on the belt buckle). Finally, we have hunger and satiety hormones that control the amount of food we eat (Sumithran et al., 2011). Ghrelin is a common hormone that increases hunger, and its opposing hormone, leptin, increases satiety so we eat less. Dieting can significantly affect these hormones: ghrelin can go up while leptin can go down.

Obesity is associated with an impaired regulation of the processes that normally reduce the desire to consume more food (MacLean et al., 2011). This may be one reason why traditional low-fat, low-calorie diets fail for overweight or obese individuals. An impaired ability to control food intake results in a chaotic and nearly uncontrollable rebound after weight has been lost (MacLean et al., 2011). Theoretically, if we could find a way to diet without negatively altering appetite or hunger and satiety hormones (ghrelin and leptin), long-term changes in fat loss and overall body composition could be sustained.

There is hope. One study found that after following a very-low-calorie carbohydrate-based diet for eight weeks, individuals' hunger and hunger hormones remained elevated for more than a year

CAN KETOGENIC DIETING STOP HUNGER PAINS? YES!

Hunger Hormones After Diet

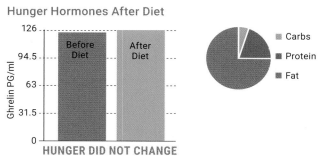

Figure 5.1.2. *Changes in hunger hormones following 8 weeks on a ketogenic diet.*

Source: Adapted from Sumithren et al., 2013.

(Sumithran et al., 2011). However, following a very-low-calorie *ketogenic* diet for the same amount of time did not increase hunger hormones or boost hunger, despite the drastic decline in food intake (Sumithran et al., 2013). Beyond this, a number of studies have found that individuals adhering to a ketogenic diet without restricting calories experience less hunger—and therefore may inadvertently eat fewer calories. Think about that for a moment: *people aren't as hungry as they were before they decreased their caloric intake.* In addition, the level of ketones needed to suppress hunger is likely to be small, as studies show no difference in appetite between ketone levels of 0.5 mmol/L and more than 3 mmol/L (Rosen et al., 1985; Krotkeiwski et al., 2001).

Our good friend Dr. Dominic D'Agostino once said that ketogenic dieting "puts appetite back into our control." There are several potential reasons for this. First, the ketogenic diet prevents drops in blood glucose, slightly elevates fatty acids, and robustly raises ketones, so our nutrient stat may recognize that we don't need to eat (Paoli et al., 2015). This contrasts with low-fat diets, which promote between-meal drops in blood glucose, suppress fatty acids, and prevent the formation of ketones (Gibson et al., 2015). Second, ketosis prevents hunger hormones like ghrelin from rising, while some satiety hormones, like cholecystokinin (CCK), do not drop as they do with low-calorie diets (Sumithran et al., 2013). Finally, on a well-formulated ketogenic diet, the carbohydrates we do take in, ideally from high-fiber leafy green vegetables, can trigger greater mechanical signals of satiety due to their sheer volume (Ard et al., 2016).

Study	Diet Intervention	Outcome (Low-Carbohydrate)
Young et al., 1971	104g, 60g, or 30g carbs; amount of protein was the same in each dietary intervention	↓ hunger in all three groups
Evans et al., 1974	80g carbs, unlimited protein and fat	↓ caloric intake (30% lower)
Boden et al., 2005	21g carbs, 151g protein, 164g fat	↓ caloric intake (about 950 fewer calories) ↓ 2kg in 14 days
Nickols-Richardson et al., 2005	20–40g carbs, 90–100g protein, 95–105g fat	↓ hunger ↓ body weight
Vander Wal et al., 2005	Egg or bagel breakfast	↓ caloric intake at lunch and for the remainder of the day after eating the egg breakfast
Wood et al., 2006	Low-carbohydrate diet with 10% of calories from carbs and no caloric restrictions	↓ caloric intake (30% lower)
McClerno et al., 2007	< 20g carbs	↓ hunger
Johnstone et al., 2008	4% calories from carbs, no caloric restrictions on protein and fat	↓ caloric intake ↓ hunger
Martin et al., 2011	20g carbs, no caloric restrictions on protein and fat	↓ cravings ↓ hunger ↓ appetite
Veldhorst et al., 2012	30% protein, 70% fat	↓ appetite

Maximizing Weight Loss: Low-Fat or Ketogenic?

While ketogenic dieting may help with hunger and satiety, the bigger questions are, can you adhere to it, and how does it fare in terms of weight loss? An extensive review of several studies found that in nearly 70 percent of those lasting from six to thirty-six months, overweight individuals had a greater adherence to a ketogenic diet than to a low-fat diet (Hession et al., 2009). The satiating effects of the ketogenic diet make it easier to stay on it—because you're not hungry all the time, you're more likely to stick to this way of eating. What's unique about ketogenic dieting is that you can lose fat even without being told to reduce the number of calories you consume (Volek et al., 2004; Sondike, 2003; Brehm, 2003; Holland et al., 2016; Kennedy et al., 2007).

> "Telling someone that weight loss is just eating less calories than you burn is like telling an athlete that all they have to do to win the game is score. Sounds simple, but it's really not."
>
> —Unknown

Studies consistently show that ketogenic diets result in more lost weight than low-fat diets. For example, in one study, after six months, weight loss was greater among those following a ketogenic diet than those following a low-fat diet (Hession et al., 2009). However, in most of these studies protein intake is greater in the ketogenic dieting group. This makes it unclear whether it's the ketogenic diet or the higher protein intake driving the increased weight loss. Recent research from our lab (Wilson et al., 2017) found that eight weeks of resistance training combined with ketogenic dieting resulted in a loss of about 9 pounds of body fat, while the same exercise combined with a traditional low-fat diet resulted in a loss of about 4

Attrition Rate for Low-Carb and Low-Fat Diets

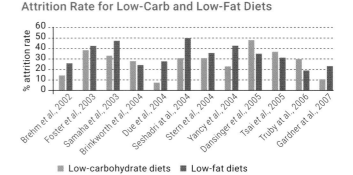

■ Low-carbohydrate diets ■ Low-fat diets

Figure 5.1.3. *Studies of low-carbohydrate diets show lower dropout rates than studies of low-fat diets.*

Source: Hession et al., 2009.

pounds of body fat. One key element of our study: protein intake was the same in both groups.

In another study (Young et al., 1971), sedentary, overweight college students were divided into three groups that consumed either 100, 60, or 30 grams of carbohydrates per day. Protein intake was the same for all groups: 115 grams. The lowest-carbohydrate group (30 grams) had the highest ketone levels, and the highest-carbohydrate group (100 grams) had the lowest ketone levels. Weight loss was greatest and muscle mass was preserved the most in the lowest-carbohydrate group. The fact that the weight loss was primarily due to loss of body fat indicates that ketones may spare us from losing muscle when in a calorie deficit.

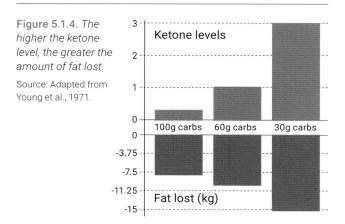

Figure 5.1.4. *The higher the ketone level, the greater the amount of fat lost.*

Source: Adapted from Young et al., 1971.

While the reasons for this advantage are uncertain, Dr. Volek (2002) postulates that ketogenic dieting creates a unique metabolic state in which fat loss can occur even as caloric intake is maintained—and possibly even with a slightly *increased* caloric intake. The reason centers around gluconeogenesis. Recall from Chapter 1 that in gluconeogenesis, glucose is produced from non-carbohydrate sources. When carbohydrate intake is low and protein intake is moderate, the body uses fatty acids and glucogenic amino acids (glucose-producing protein precursors that are not essential for building muscle). In order to make 1 gram of glucose, 10 grams of fat need to be broken down (Volek et al., 2007), so the simple fact that the ketogenic diet restricts carbs and, to a lesser extent, protein means that more fat needs to be used to create the glucose needed for certain body processes that rely on glucose.

Another potential reason why ketogenic diets may offer an advantage is related to a concept known as feed efficiency, which refers to how much fat is stored for every calorie of food consumed. For example, if you and your friend eat the same 500-calorie piece of cake, yet you store more fat from it than she does, then you are more efficient at storing calories than she is. Recently, we collaborated with Dr. Mike Roberts and Dr. Maleah Holland (Holland et al., 2016), who found that even when protein intake is similar, rats fed a ketogenic diet had a lower feed efficiency—they gained less weight per gram of food eaten—and lower fat mass than rats on a Western or low-fat diet, regardless of exercise. The mechanism behind these findings isn't entirely clear, but it could be related to an increase in brown adipose tissue (BAT) (Veech et al., 2007). We will discuss this concept further later on, but briefly, BAT raises metabolic rate—the rate at which we burn energy simply to stay alive—by converting the food we eat to heat rather than usable energy.

Several studies have shown that a ketogenic diet leads to profound decreases in body fat. In addition to those studies cited above, Dr. Volek (2004) found that despite eating nearly 300 extra calories per day, individuals on a ketogenic diet lost significantly more fat than those on a low-fat diet. Studies dating back to the 1950s show that during a 1,000-calories-per-day dieting period, the most rapid weight loss occurred with a high-fat diet, and this effect persisted when calorie intake rose to 2,600 per day (Kekwick and Pawan, 1956). Another study looked at overweight adolescents who consumed 20 to 40 grams of carbohydrates per day for twelve weeks (Sondike et al., 2003). Despite consuming 700 calories more per day than their counterparts on a low-fat diet, these adolescents lost 9.9 kilograms (21.8 pounds) compared to just 4.1 kilograms (9 pounds) in the low-fat group. This is yet another study showing that the fat loss achieved under these conditions is the result of more than just lowering calories.

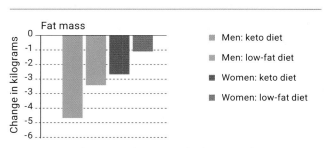

Figure 5.1.5. *Changes in fat mass in both men and women, comparing a ketogenic diet to a low-fat diet.*

Source: Volek et al., 2004.

How Much Will You Lose?
It Depends on You

People often ask us, "How much weight can I expect to lose on the keto diet?" Honestly, it varies from person to person, depending not just on how your particular body works but also on your starting weight, your caloric intake, and ultimately your goals. However, one study found that subjects on a high-fat, low-carbohydrate diet (no more than 50 to 60 grams of carbs and approximately 150 grams of fat per day) lost an average of 0.3 kilogram (0.66 pound) per day over a forty-five-day period (Kasper et al., 1973).

It might take longer for individuals who are insulin resistant to see the same metabolic benefits of a ketogenic diet as those who are insulin sensitive. Research shows that people who are overweight and insulin resistant tend to have impaired mitochondrial function and fewer mitochondria overall (Short et al., 2004). Mitochondria are responsible for breaking down fat for fuel and thus play a significant role in the formation and utilization of ketones (Hyatt et al., 2016), so problems with mitochondria automatically put those individuals at a disadvantage for becoming

keto-adapted. Fortunately, ketogenic dieting itself appears to improve both the number of mitochondria and their function, so the disadvantage can be overcome over time (Hyatt et al., 2016). Therefore, individuals who are overweight or obese (and likely insulin resistant) would likely see beneficial effects from decreasing carbohydrate intake and turning to an alternative fuel source (i.e., ketones). On the other hand, insulin-sensitive people, like that friend who can eat a piece of cake every night and stay lean, would likely do well on any diet as long as he has the ability to properly digest, absorb, and metabolize any ratio of macronutrients and maintain a healthy body composition.

Keep in mind that the process of adapting to a ketogenic diet takes time. If you are overweight and insulin resistant, the true metabolic advantages of ketogenic dieting likely will not manifest themselves fully until you've been on the diet for at least several weeks.

The notion that it generally takes overweight and insulin-resistant people longer to adapt to a ketogenic diet was recently supported in a study of obese individuals ranging from eighteen to fifty years of age (Hall et al., 2016). The eight-week trial consisted of two phases: For the first four weeks, the subjects were placed on a low-fat, high-carbohydrate diet. Although the researchers attempted to set calories

Figure 5.1.6. *An individual's metabolic flexibility can determine how well he or she is able to utilize fat when needed.*
Source: Kelley, 2005.

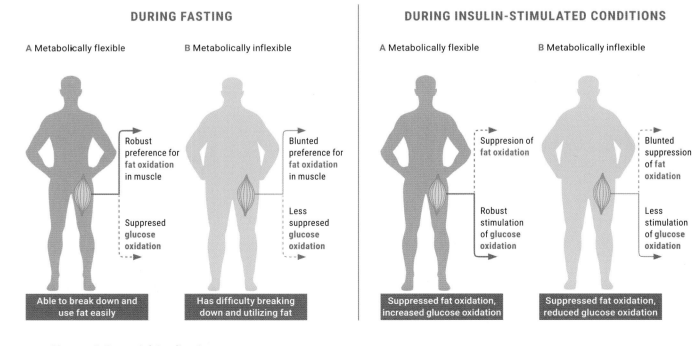

DURING FASTING

A Metabolically flexible   B Metabolically inflexible

Robust preference for fat oxidation in muscle

Suppresed glucose oxidation

Blunted preference for fat oxidation in muscle

Less suppressed glucose oxidation

Able to break down and use fat easily

Has difficulty breaking down and utilizing fat

DURING INSULIN-STIMULATED CONDITIONS

A Metabolically flexible   B Metabolically inflexible

Suppresion of fat oxidation

Robust stimulation of glucose oxidation

Blunted suppression of fat oxidation

Less stimulation of glucose oxidation

Suppressed fat oxidation, increased glucose oxidation

Suppressed fat oxidation, reduced glucose oxidation

for maintenance, the subjects lost approximately 2 pounds during that time, indicating that they were consuming about 300 fewer calories a day than usual. For the second four weeks, the subjects were placed on a not-well-formulated ketogenic diet for fat loss. We say "not-well-formulated" because protein intake, at 15 percent of total calories or 1 gram per kilogram of body weight, was suboptimal for the maintenance of muscle mass. The recommendation to prevent muscle wasting is 1.6 grams of protein per kilogram of body weight (Phinney et al., 2004). In addition, fiber intake was far less than what is recommended for health—roughly 12 grams per day.

The researchers found that when the subjects switched from a high-carbohydrate, calorie-restricted diet to a ketogenic diet, their metabolic rate increased by 100 calories in the first week but returned to normal for the remainder of the study. They concluded that "there was no metabolic advantage of a ketogenic diet compared to a low-fat diet."

There are a number of problems with this statement. Principally, it is impossible to compare a diet that restricts calories for four weeks to a subsequent dieting period. This is because the initial diet will likely result in adaptations that impede fat loss. Respiratory quotient (RQ) values, which represent the ratio of the volume of carbon dioxide produced to the volume of oxygen consumed on a cellular level, can be used to measure whether someone is burning primarily fat or carbohydrates as fuel. When we're utilizing glucose for fuel, RQ equals 1.0 because we are consuming six O_2s and expelling six CO_2s. When we're burning pure fat, RQ drops to 0.7, as more oxygen is required to oxidize fat. In this study, RQ dropped only a little, from 0.87 to 0.78. Though this decrease was slight, RQ likely isn't the best measure of whether someone is keto-adapted. Because the metabolic measures lacked the sensitivity necessary to maintain body weight, the short duration of the trial did not allow the subjects to become fully adapted, and the protein intake was suboptimal, we are unable to make definitive conclusions. Lastly, a diet's metabolic advantage may be indicated not by the total resting calories expended per day but by long-term metabolic changes, such as a lowered ability to efficiently store energy (feed efficiency). While the study didn't explore this area, it is a main advantage of the ketogenic diet when it comes to weight loss.

Is the Ketogenic Diet Better for Me or for My Friend?

Do some people respond better to a ketogenic diet than others? A study by McClain et al. (2013) divided subjects into two groups: insulin sensitive and insulin resistant. Think of insulin-sensitive people (see page 77) as those who can consume a high-carbohydrate meal and use the resulting glucose for fuel with low amounts of insulin. Those who are insulin resistant must use excessive amounts of insulin to do the same job, which means that their blood glucose is typically higher. McClain's study found that insulin-resistant individuals placed on a low-fat diet lost minimal weight. When placed on a ketogenic diet, however, they lost more weight. In contrast, those who were insulin sensitive did equally well on both diets.

One way to test yourself is to examine your blood glucose level after fasting and before and after meals. Fasting blood glucose tests typically are taken eight to twelve hours after eating a meal. For example, if you stop eating at 7 p.m. and wake up at 7 a.m., that constitutes a twelve-hour fast. Normal fasting (pre-meal) blood glucose levels in non-diabetic individuals are around 70 to 99 mg/dL, and glucose levels two hours post-meal should be less than 140 mg/dL. If your levels remain higher than 140 mg/dL, you may want to have your doctor check you for insulin resistance. Robb Wolf's book *Wired to Eat* is an excellent resource for this.

SHOULD INSULIN SENSITIVITY DETERMINE YOUR DIET?

Possibly! Insulin sensitivity can account for one's ability to take in and utilize carbohydrates. A quick way to measure insulin sensitivity is a glucose tolerance test.

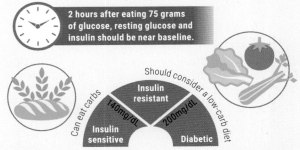

2 hours after eating 75 grams of glucose, resting glucose and insulin should be near baseline.

Can eat carbs — 140mg/dL — Insulin sensitive — Insulin resistant — 200mg/dL — Should consider a low-carb diet — Diabetic

If it doesn't, you likely won't tolerate carbs well and might need to use a low-carb, ketogenic diet to lower insulin and improve sensitivity.

Figure 5.1.7. *A glucose tolerance test carried out for a couple hours is a simple way to generalize a person's insulin sensitivity level.*

Can Weight Loss Be Sustained on a Ketogenic Diet?

Because of its satiating effects and the resulting decrease in hunger, the ketogenic diet can be easier to incorporate into a more permanent lifestyle change than a low-fat diet, making it a unique tool for long-term weight loss.

In a six-month study, researchers counseled subjects on what to consume while on the ketogenic diet. After six months, they encouraged the subjects to sustain the diet on their own without further guidance. The researchers then followed up three years later to see whether the subjects were able to maintain their weight loss. The average weight at the start of the study was 221 pounds. At the end of the six-month period, the average had dropped to 196 pounds—a loss of 25 pounds. Three years later, the subjects had gained, on average, about 9 pounds—so they'd maintained 16 pounds of the initial weight loss (Nielsen et al., 2008). However, of the sixteen patients, five had either remained at the same weight they'd reached at the end of the study or had lost *even more* weight, and all but one had a lower weight than at the start of the study.

If you still don't think that a ketogenic diet is sustainable, skip ahead to Chapter 8, which offers more than seventy-five keto-friendly recipes. Believe us, there is plenty to eat on this diet!

> "I'm not telling you it's going to be easy—I'm telling you it's going to be worth it."
> —Art Williams

We don't want to underplay the challenges that some people face when attempting to implement a ketogenic diet. There are often trials and hurdles to overcome. Let's face it: every day we are bombarded with temptations from sugar-filled foods and fast-food restaurants on every corner. Our goal is to show you that there are alternatives and that this style of eating is sustainable in the long run. Once you are educated on the diet itself, you will look at foods and nutrition labels much differently.

Cyclic Ketogenic Dieting: Can You Have Your Cake and Eat It, Too?

Cyclic ketogenic dieting consists of alternating periods of ketogenic dieting with periods of eating a low-fat, high-carbohydrate diet. Usually, this means eating ketogenic five days a week and "carbing up" on weekends. The general premise is that cyclic dieting allows people to reap the fat-loss benefits of the ketogenic diet while still being allowed to enjoy carbs on weekends. Cyclic dieting with various protocols has been popular for decades (McDonald, 1998).

Our lab examined the impact of a calorie deficit (eating fewer calories than previously) combined with resistance training and high-intensity endurance exercise on fat and muscle tissue (Lowery et al., in prep). Subjects either followed a ketogenic diet seven days a week or ate ketogenic five days a week and increased carbs on weekends. Calories and protein were the same in both groups, and both were put on a calorie deficit. We found that while both groups lost the same amount of weight over several weeks, the majority of mass lost in the ketogenic group was fat, while the cyclic group lost primarily muscle. Why was this the case? Being that both groups were in a calorie deficit, the ketogenic diet (likely due to the elevation in ketones) was able to spare lean body mass, while the individuals who carbed up on weekends had low ketone levels all week. In fact, individuals in the cyclic group did not achieve ketosis until Thursday after carbing up on the weekend, while the traditional group sustained ketosis throughout the week.

More recently, we have found that increased ketones are associated with proportional increases in muscle protein synthesis (unpublished). Therefore, ketones may have a unique benefit, and because the individuals who carbed up on weekends had low levels of ketones, this increase in muscle protein synthesis (and the protein-sparing effect of ketones) likely didn't occur. Another study found that subjects who switched from a ketogenic to a low-fat diet regained both weight and fat mass (Volek et al., 2004). Therefore, a cyclic ketogenic diet, which does not allow for fat adaptation, may be disadvantageous for fat loss.

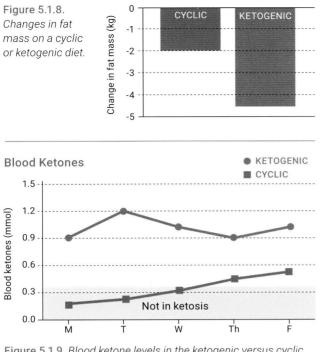

Figure 5.1.8. *Changes in fat mass on a cyclic or ketogenic diet.*

Figure 5.1.9. *Blood ketone levels in the ketogenic versus cyclic groups.*

No studies have examined the use of less-severe carb-ups or whether carb-ups can be used once individuals have been fat-adapted for a long time. For example, we don't know the implications for someone who carbs up for just one meal or even just one day rather than two straight days, as they did in our study. In addition, we feel that the longer a person is fat-adapted, the easier it is to get back into ketosis. Thus individuals who have been on a ketogenic diet for a longer period and are truly fat-adapted might be able to get away with a higher-carbohydrate meal or day occasionally. More studies and more data are needed to truly determine whether carbohydrates can be utilized as a strategic tool and whether "cheat days" can be mitigated by exercise.

Recently, Paoli et al. (2013) proposed a less-frequent cyclic approach to fat loss. These researchers had subjects follow a ketogenic diet (less than 10 percent carbohydrate) for twenty days and then transition to twenty days of a high-protein, fairly low-carbohydrate diet (30 percent fat, 20 to 25 percent carbohydrate), in which carbs were derived from salads, with the remainder of calories derived from fat. Then, for six months, subjects ate a Mediterranean diet rich in olive oil and other monounsaturated fats, wine, milk, and higher in fiber. Then they repeated the experiment: twenty more days on a ketogenic diet, high protein

and low carbs for twenty days, and six months on a Mediterranean diet. These individuals continuously lost body fat on the ketogenic and low-carb diets and were able to maintain that fat loss on a Mediterranean diet. Also of interest is that adherence to this protocol was extremely high, suggesting that slowly switching among ketogenic, low-carb/high-protein, and balanced high-fiber/moderate-carbohydrate diets may lead to long-term success for fat loss. However, it is unclear whether this approach would optimize health and longevity as much as a consistent ketogenic diet does. (See page 170 for more on longevity on the ketogenic diet.)

KETO CONCEPT

Protein-Sparing Modified Fasts

A protein-sparing modified fast involves consuming a reduced number of calories (typically fewer than 1,000 calories per day) but incorporating enough protein to maintain muscle mass. This approach can lead to a slight degree of ketosis (since you are significantly restricting calories and not consuming carbs, your body could begin producing some ketones), but it is not the same as following a ketogenic diet.

One study put obese adolescents on a protein-sparing fast (25 percent fat, 25 percent carbohydrate, 50 percent protein) for eight weeks. Over that period, the subjects lost an average of 15 kilograms (33 pounds), predominately from fat mass (Willi et al., 1998). Thus this type of modified fast may be another option to incorporate every once in a while in place of a carb-up. (See page 74 for more on carb-ups.)

Exogenous Ketones for Weight Loss

One question we consistently get is whether supplementing with exogenous ketones will lead to fat loss. Ketones certainly are not a magic weight-loss supplement, and they are unlikely to directly cause fat loss—they are an energy source. However, ketones may have indirect effects that can induce fat loss through a multitude of mechanisms, such as:

- Increasing brown adipose tissue, which is the kind of fat we want on our bodies

- Improving insulin sensitivity (discussed on page 77), which allows us to use glucose more efficiently rather than just store it

- Suppressing appetite, which leads to a decrease in overall calorie consumption

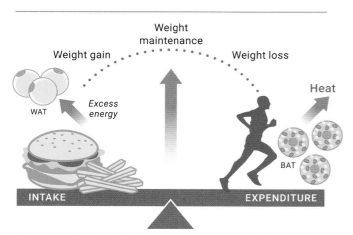

Figure 5.1.10. *Several factors play into the "calories in, calories out" equation. It is much more complex than we traditionally think.*

Increasing Brown Adipose Tissue

We have distinct types of fat, or adipose tissue, in our bodies. When most people think of fat tissue, they are thinking of white adipose tissue (WAT): that's what tends to be stored around the waist, hips, and butt. However, we also have brown adipose tissue (BAT). BAT's function is to generate body heat, especially in newborn babies. BAT cells are high in unique proteins called uncoupling proteins, specifically UCP1, which make it more difficult for our bodies to produce ATP (cellular energy). Because our bodies have to work extra-hard to produce energy in the presence of UCP1, we end up burning more calories in order to generate heat in BAT cells (Seale and Lazar, 2009). One way to think of this is that consuming food increases the amount of fuel in our bodies. This fuel can be either stored or burned to produce energy, which generates heat. BAT cells do not store or produce energy, but rather generate heat directly by utilizing lipids in the body to fuel the fire. So increasing the amount of BAT cells is ideal for weight loss because it means that we burn more calories.

Our bodies are smart biological systems that respond to the stimuli we present them with. Overeating tends to increase BAT levels to prevent us from storing too much fat, while caloric restriction tends to decrease BAT levels to ensure that we have enough fat stored for regular bodily functions (Rothwell and Stock, 1979). However, overeating also causes a host of health problems, and even with a slight increase in BAT, the adverse effects of overeating likely far outweigh any benefits. But if BAT could be increased without overeating, there is a chance that it could have a beneficial effect on weight loss and overall health.

Dr. Veech and his lab performed one of the first studies examining the effects of exogenous ketones on BAT. His lab divided mice into two groups. Both groups were fed the same amounts of fat, protein, and total calories, but one group was also administered a ketone ester; the other group was provided carbohydrates with the same number of calories as the ketone ester. The researchers found that in the ketone ester group, the number of mitochondria increased and the amount of UCP1 in BAT and mitochondria-promoting proteins had doubled (Srivastava et al., 2012). In addition, the ketone ester group burned 14 percent more calories at rest and had improved insulin sensitivity, indicating that ketone supplementation may be beneficial for weight loss.

Recently, we teamed up with researchers at Auburn University to investigate supplementation with ketone salts. Exercising animals were fed the same number of calories on either a low-carbohydrate ketogenic diet or a Western diet; half of each dietary group was provided ketone salt supplements. At the end of six weeks, the animals who had received

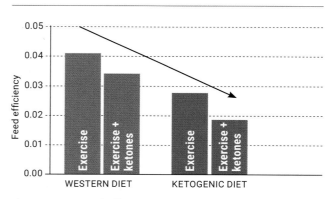

Figure 5.1.11. *Feed efficiency was lower in animals supplementing with ketone salts, both on a Western diet and a ketogenic diet.*

Source: Roberts et al., 2017 (in review).

ketone salts weighed less than those who had not, whether they had been fed a ketogenic diet or a Western diet. In addition, in the ketogenic diet group that received ketone supplements, BAT was elevated by 41 percent compared to the group on the ketogenic diet alone. Feed efficiency—the amount of weight gained per calorie consumed—was reduced in both groups receiving ketone salts. In other words, ketone salt supplementation increased BAT significantly and made the animals' bodies less efficient at storing calories. Imagine that: being able to eat the same number of calories and weigh less. You may find yourself asking, "But I thought losing weight was all about cutting calories?" While it's often said that to lose weight we have to consume fewer calories than we use, it just isn't that cut-and-dried. By way of things like BAT, our bodies can help us burn more calories without having to "eat less."

Improving Insulin Sensitivity

Insulin sensitivity can be defined as the amount of insulin the pancreas needs to produce in order to deposit a certain amount of glucose. For example, someone who is insulin sensitive might need to secrete only a small amount of insulin to deposit a certain amount of glucose, while someone who is insulin resistant would need to secrete a lot of insulin to deposit the same amount of glucose.

One of the first studies to examine ketone infusion in dogs found that ketones resulted in a significant improvement in glucose tolerance (Felts et al., 1964). Years later, Dr. Veech's group found that supplementing the diets of mice with ketone esters improved insulin sensitivity by 73 percent, despite ketones being elevated to 4 to 7 mmol/L (Srivastava et al., 2012). Other studies have shown similar results, including one in which researchers infused BHB into human subjects and found that it led to a 40 percent increase in insulin sensitivity by raising ketones to 3.5 mmol/L (Amiel et al., 1991). More recently, Dr. D'Agostino's lab investigated various ketone supplements (ketone mineral salts alone and in combination with MCT oil and even ketone esters) on blood glucose levels in rats. They found that supplementing with ketone salts alone, ketone salts in combination with MCT oil, and ketone salts in combination with ketone esters all significantly lowered blood glucose for up to twelve hours after ingestion. This could indicate an improvement in insulin sensitivity in the animals. Lastly, we have done numerous pilot experiments in our lab confirming the findings that ketones seem to decrease blood glucose consistently in a wide range of populations. Therefore, improving insulin sensitivity and decreasing blood glucose has big implications for individuals with impaired glucose metabolism (people with diabetes, obesity, metabolic syndrome, etc.).

Suppressing Appetite

Eat less and move more: that's the advice that we have been hearing for years. On paper it sounds great, but in reality the issue is much more complex. There are several factors at play in weight gain and loss, such as genetics, metabolism, hunger and satiety signals, gut microbiome, physical activity, and of course food consumption. Once we were at an event with hundreds of people selling fitness equipment, and the topic of obesity came up. One person said, "The solution is easy. Put down the candy bar and pick up some weights!" His statement was incredibly rude, of course, but we also found it quite interesting how ignorant it was. It made us think of this quote:

> "Telling an obese person to eat less and move more is like telling a depressed person to quit being sad."

The ability to control and regulate hunger and satiety signals is of extreme importance when it comes to weight loss, so much so that several food companies attempt to override those signals by using various sweeteners, colors, and textures to ensure that "you can't eat just one." Companies literally create food items with the goal of making us become addicted to them. Ever wonder why the combination of sugar and salt makes it so tough to have only "one serving" of chips or pretzels?

Appetite-suppressing drugs are becoming increasingly popular as a strategy to help individuals avoid overeating throughout the day. These drugs aim to shut down hunger cravings by increasing certain neurotransmitters in the brain; without feelings of hunger, people can eat less. We know from studies that people on a ketogenic diet often feel more satiated or full, which is largely attributed to the diet's high fat content (Paoli et al., 2015). But is it possible that ketones themselves affect appetite and hunger?

One study looked at direct infusion of BHB and found that it reduced food intake (and ultimately body weight) in rats eating a low-fat or low-carbohydrate diet (Arase et al., 1988). Years later, an interesting study looked at injections of ketones in pygmy goats. The injections decreased food intake per meal, characterized by a significant decrease in the number of times the goats ate per day (Rossi et al., 2000). These results seem to indicate that the appetite suppression that occurs on a ketogenic diet may be related to elevated levels of BHB.

Both Dr. Veech's and Dr. Roberts's labs saw similar results in their experimental trials with ketone esters and ketone salts. Dr. Veech's lab found that the greater the level of ketones, the more food consumption was reduced. The levels of leptin, the hormone that makes us feel full, in the ketone ester group were more than twice those of the control group not consuming ketone esters. Also, the increased leptin levels in the ketone ester group were associated with increased activity of brown adipose tissue—possibly meaning more heat-producing activity of BAT (Srivastava et al., 2012). Similarly, Dr. Roberts's lab noted that animals given ketone salts tended to eat less, and even though the researchers made sure the control group ate the same number of calories, the ketone salt subjects weighed less (Kephart et al., 2016).

The exact mechanisms by which ketones can suppress appetite are still to be determined. However, researchers (Paoli et al., 2015) have proposed some possibilities:

- By maintaining normal glucose meal response, which would reduce blood glucose spikes and crashes that lead to increased hunger.

- By maintaining post-meal cholecystokinin secretion, which is responsible for both stimulating the digestion of fat and protein and increasing satiety. (Weight loss typically leads to a reduction in post-meal cholecystokinin secretion.)

- By decreasing circulating ghrelin, the hunger hormone.

Lastly, it is possible that ketone supplementation directly affects brain signals and processes that help regulate hunger and satiety controls. For instance, feeding animals a ketone ester and allowing them to eat freely (buffet style) resulted in a significant decrease in voluntary food intake (Kashiwaya et al., 2010). This could be attributed to an increase in brain malonyl-CoA, a component of a fuel-sensing and signaling mechanism that responds to changes in glucose availability and energy expenditure. However, more research is needed to investigate how ketones might affect appetite and hunger.

CHAPTER SUMMARY

Both ketogenic diets and ketones themselves appear to have a strong effect on appetite, which, in combination with their other metabolic effects, such as increased BAT, feed efficiency, and improved insulin sensitivity, could make them helpful for weight loss. Individuals who have been on a ketogenic diet for a long period often get to a point where they can eat to satiety without much concern for gaining weight since they know they aren't likely to overeat. When it comes to increasing carbohydrates, as on a cyclic ketogenic diet, we need more data to determine the best approach for maintaining muscle mass while losing fat. It will likely vary from person to person—some individuals can get away with a small carbohydrate meal, while others cannot. If you want to experiment with these approaches, make sure that you are completely fat-adapted first (don't start increasing carbs during your first couple of weeks on the diet), incorporate the extra carbs on an exercise/training day, and minimize the glucose load as much as possible (don't hit a buffet and wipe out all the desserts!). If your goal is specifically to lose body fat while maintaining muscle mass, remember that it is important to consume at least 0.8 gram of protein per pound of body weight. Finally, we do not recommend carbing up frequently, but if you plan to, it may be more beneficial to slowly transition from a low-carbohydrate ketogenic diet to a low- to moderate-carbohydrate, higher-protein diet. Whatever you do, don't go straight from a ketogenic diet to a low-fat, high-carbohydrate diet for an extended period.

References

Amiel, S. A., et al. "Ketone infusion lowers hormonal responses to hypoglycaemia: evidence for acute cerebral utilization of a non-glucose fuel." *Clinical Science* 81, no. 18 (1991): 189–94.

Arase, K., J. S. Fisler, N. S. Shargill, D. A. York, and G. A. Bray. "Intracerebroventricular infusions of 3-OHB and insulin in a rat model of dietary obesity." *American Journal of Physiology-Regulatory, Integrative and Comparative Physiology* 255, no. 6 (1988): R974–81.

Ard, J. D., G. Miller, and S. Kahan. "Nutrition Interventions for Obesity." *Medical Clinics of North America* 100, no. 6 (2016): 1341–56.

Boden, G., K. Sargrad, C. Homko, M. Mozzoli, and T. P. Stein. "Effect of a low-carbohydrate diet on appetite, blood glucose levels, and insulin resistance in obese patients with type 2 diabetes." *Annals of Internal Medicine* 142, no. 6 (2005): 403–11.

Brehm, B. J., R. J. Seeley, S. R. Daniels, and D. A. D'Alessio. "A randomized trial comparing a very low carbohydrate diet and a calorie-restricted low fat diet on body weight and cardiovascular risk factors in healthy women." *Journal of Clinical Endocrinology & Metabolism* 88, no. 4 (2003): 1617–23.

Cecil, J. E., R. Tavendale, P. Watt, M. M. Hetherington, and C. N. Palmer. "An obesity-associated FTO gene variant and increased energy intake in children." *New England Journal of Medicine* 359, no. 24 (2008): 2558–66.

Corpeleijn, E., W. H. Saris, and E. E. Blaak. "Metabolic flexibility in the development of insulin resistance and type 2 diabetes: effects of lifestyle." *Obesity Reviews* 10, no. 2 (2009): 178–93.

Doucet, E., P. Imbeault, S. St-Pierre, N. Almeras, P. Mauriege, D. Richard, and A. Tremblay. "Appetite after weight loss by energy restriction and a low-fat diet-exercise follow-up." *International Journal of Obesity* 24, no. 7 (2000): 906–14.

Evans, E., A. L. Stock, and J. Yudkin. "The absence of undesirable changes during consumption of the low carbohydrate diet." *Annals of Nutrition and Metabolism* 17, no. 6 (1974): 360–7.

Fothergill, E., J. Guo, L. Howard, J. C. Kerns, N. D. Knuth, R. Brychta, ... and K. D. Hall. "Persistent metabolic adaptation 6 years after 'The Biggest Loser' competition." *Obesity* 24, no. 8 (2016): 1612–9.

Gibson, A. A., R. V. Seimon, C. M. Y. Lee, J. Ayre, J. Franklin, T. P. Markovic, ... and A. Sainsbury. "Do ketogenic diets really suppress appetite? A systematic review and meta-analysis." *Obesity Reviews* 16, no. 1 (2015): 64–76.

Hall, K. D., K. Y. Chen, J. Guo, Y. Y. Lam, R. L. Leibel, L. E. Mayer, ... and E. Ravussin. "Energy expenditure and body composition changes after an isocaloric ketogenic diet in overweight and obese men." *American Journal of Clinical Nutrition* 104, no. 2 (2016): 324–33.

Hession, M., C. Rolland, U. Kulkarni, A. Wise, and J. Broom. "Systematic review of randomized controlled trials of low-carbohydrate vs. low-fat/low-calorie diets in the management of obesity and its comorbidities." *Obesity Reviews* 10, no. 1 (2009): 36–50.

Holland, A. M., W. C. Kephart, P. W. Mumford, C. B. Mobley, R. P. Lowery, J. J. Shake, ... and K. W. Huggins. "Effects of a ketogenic diet on adipose tissue, liver and serum biomarkers in sedentary rats and rats that exercised via resisted voluntary wheel running." *American Journal of Physiology-Regulatory, Integrative and Comparative Physiology* 311, no. 2 (2016): R337–51.

Hyatt, H. W., W. C. Kephart, A. M. Holland, P. W. Mumford, C. B. Mobley, R. P. Lowery, ... and A. N. Kavazis. "A ketogenic diet in rodents elicits improved mitochondrial adaptations in response to resistance exercise training compared to an isocaloric western diet." *Frontiers in Physiology* 7 (2016): 533.

Imes, C. C., and L. E. Burke. "The obesity epidemic: the USA as a cautionary tale for the rest of the world." *Current Epidemiology Reports* 1, no. 2 (2014): 82–8.

Johnston, Carol S., et al. "Ketogenic low-carbohydrate diets have no metabolic advantage over nonketogenic low-carbohydrate diets." *American Journal of Clinical Nutrition* 83, no. 5 (2006): 1055–61.

Johnstone, A. M., G. W. Horgan, S. D. Murison, D. M. Bremner, and G. E. Lobley. "Effects of a high-protein ketogenic diet on hunger, appetite, and weight loss in obese men feeding ad libitum." *American Journal of Clinical Nutrition* 87, no. 1 (2008): 44–55.

Kashiwaya, Y., R. Pawlosky, W. Markis, M. T. King, C. Bergman, S. Srivastava, ... and R. L. Veech. "A ketone ester diet increases brain malonyl-CoA and uncoupling proteins 4 and 5 while decreasing food intake in the normal Wistar rat." *Journal of Biological Chemistry* 285, no. 34 (2010): 25950–6.

Kasper, H., H. Thiel, and M. Ehl. "Response of body weight to a low carbohydrate, high fat diet in normal and obese subjects." *American Journal of Clinical Nutrition* 26, no. 2 (1973): 197–204.

Kekwick, A., and G. L. S. Pawan. "Calorie intake in relation to body-weight changes in the obese." *The Lancet* 268, no. 6935 (1956): 155–61.

Kennedy, A. R., et al. "A high-fat, ketogenic diet induces a unique metabolic state in mice." *American Journal of Physiology-Endocrinology and Metabolism* 292, no. 6 (2007): E1724–39.

Kephart, W., M. Holland, P. Mumford, B. Mobley, R. Lowery, M. Roberts, and J. Wilson. "The effects of intermittent ketogenic dieting as well as ketone salt supplementation on body composition and circulating health biomarkers in exercising rodents." *FASEB Journal* 30, suppl 1 (2016): lb383.

Krotkiewski, M. "Value of VLCD supplementation with medium chain triglycerides." *International Journal of Obesity Related Metabolic Disorders* 25, no. 9 (2001): 1393–400.

Liu, Y., W. Yang, and Y. Chiang. "How to reduce 500 kcal intake per day–My Plate." *Obesity Reviews* 15, no. 7 (2014): e10.

Llewellyn, C. H., M. Trzaskowski, C. H. van Jaarsveld, R. Plomin, and J. Wardle. "Satiety mechanisms in genetic risk of obesity." *JAMA Pediatrics* 168, no. 4 (2014): 338–44.

MacLean, P. S., A. Bergouignan, M. A. Cornier, and M. R. Jackman. "Biology's response to dieting: the impetus for weight regain." *American Journal of Physiology-Regulatory, Integrative and Comparative Physiology* 301, no. 3 (2011): R581–600.

Malik, V. S., W. C. Willett, and F. B. Hu. "Global obesity: trends, risk factors and policy implications." *Nature Reviews Endocrinology* 9, no. 1 (2013): 13–27.

Martin, C. K., D. E. Bellanger, K. K. Rau, S. Coulon, and F. L. Greenway. "Safety of the Ullorex® oral intragastric balloon for the treatment of obesity." *Journal of Diabetes Science and Technology* 1, no. 4 (2007): 574–81.

Martin, C. K., D. Rosenbaum, H. Han, P. J. Geiselman, H. R. Wyatt, J. O. Hill, ... and S. Klein. "Change in food cravings, food preferences, and appetite during a low-carbohydrate and low-fat diet." *Obesity* 19, no. 10 (2011): 1963–70.

McClain, A. D., J. J. Otten, E. B. Hekler, and C. D. Gardner. "Adherence to a low-fat vs. low-carbohydrate diet differs by insulin resistance status." *Diabetes, Obesity, and Metabolism* 15, no. 1 (2013): 87–90.

McClernon, F. J., W. S. Yancy, J. A. Eberstein, R. C. Atkins, and E. C. Westman. "The effects of a low-carbohydrate ketogenic diet and a low-fat diet on mood, hunger, and other self-reported symptoms." *Obesity* 15, no. 1 (2007): 182–7.

McDonald, L. *The Ketogenic Diet: A Complete Guide for the Dieter and Practitioner.* Austin, Texas: Morris Publishing, 1998.

Nickols-Richardson, S. M., M. D. Coleman, J. J. Volpe, and K. W. Hosig. "Perceived hunger is lower and weight loss is greater in overweight premenopausal women consuming a low-carbohydrate/high-protein vs high-carbohydrate/low-fat diet." *Journal of the American Dietetic Association* 105, no. 9 (2005): 1433–7.

Nielsen, J. V., and E. A. Joensson. "Low-carbohydrate diet in type 2 diabetes: stable improvement of bodyweight and glycemic control during 44 months follow-up." *Nutrition & Metabolism* (London) 5 (2008): 14.

Obici, S., Z. Feng, K. Morgan, D. Stein, G. Karkanias, and L. Rossetti. "Central administration of oleic acid inhibits glucose production and food intake." *Diabetes* 51, no. 2 (2002): 271–5.

Paoli, A., G. Bosco, E. M. Camporesi, and D. Mangar. "Ketosis, ketogenic diet and food intake control: a complex relationship." *Frontiers in Psychology* 6 (2015): 27.

Paoli, A., et al. "Long term successful weight loss with a combination biphasic ketogenic Mediterranean diet and Mediterranean diet maintenance protocol." *Nutrients* 5, no. 12 (2013): 5205–17.

Phinney, S. D., B. R. Bistrian, W. J. Evans, E. Gervino, and G. L. Blackburn. "The human metabolic response to chronic ketosis without caloric restriction: preservation of submaximal exercise capability with reduced carbohydrate oxidation." *Metabolism* 32, no. 8 (1983): 769–76.

Phinney, S. D. "Ketogenic diets and physical performance." *Nutrition & Metabolism* 1, no. 1 (2004): 2.

Roberts, M. D., A. M. Holland, W. C. Kephart, C. B. Mobley, P. W. Mumford, R. P. Lowery, ... and R. K. Patel. "A putative low-carbohydrate ketogenic diet elicits mild nutritional ketosis but does not impair the acute or chronic hypertrophic responses to resistance exercise in rodents." *Journal of Applied Physiology* 120, no. 10 (2016): 1173–85.

Rosen J. C., J. Gross, D. Loew, and E. A. Sims. "Mood and appetite during minimal-carbohydrate and carbohydrate-supplemented hypocaloric diets." *American Journal of Clinical Nutrition* 42, no. 3 (1985): 371–9.

Rossi, R., S. D. Örig, E. Del Prete, and E. Scharrer. "Suppression of feed intake after parenteral administration of d-ββ-hydroxybutyrate in pygmy goats." *Journal of Veterinary Medicine* Series A, 47, no. 1 (2000): 9–16.

Seale, P., and M. A. Lazar. "Brown fat in humans: turning up the heat on obesity." *Diabetes* 58, no. 7 (2009): 1482–4.

Sharp, M. H., R. P. Lowery, K. A. Shields, D. W. Hayes, J. R. Lane, J. T. Rauch, J. M. Partl, C. A. Hollmer, J. R. Minevich, J. Gray, E. O. DeSouza, and J. M. Wilson. "The effects of weekly carbohydrate reintroduction vs strict very low carbohydrate dieting on body composition." National Strength and Conditioning Association Conference (2015).

Short, K. R., K. S. Nair, and C. S. Stump. "Impaired mitochondrial activity and insulin-resistant offspring of patients with type 2 diabetes." *New England Journal of Medicine* 350, no. 23 (2004): 2419–21.

Sondike, S. B., N. Copperman, and M. S. Jacobson. "Effects of a low-carbohydrate diet on weight loss and cardiovascular risk factor in overweight adolescents." *Journal of Pediatrics* 142, no. 3 (2003): 253–8.

Speliotes, E. K., C. J. Willer, S. I. Berndt, et al; MAGIC; Procardis Consortium. "Association analyses of 249,796 individuals reveal 18 new loci associated with body mass index." *Nature Genetics* 42, no. 11 (2010): 937–48.

Srivastava, S., Y. Kashiwaya, M. T. King, U. Baxa, J. Tam, G. Niu, ... and R. L. Veech. "Mitochondrial biogenesis and increased uncoupling protein 1 in brown adipose tissue of mice fed a ketone ester diet." *FASEB Journal* 26, no. 6 (2012): 2351–62.

Sumithran, P., and J. Proietto. "The defence of body weight: a physiological basis for weight regain after weight loss." *Clinical Science* 124, no. 4 (2013): 231–41.

Sumithran, P., L. A. Prendergast, E. Delbridge, K. Purcell, A. Shulkes, A. Kriketos, et al. "Ketosis and appetite-mediating nutrients and hormones after weight loss." *European Journal of Clinical Nutrition* 67(7) (2013): 759–64.

Sumithran, P., L. A. Prendergast, E. Delbridge, K. Purcell, A. Shulkes, A. Kriketos, and J. Proietto. "Long-term persistence of hormonal adaptations to weight loss." *New England Journal of Medicine* 365 (2011): 1597–604.

Swinburn, B. A., et al. "The global obesity pandemic: shaped by global drivers and local environments." *The Lancet* 378, no. 9793 (2011): 804–14.

Vander Wal, J. S., J. M. Marth, P. Khosla, K. C. Jen, and N. V. Dhurandhar. "Short-term effect of eggs on satiety in overweight and obese subjects." *Journal of the American College of Nutrition* 24, no. 6 (2004): 510–5.

Veech, R. L. "Ketone esters increase brown fat in mice and overcome insulin resistance in other tissues in the rat." *Annals of the New York Academy of Sciences* 1302, no. 1 (2013): 42–8.

Veldhorst, M. A., K. R. Westerterp, and M. S. Westerterp-Plantenga. "Gluconeogenesis and protein-induced satiety." *British Journal of Nutrition* 107, no. 04 (2012): 595–600.

Volek, J. S., D. J. Freidenreich, C. Saenz, L. J. Kunces, B. C. Creighton, J. M. Bartley, ... and E. C. Lee. "Metabolic characteristics of keto-adapted ultra-endurance runners." *Metabolism* 65, no. 3 (2016): 100–10.

Volek, J. S., M. J. Sharman, D. M. Love, N. G. Avery, T. P. Scheett, and W. J. Kraemer. "Body composition and hormonal responses to a carbohydrate-restricted diet." *Metabolism* 51, no. 7 (2002): 864–70.

Volek, J., M. J. Sharman, A. Gomez, D. A. Judelson, M. R. Rubin, G. Watson, ... and W. J. Kraemer. "Comparison of energy-restricted very low-carbohydrate and low-fat diets on weight loss and body composition in overweight men and women." *Nutrition & Metabolism* (London) 1, no. 1 (2004): 13.

Willi, S. M., M. J. Oexmann, N. M. Wright, N. A. Collop, and L. L. Key. "The effects of a high-protein, low-fat, ketogenic diet on adolescents with morbid obesity: body composition, blood chemistries, and sleep abnormalities." *Pediatrics* 101, no. 1 (1998): 61–67.

Wilson J., R. Lowery, M. Roberts, M. Sharp, J. Joy, K. Shields, E. De Souza, J. Rauch, J. Partl, J. Volek, and D. D'Agostino. "The effects of ketogenic dieting on body composition, strength, power, and hormonal profiles in resistance training males." Accepted and in press at the *Journal of Strength and Conditioning Research*, 2016.

Wood, R. J., J. S. Volek, S. R. Davis, C. Dell'Ova, and M. L. Fernandez. "Effects of a carbohydrate-restricted diet on emerging plasma markers for cardiovascular disease." *Nutrition & Metabolism* 3, no. 1 (2006): 19.

Yancy Jr., W. S., M. K. Olsen, J. R. Guyton, R. P. Bakst, and E. C. Westman. "A low-carbohydrate, ketogenic diet versus a low-fat diet to treat obesity and hyperlipidemia: a randomized, controlled trial." *Annals of Internal Medicine* 140, no. 10 (2004): 769–77.

Young, C. M., S. S. Scanlan, H. S. Im, and L. Lutwak. "Effect on body composition and other parameters in obese young men of carbohydrate level of reduction diet." *American Journal of Clinical Nutrition* 24, no. 3 (1971): 290–6.

Section 2:
Diabetes, Cholesterol, and Heart Health

Years ago, we walked into a meeting with a colleague. He was overweight, had just been diagnosed with type 2 diabetes, had high cholesterol, and truly wanted to make a change to help not only himself, but also his family. He ordered lunch for us but had to excuse himself to go inject himself with insulin just prior to the meal—a nuisance he was new to but already disliked tremendously. Upon returning, he sat down to what he perceived to be a healthy meal: apple juice, a granola bar, and a turkey wrap (whole grain, of course). He was blind to the fact that the meal in front of him was contributing to his need to make that earlier trip to take insulin.

When we took the lunch meat out of the wrap and asked for a side of ranch dressing, our colleague seemed perplexed. "But how can that be healthy?" he asked. The assumption that a high-fat diet is inevitably bad for our cholesterol is not grounded in science. By the end of our hour-long lunch meeting, he had decided to try out the ketogenic way of eating, even though it ran counter to his physician's advice.

Twelve weeks later, we met up again. Not only had our colleague lost a significant amount of weight, but he was no longer taking insulin, and his doctor had taken him off of statin medication since his cholesterol had significantly improved. This man had gotten his life back, and he couldn't believe that the small amount of education we had given him combined with some trial and error on his part had allowed him such freedom, both physically and emotionally. The experience played a big part in developing our passion for this area.

Throughout this chapter, we will expand on what diabetes and cholesterol are and explain how a ketogenic lifestyle could play a positive role in managing glucose, insulin, and cholesterol levels.

> "The secret of change is to focus all of your energy, not on fighting the old, but on building the new."
> —Socrates

Sugar is one of the world's most popular ingredients, and it is no surprise how abundant it is in the American diet. This ingredient, once exclusive to desserts, has made its way into nearly all of our prepackaged food items. Sugar has been demonstrated to have a euphoric effect and produce behaviors and biological responses similar to drug addictions (Avena, 2009; see Figure 5.2.1); this has resulted in excessive consumption of sugar-laden foods, drinks, and candy. But chronic overconsumption of sugar may lead to a slew of metabolic issues, such as dyslipidemia (an abnormal amount of circulating blood lipids) or hyperinsulinemia (a high amount of insulin circulating in the blood). These metabolic issues are the driving forces behind many chronic diseases, particularly type 2 diabetes. In order to halt this alarming and growing pandemic, our most effective treatment is to educate people about the detrimental health consequences of excessive sugar consumption.

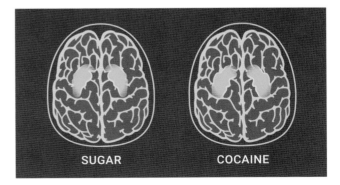

Figure 5.2.1. *The same areas of the brain that light up when certain drugs are taken also light up when sugar is eaten.*

Diabetes

Diabetes is a metabolic disorder that occurs due to a dysfunction with the hormone insulin. There are two main types of diabetes, types 1 and 2, along with another, less-discussed type called gestational diabetes. According to the International Diabetes Federation, 382 million adults are diabetic, and that number is expected to rise to 592 million by 2035. It's also estimated that as many as 183 million people are unaware they have diabetes (Ogurtsova et al., 2017). According to the Centers for Disease Control and Prevention (CDC), types 1 and 2 diabetes affect 9.3 percent of the U.S. population, or one out of every eleven people; however, 27.8 percent of those individuals are estimated to be living with *undiagnosed* diabetes. Obesity is the primary risk factor for type 2 diabetes (Westman et al., 2016), and the risk of developing type 2 diabetes increases as body mass index (BMI) increases (Clark et al., 2004). In addition to its many health consequences, diabetes can be accompanied by hypertension, dyslipidemia, glaucoma, and insulin resistance.

What Is Insulin?

Insulin is a hormone that is produced and secreted by the beta cells of the pancreas following the consumption of carbohydrates. The process goes like this: After we consume carbohydrates, they are broken down into glucose, which raises the amount of glucose circulating throughout the bloodstream. To restore the now-elevated blood glucose to normal levels, the pancreas secretes insulin, which moves glucose from the bloodstream to inside cells. Insulin does so by triggering membrane proteins (similar to tunnels) to the cell's surface (GLUT) in order to allow glucose to travel into the cell. Insulin also suppresses fat-burning and regulates gluconeogenesis in the liver.

While dysfunctional insulin is the hallmark of all kinds of diabetes, each type has its own pathology.

Type 1 Diabetes

Type 1 diabetes is rare, affecting approximately 1 in every 5,000 people (Cooke et al., 2008). In this disease, the beta cells of the pancreas, which produce insulin, are destroyed by the body's immune system, resulting in insulin deficiency. The lack of insulin wreaks havoc on glucose metabolism: cells are unable to take up glucose, leading to "starvation in the face of plenty," since blood sugar is high but it can't get into cells. This can lead to dehydration, weight loss, tissue damage, and diabetic ketoacidosis, which is not the type of ketosis we want (for more details, see page 17.)

Type 1 diabetes is generally treated with insulin injections, which provide the insulin that the body can't make on its own. As such, this type of diabetes is often referred to as *insulin-dependent diabetes*, since individuals with type 1 diabetes rely on external insulin to handle their condition. Rather than their own bodies being able to release insulin when they consume carbohydrates, these individuals need an external pump or pen to do it for them. This creates a need to balance blood glucose levels with insulin injections throughout the day.

Figure 5.2.2. *The process of insulin being released following carbohydrate consumption.*

Source: www.clinicians.co.nz/chromium

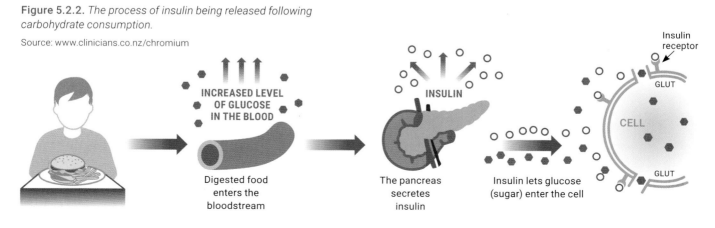

INCREASED LEVEL OF GLUCOSE IN THE BLOOD

Digested food enters the bloodstream

INSULIN

The pancreas secretes insulin

Insulin lets glucose (sugar) enter the cell

Insulin receptor

GLUT

CELL

GLUT

The Ketogenic Diet for Type 1 Diabetes

One of the biggest concerns regarding the use of the ketogenic diet for type 1 diabetes is diabetic ketoacidosis (DKA). When insulin is low and subsequent cell starvation (i.e., glucose not getting into the cells) occurs, the rate of lipolysis (the breakdown of fat) increases, which, in turn, may lead to rapid and uncontrolled ketone production and thus toxic ketoacidosis.

Because of the danger of DKA, it sounds ludicrous to recommend that type 1 diabetics intentionally pursue an increase in ketone production. It is plausible, however, that a low-carbohydrate ketogenic diet could reduce the amount of insulin a person with type 1 diabetes requires. We have heard many case reports of type 1 diabetics utilizing this approach under the supervision of their doctors, and as long as the diet is properly implemented and insulin load is closely monitored, this approach can be effective.

Dr. Richard Bernstein, a type 1 diabetic himself, opened a clinic specifically to use low-carbohydrate diets for people with type 1 diabetes. Today, several of our colleagues—including Dr. Jason Fung, Dr. Adam Nally, Dr. Eric Westman, and Dr. Andreas Eenfeldt—encourage a low-carb, high-fat approach for certain type 1 diabetics. Dr. Eenfeldt found that in a patient with type 1 diabetes, the application of a ketogenic diet led to a decreased dependence on insulin as well as improvements in gastrointestinal problems, headaches, leg pain, throat infections, and yeast infections. Despite these promising results, research on the topic is still in its infancy, and further investigation must be performed before the ketogenic diet as a treatment option for type 1 diabetes becomes widely accepted.

Individuals with type 1 diabetes should consult with their doctors before making any dietary changes. Reducing carbohydrates may require a reduction in glucose-lowering medications to prevent hypoglycemia. Also, it is crucial for these patients to be monitored for DKA.

Type 2 Diabetes

In contrast to type 1 diabetes, type 2 diabetes is an all-too-common disease: it affects approximately 170 million people worldwide (Wild et al., 2004). While both type 1 and type 2 stem from insulin dysfunction, individuals with type 2 diabetes are still able to secrete insulin from the pancreas, but its signaling ability is impaired: cells are unable to respond to insulin and therefore don't allow glucose to enter. This is known as insulin resistance, and it's a hallmark of type 2 diabetes. It's essentially the opposite of insulin sensitivity, in which insulin easily moves glucose into cells. Individuals with type 2 diabetes should aim to improve their insulin resistance.

Have you ever had a friend who somehow is able to eat all the cake, cookies, and brownies she wants while staying lean? It is likely because she is particularly insulin sensitive. Someone who is insulin sensitive might need only a small amount of insulin to move a certain amount of glucose into a cell, while someone who is insulin resistant would need a lot of insulin to move the same amount of glucose. That's why people who are insulin sensitive are more likely to stay lean even if they eat a lot of sweets: the carbs

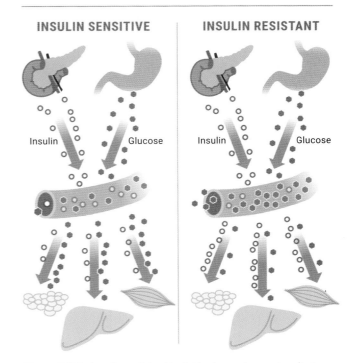

INSULIN SENSITIVE   **INSULIN RESISTANT**

Insulin   Glucose   Insulin   Glucose

Figure 5.2.3. *Insulin-resistant individuals need more insulin to dispose of glucose than insulin-sensitive people do.*

Source: www.mangomannutrition.com/fat-kills-insulin-producing-beta-cells/

they eat are more likely to be moved into cells to be used for fuel than they are in those who are insulin resistant, who have to release a large amount of insulin just to get some of that glucose into the cells. This can turn off the breakdown of fat, in which case the glucose is stored as body fat instead.

Because insulin-resistant cells do not respond efficiently to insulin's signal to take up excess glucose, the beta cells of the pancreas secrete more and more insulin to compensate for insulin resistance and manage blood glucose levels: if a little insulin doesn't work, maybe an abundant amount will allow glucose to enter the cells. Over time, this taxing biological response can lead to dysfunction of the pancreas's insulin-producing beta cells, exhausting their ability to produce and release appropriate levels of insulin to maintain healthy blood sugar levels. Glucose then accumulates in the bloodstream, which may lead to type 2 diabetes.

Remember when we talked about insulin resistance and related it to green sludge in the streets (see page 19)? Imagine that constant influx of sludge (glucose) pouring into the street (your bloodstream) and then pounding on the door of a house (a cell in the body) day in and day out. Yet rather than opening, the door stays shut until the sludge accumulates to the point where it *forces* its way in.

At its core, insulin resistance is also like an elderly man with a hearing impairment. Perhaps he blasted music through headphones every day throughout his youth. Over time, his hearing would have become progressively worse, and eventually, a message that once might have been whispered would have to be shouted so that he could hear it. Similarly, in a person with insulin resistance, cells need insulin to "shout" and send a big signal in order for them to open up and take in glucose.

HbA1c

To diagnose and monitor diabetes, blood tests look at a marker called glycated hemoglobin, or HbA1c. This form of hemoglobin develops when glucose molecules bind to hemoglobin, a protein within red blood cells. Because red blood cells live for three months, a person's HbA1c level gives an average of blood sugar levels over the previous three months.

The Problems with Insulin

For all types of diabetes, insulin injections are a treatment option. These injections are often paired with drugs that lower blood glucose. However, although the use of drugs has been the preferred form of treatment, we can't stress enough the importance of making healthy lifestyle changes, including exercise and diet. Even walking can positively affect insulin sensitivity.

Insulin is an important hormone that has many functions—and injections are completely necessary and life-saving for those with type 1 diabetes, who cannot make insulin on their own. However, insulin is often relied on too heavily for the treatment of type 2 diabetes, and the resulting hyperinsulinemia (excess circulating insulin relative to circulating glucose) and resistance to insulin's effects are plaguing our society with detrimental health outcomes. Although it has yet to be established whether a low-carbohydrate diet or drug-based therapies are more advantageous for type 2 diabetes (Westman et al., 2016), the physiological understanding of diabetes suggests that insulin treatment alone is just a bandage that does not address the root cause of the problem: resistance to insulin and intolerance of carbohydrates. Insulin treatment still allows individuals to consume sugar; they just have to inject themselves with insulin to allow cells to take up that sugar.

Imagine you have a bike that has a tire with a small cut in it, causing the tire to leak air. Rather than patch the tire, you carry an air pump with you all the time. Similar to pumping air into a leaking tire, insulin injections provide a temporary fix to a much larger problem, which is insulin resistance. Therefore, it is worth considering alternative therapies, including dietary modifications, as treatment for type 2 diabetes. In fact, prior to the discovery of insulin, non-drug modalities were the only available forms of treatment. A textbook from the late 1800s recommended that individuals with diabetes exclude sugary and starchy foods from their diet and stated, "There are few diseases which present the practitioner so clean an indication of what is to be done" (Morgan et al., 1877).

While genetics seem to play a role in the development of type 2 diabetes, genetics are too often used as a scapegoat; more often, poor dietary choices and physical inactivity are to blame. The addictive nature of sugar leads to frequent consumption of foods that are high in carbs, which leads to a continuous amplification of insulin output. Over time, this can make cells resistant to insulin's signals. Moreover, chronic overstimulation of insulin secretion gradually diminishes and eventually results in beta cell dysfunction, leading to a change in the way the body converts food to energy—a process that does not function optimally with a high dietary carbohydrate intake (Dey et al., 2011).

Education must be our first line of defense against diseases like type 2 diabetes that stem from lifestyle and dietary factors. Although glucose-lowering agents like metformin and insulin injections may be helpful in the short term, they treat the symptom (high blood sugar) rather than the root cause (insulin resistance). Once we realize that lifestyle and eating habits are the source of the problem, it becomes obvious that the most powerful and effective way to prevent and treat chronic metabolic diseases, including type 2 diabetes, is through dietary means.

Restricting Glucose in Type 2 Diabetes

Remember that insulin resistance and eventually type 2 diabetes develop in response to chronically elevated insulin, which is caused by chronic overconsumption of carbohydrates, lack of exercise, etc. Therefore, it's logical that restricting carbohydrates can provide therapeutic benefits (despite the fact that the standard care is to recommend a high-carb diet). Treating type 2 diabetes is essentially about controlling blood glucose levels, which in turn controls insulin levels. One important factor is to try to keep fasting blood glucose levels—first thing in the morning, before food or exercise—within a normal range (between 80 and 120 mg/dL). And what we eat has a profound effect on our blood glucose levels.

Glycemic index and glycemic load are two powerful measurements that classify how much a particular food raises blood glucose. While there are limitations to these measurements, low-glycemic diets—those that don't significantly raise blood sugar—have demonstrated improvements in normalizing blood sugar levels in diabetics (Brand-Miller et al., 2003; Westman et al., 2016). However, low-glycemic diets that are still high in carbohydrates aren't much better than high-glycemic diets (Westman et al., 2016). The most effective form of glycemic control is to couple a low-glycemic diet with carbohydrate restriction. Several studies have found that when a low-carbohydrate diet was implemented, glucose and insulin levels following a meal mimic the levels seen during fasting—in other words, they barely change (Nuttall et al., 2015). Low-carbohydrate studies have demonstrated improvements not only in fasting blood glucose levels but also in HbA1c levels (Heilbronn et al., 2002; Rizkalla et al., 2004; Gannon et al., 2004). In one study, people with type 2 diabetes followed a low-carbohydrate diet for sixteen weeks and saw their HbA1c decrease by 15 percent; as a result, seventeen of twenty-two subjects were able to reduce or even discontinue their diabetes medications (Yancy et al., 2003).

However, these studies didn't restrict carbohydrates enough for ketogenesis to occur. This prompts the question: would lowered blood glucose in the presence of ketosis have an even greater efficacy?

KETO CONCEPT

How Does Your Body Respond to Ice Cream?

One message we hope to get across with this book is that every person is different. For instance, studies have shown that some individuals see a huge glucose and insulin spike after eating ice cream, while others don't. If you truly want to take your awareness of your body to another level, measure your blood glucose after eating some of your favorite foods. You will be surprised at how much certain foods increase your blood glucose while others don't. Even on a ketogenic diet, knowing how your body responds to different foods can help you tailor your diet even more specifically to what works best for you.

The Ketogenic Diet for Type 2 Diabetes

The use of the ketogenic diet as a treatment for type 2 diabetes has been met with much skepticism due to its high-fat nature. Obesity, high cholesterol, and elevated triglycerides are all risk factors for type 2 diabetes, and unfortunately, a common misperception is that dietary fat contributes to these risk factors. (See pages 70 and 88 for more on this misconception.) Therefore, the use of a high-fat ketogenic diet as a treatment option for most diseases, including diabetes, has not been favored thus far. However, the physiological changes induced by a state of ketosis may prove beneficial for those suffering from type 2 diabetes (and may improve cholesterol and triglyceride levels, too—see page 89). Keep in mind that nutritional ketosis is completely different from ketoacidosis, a by-product of uncontrolled diabetes. (See page 17 for more on ketoacidosis.)

With that in mind, there are several potential mechanisms by which the ketogenic diet may act as an effective therapy for type 2 diabetes.

Weight Loss: Obesity is a huge risk factor for diabetes. In fact, 85 percent of type 2 diabetics are overweight and 55 percent are obese (Campbell et al., 2009). Although the ketogenic diet has many applications and benefits, one of its most common is weight loss. Studies have shown that the ketogenic diet is up to three times more effective for weight loss than a low-fat diet (Samaha et al., 2003).

Weight loss in diabetic patients tends to be slower than in individuals suffering from obesity alone. Furthermore, unpublished data from a friend and colleague of ours found that individuals suffering from both obesity and diabetes initially lost less weight on a ketogenic diet than individuals who were only obese (Maguire, unpublished observations). However, after twelve months of adherence to the ketogenic diet, both groups had lost the same amount of weight, on average. More recently, a new study compared the ketogenic diet to a diet based on the American Diabetes Association's "Create Your Plate" program in individuals with type 2 diabetes (Saslow et al., 2017). After thirty-two weeks, the subjects who followed the ketogenic diet lost significantly more weight—12.7 kilograms (27.9 pounds)—than those subjects on the ADA program, who lost just 3 kilograms (6.6 pounds).

Nonetheless, research clearly supports that the ketogenic diet is a safe and effective weight-loss strategy in obese individuals with type 2 diabetes (Leonetti et al., 2015). Although low-calorie diets that target weight loss may be effective for improving diabetic risk factors, such as high blood pressure and dyslipidemia, low-carbohydrate diets appear to be more effective (Hussain et al., 2012).

Insulin Sensitivity and Blood Sugar Regulation: Glycated hemoglobin (HbA1c) is formed when hemoglobin located within red blood cells combines with glucose. Measures of HbA1c indicate average blood sugar levels over the previous eight to twelve weeks. HbA1c levels of 6.5 percent and above are indicative of type 2 diabetes, whereas levels lower than 6 percent are considered normal. How does a ketogenic diet affect these values?

One study found that an unrestricted ketogenic diet (i.e., the subjects could eat as much as they wanted) improved insulin sensitivity and reduced HbA1c (Boden et al., 2005). It also led the subjects to unintentionally reduce their calorie intake, which has important implications for weight loss. An additional study examining obese subjects with diabetes found that the use of the ketogenic diet, in combination with a reduction in diabetes medication (because following a ketogenic diet means eating fewer carbs, it's necessary to reduce medication that lowers blood glucose in order to prevent hypoglycemia, or low blood sugar), led to a reduction in HbA1c values, body weight, triglyceride levels, and, for some individuals, even further reductions in the need for medication (Yancy et al., 2004). Furthermore, Dr. Eric Westman performed a case study on a sixty-year-old male with newly onset type 2 diabetes. Within just one month of being on a carbohydrate-restricted diet (less than 20 grams of carbs per day) and in the

---

KETO CONCEPT

As mentioned above, we tend to see a decrease in blood glucose levels while on the ketogenic diet, especially in people with diabetes. Most patients who are seeking medical care are likely taking blood glucose–lowering medications, such as metformin; therefore, it is important to inform your doctor of any dietary change you make so that your needs and medications can be monitored.

absence of insulin treatment, the subject's HbA1c fell from 10.5 percent to 6.4 percent. After two years on the diet, it had dropped to 5.5 percent (Masino, 2016). Finally, in a recent study, six of the eleven participants in the intervention group lowered their HbA1c to less than 6.5 percent, while none of the eight participants in the control group did (Saslow et al., 2017).

Heart Disease (Cardiomyopathy) Management: Heart disease is common in individuals with diabetes. Our hearts are composed of energy-demanding cardiac tissue, and insulin resistance only increases this demand as cells struggle to obtain glucose. Emerging research has shown that even in a severely failing human heart, ketones can provide an alternative fuel source to glucose, thereby improving cardiac efficiency (Bedi et al., 2016).

Exogenous Ketones for Type 2 Diabetes

Although the low-carb, high-fat makeup of the ketogenic diet clearly has benefits for people with type 2 diabetes, research suggests that ketones themselves may also have benefits—which means that supplementing with ketones may be worth exploring, either on its own or in combination with a ketogenic diet.

One of the first studies to examine ketone infusion in dogs found that supplementing with ketones resulted in a significant improvement in glucose tolerance (Felts et al., 1964). Years later, Dr. Veech's group found that supplementing with a ketone ester in mice improved insulin sensitivity by 73 percent (Srivastava et al., 2012). Other studies have shown similar results, including one in which BHB was infused into human subjects, raising blood ketones to 3.5 mmol/L and resulting in a 40 percent increase in insulin sensitivity (Amiel et al., 1991).

More recently, Dr. D'Agostino's group investigated the effects of various ketone supplements on blood glucose levels in rats. They looked at three different conditions: ketone mineral salts, a combination of ketone salts and MCT oil, and ketone esters. They found that all three of these conditions significantly lowered blood glucose for up to twelve hours following ingestion, potentially indicating an improvement in insulin sensitivity in the rats (Kesl et al., 2016). (It's interesting to note that the rats consumed a human equivalent dose of more than 50 grams of ketone salts. So, contrary to what some people may think, ketones don't seem to significantly elevate blood glucose levels, even at extremely high doses.) Lastly, our lab has done numerous human pilot experiments that confirm ketones decrease blood glucose consistently in a wide range of populations, from athletes to everyday individuals. Improving insulin sensitivity and decreasing blood glucose have huge implications for people with impaired glucose metabolism, as in diabetes, obesity, and other metabolic diseases.

Ketones also seem to be beneficial in treating nephropathy, a kidney disease related to damaged capillaries that is common in diabetics. One study found that as levels of BHB increased, diabetic nephropathy was reversed (Poplawski et al., 2011). This compelling example further supports why being in a state of ketosis, whether through taking exogenous ketones, following a ketogenic diet, or both, in combination with an active lifestyle, could provide more benefits than calorie restriction alone. Our colleague Dr. Antonio Paoli (2013) put perfectly: "In studies that have evaluated well-formulated very-

Virta Health

A new company called Virta Health has taken the bull by the horns and is actively pursuing this area with a bold mission to "reverse type 2 diabetes without medications or surgery." This online specialty medical clinic has many brilliant minds behind it, including Dr. Jeff Volek and Dr. Stephen Phinney, both of whom we have mentioned previously. Utilizing this system, participants get access to a health coach and physician, online peer support, and ongoing information and feedback on their health while utilizing a low-carbohydrate ketogenic diet. Just recently, the team published some of its findings (McKenzie et al., 2017): over just ten weeks, the average participant saw A1c drop by 1 percent and experienced a weight loss of 12 percent. What is even more impressive is that more than half of the participants reduced or eliminated their use of at least one diabetes medication, and 87 percent of those using insulin either decreased their dose or eliminated their use of insulin altogether. To say that these results are promising is an understatement, and we are very excited about the future of this company and what it is doing to move the field forward for people with type 2 diabetes.

low-carbohydrate diets and documented high rates of compliance in individuals with T2D, results have been nothing short of remarkable." These studies have shown dramatic improvements in glycemic control, insulin sensitivity, and body weight.

Gestational Diabetes

Gestational diabetes occurs in some women during pregnancy. Most of them have few symptoms other than high blood glucose. However, complications emerge during birth for both mother and baby, especially if the diabetes has not been diagnosed or treated. The consequences of gestational diabetes for the baby include macrosomia (a term used to describe a fetus or newborn who is significantly larger than average), preterm birth, low blood sugar at birth, temporary respiratory problems, jaundice, and increased risk of developing obesity later in life. The consequences for the mother include increased risk for miscarriage, preterm birth, increased risk for needing a C-section, and increased risk for developing high blood pressure and type 2 diabetes.

As with type 2 diabetes, several factors may increase the risk for gestational diabetes, including obesity and a family history of type 2 diabetes. It has been advocated that gestational diabetes can be prevented by avoiding excessive weight gain before and during pregnancy (Hedderson et al., 2010). As with other types of diabetes, gestational diabetes is often treated with dietary modifications and/or insulin injections.

Finding ways to lower blood glucose and improve insulin resistance could be an effective method for overcoming gestational diabetes. If you plan on making a dietary change during pregnancy, we recommend that you consult with your physician. To date, there is limited human research on ketogenic dieting during pregnancy; therefore, you should work with your healthcare team to find the approach that you feel is right for you.

Cholesterol and Triglycerides

A friend of ours recently went to the doctor, and he told us about his visit. Over the past few years, he has gained a couple of pounds, but nothing extreme. After asking him about his diet, the doctor ordered a series of tests to measure our friend's cholesterol and triglyceride levels, or, as the doctor termed them, "the silent killers." Because heart attacks are prevalent in our friend's family, the doctor was especially concerned. Upon receiving the results and seeing high levels of both cholesterol and triglycerides, the doctor raised an alarm. "You have to cut the bacon, red meat, oils, and butter from your

PCOS

Type 2 diabetes and obesity have been identified as risk factors for polycystic ovary syndrome (PCOS), as have certain endocrine disruptors, such as pesticides and other harmful chemicals. PCOS is characterized by excess androgens (a type of hormone), ovarian cysts, and the absence of ovulation. A vast array of complications can arise, including insulin resistance, dyslipidemia (abnormal blood lipid levels), anxiety, and depression. Several medications may be prescribed for PCOS to normalize hormones and reduce blood glucose, but because insulin resistance plays a major role in PCOS, changes in dietary habits may be an effective tool for managing it. The medications prescribed for PCOS often lead to weight gain and further hormonal imbalances, which only fuel the pathology of the disease. One pilot study monitored five women with PCOS on a ketogenic diet (20 grams of carbohydrates or less per day for twenty-four weeks) and noted decreases in body weight (12 percent), percent free testosterone (the available testosterone not bound to albumin, which is more bioavailable) (22 percent), LH/FSH ratio (two important hormones for ovulation) (36 percent), and fasting insulin (54 percent). Two women actually became pregnant during the study despite previous infertility problems (Mavropoulos et al., 2005).

diet. Stick to whole grains, vegetables, and fruits, and even do some occasional juicing," the doctor proclaimed.

Unfortunately, this is a conversation that many physicians have with their patients every day. The majority of healthcare professionals still believe that dietary cholesterol intake is related to high levels of cholesterol in the blood and can lead to health problems. In this section, we will discuss how cholesterol is not the enemy and explain that a properly formulated ketogenic diet can not only improve triglyceride levels, but also positively impact blood cholesterol levels.

HDL versus LDL Cholesterol

Lipoproteins are molecules that are responsible for carrying lipids—fats—in the blood. Two kinds of lipoproteins carry cholesterol: LDL and HDL. LDL is often demonized as the "bad" cholesterol; high levels of LDL are associated with cholesterol buildup in the arteries (Grundy, 1997), which may develop into atherosclerosis and increase risk for cardiovascular disease. HDL, commonly known as the "good" cholesterol, is responsible for moving cholesterol from the blood to the liver, where it is metabolized, preventing blood cholesterol levels from becoming too high. When a blood test indicates that total blood cholesterol is elevated, it generally means that LDL is high and HDL is low, and that is said to increase the risk of coronary heart disease (CHD)—a fundamental feature and convergence point of many metabolic diseases, including diabetes. However, as we will soon discuss, linking high cholesterol levels to an increased risk of CHD is not so simple.

Dietary cholesterol (present in high-fat foods) has traditionally been targeted as the culprit for elevated blood cholesterol. But, as we explored in Chapter 2, one of the positive things that Ancel Keys did was to disprove the theory that dietary cholesterol directly contributes to blood cholesterol.

Misconceptions regarding the ketogenic diet are compounded by conflicting literature on the effect of dietary fat on blood cholesterol. Some studies comparing low-carbohydrate and low-fat diets report that low-carb diets actually lead to *increases* in total cholesterol (LDL plus HDL). However, we are beginning to realize the importance of the composition of blood cholesterol and what that composition really means. For example, low-carbohydrate diets have been shown to increase HDL to a greater extent than low-fat diets (Sparks et al., 2006). This increase in HDL may increase total cholesterol levels, but the ratio of total cholesterol to HDL improves, and this ratio has been shown to be a better predictor for heart disease risk than the ratio of LDL to HDL (Lemieux et al., 2001). Therefore, the ratio of total cholesterol to HDL should be analyzed in addition to total cholesterol itself as a predictor for heart disease risk. Low-fat diets have been shown to lower total cholesterol, but they do so primarily by decreasing HDL (Volek et al., 2005), which moves the total-cholesterol-to-HDL ratio in the wrong direction—potentially indicating a greater risk of heart disease.

Numerous studies have shown that a low-carbohydrate, high-fat diet has positive effects on the ratio of LDL to HDL. One study showed that the diets with the greatest overall fat intake and lowest carbohydrate intake resulted in higher HDL levels (Garg et al., 1988). In another study, overweight subjects were placed on a ketogenic diet with no limit on calorie intake. These individuals saw lowered total cholesterol levels, decreased LDL, increased HDL, and improvements in their ratios of total cholesterol to HDL (Westman et al., 2002).

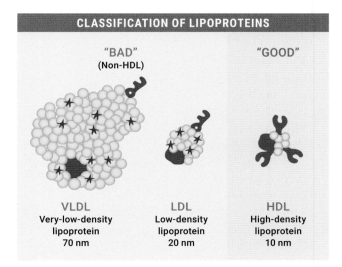

CLASSIFICATION OF LIPOPROTEINS

"BAD"
(Non-HDL)

"GOOD"

VLDL
Very-low-density
lipoprotein
70 nm

LDL
Low-density
lipoprotein
20 nm

HDL
High-density
lipoprotein
10 nm

Figure 5.2.4. *"Bad" versus "good" cholesterol.*
Source: German, Smilowitz, and Zivokovic, 2006.

Does Size Matter?

In addition to HDL and LDL ratio, there is another important consideration: LDL particle size. Currently, most people undergo a standard lipid panel that examines total cholesterol, triglycerides, and HDL-C. LDL-C is often estimated based on other numbers. Thus, even though many doctors worry about a high LDL, this number is just an estimation unless you get more detailed testing (such as an NMR LipoProfile). There are both large and small LDL particles, each with different functions and capabilities. Several studies have shown that the ketogenic diet causes a shift toward larger LDL particles, which is exactly what we want (Volek et al., 2004).

Let's say that two people both have a cholesterol level of 140 mg/dL. One of these individuals might be at risk while the other is not. Imagine large and small LDL particles are boats floating in the ocean of your bloodstream. Large particles are cruise ships, while small ones are speedboats. One of the individuals might have two large cruise ships carrying seventy cholesterol passengers each. The other might have 140 speedboats with one cholesterol passenger each. In both cases, the person's LDL is 140, but crashes and traffic jams (atherosclerosis and other complications) are much more likely with 140 speedboats. Thus, it's important to know what our LDL particle size is, so that we know how much traffic we can expect. The lower the particle number and size, the less likely it is that we would see any cardiovascular complications.

Triglycerides

Elevated triglycerides are a common characteristic of metabolic syndrome and thus diabetes. Triglycerides are the fats found in the blood, and research indicates that high triglyceride levels are a risk factor for cardiovascular disease (Hokanson and Austin, 1996).

Because the fat that we consume is made up of triglycerides, the traditional thought is that eating more fat elevates triglyceride levels and therefore increases the risk of cardiovascular and metabolic diseases—thus the recommendation to follow a low-fat diet. Despite this seemingly reasonable chain of thought, the data tells a very different story.

Research directly comparing the effects of ketogenic diets and low-fat diets shows that ketogenic diets either have no adverse effect on triglycerides or significantly lower triglyceride levels (Volek et al., 2005; Samaha et al., 2003). Low-fat diets, on the other hand—even in conjunction with weight loss or exercise—may *increase* triglyceride levels (Ginsberg et al., 1998; Yu-Poth et al., 1999).

Research from the early 1970s showed that obese individuals placed on a ketogenic diet saw a spike in triglycerides at the beginning of the experiment, but triglycerides normalized and then declined below the original levels once the individuals became keto-adapted (Kasper et al., 1973). Another study found that one week of 12 grams of carbohydrates per day lowered triglycerides, whereas 390 grams of carbohydrates per day significantly increased triglycerides within two days (Fujita et al., 1975). Another interesting study placed one group of endurance runners on a high-fat, low-carbohydrate diet and another group on a high-carbohydrate diet for fourteen days. The high-fat, low-carb group saw decreased triglycerides (despite consuming more than 110 grams of saturated fat), while the high-carb group saw significantly increased triglycerides (Thompson et al., 1984). Similarly, Dr. Jeff Volek's lab reported that calorie restriction on a ketogenic diet led to more favorable changes in triglyceride levels than calorie restriction on a low-fat diet (Volek et al., 2009). In a recent study over thirty-two weeks, participants on a ketogenic diet lowered their triglyceride levels more than participants on a low-fat, high-carbohydrate diet (traditionally recommended by the American Diabetes Association and known as the ADA diet). Triglycerides in the ketogenic group fell

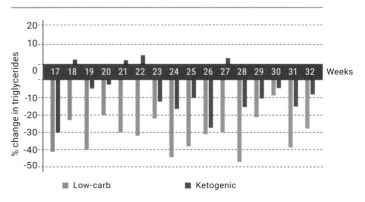

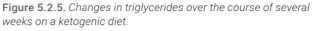

Figure 5.2.5. *Changes in triglycerides over the course of several weeks on a ketogenic diet.*

Source: Kasper et al., 1973.

by 60.1 mg/dL, while in the ADA group they dropped only 6.2 mg/dL (Saslow et al., 2017). The topper is the fact that on a high-carbohydrate diet, triglycerides increased significantly after one week and remained elevated throughout the entire six weeks of the study (Coulston et al., 1989).

While some studies show that a high-fat diet may increase triglyceride levels, it is important to note that several of these studies failed to restrict carbohydrates, thus discussing a Western-type diet that is high in both fat *and* carbohydrates. Consumption of foods high in glucose has been associated with the activation of genes that promote the production of fat, while consumption of foods high in fructose has been associated with elevated circulating blood lipids after a meal (Chong et al., 2007). When taken together, research and these associations suggest that it is the consumption of excess carbohydrates that is responsible for elevated triglycerides (Retzlaff et al., 1995).

Additionally, many studies demonstrating the adverse effects of a high-fat dieting were not performed over a long enough period; therefore, the findings should not be deemed conclusive. Triglyceride levels are likely to be elevated immediately following a high-fat meal, but only for a short time. Furthermore, as the body is becoming keto-adapted and adjusting to better utilizing and breaking down fat for fuel, triglyceride levels may be elevated, but they return to normal shortly thereafter and then continue to drop. Due to the fact that insulin is low, there may be more free fatty acids in the blood; these fatty acids can quickly get taken up into the mitochondria and broken down to be utilized as fuel—which doesn't happen when insulin is higher.

CHAPTER SUMMARY

It is evident from many research studies that the ketogenic diet is a safe and highly effective treatment option for individuals suffering from diabetes, particularly type 2 diabetes. Elevated ketone levels seem to provide additional benefits on top of reducing carbohydrates with a ketogenic diet, including lower blood glucose levels and improved glucose tolerance and insulin sensitivity. Unfortunately, the high-fat nature of the ketogenic diet has caused a misperception that it leads to high blood cholesterol and high triglycerides, when in fact a well-formulated ketogenic diet has been shown to improve cholesterol levels over the long term by increasing the number of HDL particles while simultaneously decreasing triglycerides, VLDL, and the smaller, more damaging small LDL particles. When discussing this with your physician, ask for a cholesterol panel that measures not only particle number but also particle size, in order to get a better idea of what your cholesterol actually is.

References

Aarsland, A., D. Chinkes, and R. R. Wolfe. "Contributions of de novo synthesis of fatty acids to total VLDL-triglyceride secretion during prolonged hyperglycemia/hyperinsulinemia in normal man." *Journal of Clinical Investigation* 98, no. 9 (1996): 2008–17.

Allen, F. M., E. Stillman, and R. Fitz. "Total dietary regulation in the treatment of diabetes" (no. 11). Rockefeller Institute for Medical Research (1919).

Amiel, S. A., H. R. Archibald, G. Chusney, A. J. Williams, and E. A. Gale. "Ketone infusion lowers hormonal responses to hypoglycaemia: evidence for acute cerebral utilization of a non-glucose fuel." *Clinical Science* 81, no. 2 (1991): 189–94.

Austin, M. A., M. C. King, K. M. Vranizan, and R. M. Krauss. "Atherogenic lipoprotein phenotype: a proposed genetic marker for coronary heart disease risk." *Circulation* 82, no. 2 (1990): 495–506.

Avena, N. M., P. Rada, and B. G. Hoebel. "Sugar and fat bingeing have notable differences in addictive-like behavior." *Journal of Nutrition* 139, no. 3 (2009): 623–8. doi: 10.3945/jn.108.097584.

Bedi K. C., N. W. Snyder, J. Brandimarto, M. Aziz, C. Mesaros, et al. "Evidence for intramyocardial disruption of lipid metabolism and increased myocardial ketone utilization in advanced human heart failure." *Circulation* 133, no. 8 (2016): 706–16. doi: 10.1161/CIRCULATIONAHA.115.017545.

Bierman, E. L., M. J. Albrink, and R. A. Arky. "Principles of nutrition and dietary recommendations for patients with diabetes mellitus." *Diabetes* 20, no. 9 (1971): 633–4. doi: 10.2337/diab.20.9.633.

Boden, G., K. Sargrad, C. Homko, M. Mozzoli, and T. P. Stein. "Effect of a low-carbohydrate diet on appetite, blood glucose levels, and insulin resistance in obese patients with type 2 diabetes." *Annals of Internal Medicine* 142, no. 6 (2005): 403–11.

Brand-Miller, J., S. Hayne, P. Petocz, and S. Colagiuri. "Low–glycemic index diets in the management of diabetes." *Diabetes Care* 26, no. 8 (2003): 2261–7.

Brunzell, J. D., R. L. Lerner, W. R. Hazzard, D. Porte Jr., and E. L. Bierman. "Improved glucose tolerance with high carbohydrate feeding in mild diabetes." *New England Journal of Medicine* 284, no. 10 (1971): 521–4.

Buse, J. B., K. S. Polonsky, and C. F. Burant. "Type 2 diabetes mellitus." *Williams Textbook of Endocrinology,* 10th Edition. (Philadelphia: Saunders, 2003): 1427–83.

Campbell, R. K. "Type 2 diabetes: where we are today: an overview of disease burden, current treatments, and treatment strategies." *Journal of the American Pharmacists Association* 49, suppl 1 (2009): S3–S9.

Chong, M. F., B. A. Fielding, and K. N. Frayn. "Mechanisms for the acute effect of fructose on postprandial lipemia." *American Journal of Clinical Nutrition* 85, no. 6 (2007): 1511–20.

Clark, M. "Is weight loss a realistic goal of treatment in type 2 diabetes?: The implications of restraint theory." *Patient Education and Counseling* 53, no. 3 (2004): 277–83.

Cooke, D. W., and L. Plotnick. "Type 1 diabetes mellitus in pediatrics." *Pediatrics in Review* 29, no. 11 (2008): 374–84.

Coulston, A. M., C. B. Hollenbeck, A. L. Swislocki, and G. M. Reaven. "Persistence of hypertriglyceridemic effect of low-fat high-carbohydrate diets in NIDDM patients." *Diabetes Care* 12, no. 2 (1989): 94–101.

Dey, L., and A. S. Attele. "Type 2 diabetes." *Tradititional Chinese Medicine* 231, no. 1 (2011): 1–16.

Donnelly, K. L., C. I. Smith, S. J. Schwarzenberg, J. Jessurun, M. D. Boldt, and E. J. Parks. "Sources of fatty acids stored in liver and secreted via lipoproteins in patients with nonalcoholic fatty liver disease." *Journal of Clinical Investigation* 115, no. 5 (2005): 1343–51.

Dreon, D. M., H. A. Fernstrom, B. Miller, and R. M. Krauss. "Low-density lipoprotein subclass patterns and lipoprotein response to a reduced-fat diet in men." *FASEB Journal* 8, no. 1 (1994): 121–6.

Dreon, D. M., H. A. Fernstrom, P. T. Williams, and R. M. Krauss. "A very-low-fat diet is not associated with improved lipoprotein profiles in men with a predominance of large, low-density lipoproteins." *American Journal of Clinical Nutrition* 69, no. 3 (1999): 411–8.

Dumesic, D. A., S. E. Oberfield, E. Stener-Victorin, J. C. Marshall, J. S. Laven, and R. S. Legro. "Scientific statement on the diagnostic criteria, epidemiology, pathophysiology, and molecular genetics of polycystic ovary syndrome." *Endocrine Reviews* 36, no. 5 (2015): 487–525.

Felts, P. W., O. B. Crofford, and C. R. Park. "Effect of infused ketone bodies on glucose utilization in the dog." *Journal of Clinical Investigation* 43, no. 4 (1964): 638–46.

Fujita, Y., A. M. Gotto, and R. M. Unger. "Basal and postprotein insulin and glucagon levels during a high and low carbohydrate intake and their relationships to plasma triglycerides." *Diabetes* 24, no. 6 (1975): 552–8.

Gannon, M. C., F. Q. Nuttall, A. Saeed, K. Jordan, and H. Hoover. "An increase in dietary protein improves the blood glucose response in persons with type 2 diabetes." *American Journal of Clinical Nutrition* 78, no. 4 (2003): 734–41.

Gannon, M. C., and F. Q. Nuttall. "Effect of a high-protein, low-carbohydrate diet on blood glucose control in people with type 2 diabetes." *Diabetes* 53, no. 9 (2004): 2375–82.

Garg, A., A. Bonanome, S. M. Grundy, Z. J. Zhang, and R. H. Unger. "Comparison of a high-carbohydrate diet with a high-monounsaturated-fat diet in patients with non-insulin-dependent diabetes mellitus." *New England Journal of Medicine* 319, no. 13 (1988): 829–34.

German, J. B., J. T. Smilowitz, and A. M. Zivkovic. "Lipoproteins: When size really matters." *Current Opinion in Colloid & Interface Science* 11, no. 2 (2006): 171–83.

Ginsberg, H. N., P. Kris-Etherton, B. Dennis, P. J. Elmer, A. Ershow, M. Lefevre, ... and K. Stewart. "Effects of reducing dietary saturated fatty acids on plasma lipids and lipoproteins in healthy subjects." *Arteriosclerosis, Thrombosis, and Vascular Biology* 18, no. 3 (1998): 441–9.

Grundy, S. M. "Small LDL, atherogenic dyslipidemia, and the metabolic syndrome." *Circulation* 95, no. 1 (1997): 1–4.

Haffner, S., and H. B. Cassells. "Metabolic syndrome—a new risk factor of coronary heart disease?" *Diabetes Obesity and Metabolism* 5, no. 6 (2003): 359–70.

Hedderson, M. M., E. P. Gunderson, and A. Ferrara. "Gestational weight gain and risk of gestational diabetes mellitus." *Obstetrics and Gynecology* 115, no. 3 (2010): 597–604.

Heilbronn, L. K., M. Noakes, and P. M. Clifton. "Effect of energy restriction, weight loss, and diet composition on plasma lipids and glucose in patients with type 2 diabetes." *Diabetes Care* 22, no. 6 (1999): 889–95.

Heilbronn, L. K., Noakes, M., and Clifton, P. M. "The effect of high- and low-glycemic index energy restricted diets on plasma lipid and glucose profiles in type 2 diabetic subjects with varying glycemic control." *Journal of the American College of Nutrition* 21, no. 2 (2002): 120–7.

Hokanson, J. E., and M. A. Austin. "Plasma triglyceride level is a risk factor for cardiovascular disease independent of high-density lipoprotein cholesterol level: a metaanalysis of population-based prospective studies." *Journal of Cardiovascular Risk* 3, no. 2: (1996): 213–9.

Hussain, T. A., T. C. Mathew, A. A. Dashti, S. Asfar, N. Al-Zaid, and H. M. Dashti. "Effect of low-calorie versus low-carbohydrate ketogenic diet in type 2 diabetes." *Nutrition* 28, no. 10 (2012): 1016–21. doi: 10.1016/j. nut.2012.01.016.

Joslin, E. P. *A Diabetic Manual for the Mutual Use of Doctor and Patient.* Philadelphia and New York: Lea & Febiger, 1919.

Kasper, H., H. Thiel, and M. Ehl. "Response of body weight to a low carbohydrate, high fat diet in normal and obese subjects." *American Journal of Clinical Nutrition* 26, no. 2 (1973): 197–204.

Katzel, L. I., M. J. Busby-Whitehead, E. M. Rogus, R. M. Krauss, and A. P. Goldberg. "Reduced adipose tissue lipoprotein lipase responses, postprandial lipemia, and low high-density lipoprotein-2 subspecies levels in older athletes with silent myocardial ischemia." *Metabolism* 43, no. 2 (1994): 190–8.

Kesl, S. L., A. M. Poff, N. P. Ward, T. N. Fiorelli, C. Ari, A. J. Van Putten, ... and D. P. D'Agostino. "Effects of exogenous ketone supplementation on blood ketone, glucose, triglyceride, and lipoprotein levels in Sprague–Dawley rats." *Nutrition & Metabolism* 13, no. 1 (2016): 9.

Klein, S., and Wolfe, R. R. "Carbohydrate restriction regulates the adaptive response to fasting." *American Journal of Physiology-Endocrinology and Metabolism* 262, no. 5 (1992): E631–6.

Lemieux, I., B. Lamarche, C. Couillard, A. Pascot, B. Cantin, J. Bergeron, ... and J. P. Després. "Total cholesterol/HDL cholesterol ratio vs LDL cholesterol/HDL cholesterol ratio as indices of ischemic heart disease risk in men: the Quebec Cardiovascular Study." *Archives of Internal Medicine* 161, no. 22 (2001): 2685–92.

Leonetti, F., F. Campanile, F. Coccia, D. Capoccia, L. Alessandroni, et al. "Very low-carbohydrate ketogenic diet before bariatric surgery: prospective evaluation of a sequential diet." *Obesity Surgery* 25, no. 1 (2015): 64–71. doi: 10.1007/s11695-014-1348-1.

Masino, S. A. (Ed.). *Ketogenic Diet and Metabolic Therapies: Expanded Roles in Health and Disease.* New York: Oxford University Press, 2016.

Mavropoulos, J. C., W. S. Yancy, J. Hepburn, and E. C. Westman. "The effects of a low-carbohydrate, ketogenic diet on the polycystic ovary syndrome: a pilot study." *Nutrition & Metabolism* 2, no. 1 (2005): 35. doi: 10.1186/1743-7075-2-35.

McKenzie, A. L., S. J. Hallberg, B. C. Creighton, B. M. Volk, T. M. Link, M. K. Abner, ... and S. D. Phinney. "A novel intervention including individualized nutritional recommendations reduces hemoglobin A1c level, medication use, and weight in type 2 diabetes." *JMIR Diabetes* 2, no. 1 (2017): e5.

McLaughlin, T., G. Reaven, F. Abbasi, C. Lamendola, M. Saad, D. Waters, ... and R. M. Krauss. "Is there a simple way to identify insulin-resistant individuals at increased risk of cardiovascular disease?" *American Journal of Cardiology* 96, no. 3 (2005): 399–404.

Morgan, W. *Diabetes Mellitus: Its History, Chemistry, Anatomy, Pathology, Physiology, and Treatment and Cases Successfully Treated.* Sett Dey & Co., 1973.

Nuttall, F. Q., R. M. Almokayyad, and M. C. Gannon. "Comparison of a carbohydrate-free diet vs. fasting on plasma glucose, insulin and glucagon in type 2 diabetes." *Metabolism* 64, no. 2 (2015): 253–62. doi: 10.1016/j.metabol.2014.10.004.

Ogurtsova, K., J. D. da Rocha Fernandes, Y. Huang, U. Linnenkamp, L. Guariguata, N. H. Cho, ... and L. E. Makaroff. "IDF Diabetes Atlas: Global estimates for the prevalence of diabetes for 2015 and 2040." *Diabetes Research and Clinical Practice* 128 (2017): 40–50.

Paoli, A. "Ketogenic diet for obesity: friend or foe?" *International Journal of Environmental Research and Public Health* 11, no. 2 (2014): 2092–107. doi: 10.3390/ijerph110202092.

Paoli, A., A. Rubini, J. S. Volek, and K. A. Grimaldi. "Beyond weight loss: a review of the therapeutic uses of very-low-carbohydrate (ketogenic) diets." *European Journal of Clinical Nutrition* 67, no. 8 (2013): 789–96.

Parks, E. J. "Changes in fat synthesis influenced by dietary macronutrient content." *Proceedings of the Nutrition Society* 61, no. 2 (2002): 281–6. doi: 10.1079/PNS2002148.

Poplawski, M. M., J. W. Mastaitis, F. Isoda, F. Grosjean, F. Zheng, et al. "Reversal of diabetic nephropathy by a ketogenic diet." *PLOS ONE* 6, no. 4 (2011): e18604. doi: 10.1371/journal.pone.0018604.

Retzlaff, B. M., Walden, C. E., Dowdy, A. A., McCann, B. S., Anderson, K. V., and R. H. Knopp. "Changes in plasma triacylglycerol concentrations among free-living hyperlipidemic men adopting different carbohydrate intakes over 2 y: the Dietary Alternatives Study." *American Journal of Clinical Nutrition* 62, no. 5 (1995): 988–95.

Rizkalla, S. W., Taghrid, L., Laromiguiere, M., Huet, D., Boillot, J., Rigoir, A., ... and G. Slama. "Improved plasma glucose control, whole-body glucose utilization, and lipid profile on a low-glycemic index diet in type 2 diabetic men." *Diabetes Care* 27, no. 8 (2004): 1866–72.

Samaha, F. F., N. Iqbal, P. Seshadri, K. L. Chicano, D. A. Daily, et al. "A low-carbohydrate as compared with a low-fat diet in severe obesity." *New England Journal of Medicine* 348 (2003): 2074–81. doi: 10.1056/NEJMoa022637.

Sansum, W. D., N. R. Blatherwick, and R. Bowden. "The use of high carbohydrate diets in the treatment of diabetes mellitus." *Journal of the American Medical Association* 86, no. 3 (1926): 178–81.

Saslow, L. R., A. E. Mason, S. Kim, V. Goldman, R. Ploutz-Snyder, H. Bayandorian, ... and J. T. Moskowitz. "An online intervention comparing a very low-carbohydrate ketogenic diet and lifestyle recommendations versus a plate method diet in overweight individuals with type 2 diabetes: a randomized controlled trial." *Journal of Medical Internet Research* 19, no. 2 (2017): e36. doi: 10.2196/jmir.5806.

Sharman, M. J., A. L. Gómez, W. J. Kraemer, and J. S. Volek. "Very low-carbohydrate and low-fat diets affect fasting lipids and postprandial lipemia differently in overweight men." *Journal of Nutrition* 134, no. 4 (2004): 880–5.

Sharman, M. J., W. J. Kraemer, D. M. Love, N. G. Avery, A. L. Gómez, T. P. Scheett, and J. S. Volek. "A ketogenic diet favorably affects serum biomarkers for cardiovascular disease in normal-weight men." *Journal of Nutrition* 132, no. 7 (2002): 1879–85.

Sparks, L. M., H. Xie, R. A. Koza, R. Mynatt, G. A. Bray, and S. R. Smith. "High-fat/low-carbohydrate diets regulate glucose metabolism via a long-term transcriptional loop." *Metabolism* 55, no. 11 (2006): 1457–63.

Srivastava, S., U. Bedi, and P. Roy. "Synergistic actions of insulin-sensitive and Sirt1-mediated pathways in the differentiation of mouse embryonic stem cells to osteoblast." *Molecular and Cellular Endocrinology* 361, no. 1 (2012): 153–64. doi: 10.1016/j.mce.2012.04.002.

Stone, D. B., and W. E. Connor. "The prolonged effects of a low cholesterol, high carbohydrate diet upon the serum lipids in diabetic patients." *Diabetes* 12, no. 2 (1963): 127–32.

Thompson, P. D., E. M. Cullinane, R. Eshleman, M. A. Kantor, and P. N. Herbert. "The effects of high-carbohydrate and high-fat diets on the serum lipid and lipoprotein concentrations of endurance athletes." *Metabolism* 33, no. 11 (1984): 1003–10.

Volek, J. S., M. J. Sharman, A. L. Gómez, C. DiPasquale, M. Roti, A. Pumerantz, and W. J. Kraemer. "Comparison of a very low-carbohydrate and low-fat diet on fasting lipids, LDL subclasses, insulin resistance, and postprandial lipemic responses in overweight women." *Journal of the American College of Nutrition* 23, no. 2 (2004): 177–84.

Volek, J. S., and R. D. Feinman. "Carbohydrate restriction improves the features of Metabolic Syndrome. Metabolic Syndrome may be defined by the response to carbohydrate restriction." *Nutrition & Metabolism* 2, no. 1 (2005): 31.

Volek, J. S., M. L. Fernandez, R. D. Feinman, and S. D. Phinney. "Dietary carbohydrate restriction induces a unique metabolic state positively affecting atherogenic dyslipidemia, fatty acid partitioning, and metabolic syndrome." *Progress in Lipid Research* 47, no. 5 (2008): 307–18.

Volek, J. S., S. D. Phinney, C. E. Forsythe, E. E. Quann, R. J. Wood, M. J. Puglisi, ... and R. D. Feinman. "Carbohydrate restriction has a more favorable impact on the metabolic syndrome than a low fat diet." *Lipids* 44, no. 4 (2009): 297–309. doi: 10.1007/s11745-008-3274-2.

Volek, J. S., M. J. Sharman, and C. E. Forsythe. "Modification of lipoproteins by very low-carbohydrate diets." *Journal of Nutrition* 135, no. 6 (2005): 1339–42.

Westman, E. C., W. S. Yancy, J. S. Edman, K. F. Tomlin, and C. E. Perkins. "Effect of 6-month adherence to a very low carbohydrate diet program." *American Journal of Medicine* 113, no. 1 (2002): 30–36.

Yancy Jr., W. S., M. C. Vernon, and E. C. Westman. "A pilot trial of a low-carbohydrate, ketogenic diet in patients with type 2 diabetes." *Metabolic Syndrome and Related Disorders* 1, no. 3 (2003): 239–43.

Yancy, W. S., M. K. Olsen, J. R. Guyton, R. P. Bakst, and E. C. Westman. "A low-carbohydrate, ketogenic diet versus a low-fat diet to treat obesity and hyperlipidemia: a randomized, controlled trial." *Annals of Internal Medicine* 140, no. 10 (2004): 769–77.

Yu-Poth, S., G. Zhao, T. Etherton, M. Naglak, S. Jonnalagadda, and P. M. Kris-Etherton. "Effects of the national cholesterol education program's step I and step II dietary intervention programs on cardiovascular disease risk factors: a meta-analysis." *American Journal of Clinical Nutrition* 69, no. 4 (1999): 632–46.

Section 3:
Neurodegenerative Diseases

Mary and Steve Newport were happily married. Mary was a physician and Steve was a skilled accountant—a wizard with numbers. In his early fifties, Steve began showing signs of dementia. Soon thereafter, he began having trouble with numbers and eventually had to give up the job he loved so much. Steve had Alzheimer's disease.

Years later, Mary attempted to enroll Steve in a clinical trial, but unfortunately, his disease was too far advanced and he did not qualify. Upon further research, Mary discovered that coconut oil was high in MCTs, which are rapidly broken down into ketones and therefore could be a source of fuel for Steve's brain. In a last-ditch effort to help Steve, she decided to give it a try. Within days of beginning to take coconut oil, Steve's cognitive function significantly improved. He began to read again, and Mary felt that she had regained quality time with her husband. Mary was on to something, and she knew she needed to share her discovery with the world.

Mary's story is the driving motivation behind this chapter, which addresses the impact of ketones on major cognitive disorders: Parkinson's disease, epilepsy, Alzheimer's disease, and traumatic brain injury.

Parkinson's Disease

Parkinson's disease occurs in 1 percent of individuals over the age of sixty. It affects 53 million people worldwide and causes more than 100,000 deaths annually (Sveinbjornsdottir et al., 2016). The primary symptoms are shaking, rigid muscles, slowed movements, difficulty maintaining posture, difficulty walking, dementia, emotional problems, and depression. The primary area of the brain affected is the basal ganglia, which plays an important role in motor learning and planning, voluntary motor movements, routine behaviors, and eye movements (Purves et al., 2001). The specific area impacted is the substantia nigra, which produces the neurotransmitter dopamine and is responsible for emotion, movement, pleasure, and pain (Purves et al., 2001). Patients with Parkinson's disease typically lose as much as 70 percent of the neurons in their substantia nigra, and with those neurons goes the ability to produce enough dopamine to maintain normal function.

Difference in Dopamine Secretion in Normal and Parkinson's Affected

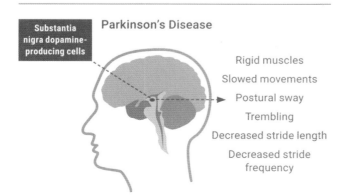

Figure 5.3.1. *The impact of dopamine loss on motor function.*

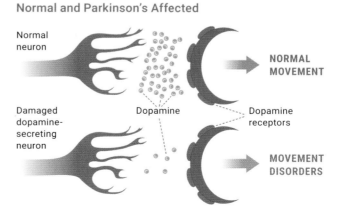

Figure 5.3.2. *Damaged dopamine signaling in patients with Parkinson's affects movement.*

Levodopa (L-DOPA) has been the most common treatment for Parkinson's for more than thirty years. L-DOPA is a precursor to dopamine and therefore helps increase the amount of dopamine produced. Although it certainly helps alleviate symptoms, it does not halt the progressive loss of dopamine-producing neurons in the brain (Yokoyama et al., 2008). Like many drug therapies, L-DOPA treats the symptoms of Parkinson's, not the root cause. While the underlying causes of Parkinson's remain to be fully elucidated, one theory is that the dopamine-producing cells in the substantia nigra deteriorate and die due to a lack of energy. That lack of energy stems primarily from impaired mitochondrial function. Whether mitochondrial dysfunction is the cause or a by-product of the disease is still being debated; however, it is an essential part of understanding how to treat the disease.

Impaired Mitochondrial Function

The most prominent theory for what underlies Parkinson's disease is that mitochondrial function is impaired. Mitochondria are the cells' energy powerhouses, and they are responsible for turning carbohydrates, amino acids, fatty acids, and ketones into usable energy known as ATP. Mitochondria also play a role in autophagy, the process of breaking down and recycling damaged or unnecessary proteins in a cell, which is essential for proper cell function. They are essential for insulin sensitivity; when mitochondria are impaired, the result is an impairment in the ability to use glucose. Finally, mitochondria produce reactive oxygen species (ROS), highly unstable oxygen-containing molecules that can serve several positive signaling effects in the cell. However, an overproduction of ROS can damage tissue and DNA (Balaban et al., 2005).

While it's not known exactly what causes Parkinson's to develop, it's clear that patients with Parkinson's have impaired mitochondrial function and the problems that accompany it—most importantly, an energy crisis. Research has shown that when a substance called MPTP (1-methyl-4-phenyl-1,2,3,6-tetrahydropyridine) inhibits the energy production process in mitochondria, dopamine-producing cells in the substantia nigra die (Betarbet et al., 2000). Another inhibitor of energy production, called

rotenone, has caused Parkinson's in rats (Betarbet et al., 2000). Additionally, it is well established that individuals with Parkinson's have a pronounced reduction in brain glucose metabolism compared to normal subjects—their brains aren't taking up glucose effectively (Polito et al., 2012). Laboratories have seen impaired energy production in the mitochondria of brain and skeletal muscle cells in patients with Parkinson's (Parker et al., 1989; Schapira et al., 1990). In addition, in patients with Parkinson's, impaired autophagy leads to an accumulation of damaged proteins called Lewy bodies. This accumulation disrupts the cells and leads to neurodegeneration and cell death (Ferracci et al., 2008).

Individuals diagnosed with Parkinson's disease also display elevated levels of inflammation in the brain (Hunot et al., 2003), likely due to energy deprivation and an inability to clear damaged proteins, both resulting in impaired mitochondrial function.

Ketosis may benefit mitochondrial function in several ways. Research indicates that ketogenic dieting and exogenous ketones may improve mitochondrial energy production when components of the mitochondria that normally produce energy from glucose are damaged. Additionally, ketones themselves may increase the formation of new mitochondria in various neurological disorders (Kim et al., 2010; Bough et al., 2006). One study induced Parkinson's in animals by inhibiting part of the energy production process. When the animals were administered the ketone body D-beta-hydroxybutyrate (D-BHB), ATP levels in the brain were restored, the substantia nigra was protected from further neuron degradation, and motor function was maintained (Tieu et al., 2003). In essence, D-BHB may not only increase the formation of new mitochondria but also bypass the damaged part of the energy-producing process in impaired mitochondria, helping to maintain normal ATP/energy levels.

The Ketogenic Diet for Parkinson's

Fascinating research in animals with Parkinson's has demonstrated that ketogenic diets drastically alleviated impaired motor symptoms, reduced the loss of neurons, decreased dopamine loss, and cut inflammation virtually in half (Hirsch et al.,

1998). Another study found that a ketogenic diet improved motor function and reduced levels of pro-inflammatory cells in the brain (Yang and Cheng, 2010). More recently, animals with Parkinson's disease that were placed on a ketogenic diet did not demonstrate the notable decline in stride length typically seen in Parkinson's (Rubin et al., 2016; Raiff et al., 2015). Lastly, the ketogenic diet not only prevented cell death in mice but also resulted in nearly 150 percent more neurons than in animals with Parkinson's fed a normal diet.

To date, one landmark study has been conducted in human Parkinson's patients (Vanitallie et al., 2005). In this study, five patients adhered to a ketogenic diet for twenty-eight days. The subjects' Unified Parkinson's Disease Rating Scale (UPDRS) scores were determined at the beginning of the study and at weekly intervals thereafter. These scores gauge the progression of Parkinson's, with the highest score of 199 indicating total disability and the lowest score of 0 indicating no disability. In the three subjects who were best able to comply with a ketogenic diet, periodic blood ketone concentrations ranged from 4.8 to 8.9 mmol/L throughout the twenty-eight days, and urinary ketones, measured daily, were always strongly positive. The five subjects who completed the study reduced their UPDRS scores by an average of 10.72 points, which represented an average decrease of nearly 45 percent (a range from 21 to 81 percent) in just twenty-eight days. Resting tremors, balance, gait, mood, and energy level all improved.

In another study, twenty healthy elderly subjects (older than sixty years of age) who didn't have Parkinson's were fed a ketogenic meal with 20 grams of medium-chain triglycerides (Ota et al., 2016). Improvements in cognition were measured after the meal, and the changes positively correlated with plasma ketone levels—that is, when ketone levels rose, cognitive function improved. Intriguingly enough, the cognitive-enhancing effect was observed predominantly in individuals who had a relatively low score at the beginning of the study, lending further support to why this might be applicable for individuals with Parkinson's.

In addition to the benefits of ketones, ketogenic dieting may be helpful for Parkinson's because it improves insulin resistance. Research demonstrates that more than 60 percent of Parkinson's patients have impaired insulin signaling and cannot effectively utilize glucose for energy (Lipman et al., 1974; Sandyk, 1993)—another effect of impaired mitochondrial function. Sadly, L-DOPA has been shown to make patients even more glucose intolerant (Lipman et al., 1974). In addition, individuals with type 2 diabetes demonstrate a nearly 40 percent higher risk of developing Parkinson's disease (Santiago et al., 2013). It is likely that Parkinson's is an extension of insulin resistance and that those who have it are "starving" for an alternative energy source because they are unable to use glucose effectively. Ketogenic diets may be able to overcome this deficit by improving insulin sensitivity and providing an alternative energy source (Borghammer et al., 2010).

Exogenous Ketones for Parkinson's

The landmark study mentioned above used exogenous ketones to treat Parkinson's in animals, so its positive results speak to the efficacy of an alternative fuel source: directly administering ketones improved the energy of the cell and protected dopamine-producing neurons in animals with Parkinson's (Tieu et al., 2003). Additionally, a diet containing ketone esters fed to healthy mice increased the total number of mitochondria and increased a kind of protein that is thought to reduce ROS production in the mitochondria (Srivastava et al., 2012), helping to protect cells and DNA from damage.

Other studies have confirmed that exogenous ketones can benefit neurons. One of the first studies looking at neuronal damage from deprivation of glucose found that the ketone body D-BHB not only was able to substitute for glucose as an energy source but also preserved neuronal integrity and stability (Izumi et al., 1998). In addition, studies examining D-BHB have found that it prevented motor deficits and cell death and protected dopamine-producing neurons in mice (Tieu et al., 2003). Animals treated with the highest dose of sodium BHB showed increased cell survival even at plasma levels of just 0.9 mmol/L.

Finally, we recently looked at exogenous ketone supplementation (10 grams of D-BHB) in an individual who has had Parkinson's for more than two decades. The subject was examined with an eye-tracking device, which measures the abnormal eye movement that is characteristic in patients with Parkinson's.

BEFORE

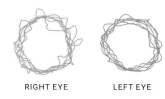

RIGHT EYE   LEFT EYE

Metrics	RIGHT EYE		LEFT EYE		BOTH	
	Actual	Population	Actual	Population	Actual	Population
Smooth pursuit (%)	87.14	90 (+/-7)	91.27	90 (+/-7)	90.53	92 (+/-6)
Saccade (%)	7.62	6 (+/-5)	4.55	6 (+/-5)	5.50	5 (+/-4)
Fixation (%)	5.24	4 (+/-3)	4.18	4 (+/-3)	3.97	3 (+/-3)
Eye target velocity error (%)	14.92	15 (+/-2)	15.11	15 (+/-2)	16.16	15 (+/-2)
Horizontal synchronization SP (0-1)	0.87	0.89 (+/-0.06)	0.86	0.89 (+/-0.06)	0.90	0.91 (+/-0.05)
Vertical synchronization SP (0-1)	0.62	0.85 (+/-0.07)	0.76	0.85 (+/-0.07)	0.89	0.87 (+/-0.06)

30 MINUTES AFTER KETONES

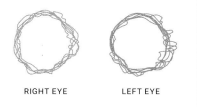

RIGHT EYE   LEFT EYE

Metrics	RIGHT EYE		LEFT EYE		BOTH	
	Actual	Population	Actual	Population	Actual	Population
Smooth pursuit (%)	94.29	90 (+/-7)	91.75	90 (+/-7)	96.25	92 (+/-6)
Saccade (%)	4.81	6 (+/-5)	4.81	6 (+/-5)	3.80	5 (+/-4)
Fixation (%)	0.90	4 (+/-3)	3.44	4 (+/-3)	0.95	3 (+/-3)
Eye target velocity error (%)	14.09	15 (+/-2)	14.61	15 (+/-2)	14.45	15 (+/-2)
Horizontal synchronization SP (0-1)	0.89	0.89 (+/-0.06)	0.92	0.89 (+/-0.06)	0.90	0.91 (+/-0.05)
Vertical synchronization SP (0-1)	0.91	0.85 (+/-0.07)	0.81	0.85 (+/-0.07)	0.91	0.87 (+/-0.06)

Figure 5.3.3. Cognitive tracking of a Parkinson's subject before and thirty minutes after being given exogenous ketones. His baseline was 87.1 percent (below normal average); after D-BHB, he scored 94.3 percent (slightly above normal average).

The average score for a person his age is 17 targets. Before treatment, the subject scored a 6. However, after supplementing with exogenous ketones, he scored above average (18) and his hands had stopped shaking. For the first time since the disease had taken hold, this man felt like he had control over his life, without tremors getting in his way. These results all demonstrate that ketones show promise in the realm of Parkinson's.

In conclusion, Parkinson's disease is characterized by the substantial death of dopamine-producing cells in the substantia nigra, dysfunctional proteins called Lewy bodies, inflammation, impaired mitochondrial function, increased ROS, and a resulting dysregulation of motor function. Ketogenic dieting and exogenous ketones have been demonstrated to improve symptoms in humans by about 45 percent in as little as twenty-eight days. Moreover, animal models have demonstrated that exogenous ketones and/or a ketogenic diet prevent declines in ATP, increase mitochondrial function, lower inflammation, and improve motor function. Thus it is possible that ketogenic dieting and/or exogenous ketones may be a viable treatment option for individuals with Parkinson's.

Epilepsy

Epilepsy is a neurological disorder characterized by recurrent spontaneous seizures. It can occur in people of all ages. About 22 million people worldwide have epilepsy, and in 2013, it resulted in 116,000 deaths (Global Burden of Disease Study, 2013).

Throughout history, epilepsy has been viewed as a mystery. In fact, in the ancient world, seizures were attributed to demonic possession and seen as a sign that a person was a witch. One of the earliest documented treatments for epilepsy was by Hippocrates, who prescribed fasting as a cure (Magiorkinis et al., 2010). As discussed in Chapter 2, research has long looked at fasting and, later, the ketogenic diet as treatments for epilepsy, for good reason: they've been proven effective.

The introduction of anticonvulsant drugs in the late 1930s did not cure epilepsy. In fact, at least one-third of patients are fully resistant to drug treatment (Lutas et al., 2013). One brave father, Jim Abrahams, wouldn't take no for an answer when his two-year-old son, Charlie, didn't respond to anticonvulsant drugs. Instead, he sought out experts at Johns Hopkins

Types of Effective Ketogenic Diets

Researchers have identified three variations of the ketogenic diet that have been utilized with success in children with epilepsy:

MCT diet: One study showed that consuming 60 percent of total calories as MCTs led to a 50 percent reduction in seizures (Huttenlocher et al., 1971). In 2012, Dr. Elizabeth Neal published her book *Dietary Treatment of Epilepsy: Practical Implementation of Ketogenic Therapy*, in which she outlines the MCT protocol that is now recommended: 60 to 70 percent of calories from fat, with 40 to 50 percent of those fat calories coming from MCT supplementation, 10 to 12 percent of calories from protein, and 15 to 18 percent of calories from carbohydrates, along with vitamin and mineral supplementation. One limitation, however, is that MCT supplements can wreak havoc on the gastrointestinal system.

Low-glycemic-index treatment (LGIT): As discussed in Chapter 3, the glycemic index measures how a particular food affects blood sugar. Because uncontrolled glucose levels can provoke seizures, this treatment attempts to control glucose levels without being as restrictive as a traditional ketogenic diet. Dr. Heidi Pfeifer did a lot of the early work on this approach and has suggested that 10 percent of calories should come from carbohydrates with a glycemic index of under 50 (distributed throughout the day and eaten with fat), 30 percent of calories from protein, and 60 percent of calories from fat. Success has been achieved, with 66 percent of the children studied seeing seizure reductions after twelve months (Muzykewicz et al., 2009).

Modified Atkins diet (MAD): Dr. Eric Kossof has led the way in developing the MAD approach after finding that thirteen of twenty children saw a 50 percent reduction in seizures after six months, with four children becoming seizure free while on the diet. The MAD approach is much looser than the traditional ketogenic diet in that carbohydrates are strictly controlled (10 to 15 grams per day), but protein and calories are consumed freely. This diet has been used worldwide for years with promising results; trials consistently show that more than 50 percent of children placed on a MAD see a 50 percent decrease in seizures, with a percentage of those children becoming seizure free (Kossof et al., 2013).

When choosing a type of ketogenic diet to treat epilepsy, consult with your physician and think about practicality and feasibility. Some experts suggest that a stricter ketogenic diet is more effective at reducing seizures than a modified Atkins diet (El Rashidy et al., 2013), but the initiation period seems to be most crucial in the overall success of any diet, and after three to four months, it may be possible to be less restrictive. Therefore, you might consider beginning with a stricter approach—for instance, fasting followed by a traditional ketogenic diet, with MCTs or exogenous ketone supplementation—and then transitioning to the more flexible MAD with consistent monitoring to ensure success and long-term adherence.

for help with his son's recurring seizures. Within days of being placed on a ketogenic diet, Charlie began to have seizure control. (Read more about the Abrahamses and their efforts to help educate others on the use of the ketogenic diet for the treatment of epilepsy in Chapter 2.)

In recent years, doctors have returned to using the ketogenic diet as a treatment. Research demonstrates that the diet can reduce seizures by more than 50 percent in up to 55 percent of patients (Klein et al., 2014), and up to 27 percent of patients experience a greater than 90 percent reduction in the number of seizures, with many entering into

complete remission (Schoeler et al., 2014; Klein et al., 2010). Clearly, ketogenic dieting or a combination of the diet and fasting is a viable option for epilepsy patients.

To understand how ketogenic dieting may affect epilepsy, it is important to understand the underlying mechanisms of the disease. Neurons fire by rapidly reversing their polarization from positive to negative and vice versa. Changing from a negative charge to a positive charge on the inside of the cell membrane is called depolarization.

Imagine it is Black Friday, and outside your favorite store is a huge line of people waiting to rush in as soon as the doors open. Then, when the number of people in the store reaches a certain limit, the doors shut again to prevent overcrowding. Similarly, depolarization involves opening channels in the neuron to positively charged ions, carrying a positive charge along the length of the neuron—this is how the nerve sends a signal. At a certain point, the channels close, stopping the flood of positively charged ions and ending the nerve's signal. But in some cases of epilepsy, the channels don't fully close (Strafstrom et al., 2007; Powell et al., 2014)—the store is packed on Black Friday, but the doors are never locked, giving people the opportunity to cram in, even after the store reaches maximum capacity. During these epileptic events, the neuron depolarizes more easily than usual, causing abnormal firing and spreading of excitation throughout the brain (Strafstrom et al., 2007).

Seizures also can be caused by a general imbalance between excitatory neurotransmitters like glutamate that trigger nerves to fire and inhibitory neurotransmitters like GABA that stop nerves from firing (Powell et al., 2014). Standard drug treatments for epilepsy act on the ion channels, blocking more ions from entering the neuron and thereby preventing the nerve from firing, or balancing the neurotransmitters (Powell et al., 2014).

The ketogenic diet targets multiple mechanisms that may be the cause of impaired neuronal firing (Yudkoff et al., 2007). Data shows that the ketone bodies acetoacetate (AcAc) and acetone have anticonvulsant effects. AcAc has been shown to impair the release of glutamate in neurons (Judge et al., 2010). Too much glutamate is associated with neurological disorders. It also has been suggested that ketone bodies may increase the synthesis of GABA. The net result would be a decrease in the probability of an unpredictable excitatory event, such as a seizure, occurring in the future (Yudkoff et al., 2007). Additionally, research indicates that ketone bodies may activate potassium (K+) channels (Bough et al., 2007). K+ has a positive charge, and if its respective channels are opened, that positive charge leaks out of the neuron, thereby reducing the positive charge inside the cell and causing it to be hyperpolarized. The result is increased difficulty in depolarizing the neurons and therefore a decreased likelihood of seizure (Bough et al., 2007).

The Ketogenic Diet for Epilepsy

In addition to the general benefits of ketones, a ketogenic diet may have anticonvulsant effects because it lowers blood glucose levels. It is thought that a neuron's capacity to trigger activity is highly dependent on glucose, so a general restriction of glucose may limit a neuron's ability to reach and maintain the high levels of synaptic activity necessary for seizures to occur (Bough et al., 2007; Greene et al., 2003).

Ketogenic diets have been studied extensively in both children and adults with epilepsy. One of the first documented cases of treating patients with a long-term ketogenic diet came in the 1930s (Barborka, 1930); 12 percent of the individuals placed on a ketogenic diet experienced full remission, while 50 to 90 percent saw a reduction in seizures (Bastible et al., 1931). One of the most highly cited studies investigated the implementation of a ketogenic diet in children who were resistant to anti-epileptic drugs (Vining et al., 1998). After three months on a 4:1 ketogenic diet (90 percent fat, 10 percent protein, and carbs), 54 percent of these young patients experienced a greater than 50 percent decrease in the frequency of seizures. After a year on the diet, 10 percent of them became seizure free.

KETO CONCEPT

Dravet Syndrome

Dravet syndrome (previously known as severe myoclonic epilepsy in infancy, or SMEI) is a rare genetic epileptic dysfunction of the brain that begins in infancy. It is usually the result of a mutation in the SCN1A gene. It is characterized by prolonged and frequent seizures, developmental delays, movement disorders, and other difficulties. One study (Caraballo et al., 2005) found that after a year on a ketogenic diet, two patients (15 percent) became seizure-free, eight (62 percent) saw a 75 to 99 percent decrease in seizures, and the remaining three (23 percent) saw a 50 to 74 percent decrease in seizures. In other words, 77 percent of the children achieved a greater than 75 percent decrease in seizures. In addition, all the subjects reported improvement in quality of life.

Another study (Neal et al., 2008) compared seizure activity in children with epilepsy on a ketogenic diet to those in a control group that did not consume the diet. No other changes in treatment were made in either group. After three months, the occurrence of seizures in the ketogenic diet group decreased by 38 percent, while seizure frequency in the control group increased by 37 percent. Twenty-eight children in the ketogenic diet group (38 percent) had a greater than 50 percent seizure reduction, compared with just four children in the control group (6 percent). Furthermore, five children in the ketogenic diet group (7 percent) had a greater than 90 percent seizure reduction; no one in the control group saw a reduction that significant.

More recently, a study comparing the modified Atkins diet (MAD) to no intervention in children with epilepsy (Sharma et al., 2013) found that with the MAD intervention, the occurrence of seizures decreased by 41 percent after three months, while there was no significant change in the control group. In the MAD group, 30 percent of children saw seizure frequency drop by more than 90 percent, and five of them became seizure free.

The results speak for themselves. When a ketogenic diet is properly implemented, children with epilepsy can achieve remarkable results. Often, children can be more "loose" with the diet after they become seizure-free. However, with less restriction, there is a higher risk of seizure recurrence. Thus many physicians recommend maintaining a ketogenic diet with as few variations as possible in order to prevent recurrence in the long run. As you can imagine, however, sticking to a strict ketogenic diet can be tough for young children. We once had a great conversation with a doctor who often prescribes the ketogenic diet for children with epilepsy, and she told us that the biggest limiting factor is adherence. When children go to school, it's hard to know what they may be eating. Think about how often teachers hand out candy or how easy it is to buy a bag of chips at lunch. In addition, some of the strict ketogenic diets on which epileptic children are placed may affect growth maturation; therefore, these children need to be monitored very closely (Williams et al., 2002).

Exogenous Ketones for Epilepsy

One of the first studies to look at ketone supplementation and epilepsy dates back to the 1930s. Researchers found that AcAc protected against seizures in rabbits (Keith, 1933; Keith et al., 1936). More recently, researchers have tried to isolate which ketone bodies have a direct effect on seizure activity and possess the greatest anticonvulsant properties. In one study, mice were injected with various kinds of ketone bodies and then exposed to loud sounds that induced seizures. The researchers found that both acetone and AcAc protected against seizures. Thus acetone and AcAc appear to be the driving forces behind the anticonvulsant properties of ketone bodies. This was confirmed by other studies in which acetone, AcAc, or both were shown to exhibit anticonvulsant properties (Thio et al., 2000; Gasior et al., 2007; Likhodii et al., 2002).

Studies have also looked at seizures caused by oxygen toxicity in simulations of Navy SEAL dive missions—breathing 100 percent oxygen at the increased levels of pressure experienced deep under water increases the likelihood of seizures. Researchers found that supplementing with ketone esters caused rapid and sustained elevations of BHB, AcAc, and acetone and increased resistance to seizures by more than 500 percent (D'Agostino et al., 2013).

The exact mechanism by which ketone supplements affect seizure control or activity remains unclear. More studies on the anticonvulsant effects of various ketone supplements are needed for us to develop a better understanding of the specific effects that ketone bodies have on seizure control and the levels of ketones that are needed to create these effects. In the meantime, for children with epilepsy who may be struggling to follow a strict ketogenic diet, combining exogenous ketones with a low-carbohydrate diet may be helpful. This approach restricts their dietary practices less while still potentially preventing seizures.

In summary, epilepsy is a chronic and persistent recurrence of seizures. Epilepsy emerges from abnormal activity of neuronal networks. In particular, hyperexcitability on many levels, including altered ion channel function, contributes to the seizure-prone state. It is postulated that epilepsy may be caused by a dysfunction of ion channels or an imbalance between excitatory (glutamate) and inhibitory (GABA) neurotransmitters. Anticonvulsant drugs are used to target these mechanisms, but they often fail. Moreover, these drugs come with side effects that can detract even more from quality of life than the seizures themselves. We argue that ketogenic dieting should be the first line of treatment for epilepsy. In the majority of cases, the diet leads to a greater than 50 percent improvement in epileptic outbreaks and often complete remission from the disease. While the mechanisms are not fully understood, it is believed that the ketogenic diet improves ion channel function, blunts the release of glutamate, and lowers general glucose utilization. Therefore, the approach should be individualized based on goals and adherence. However, it could be beneficial to begin with a stricter approach (i.e., fasting followed by traditional ketogenic dieting with the incorporation of MCTs or exogenous ketone supplements) and then transition to the more flexible modified Atkins diet, with consistent monitoring to ensure success and long-term adherence.

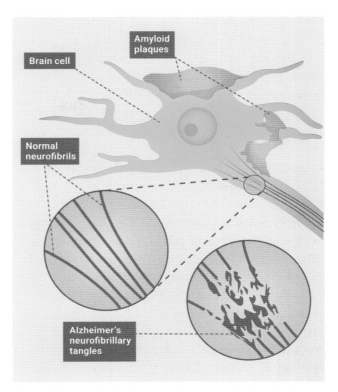

Figure 5.3.4. *Amyloid plaques and brain tangles found in the brains of Alzheimer's patients.*

Source: www.webmd.com/alzheimers/guide/understanding-alzheimers-disease-basics

Alzheimer's Disease

Auguste was born in Germany in May 1850. While her maiden name is unknown, she married Karl Deter in her thirties and they started a family. She lived a normal life until her mid-forties, when she began developing signs of dementia. Her dementia progressively worsened, ultimately impairing her ability to remember events. She soon began experiencing delusions and started screaming during the night. Eventually Auguste was committed to a mental institution, where she was treated by psychiatrist Alois Alzheimer until Auguste passed away in 1906. After Auguste died, Dr. Alzheimer performed an autopsy on her brain. Under a microscope he identified two horrifying characteristics: a buildup of amyloid plaques that inhibited neuron function and clumps of proteins called neurofibrillary tangles. This was the first documented case of the neurodegenerative condition that came to be known as Alzheimer's disease, the leading cause of dementia.

Today, approximately 37 million people worldwide have Alzheimer's disease, the majority of whom are over sixty-five years old. The prevalence of Alzheimer's is rising at an alarming rate. With the Baby Boomer generation aging, this number is only expected to climb; one new case of Alzheimer's is expected to develop every thirty-three seconds, resulting in nearly a million new cases per year. If that isn't alarming enough, it is estimated that in 2014, family members and other caregivers spent more than 17.9 billion hours caring for people with Alzheimer's. Not to mention the financial burden: well over $200 billon for costs associated with medical and informal care.

The most noticeable symptoms of Alzheimer's disease are life-affecting memory loss, difficulty performing normal activities of daily living, confusion, impaired judgment, and withdrawal from social and work-related activities. Alzheimer's primarily impacts the areas of the brain associated with memory (the temporal lobe); intelligence, judgment, and behavior (the frontal cortex); and language (the parietal cortex/lobe). The brains of

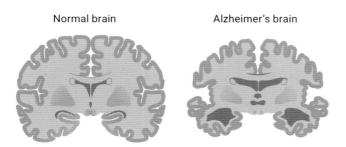

Normal brain   Alzheimer's brain

Figure 5.3.5. *Shrinkage in certain areas of the brain is common in Alzheimer's patients.*

Alzheimer's patients are atrophied in these areas (Cipriani et al., 2011) and display a buildup of amyloid plaques and neurofibrillary tangles.

Amyloid plaques are formed from amyloid precursor protein, which is thought to help repair injured neurons in the brain (Panza et al., 2014). When this protein isn't broken down properly, sticky fragments clump together on the outsides of neurons, forming plaques. The result is impaired neuronal communication, heightened inflammatory responses, blood vessel hemorrhage, and ultimately neuron death (Castello et al., 2014).

The buildup of plaques is thought to initiate the formation of neurofibrillary tangles. These tangles are made of a protein called tau. Tau forms part of the framework of neurons and is essential for nutrient and signal transfer across the cell (Castello et al., 2014). The buildup of plaques changes the shape of the tau protein, causing it to clump up and tangle together. This tangling damages the integrity of the neuron, and cell death ensues.

Individuals who have a genetic propensity toward the accumulation of amyloid plaques are more susceptible to developing Alzheimer's disease because this accumulation can lead to neuronal cell death. Thus many therapies are designed to remove these plaques (Panza et al., 2014). However, there is no evidence that these treatment strategies will be effective anytime soon (Rafii and Aisen, 2009). Treatment options for advanced Alzheimer's that has progressed to its later stages have generally been unsuccessful, so scientists are attempting to find strategies to prevent the buildup of amyloid plaques, which may stop Alzheimer's from developing in the first place. Preventative strategies begin with alternative energy sources to glucose because, similar to Parkinson's, the underlying cause of Alzheimer's may be an energy crisis in the brain.

Alzheimer's Disease as Type 3 Diabetes

Alarming epidemiological studies have shown that individuals with diabetes are ten times more likely to develop Alzheimer's disease (Talbot et al., 2012). This may be because, like Parkinson's disease, Alzheimer's has several commonalities with type 2 diabetes (Talbot et al., 2012).

With both type 2 diabetes and Alzheimer's disease, insulin resistance is present: insulin is unable to move glucose from the bloodstream into the cells. In type 2 diabetes, this occurs primarily in the muscles and liver. In Alzheimer's patients, it occurs primarily in the brain (Zhao et al., 2009; Kleinridders et al., 2014). (The idea that the cause of Alzheimer's disease is an impairment in glucose uptake and utilization in the brain was first supported nearly thirty years ago, when scientists found that individuals in the very early stages of Alzheimer's had a 45 percent lower brain glucose uptake [Hoyer et al., 1988]. This means that people who are more susceptible to Alzheimer's may have insulin resistance in the brain long before they are diagnosed with Alzheimer's.) In fact, the transporters that are responsible for moving glucose into neurons are decreased in the brain of a person with Alzheimer's disease (Simpson et al., 1994; Liu et al., 2008). In other words, plenty of blood glucose is available; it just can't be taken up and utilized. This has led some people to call Alzheimer's "type 3 diabetes."

When the brain isn't able to use available glucose effectively, the brain's ATP (cell energy) levels decrease, which leads to an impaired ability to handle and dispose of amyloid precursor protein—ultimately leading to the formation of amyloid plaques (Hoyer et al., 2004) and neurofibrillary tangles. Consequently, if we could either

1) enhance glucose uptake in the brain, or
2) provide an alternative source of fuel that could be taken up and used by the brain,

then it is conceivable that the brain wouldn't face "starvation in the face of plenty," thus preventing the development of the plaques and neurofibrillary tangles that characterize Alzheimer's.

Glucose may be the brain's primary fuel source in individuals on a carbohydrate-based diet, but research in fasting studies has shown that the brain can get as much as 85 percent of its fuel

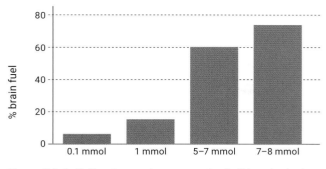
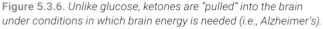

Figure 5.3.6. *Unlike glucose, ketones are "pulled" into the brain under conditions in which brain energy is needed (i.e., Alzheimer's).*

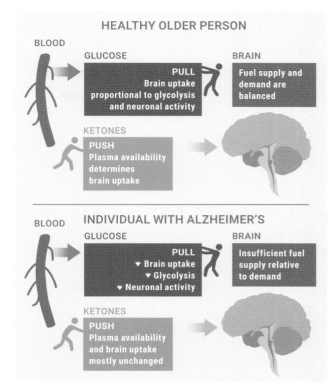

Figure 5.3.7. *The Alzheimer's brain cannot efficiently take up and utilize glucose as fuel.*

from ketones (Castellano et al., 2015). Blood ketone concentrations increase the utilization of ketones by the brain in a dose-dependent fashion, meaning that the higher the concentration of ketones in the blood, the better the brain is able to take them up and utilize them for fuel (Cunnane et al., 2016). Rather than trying to "push" glucose into a brain that is inefficient at taking it up, ketones are "pulled" into the brain as dictated by their levels in the blood and the transporters' ability to take them up into the brain. This has important implications for Alzheimer's disease because landmark studies have confirmed that, unlike glucose, ketone uptake and utilization in the brain are not impaired in individuals with Alzheimer's (Ogawa et al., 1996; Tunell et al., 1981). Recently, a study found that individuals with early Alzheimer's saw a 14 percent decline in blood glucose utilization but were able to fully utilize ketones (Castellano et al., 2015). So it is plausible that a ketogenic diet may stave off and slow the progression of Alzheimer's, particularly when implemented early, by preventing this energy deficit.

Unlike glucose, the transportation and uptake of ketones in the brain are not decreased in Alzheimer's patients. Think about that. We have the ability to provide an alternative fuel source to these individuals' brains, yet this option is often overlooked (Hashim and VanItallie, 2014). Imagine you are driving a hybrid car and accidently back into a pole, damaging the gas tank so it can't be refilled. Fortunately, because the car is a hybrid, you have a second, unaffected fuel source (a battery), so you can still get to your destination. The same logic seems to apply to the Alzheimer's brain, in which glucose metabolism is impaired. Instead of trying to force in bits of glucose here and there, we should explore providing an alternative source of fuel—ketones—that the brain can use.

Impaired Mitochondrial Function in Alzheimer's Disease

As with Parkinson's disease, extensive research has shown impaired mitochondrial function in patients with Alzheimer's disease. Along with changes in mitochondrial function, individuals with Alzheimer's tend to have elevated levels of oxidative stress (an accumulation of free radicals that may result in cell damage) and inflammation. When the ability of mitochondria to produce energy is impaired, it causes inflammation, increases amyloid plaque formation, and ultimately results in the deterioration of cognitive function. In fact, just as giving rats Rotenone, a substance that inhibits the production of energy in mitochondria, induces Parkinson's, it also causes inflammation, and the resulting symptoms resemble those seen in Alzheimer's patients. A ketogenic diet has been shown to increase the production of ATP—the form of energy used by cells—produce new mitochondria, decrease oxidative stress, and lower inflammation in the brains of animals, so it may be a viable way to overcome the impaired mitochondrial function seen in Alzheimer's patients (Gasior et al., 2006).

The Ketogenic Diet for Alzheimer's Disease

The first research study to investigate ketosis in patients with memory impairment (Reger et al., 2004) gave subjects a ketogenic meal consisting of 40 milliliters of MCTs and roughly 200 milliliters of whipping cream blended together. After the meal, the subjects' scores on a memory test increased significantly. This improvement was directly proportional to the rise in blood ketones (i.e., the higher their blood ketones, the better their score). These results were later supported in a ninety-day trial with daily MCT supplementation that also found positive results (Henderson et al., 2009). However, in both studies, subjects who had a gene associated with late-onset Alzheimer's disease did not improve as much as those who did not have this gene; it seems that the earlier Alzheimer's is detected and a ketogenic diet is initiated, the better the chance for improvements. This gene—the E4 allele—is associated with a greater buildup of plaque in the brain; because plaque impairs the ability to use glucose, it is conceivable that MCTs cannot raise ketone levels high enough to overcome this deficit (Reger et al., 2004).

More recently, scientists found that individuals with mild cognitive impairment, specifically memory decline, saw fairly robust improvements in memory following only six weeks of ketogenic dieting (Krikorian et al., 2012). These changes in performance were directly related to the levels of ketones in their urine. The authors of the study speculated that in addition to improved energy status of the brain, the ketogenic diet may have countered neuroinflammation (inflammation in the brain).

Lastly, laboratory mice with Alzheimer's disease have demonstrated a buildup of amyloid plaques that is similar to what is seen in humans (Van der Auwera et al., 2005). However, in the rats adapted to a ketogenic diet, fewer neurons died than in the rats on a carbohydrate-based diet (Yamada et al., 2005). While these results are preliminary, ketogenic diets and supplements show promise for overcoming the energy deficiency that results from impaired glucose uptake in Alzheimer's.

KETO CONCEPT

Early Intervention Is Key

By the time cognitive impairments due to Alzheimer's disease are apparent and a patient receives a diagnosis of Alzheimer's, a great deal of atrophy in the brain has already occurred. Therefore, those individuals with a family history of the disease and with medical conditions highly associated with Alzheimer's should consider ketogenic therapies early on. This may prevent the energy deficits due to impaired glucose uptake that seem to be behind the damage typically seen in Alzheimer's. Monitor both your and your loved ones' cognitive health, and remember that you shouldn't consistently be forgetting where you put your car keys *every day*.

Exogenous Ketones for Alzheimer's Disease

To investigate whether exogenous ketones outside of a ketogenic diet would be beneficial for Alzheimer's disease, researchers looked at animal brain cells. They found that the addition of sodium D-BHB doubled neuron survival and protected against amyloid plaque buildup associated with memory loss (Kashiwaya et al., 2000). Therefore, it is plausible that ketosis via supplementation might serve as a potential therapy for Alzheimer's.

Further studies have shown that mice fed a ketone ester had less anxiety and performed better on learning and memory tests (Kashiwaya et al., 2013). Moreover, they showed reduced levels of tau proteins, which make up the neurofibrillary tangles that characterize Alzheimer's disease in the brain. Adding BHB to a standard animal diet reversed the energy deficits in a mouse model of Alzheimer's disease (Zilberter et al., 2013). Researchers concluded that adding BHB to the diet could reverse the impaired brain energy metabolism observed in Alzheimer's.

In one of the first studies to analyze the effects of ketones in people with Alzheimer's, individuals with mild cognitive impairment or probable Alzheimer's were given 40 grams of a unique MCT blend, which slightly elevated serum BHB levels to between 0.5 and 0.8 mmol/L. Even with just a slight bump in blood ketone levels, there was a significant improvement

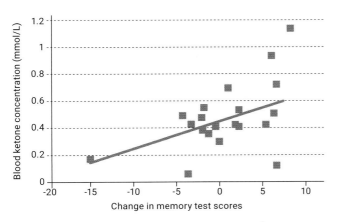

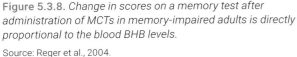

Figure 5.3.8. *Change in scores on a memory test after administration of MCTs in memory-impaired adults is directly proportional to the blood BHB levels.*

Source: Reger et al., 2004.

in scores on memory tests and other cognitive tasks (Reger et al., 2004). However, as mentioned earlier, taking too much MCTs can cause gastrointestinal distress, so this kind of supplementation needs to take that effect into account. Additionally, ketone salts and ketone esters can raise serum BHB levels to anywhere from 1.0 to 6.0 mmol/L—so their effects may be significantly greater.

Recently, our friend and colleague Dr. Mary Newport published a paper in which she talks about using a ketone ester for her husband, Steve, who had Alzheimer's disease. (We brought up their story at the beginning of this chapter.) Steve was in the late stages of the disease and demonstrated dementia, severe memory loss, poor concentration, a lack of organization, a tendency to misplace items, an inability to carry out activities of daily living, and an inability to spell and read.

During the first two days of supplementation, Steve received 21.5 grams of the D-BHB ketone ester three times a day, allowing his blood ketone levels to eventually reach 3 to 7 mmol/L. Dr. Newport noted a significant improvement in his mood and in his ability to recite and write out the alphabet, which he had been unable to do for many months. When the dose was increased to 28.7 grams, his ability to perform activities of daily life, such as showering, shaving, brushing his teeth, finding his way around the house, ordering food from a menu, and putting away utensils from the dishwasher, markedly improved. He had been unable to perform these kinds of tasks for several months prior to supplementation (Newport et al., 2015).

One of the greatest aspects of this case study was that the patient said he had more energy and was happier, and he felt that it was easier to accomplish various tasks. The treatment improved not only his Alzheimer's symptoms but also his quality of life. After several weeks of this supplementation protocol, Steve began to exhibit improvement in memory retrieval and other complex tasks such as yard work.

Steve tolerated the ketone ester well throughout the twenty-month treatment period. During this time, Dr. Newport indicated that "noticeable improvements in performance (conversation, interaction) were observed at higher, post-dose BHB levels," indicating that higher blood ketone levels resulted in further improvements. As shown in Figure 5.3.9, she examined doses of 25, 35, and 50 grams taken on separate days. At 25 grams, Steve's blood ketone levels reached anywhere from 3 to 5 mmol/L, while 50 grams yielded upwards of 7 mmol/L (Newport et al., 2015).

In another recent study, researchers discovered a neuroprotective mechanism in which the ketone bodies BHB and AcAc may block an amyloid protein from entering neurons, which improved mitochondrial energy production, synaptic plasticity (the ability to strengthen signals between neurons), learning,

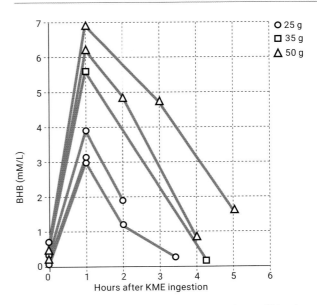

Figure 5.3.9. *The D-BHB ketone monoester elevated blood ketones in a dose-dependent fashion, and they remained elevated for several hours after administration. It is also worth noting that over twenty months of treatment, total cholesterol fell from 244 to 163 mg/dL, LDL fell from 145 to 81 mg/dL, and HDL fell from 85 to 68 mg/dL.*

Source: Newport et al., 2015.

and memory and reduced oxidative stress in mice with Alzheimer's symptoms (Yin et al., 2016). It's almost as if ketones act as a sort of bouncer, preventing this bad protein from entering the neurons of the brain and thus protecting the brain from the harmful effects that the protein could have. These observations and Dr. Newport's case study are profound examples of the potential for ketone supplements in treating Alzheimer's patients. We have received numerous anecdotal reports from individuals who are supplementing with exogenous ketones, with findings similar to Dr. Newport's. The future is bright for ketone supplementation and its potentially wide-reaching effects for this population.

In summary, Alzheimer's disease results in atrophy of the brain and accumulation of amyloid plaques and neural tangles. Failure to treat these outcomes by removing plaques has led scientists to believe that these are symptoms rather than the underlying cause of Alzheimer's. For the past three decades, research has demonstrated a strong link between insulin resistance in muscle and brain tissue and symptoms of Alzheimer's. Specifically, brain insulin resistance and impaired glucose uptake and utilization are thought to cause an energy crisis in the brain. This crisis leads to the improper disposal of amyloid, which leads to the formation of plaques, neural tangles, inflammation, and oxidative stress. The end result is atrophy and dementia in the latter stages of Alzheimer's. The ketogenic diet and/or ketone supplementation hold promise for overcoming this energy deficit and providing the brain with an alternative fuel source that can be utilized even under these conditions.

Traumatic Brain Injury

"Iron Mike" Webster is regarded by many as the greatest center ever to have played in the National Football League. He protected quarterback Terry Bradshaw as the Pittsburgh Steelers won four Super Bowls. He was also a nine-time Pro Bowler and seven-time All Pro, and he made the NFL's seventy-fifth anniversary all-time team. However, in 2002, tragedy struck: the fifty-year-old Pittsburgh

KETO CONCEPT

Headers Among Youth

Recently, a study was published that looked at repetitive head impacts (RHI) and cognitive function in youth athletes. To put this in perspective, more than 22 million children and adolescents worldwide are exposed to RHI in soccer alone. On average, soccer players perform six to twelve headers per game and many more during practice, resulting in thousands of headers over a player's career (Koerte et al., 2017). This study looked at cognitive function in a group of fifteen-year-old male soccer players throughout an entire season. The researchers found an association between exposure to specific RHI (long headers) and a lack of improvement in cognitive performance in the young athletes over time. Additionally, the kids who performed the most long headers saw the least improvement in reaction time over the course of the study. This indicates that even children in "noncontact" sports see cognitive impairment over the course of a season.

legend was found dead from a heart attack. Bennet Omalu, the forensic pathologist profiled in the movie *Concussion*, performed Webster's autopsy. Puzzled by the fact that Webster had died at such a young age, Dr. Omalu closely examined Webster's brain and discovered severe damage, similar to what is found in people with Alzheimer's disease. For example, Webster had a buildup of amyloid plaques and neurofibrillary tangles (Omalu et al., 2005). Dr. Omalu diagnosed Webster and another former Steeler, Terry Long, with chronic traumatic encephalopathy (CTE). Four years later, Andre Waters, a hard-hitting NFL safety from 1984 to 1995, became the third NFL player found to have CTE after his death (Cantu et al., 2007).

All three players who to this point had been documented to have died having suffered from CTE were known as "iron men." These athletes were hard hitters who never came out of the game, continuing to play through countless injuries, including concussions. Could playing contact sports like football lead to serious cognitive disorders later on? The answer appears to be a resounding yes, and the underlying cause appears to be repeated concussions (Cantu et al., 2007).

> "The concept that blunt-force trauma of the head causes brain damage is a generally accepted principle of medicine."
> —Dr. Bennet Omalu

Concussions are on the rise not only among professional athletes but also among youth. According to the U.S. Centers for Disease Control and Prevention (CDC), the number of reported concussions in people of all ages has doubled in the last ten years. The American Academy of Pediatrics reports that emergency room visits for concussions in kids ages eight to nineteen have doubled in the last decade (Head Case). Let's look at some other alarming statistics:

- One in five high school athletes sustains a concussion during the regular season each year.

- 90 percent of diagnosed concussions do not involve a loss of consciousness and often go undetected initially.

- Cumulative sports concussions have been shown to increase the likelihood of permanent neurologic disability by 39 percent.

- 47 percent of all reported sports concussions occur in high school football, followed by wrestling, ice hockey, and women's soccer.

When we think about traumatic brain injury (TBI) in sports, we often think about football; however, the prevalence of concussions in women's sports is just as high as, if not higher than, the prevalence of concussions in men's athletics (Hootman, 2007). And the problem isn't unique to athletes. According to the CDC, an estimated 5.3 million Americans live with a disability related to TBI. The top three causes are car accidents, blast waves generated by firearms, and falls.

A concussion, defined as a short-term dysfunction of the brain caused by blunt or mechanical force, is considered a mild TBI. Signs of mild TBI include confusion, disorientation, dizziness, and headache.

As with other cognitive disorders, the root cause of TBI symptoms seems to be a cellular energy crisis. Following a concussion or blow to the head, a cascade of events occurs that causes a robust increase in energy needs in the brain. At the same time, TBI impairs the brain's ability to use glucose.

Think about that for a moment: the brain needs more energy than it usually does, yet it has an impaired ability to use glucose as an energy source. This results in an energy crisis that causes secondary injury to the brain (Barkhoudarian et al., 2011).

> "Please, see that my brain is given to the N.F.L.'s brain bank."
> —former Chicago Bears safety Dave Duerson, in his suicide note

KETO CONCEPT

Football, TBI, and Ketones

Think about what traditionally happens in a football game. Let's say Player A, a running back, ran the ball twenty-five times in the game. Like most running backs, he was frequently hit by hefty linemen and linebackers. The running back was expected to continue to perform play after play, despite repeated blows to the head. Now let's look at his teammate, Player B, a wide receiver who ran a slant route across the middle of the field and got demolished by a middle linebacker. He lay motionless on the ground and was helped off the field. Believe it or not, both of these athletes are at risk for CTE and may have varying degrees of TBI. Yet they walk to the sideline and grab sugar-filled sports drinks to replenish their bodies (or so they think) before going back out onto the field.

It's as if you blew out two tires, and the stranger who stopped by your stranded car to help dropped off a couple gallons of gas and then sped off. It was a nice gesture, but the gas wouldn't help you—what you really needed was new tires. Similarly, if our brains are unable to effectively use the fuel we provide, then what good is that fuel? This is what happens when athletes at risk for TBI rely on sugar to fuel their brains and bodies. When glucose uptake in the brain is impaired, sugar can't adequately fuel the brain, no matter how much sugar is ingested.

> "If I didn't know anything about this case and I looked at the slides, I would have asked, 'Was this patient a boxer?'"
> —Dr. Ronald Hamilton, physician to former Pittsburgh Steelers tackle Justin Strzelczyk

Here's what happens on a cellular level: During a traumatic impact, neurons in the brain are stretched, triggering a robust release of neurotransmitters. These neurotransmitters trigger the release of potassium ions from the neuron, disrupting the ratio of sodium ions outside the neuron and potassium ions inside the neuron, which damages the neuron's ability to communicate with other neurons. (Remember our Black Friday example with people going in and out of the store? In this case, the release of people leaving the store messes with the doors' ability to open and close, and poor communication leads to chaos.) To re-establish the proper balance of sodium and potassium, a pump begins working overtime to drive potassium back into the neuron. However, the pump requires a great deal of energy, which normally comes from glucose. Unfortunately, following a TBI, blood flow to the brain is initially decreased (Yamakami et al., 1989; Velarde et al., 1992). Thus, while glucose is being used at rapid rates, glucose delivery to the brain is impaired. To compound the situation, the neurotransmitters also cause a large release of calcium into the neurons; calcium then accumulates in the mitochondria, further impairing energy production. After a TBI, brain glucose use is diminished for twenty-four hours and remains low for an average of five to fourteen days, and at times for months, depending on the severity of the injury (Hovda et al., 1994). The level of depressed glucose metabolism is strongly associated with cognitive impairments, indicating that the longer the brain can't take up

that glucose, the worse cognitive function will be (Barkhoudarian et al., 2011).

Chronic repeated TBI and the energy crises that ensue are thought to underlie chronic traumatic encephalopathy (CTE), a neurodegenerative disease that shares several characteristics with Alzheimer's. Remember when we discussed former NFL athletes and the complications of life after the game? Those individuals had developed CTE. Behavioral symptoms denoting the onset of CTE occur, on average, eight years after retirement from sports known for causing head trauma, such as football, hockey, and boxing. The average age at which symptoms begin to appear is forty-two years; symptoms include suicidality, memory loss, impaired decision-making abilities, loss of emotion, and signs of Parkinson's disease, such as movement, speech, and ocular abnormalities. Like those with Alzheimer's, individuals with CTE have large amounts of neurofibrillary tangles in their brains, as well as amyloid plaques (Raiff et al., 2015). However, in patients with CTE, these tangles and plaques are localized in specific regions of the brain (the frontal and temporal cortices), which may be where blunt force trauma has its greatest impacts.

> "I think it's important for everyone to know that Junior did indeed suffer from CTE. It's important that we take steps to help these players."
> —Gina Seau, ex-wife of Junior Seau, former NFL linebacker

There are at least five different ways in which being in a state of ketosis may either be beneficial as a "prehab" to prevent CTE or aid in recovery after a traumatic brain injury:

- Because TBI results in impaired glucose uptake by the brain, providing an alternative energy source—ketones—may be beneficial. Moreover, ketones are more than 25 percent more efficient than glucose as a fuel, thus they yield more ATP per molecule (Veech et al., 2001). Research has shown that following a TBI, the number of transporters that move ketones into cells increases by more than 85 percent (Prins and Giza, 2006). With this increase in transport activity, cerebral uptake of ketones is even higher, potentially indicating the absolute

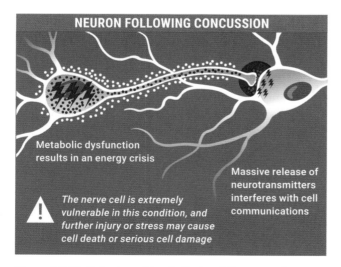

NEURON FOLLOWING CONCUSSION

Metabolic dysfunction results in an energy crisis

Massive release of neurotransmitters interferes with cell communications

⚠ *The nerve cell is extremely vulnerable in this condition, and further injury or stress may cause cell death or serious cell damage*

Figure 5.3.10. *Following a blow to the head, the neuron faces an energy crisis..*

Source: www.slideshare.net/forefront/saint-brigidimpact-concussion-seminar.

need for an elevation in ketones during this time. In addition, an enzyme involved in the metabolism of BHB is increased following a head injury (Tieu et al., 2003). All this suggests that the inability to use glucose triggers the body to increase its ability to use ketones following a TBI (Prins et al., 2006).

- Ketones lower free radical production, first by improving mitochondrial function and then by increasing antioxidant enzymes that counter oxidative stress (Ziegler et al., 2003). This reduction in oxidative stress helps spare neurons from further damage.

- Ketones improve mitochondrial function and number, another way of increasing energy production (Veech et al., 2001).

- Ketones lower inflammation (Youm et al., 2015). Chronic inflammation can harm healthy tissues; therefore, reducing inflammation in people with TBI can help maintain healthy neurons.

- Ketogenic diets lower apoptosis, or cell death, which is the main pathway through which TBI lesions spread. Studies have shown that animals fed a ketogenic diet around the time of receiving a TBI had decreased brain swelling and less apoptosis (Hu et al., 2009).

The Ketogenic Diet for Traumatic Brain Injury

The potential application for ketogenic diets in individuals with TBI is promising. In studies in which adolescent and adult rats underwent experimentally induced TBI, rats put on a ketogenic diet immediately after the TBI saw improvements in cognitive and motor function as compared to the control group. Moreover, brain tissue showed improved energy production twenty-four hours after the injury (Biros et al., 1996).

Putting adolescent animals on a ketogenic diet immediately following a TBI decreased the size of the lesions in the brain and decreased cell death (Appelberg et al., 2009). Adolescent rats may have had better results than their adult counterparts because they had 80 percent more ketone transporters (Prins et al., 2014). Generally, younger animals—and humans—are more fat-adapted than older adults (Prins et al., 2005; Deng-Bryant et al.,

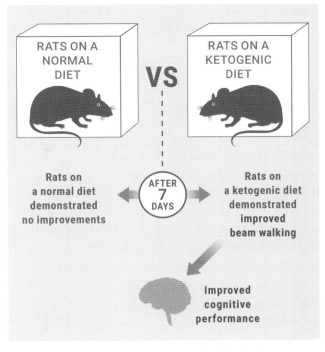

Figure 5.3.11. *Rats put on a ketogenic diet following injury saw improvements in cognitive and motor function.*

Source: Appelberg et al., 2009.

2011; Prins et al., 2014). At older ages, a combination of ketogenic dieting, exercise, and exogenous ketones may be necessary to elevate ketones enough to overcome the energy deficit and increase ketone transports in order to allow the brain to effectively take them up and use them as fuel.

As a protective measure, adults may need to keto-adapt for a longer period prior to receiving a TBI. And since we cannot predict when or how frequently TBI will occur, athletes in contact sports may find it effective to be on a ketogenic diet permanently, with periods of intermittent fasting (or to utilize supplemental ketones strategically, as we'll discuss in the next section). The keto adaptation process increases ketone-transporting capacity (Leino et al., 2001). It is also plausible that adult athletes may have a greater amount of ketone transporters than the sedentary animals traditionally used in these studies, as exercise training itself has been shown to increase ketone transporter expression in animal brains, specifically in the hippocampus and cortex regions (Aveseh et al., 2014). Though speculative at this point, it is conceivable that adult athletes may respond similarly to adolescents in their ability to take up and utilize ketones quickly and effectively.

Exogenous Ketones and Traumatic Brain Injury

One of the first studies done on ketones and TBI demonstrated that infusing BHB following a TBI in an adult rat resulted in improved ATP concentrations (Massieu et al., 2003; Prins et al., 2004). More recently, a study found that BHB decreased the generation of reactive oxygen species (ROS), which are molecules that can damage tissue and DNA, and protected against cell damage and death (Wang et al., 2016).

Several studies that have been done with ketone supplementation have looked at glutamate neurotoxicity, a marker of oxidative stress that can be toxic to neurons at high concentrations and is highly associated with brain trauma. Ketones can protect against this neurotoxicity and limit the neuronal damage (Maalouf et al., 2007; Mejía-Toiber et al., 2006). TBI can also lead to conditions of decreased oxygen availability due to a decrease in metabolism, and BHB has been shown to significantly reduce cerebral swelling, dead tissue area size, and defective functioning of the nervous system by improving brain energy metabolism (Suzuki et al., 2002).

We look forward to the day when athletes from various contact sports are encouraged to consume exogenous ketones before, during, and after competition in order to provide their brains with the necessary fuel to function optimally. We wouldn't be surprised if, in the next couple of years, we started seeing ketone supplementation implemented as part of the concussion treatment protocol. More research needs to be done in this area, but it is being investigated heavily.

> "A child who plays a game of football for one season without any documented concussion—several months after that season . . . there is evidence of brain damage."
>
> —Dr. Bennet Omalu

In conclusion, TBI results in an energy crisis in the brain and impaired glucose metabolism for several days or even months following the trauma. Research suggests that correcting the energy crisis may assist in recovery and restore cellular energy. Adolescents tend to have a greater ability to utilize ketones than adults; however, that may not be the case in adults who are physically active (i.e., athletes) and have upregulated MCT transporters. Therefore, placing individuals on a ketogenic diet immediately before and following injury, along with a strategic implementation of exogenous ketones, may provide a benefit to both adolescents and adults who have or may experience traumatic brain injury, but this remains to be determined.

CHAPTER SUMMARY

This chapter discussed neurodegenerative diseases: Parkinson's, epilepsy, Alzheimer's, and traumatic brain injury (TBI). Two common threads among these are impaired mitochondrial function and a reduced ability to utilize glucose. The result is an energy crisis that causes neuron death, inflammation, and poor cognitive function. Ketogenic dieting and ketone supplementation attempt to correct the energy crisis by providing an alternative fuel source for the brain that is more efficient than glucose and may aid in decreasing injury. A number of studies have shown that ketogenic dieting and possibly ketone supplementation are efficacious in these situations, and we encourage patients, their families, and their healthcare providers to investigate how these therapies might be of benefit.

References

Appelberg, K. S., D. A. Hovda, and M. L. Prins. "The effects of a ketogenic diet on behavioral outcome after controlled cortical impact injury in the juvenile and adult rat." *Journal of Neurotrauma* 26, no. 4 (2009): 497–506. doi: 10.1089/neu.2008.0664.

Aveseh, M., R. Nikooie, V. Sheibani, and S. Esmaeili-Mahani. "Endurance training increases brain lactate uptake during hypoglycemia by up regulation of brain lactate transporters." *Molecular and Cellular Endocrinology* 394, nos. 1–2 (2014): 29–36. doi: 10.1016/j.mce.2014.06.019.

Balaban, R. S., S. Nemoto, and T. Finkel. "Mitochondria, oxidants, and aging." *Cell* 120, no. 4 (2005): 483–95.

Barborka, C. J. "Epilepsy in adults: results of treatment by ketogenic diet in one hundred cases." *Archives of Neurology & Psychiatry* 23, no. 5 (1930): 904–14.

Barkhoudarian, G., D. A. Hovda, and C. C. Giza. "The molecular pathophysiology of concussive brain injury." *Clinics in Sports Medicine* 30, no. 1 (2011): 33–48.

Bastible, C. "The ketogenic treatment of epilepsy." *Irish Journal of Medical Science (1926–1967)* 6, no. 9 (1931): 506–20.

Bellucci, A., G. Collo, I. Sarnico, L. Battistin, C. Missale, and P. Spano. "Alpha-synuclein aggregation and cell death triggered by energy deprivation and dopamine overload are counteracted by D2/D3 receptor activation." *Journal of Neurochemistry* 106, no. 2 (2008): 560–77. doi: 10.1111/j.1471-4159.2008.05406.x.

Betarbet, R., T. B. Sherer, G. MacKenzie, M. Garcia-Osuna, A. V. Panov, and J. T. Greenamyre. "Chronic systemic pesticide exposure reproduces features of Parkinson's disease." *Nature Neuroscience* 3: (2000): 1301–6.

Biros, M. H., and R. Nordness. "Effects of chemical pretreatment on post-traumatic cortical edema in the rat." *American Journal of Emergency Medicine* 14, no. 1 (1996): 27–32. doi: 10.1016/S0735-6757(96)90008-X.

Borghammer, P. "Perfusion and metabolism imaging studies in Parkinson's disease." *European Journal of Neurology* 17, no. 2 (2012): 314–20.

Borghammer, P., M. Chakravarty, K. Y. Jonsdottir, N. Sato, H. Matsuda, K. Ito, ... and A. Gjedde. "Cortical hypometabolism and hypoperfusion in Parkinson's disease is extensive: probably even at early disease stages." *Brain Structure and Function* 214, no. 4 (2010): 303–17. doi: 10.1007/s00429-010-0246-0.

Bosco, D., et al. "Dementia is associated with insulin resistance in patients with Parkinson's disease." *Journal of Neurological Science* 315, no. 1–2 (2012): 39–43. doi: 10.1016/j.jns.2011.12.008.

Bough, K. J., and J. M. Rho. "Anticonvulsant mechanisms of the ketogenic diet." *Epilepsia* 48, no. 1 (2007): 43–58.

Cantu, R. C. "Chronic traumatic encephalopathy in the National Football League." *Neurosurgery* 61, no. 2 (2007): 223–5.

Caraballo, R. H., R. O. Cersósimo, D. Sakr, A. Cresta, N. Escobal, and N. Fejerman. "Ketogenic diet in patients with Dravet syndrome." *Epilepsia* 46, no. 9 (2005): 1539–44.

Castellano, C. A., S. Nugent, N. Paquet, S. Tremblay, C. Bocti, G. Lacombe, ... and S. C. Cunnane. "Lower brain 18F-fluorodeoxyglucose uptake but normal 11C-acetoacetate metabolism in mild Alzheimer's disease dementia." *Journal of Alzheimer's Disease* 43, no. 4 (2015): 1343–53. doi: 10.3233/JAD-141074.

Castello, M. A., and S. Soriano. "On the origin of Alzheimer's disease. Trials and tribulations of the amyloid hypothesis." *Ageing Research Reviews* 13 (2014): 10–12.

Cipriani, G., C. Dolciotti, L. Picchi, and U. Bonuccelli. "Alzheimer and his disease: a brief history." *Neurological Sciences* 32, no. 2 (2011): 275–9. doi: 10.1007/s10072-010-0454-7.

Cotter, D. G., D. A. d'Avignon, A. E. Wentz, M. L. Weber, and P. A. Crawford. "Obligate role for ketone body oxidation in neonatal metabolic homeostasis." *Journal of Biological Chemistry* 286, no. 9 (2011): 6902–10. doi: 10.1074/jbc.M110.192369.

Craft, S. "Insulin resistance syndrome and Alzheimer's disease: age- and obesity-related effects on memory, amyloid, and inflammation." *Neurobiology of Aging* 26, suppl 1 (2005): 65–69.

Cunnane, S. C., A. Courchesne-Loyer, V. St-Pierre, C. Vandenberghe, T. Pierotti, M. Fortier, ... and C. A. Castellano. "Can ketones compensate for deteriorating brain glucose uptake during aging? Implications for the risk and treatment of Alzheimer's disease." *Annals of the New York Academy of Sciences* 1367, no. 1 (2016): 12–20. doi: 10.1111/nyas.12999.

D'Agostino, D. P., R. Pilla, H. E. Held, C. S. Landon, M. Puchowicz, H. Brunengraber, ... and J. B. Dean. "Therapeutic ketosis with ketone ester delays central nervous system oxygen toxicity seizures in rats." *American Journal of Physiology-Regulatory, Integrative and Comparative Physiology* 304, no. 10 (2013): R829–R836. doi: 10.1152/ajpregu.00506.2012.

Davis, L. M., J. R. Pauly, R. D. Readnower, J. M. Rho, and P. G. Sullivan. "Fasting is neuroprotective following traumatic brain injury." *Journal of Neuroscience Research* 86, no. 8 (2008): 1812–22.

Deng-Bryant, Y., M. L. Prins, D. A. Hovda, and N. G. Harris. "Ketogenic diet prevents alterations in brain metabolism in young but not adult rats after traumatic brain injury." *Journal of Neurotrauma* 28, no. 9 (2011): 1813–25.

El-Rashidy, O. F., M. F. Nassar, I. A. Abdel-Hamid, R. H. Shatla, M. H. Abdel-Hamid, S. S. Gabr, ... and S. Y. Shaaban. "Modified Atkins diet vs classic ketogenic formula in intractable epilepsy." *Acta Neurologica Scandinavica* 128, no. 6 (2013): 402–8.

Faul M., L. Xu, M. M. Wald, and V. G. Coronado. "Traumatic brain injury in the United States: emergency department visits, hospitalizations and deaths 2002–2006." Centers for Disease Control and Prevention, National Center for Injury Prevention and Control, Atlanta, GA. (2010). Available at www.cdc.gov/TraumaticBrainInjury/.

Ferrucci, M., L. Pasquali, S. Ruggieri, A. Paparelli, and F. Fornai. "Alpha-synuclein and autophagy as common steps in neurodegeneration." *Parkinsonism & Related Disorders* 14, suppl 2 (2008): S180–4.

Gasior, M., M. A. Rogawski, and A. L. Hartman. "Neuroprotective and disease-modifying effects of the ketogenic diet." *Behavioural Pharmacology* 17, no. 5–6 (2006): 431–9.

George Jr., A. L. "Inherited channelopathiesassociated with epilepsy." *Epilepsy Currents* 4, no. 2 (2004): 65–70.

Giza, C. C., and D. A. Hovda. "The neurometaboliccascade of concussion." *Journal of Athletic Training* 36, no. 3 (2001): 228–35.

Global Burden of Disease Study 2013, Collaborators. "Global, regional, and national incidence, prevalence, and years lived with disability for 301 acute and chronic diseases and injuries in 188 countries, 1990–2013: a systematic analysis for the Global Burden of Disease Study 2013." *The Lancet* 386, no. 9995 (2015): 743–800.

Greene A. E., M. T. Todorova, R. McGowan, and T. N. Seyfried. "Caloric restriction inhibits seizure susceptibility in epileptic EL mice by reducing blood glucose." *Epilepsia* 42, no. 11 (2001): 1371–8.

Greene, A. E., M. T. Todorova, and T. N. Seyfried. "Perspectives on the metabolic management of epilepsy through dietary reduction of glucose and elevation of ketone bodies." *Journal of Neurochemistry* 86, no. 3 (2003): 529–37.

Hall, E. D., P. K. Andrus, and P. A. Yonkers. "Brain hydroxyl radical generation in acute experimental head injury." *Journal of Neurochemistry* 60, no. 2 (1993): 588–94.

Hawkins R. A., D. H. Williamson, and H. A. Krebs. "Ketone-body utilization by adult and suckling rat brain in vivo." *Biochemical Journal* 122, no. 1 (1971): 13–18.

Henderson, S. T., J. L. Vogel, L. J. Barr, F. Garvin, J. J. Jones, and L. C. Costantini. "Study of the ketogenic agent AC-1202 in mild to moderate Alzheimer's disease: a randomized, double-blind, placebo-controlled, multicenter trial." *Nutrition & Metabolism* 6 (2009): 31.

Hirsch, E. C., S. Hunot, P. Damier, and B. Faucheux. "Glial cells and inflammation in Parkinson's disease: a role in neurodegeneration?" *Annals of Neurology* 44, 3 suppl 1 (1998): S115–20.

Hootman, J. M., R. Dick, and J. Agel. "Epidemiology of collegiate injuries for 15 sports: summary and recommendations for injury prevention initiatives." *Journal of Athletic Training* 42, no. 2 (2007): 311–9.

Hovda, D. A., J. Lifshitz, J. A. Berry, H. Badie, A. Yoshino, and S. M. Lee. "Long-term changes in metabolic rates for glucose following mild, moderate, and severe concussive head injuries in adult rats." *Society for Neuroscience*. Abstract. (1994).

Hoyer, S. "Glucose metabolism and insulin receptor signal transduction in Alzheimer disease." *European Journal of Pharmacology* 490, no. 1–3 (2004): 115–25.

Hoyer, S., K. Oesterreich, and O. Wagner. "Glucose metabolism as the site of the primary abnormality in early-onset dementia of Alzheimer type?" *Journal of Neurology* 235, no. 3 (1988): 143–8.

Hu, Z. G., H. D. Wang, W. Jin, and H. X. Yin. "Ketogenic diet reduces cytochrome C release and cellular apoptosis following traumatic brain injury in juvenile rats." *Annals of Clinical & Laboratory Science* 39, no. 1 (2009): 76–83.

Huno, S., and E. C. Hirsch. "Neuroinflammatory processes in Parkinson's disease." *Annals of Neurology* 53, suppl 3 (2003): S49–58; discussion S60.

Huttenlocher, P. R., A. J. Wilbourn, and J. M. Signore. "Medium-chain triglycerides as a therapy for intractable childhood epilepsy." *Neurology* 21, no. 11 (1971): 1097–103.

Isaev, N. K., E. V. Stel'mashuk,and D. B. Zorov. "Cellular mechanisms of brain hypoglycemia." *Biochemistry* (Moscow) 72, no. 5 (2007): 471–8.

Izumi, Y., K. Ishii, H. Katsuki, A. M. Benz, and C. F. Zorumski. "Beta-hydroxybutyrate fuels synaptic function during development. Histological and physiological evidence in rat hippocampal slices." *Journal of Clinical Investigation* 101, no. 5 (1998): 1121–32.

Juge, N., et al. "Metabolic control of vesicular glutamate transport and release." *Neuron* 68 (2010): 99–211. doi: 10.1016/j.neuron.2010.09.002.

Juge, N., J. A. Gray, H. Omote, T. Miyaji, T. Inoue, C. Hara, ... and Y. Moriyama. "Metabolic control of vesicular glutamate transport and release." *Neuron* 68, no. 1 (2010): 99–112. doi: 10.1016/j.neuron.2010.09.002.

Kashiwaya, Y., T. Takeshima, N. Mori, K. Nakashima, K. Clarke, and R. L. Veech. "D-beta-hydroxybutyrate protects neurons in models of Alzheimer's and Parkinson's disease." *Proceedings of the National Academy of Sciences* 97, no. 10 (2000): 5440–4.

Kashiwaya, Y., C. Bergman, J. H. Lee, R. Wan, M. T. King, M. R. Mughal, ... and R. L. Veech. "A ketone ester diet exhibits anxiolytic and cognition-sparing properties, and lessens amyloid and tau pathologies in a mouse model of Alzheimer's disease." *Neurobiology of Aging* 34, no. 6 (2013): 1530–9. doi: 10.1016/j.neurobiolaging.2012.11.023.

Keith, H. M. "Factors influencing experimentally produced convulsions." *Archives of Neurology & Psychiatry* 29, no. 1 (1933): 148–54.

Keith, H. M., G. W. Stavraky, C. H. Rogerson, D. H. Hardcastle, and K. Duguid. "Experimental convulsions induced by administration of thujone." *Journal of Nervous and Mental Disease* 84, no. 1 (1936): 84.

Kim, D. Y., J. Vallejo, and J. M. Rho. "Ketones prevent synaptic dysfunction induced by mitochondrial respiratory complex inhibitors." *Journal of Neurochemistry* 114, no. 1 (2010): 130–41. doi: 10.1111/j.1471-4159.2010.06728.x.

Klein, P., J. Janousek, A. Barber, and R. Weissberger. "Ketogenic diet treatment in adults with refractory epilepsy." *Epilepsy & Behavior* 19, no. 4 (2010): 575–9. doi: 10.1016/j.yebeh.2010.09.016.

Kleinridders, A., H. A. Ferris, W. Cai, and C. R. Kahn. "Insulin action in brain regulates systemic metabolism and brain function." *Diabetes* 63, no. 7 (2014): 2232–43. doi: 10.2337/db14-0568.

Koerte, I. K., E. Nichols, Y. Tripodis, V. Schultz, R. Lehner, R. Igbinoba, ... and D. Kaufmann. "Impaired cognitive performance in youth athletes exposed to repetitive head impacts." *Journal of Neurotrauma* (2017): epub ahead of print. doi: 10.1089/neu.2016.4960.

Kossoff, E. H., M. C. Cervenka, B. J. Henry, C. A. Haney, and Z. Turner. "A decade of the modified Atkins diet (2003–2013): results, insights, and future directions." *Epilepsy & Behavior* 29, no. 3 (2013): 437–42.

Kossoff, E. H., and J. R. McGrogan. "Worldwide use of the ketogenic diet." *Epilepsia* 46, no. 2 (2005): 280–9.

Krikorian, R., M. D. Shidler, K. Dangelo, S. C. Couch, S. C. Benoit, and D. J. Clegg. "Dietary ketosis enhances memory in mild cognitive impairment." *Neurobiology of Aging* 33, no. 2 (2012): 425.e19–27. doi: 10.1016/j.neurobiolaging.2010.10.006.

Leino, R. L., D. Z. Gerhart, R. Duelli, B. E. Enerson, and L. R. Drewes. "Diet-induced ketosis increases monocarboxylate transporter (MCT1) levels in rat brain." *Neurochemistry International* 38, no. 6 (2001): 519–27.

Likhodi, S. S., and W. M. Burnham. "Ketogenic diet: does acetone stop seizures?" *Medical Science Monitor* 8, no. 8 (2002): HY19–24.

Lipman, I. J., M. E. Boykin, and R. E. Flora. "Glucose intolerance in Parkinson's disease." *Journal of Chronic Diseases* 27, no. 11–12 (1974): 573–9.

Liu, Y., F. Liu, K. Iqbal, I. Grundke-Iqbal, and C. X. Gong. "Decreased glucose transporters correlate to abnormal hyperphosphorylation of tau in Alzheimer disease." *FEBS Letters* 582, no. 2 (2008): 359–64.

Lutas, A., and G. Yellen. "The ketogenic diet: metabolic influences on brain excitability and epilepsy." *Trends in Neurosciences* 36, no. 1 (2013): 32–40. doi: 10.1016/j.tins.2012.11.005.

Lying-Tunell, U., B. S. Lindblad, H. O. Malmlund, and B. Persson. "Cerebral blood flow and metabolic rate of oxygen, glucose, lactate, pyruvate,

ketone bodies and amino acids." *Acta Neurologica Scandinavica* 63, no. 6 (1981): 337–50.

Maalouf, M., P. G. Sullivan, L. Davis, D. Y. Kim, and J. M. Rho. "Ketones inhibit mitochondrial production of reactive oxygen species production following glutamate excitotoxicity by increasing NADH oxidation." *Neuroscience* 145, no. 1 (2007): 256–64. doi: 10.1016/j.neuroscience.2006.11.065.

Magiorkinis, E., K. Sidiropoulou, and A. Diamantis. "Hallmarks in the history of epilepsy: epilepsy in antiquity." *Epilepsy & Behavior* 17, no. 1 (2010): 103–8.

Massieu, L., M. L. Haces, T. Montiel, and K. Hernandez-Fonseca. "Acetoacetate protects hippocampal neurons against glutamate-mediated neuronal damage during glycolysis inhibition." *Neuroscience* 120, no. 2 (2003): 365–78. doi: 10.1016/S0306-4522(03)00266-5.

Mejía-Toiber, J., T. Montiel, and L. Massieu. "D-β-hydroxybutyrate prevents glutamate-mediated lipoperoxidation and neuronal damage elicited during glycolysis inhibition in vivo." *Neurochemical Research* 31, no. 12, (2006): 1399–406.

Muzykewicz, D. A., D. A. Lyczkowski, N. Memon, K. D. Conant, H. H. Pfeifer, and E. A. Thiele. "Efficacy, safety, and tolerability of the low glycemic index treatment in pediatric epilepsy." *Epilepsia* 50, no. 5 (2009): 1118–26. doi: 10.1111/j.1528-1167.2008.01959.x.

Neal, E. (Ed.). *Dietary Treatment of Epilepsy: Practical Implementation of Ketogenic Therapy*. Hoboken, NJ: John Wiley & Sons, 2012.

Neal, E. G., H. Chaffe, R. H. Schwartz, M. S. Lawson, N. Edwards, G. Fitzsimmons, ... and J. H. Cross. "The ketogenic diet for the treatment of childhood epilepsy: a randomised controlled trial." *Lancet Neurology* 7, no. 6 (2008): 500–6. doi: 10.1016/S1474-4422(08)70092-9.

Newport, M. T., T. B. VanItallie, Y. Kashiwaya, M. T. King, and R. L. Veech. "A new way to produce hyperketonemia: use of ketone ester in a case of Alzheimer's disease." *Alzheimer's & Dementia* 11, no. 1 (2015): 99–103.

Ogawa, M., H. Fukuyama, Y. Ouchi, H. Yamauchi, and J. Kimura. "Altered energy metabolism in Alzheimer's disease." *Journal of the Neurological Sciences* 139, no. 1 (1996): 78–82.

Omalu, B. I., S. T. DeKosky, R. L. Minster, M. I. Kamboh, R. L. Hamilton, and C. H. Wecht. "Chronic traumatic encephalopathy in a National Football League player." *Neurosurgery* 57, no. 1 (2005): 128–34.

Ota, M., J. Matsuo, I. Ishida, K. Hattori, T. Teraishi, H. Tonouchi, ... and H. Kunugi. "Effect of a ketogenic meal on cognitive function in elderly adults: potential for cognitive enhancement." *Psychopharmacology* 233, no. 21–22 (2016): 3797–802.

Panza, F., V. Solfrizzi, B. P. Imbimbo, R. Tortelli, A. Santamato, and G. Logroscino. "Amyloid-based immunotherapy for Alzheimer's disease in the time of prevention trials: the way forward." *Expert Review of Clinical Immunology* 10, no. 3 (2014): 405–419. doi: 10.1586/1744666X.2014.883921.

Parker, W. D., S. J. Boyson, and J. K. Parks. "Abnormalities of the electron transport chain in idiopathic Parkinson's disease." *Annals of Neurology* 26, no. 6 (1989): 719–23.

Polito, C., V. Berti, S. Ramat, E. Vanzi, M. T. De Cristofaro, G. Pellicanò, ... and A. Pupi. "Interaction of caudate dopamine depletion and brain metabolic changes with cognitive dysfunction in early Parkinson's disease." *Neurobiology of Aging* 33, no. 1 (2012): 206.e29–39.

Powell, K. L., S. M. Cain, T. P. Snutch, and T. J. O'Brien. "Low threshold T-type calcium channels as targets for novel epilepsy treatments." *British Journal of Clinical Pharmacology* 77, no. 5 (2014): 729–39. doi: 10.1111/bcp.12205.

Prins, M. L., and J. H. Matsumoto. "The collective therapeutic potential of cerebral ketone metabolism in traumatic brain injury." *Journal of Lipid Research* 55, no. 12 (2014): 2450–7. doi: 10.1194/jlr.R046706.

Prins, M. L., Y. Deng-Bryant, S. Appelberg, and D. A. Hovda. "Changes in cerebral microvessel expression of MCT1 and GLUT1 following controlled cortical impact in juvenile and adult rats." *Society for Neurotrauma* 24, (2007): 1267.

Prins, M. L., L. S. Fujima, and D. A. Hovda. "Age-dependent reduction of cortical contusion volume by ketones after traumatic brain injury." *Journal of Neuroscience Research* 82, no. 3 (2005): 413–20.

Prins, M. L., and C. C. Giza. "Induction of monocarboxylate transporter-2 expression and ketone transport following traumatic brain injury in juvenile and adult rats." *Developmental Neuroscience* 28, no. 4–5 (2006): 447–56.

Prins, M. L., S. M. Lee, L. S. Fujima, and D. A. Hovda. "Increased cerebral uptake and oxidation of exogenous betaHB improves ATP following traumatic brain injury in adult rats." *Journal of Neurochemistry* 90, no. 3 (2004): 666–72.

Purves, D., G. J. Augustine, D. Fitzpatrick, L. C. Katz, A. S. LaMantia, J. O. McNamara, and S. M. Williams. "Circuits within the basal ganglia system." *Neuroscience.* 2nd Edition. Sunderland, MA: Sinauer Associates, 2001.

Rafii, M. S., and P. S. Aisen. "Recent developments in Alzheimer's disease therapeutics." *BMC Medicine* 7 (2009): 7. doi: 10.1186/1741-7015-7-7.

Raiff, M. C. *Traumatic Brain Injury and Neurodegenerative Disease: A Literature Review* (Doctoral dissertation, University of South Florida, St. Petersburg, 2015).

Ramirez-Bermudez, J. "Alzheimer's disease: critical notes on the history of a medical concept." *Archives of Medical Research* 43, no. 8 (2012): 595–9. doi: 10.1016/j.arcmed.2012.11.008.

Reger, M. A., S. T. Henderson, C. Hale, B. Cholerton, L. D. Baker, G. S. Watson, ... and S. Craft. "Effects of β-hydroxybutyrate on cognition in memory-impaired adults." *Neurobiology of Aging* 25, no. 3 (2004): 311–4.

Rubin, J., and W. H. Church. "An initial analysis of a long-term ketogenic diet's impact on motor behavior, brain purine systems, and nigral dopamine neurons in a new genetic rodent model of Parkinson's disease." (2016). Masters Theses.

Sandyk, R. "The relationship between diabetes mellitus and Parkinson's disease." *International Journal of Neuroscience* 69, no. 1–4 (1993): 125–30.

Santiago, J. A., and J. A. Potashkin. "Shared dysregulated pathways lead to Parkinson's disease and diabetes." *Trends in Molecular Medicine* 19, no. 3 (2013): 176–86. doi: 10.1016/j.molmed.2013.01.002.

Schapira, A. H., J. M. Cooper, D. Dexter, J. B. Clark, P. Jenner, and C. D. Marsden. "Mitochondrial complex I deficiency in Parkinson's disease." *Journal of Neurochemistry* 54, no. 3 (1990): 823–7.

Schoeler, N. E., S. Wood, V. Aldridge, J. W. Sander, J. H. Cross, and S. M. Sisodiya. "Ketogenic dietary therapies for adults with epilepsy: feasibility and classification of response." *Epilepsy & Behavior* 37 (2014): 77–81. doi: 10.1016/j.yebeh.2014.06.007.

Schöll, M., O. Almkvist, K. Axelman, E. Stefanova, A. Wall, E. Westman, ... and A. Nordberg. "Glucose metabolism and PIB binding in carriers of a His163Tyrpresenilin 1 mutation." *Neurobiology of Aging* 32, no. 8 (2011): 1388–99. doi: 10.1016/j.neurobiolaging.2009.08.016.

Senior, K. "Dosing in phase II trial of Alzheimer's vaccine suspended." *Lancet Neurology* 1, no. 1 (2002): 3.

Sharifi, H., A. MohajjelNayebi, and S. Farajnia. "8-OH-DPAT (5-HT1A agonist) attenuates 6-hydroxy-dopamine-induced catalepsy and modulates inflammatory cytokines in rats." *Iranian Journal of Basic Medical Sciences* 16, no. 12 (2013): 1270–5.

Sharma, S., N. Sankhyan, S. Gulati, and A. Agarwala. "Use of the modified Atkins diet for treatment of refractory childhood epilepsy: a randomized controlled trial." *Epilepsia* 54, no. 3 (2013): 481–6.

Simpson, I. A., K. R. Chundu, T. Davies-Hill, W. G. Honer, and P. Davies. "Decreased concentrations of GLUT1 and GLUT3 glucose transporters in the brains of patients with Alzheimer's disease." *Annals of Neurology* 35, no. 5 (1994): 546–51.

Srivastava, S., Y. Kashiwaya, M. T. King, U. Baxa, J. Tam, G. Niu, ... and R. L. Veech. "Mitochondrial biogenesis and increased uncoupling protein 1 in brown adipose tissue of mice fed a ketone ester diet." *FASEB Journal* 26, no. 6 (2012): 2351–62. doi: 10.1096/fj.11-200410.

Stafstrom, C. E. "Persistent sodium current and its role in epilepsy." *Epilepsy Currents* 7, no. 1 (2007): 15–22. doi: 10.1111/j.1535-7511.2007.00156.x.

Suzuki, M., M. Suzuki, Y. Kitamura, S. Mori, K. Sato, S. Dohi, ... and A. Hiraide. "Beta-hydroxybutyrate, a cerebral function improving agent, protects rat brain against ischemic damage caused by permanent and transient focal cerebral ischemia." *Japanese Journal of Pharmacology* 89, no. 1 (2002): 36–43. doi.org/10.1254/jjp.89.36.

Sveinbjornsdottir, S. "The clinical symptoms of Parkinson's disease." *Journal of Neurochemistry* 139, suppl 1 (2016): 318–24. doi: 10.1111/jnc.13691.

Talbot, K., H. Y. Wang, H. Kazi, L. Y. Han, K. P. Bakshi, A. Stucky, ... and Z. Arvanitakis. "Demonstrated brain insulin resistance in Alzheimer's disease patients is associated with IGF-1 resistance, IRS-1 dysregulation, and cognitive decline." *Journal of Clinical Investigation* 122, no. 4 (2012): 1316–38.

Thio, L. L., M. Wong, andK. A. Yamada. "Ketone bodies do not directly alter excitatory or inhibitory hippocampal synaptic transmission." *Neurology* 54, no. 2 (2000): 325–31.

Thomas, S., M. L. Prins, M. Samii, and D. A. Hovda. "Cerebral metabolic response to traumatic brain injury sustained early in development: a

2-deoxy-D-glucoseautoradiographic study." *Journal of Neurotrauma* 17 (2000): 649–65.

Tieu, K., C. Perier, C. Caspersen, P. Teismann, D. C. Wu, S. D. Yan, A. Naini, M. Vila, V. Jackson-Lewis, and R. Ramasamy. "D-β-hydroxybutyrate rescues mitochondrial respiration and mitigates features of Parkinson disease." *Journal of Clinical Investigation* 112, no. 6 (2003): 892–901.

Van der Auwera, I., S. Wera, F. Van Leuven, and S. T. Henderson. "A ketogenic diet reduces amyloid beta 40 and 42 in a mouse model of Alzheimer's disease." *Nutrition & Metabolism* 2 (2005): 28. doi: 10.1186/1743-7075-2-28.

Vanitallie, T. B., C. Nonas, A. Di Rocco, K. Boyar, K. Hyams, and S. B. Heymsfield. "Treatment of Parkinson disease with diet-induced hyperketonemia: a feasibility study." *Neurology* 64, no. 4 (2005): 728–30.

Veech, R. L., B. Chance, Y. Kashiwaya, H. A. Lardy, and G. F. Cahill, Jr. "Ketone bodies, potential therapeutic uses." *IUBMB Life* 51, no. 4 (2001): 241–7.

Velarde, F., D. T. Fisher, and D. A. Hovda. "Fluid percussion injury induces prolonged changes in cerebral blood flow." *Journal of Neurotrauma* 9 (1992): 402.

Veneman, T., A. Mitrakou, M. Mokan, P. Cryer, and J. Gerich. "Effect of hyperketonemia and hyperlacticacidemia on symptoms, cognitive dysfunction, and counterregulatory hormone responses during hypoglycemia in normal humans." *Diabetes* 43, no. 11 (1994): 1311–7.

Vining, E. P., J. M. Freeman, K. Ballaban-Gil, C. S. Camfield, P. R. Camfield, G. L. Holmes, ... and J. W. Wheless. "A multicenter study of the efficacy of the ketogenic diet." *Archives of Neurology* 55, no. 11 (1998): 1433–7.

Wang, Y., N. Liu, W. Zhu, K. Zhang, J. Si, M. Bi, ... and J. Wang. "Protective effect of β-hydroxybutyrate on glutamate induced cell death in HT22 cells." *International Journal of Clinical & Experimental Medicine* 9, no. 12 (2016): 23433–9.

Wilder, R. M. "The effects of ketonemia on the course of epilepsy." *Mayo Clinic Proceedings* 2 (1921): 307–308.

Williams, S., C. Basualdo-Hammond, R. Curtis, and R. Schuller. "Growth retardation in children with epilepsy on the ketogenic diet: a retrospective chart review." *Journal of the Academy of Nutrition and Dietetics* 102, no. 3 (2002): 405–7.

Yamada, K. A., N. Rensing, and L. L. Thio. "Ketogenic diet reduces hypoglycemia-induced neuronal death in young rats." *Neuroscience Letters* 385, no. 3 (2005): 210–4.

Yamakami, I., and T. K. McIntosh. "Effects of traumatic brain injury on regional cerebral blood flow in rats as measured with radiolabeled microspheres." *Journal of Cerebral Blood Flow & Metabolism* 9, no. 1 (1989): 117–24.

Yang, X., and B. Cheng. "Neuroprotective and anti-inflammatory activities of ketogenic diet on MPTP-induced neurotoxicity." *Journal of Molecular Neuroscience* 42, no. 2 (2010): 145–53.

Yin, J. X., M. Maalouf, P. Han, M. Zhao, M. Gao, T. Dharshaun, ... and E. M. Reiman. "Ketones block amyloid entry and improve cognition in an Alzheimer's model." *Neurobiology of Aging* 39 (2016): 25–37. doi: 10.1016/j.neurobiolaging.2015.11.018.

Yokoyama, H., S. Takagi, Y. Watanabe, H. Kato, and T. Araki. "Role of reactive nitrogen and reactive oxygen species against MPTP neurotoxicity in mice." *Journal of Neural Transmission* 115, no. 6 (2008): 831–42.

Youm, Y. H., K. Y. Nguyen, R. W. Grant, E. L. Goldberg, M. Bodogai, D. Kim, ... and S. Kang. "The ketone metabolite [beta]-hydroxybutyrate blocks NLRP3 inflammasome-mediated inflammatory disease." *Nature Medicine* 21, no. 3 (2015): 263–9. doi: 10.1038/nm.3804.

Yudkoff, M., Y. Daikhin, T. M. Melø, I. Nissim, U. Sonnewald, and I. Nissim. "The ketogenic diet and brain metabolism of amino acids: relationship to the anticonvulsant effect." *Annual Review of Nutrition* 27 (2007): 415–20. doi: 10.1146/annurev.nutr.27.061406.093722.

Zhao, W. Q., and M. Townsend. "Insulin resistance and amyloidogenesis as common molecular foundation for type 2 diabetes and Alzheimer's disease." *Biochimica et Biophysic* Act. 1792, no. 5 (2009): 482–96.

Ziegler, D. R., L. C. Ribeiro, D. Hagenn, I. R. Siqueira, E. Araújo, I. L. S. Torres, C. Gottfried, C. A. Netto, and C. A. Gonçalves. "Ketogenic diet increases glutathione peroxidase activity in rat hippocampus." *Neurochemistry Research* 28, no. 12 (2003): 1793–7.

Zilberter, M., A. Ivanov, S. Ziyatdinova, M. Mukhtarov, A. Malkov, A. Alpár, ... and A. Pitkänen. "Dietary energy substrates reverse early neuronal hyperactivity in a mouse model of Alzheimer's disease." *Journal of Neurochemistry* 125, no. 1 (2013): 157–71. doi: 10.1111/jnc.12127.

www.epilepsy.com/learn/types-epilepsy-syndromes/dravet-syndrome

Section 4:
Cancer

Cancer is one of the deadliest chronic diseases that people endure today. It is the second leading killer in the United States, and if the current rates of growth continue, it will soon pass heart disease as the nation's leading cause of death. Today, more 1.5 million new cases of cancer are diagnosed every year. According to the National Cancer Institute, one in two men and one in three women will develop cancer at some point in their lifetime. An estimated one in four men and one in five women (almost 600,000 people per year) will die of cancer or cancer-related issues.

In his book *The Emperor of All Maladies*, Siddhartha Mukherjee describes cancer as "a monster more insatiable than the guillotine." Its ability to fight, hide from, and adapt to every treatment that crosses its path is what gives the disease such a powerful ability to progress and metastasize (i.e., spread to other sites in the body). We are making progress in terms of treatment and prevention, but despite the enormous amount of time, effort, and funds spent on cancer research (averaging just under $5 billion per year), the disease has evaded many of our efforts.

There are many therapeutic options for fighting cancer, from surgery to radiation and chemotherapy to various holistic approaches. However, one option that is often overlooked is a nutritional intervention. Sure, it isn't sexy or highly profitable, like pharmaceutical drugs, yet it is accessible to everyone, regardless of their financial situation. We all have to eat! It's particularly odd that we commonly relate dietary choices to the development of cancer (we see headlines all the time about various foods causing cancer), yet we are afraid to address the counterpoint: what if we could help treat the disease through dietary means? For certain types of cancer and with early detection, the current standard of care is rather successful; however, this does not apply to all cases and types of cancer. Even in situations in which the disease can be managed effectively, that management often comes at the expense of poisoning healthy cells along with cancer cells, as with chemotherapy. For this reason, we must continue investigating alternative therapeutic options to treat cancer.

To gain a better understanding of the plausible benefits that could come from alternative remedies, we must first understand the history of the disease and what exactly characterizes cancer.

Life Expectancy Following Diagnosis

If the current life expectancy following a cancer diagnosis is ten years and we make an advancement in cancer detection that allows us to detect cancer five years sooner, then the life expectancy following diagnosis would be fifteen years—without any improvements in treatments. This can make it appear that current treatment options and standards of care have added five years to a cancer patient's life, but as you can see, this can be misleading.

A Brief History of Cancer

Cancer is not new. Historians have found evidence of cancer in fossilized bones as well as in human mummies from ancient Egypt. However, the term *cancer* was not coined until 400 BC, when Hippocrates called a tumor *karkinos* (Greek for "crab") because its shape reminded him of a crab (Mukherjee, 2010). This began the journey toward understanding the disease and the eventual development of various treatments. In Hippocrates's time, the only valid treatment option was to simply cut the mass out of the body. As you can imagine, sanitary conditions for surgical procedures weren't the best back then, thus the rates of infection were high and the ability to treat those infections was weak.

Centuries later, Galen of Pergamon, the famous Greek physician, described cancer as containing black bile (one of the four humors that were believed to make up the human body) and found that the black bile would still flow even after the mass was removed. Based on Galen's findings, a shift in the treatment of the disease occurred. The focus turned to ridding the body of black bile—until Andreas Vesalius, who began studying anatomy in 1533 (Mukherjee, 2010: page 51), dissected the deceased in order to redraw the medical textbooks and failed to find the black bile that Galen had reported. Following the induction of regular autopsies in 1761, Scottish physician Matthew Baillie also failed to find Galen's black bile, and with that theory finally debunked, Baillie helped develop and map out various surgical procedures for the removal of tumors. This information proved useful for Scottish surgeon John Hunter, who proposed that if cancer had failed to invade nearby tissues (a process later termed *metastasis*), then the surgical removal of tumors was the best available option (Mukherjee, 2010: page 55).

In the nineteenth century, pioneering British surgeon Joseph Lister developed the first antibacterial approach to prevent postsurgical infections. In fact, in 1869, Lister performed surgery on his sister, removing a tumor from her breast (Mukherjee, 2010). Lister's sister survived this procedure, which essentially led to an explosion of tumor-removal surgeries in the 1870s. The discovery of the X-ray in 1895 initiated a new area of research. As researchers attempted to understand X-ray technology, it was proposed that it could be used to kill cancer cells. In 1896, medical student Emil Grubbe was able to shrink a cancer tumor with radiation. As X-ray research became more popular, Pierre and Marie Curie discovered that radium, a radioactive metal, possessed a similar ability but could permeate or infiltrate tissue to a deeper level than X-rays.

At that time, it was not known that radium could be toxic to the human body. In fact, this was not discovered until Marie Curie herself developed anemia (low red blood cells) as a result of radiation leaking into her bones (Mukherjee, 2010). However, scientists eventually discovered that radium directly affects DNA, leading to the death of rapidly multiplying cells, which is a hallmark of cancer. Scientists thought this seemed like a surefire way to keep cancer cells from metastasizing or multiplying. In spite of this, the excitement behind radiation and X-ray treatment eventually waned when it was found that these methods not only killed growing cancer cells but could also negatively affect healthy cells. Doctors then turned to radiation as an "after-treatment" option: after surgery to remove the tumor, the thinking went, treating the affected area with radiation could prevent the cancer from reoccurring or spreading. Think of radiation as weed killer: after weeding the lawn, we often spray some type of weed killer to ensure that no weeds remain. Though it could affect or even kill some of the healthy grass, we still take the risk to try to limit weed growth.

Meanwhile, German physician Paul Ehrlich was having great success treating various bacterial diseases with synthetic chemicals. He proposed that if we could understand the differences between a cancerous cell and a healthy cell, then we ought to be able to fight cancer with chemicals (i.e., chemotherapy).

One of the major advances in chemotherapy came from a surprising source: war. During World War I, in 1917, British soldiers stationed in Belgium were bombarded with shells containing mustard gas, resulting in both short- and long-term complications: two years later, they were found to have depleted bone marrow cells. Then, during World War II, a fleet of American ships was attacked and went up in flames. Mustard gas leaked from one of the ships as it sank, quickly killing many of the men (Mukherjee, 2010). Autopsies found that these men also had depleted bone marrow. This led two Yale researchers to propose that if mustard gas reduces the number of healthy white blood cells (which are made in the bone marrow), it might also knock out cancerous white blood cells.

This was essentially the dawn of chemotherapy. Yes, that's right: mustard gas was one of our first proposed chemotherapy options. At that point, in the 1940s, there were essentially three treatment options for cancer: radical surgery, radiation, and chemotherapy. In the years that followed, debates over which method was best—coupled with arrogance and politics—made it difficult to see through the "red ocean" (where everyone tries to tear down and soar above everyone else). Public figures, including presidents, declared war on the disease and fought to fund different areas of research to advance the field.

Cancer Treatment Options in the 1940s	
RADICAL SURGERY	Surgically removing the tumor mass (and often some of the adjoining tissue) from the body
RADIATION	Using X-rays, gamma rays, and other charged particles to shrink tumors and kill cancer cells
CHEMOTHERAPY	Using chemicals to kill cancer cells

At the same time, many advances were made in the understanding of cancer, including the role of genetic mutations, which can be caused by chemicals, radiation, or even genetic inheritance. This development sparked a whole new area of research, and in the 1970s came the discovery of genes that can impact cancer (oncogenes) and tumor suppressor genes (anti-oncogenes). Significant focus was placed on the genetic aspect of the disease, and large amounts of research funding went to looking at the genetic makeup of cancer cells.

While we have made serious advances in the treatment of cancer over the past century, are we where we should be? Scientists and researchers have dedicated their careers and lives to this tricky disease, and still we are coming up short. Chemotherapy, one of the most common cancer therapies today, is essentially a method of introducing poison into a person's body in an attempt to kill cancer cells. Unfortunately, healthy cells are

affected along with them. For this reason, there have been numerous attempts to develop alternative treatment options, such as immunotherapy—using the immune system to fight cancer—and targeted therapy—chemotherapy that kills cancer cells but leaves healthy cells intact. While some of these options have demonstrated success, depending on the cancer type, they are not foolproof—just like radiation, chemotherapy, and surgery. Cancer's ability to spread and hide often allows it to survive in the presence of these therapeutic approaches. This means that for researchers, there is much work left to be done, but where do we go from here?

What Is Cancer?

Cancer is a disease characterized by the uncontrolled division of abnormal cells in any part of the body. The human body comprises trillions of cells, and cancer can start in any one cell. Scary to think about, right? Typically, when a cell develops genetic mutations or abnormalities, the immune system destroys it before further damage can occur. For this reason, we can assume that at some point each of us has had cancerous cells, but our immune system has recognized and destroyed them.

Not to take away from the seriousness of the disease by any means, but this battle is like many of the video games that we played when we were younger. Remember the games where you had to defend the castle and prevent the enemy from coming in and destroying it? Similarly, your immune system is constantly defending your castle (your organs and tissues), but every so often, an abnormal cell becomes immune to the regular ammo your system has been using to kill all the other potential invaders. If this cell can avoid being killed by the immune system and get inside the walls of the castle, it can begin to grow and divide, eventually spreading throughout the castle and wreaking havoc.

The majority of cancer cells have mutations that allow them to acquire certain molecular, biochemical, and cellular capabilities (Hannahan and Weinberg et al., 2000). These have become what are known today as the hallmarks of cancer.

Defining Cancer Terms

The terms associated with cancer can be overwhelming. To break down a few of the common ones for you: Tumors can be *malignant* or *benign*. A malignant tumor has the ability to spread to different areas of the body, while a benign tumor does not spread; once a benign tumor is removed, it is less likely to recur compared to a malignant tumor. Typically, the term *cancer* is reserved for malignant tumors.

Cancer can also be classified as *carcinoma* or *sarcoma*. A carcinoma is a malignant tumor of the epithelial tissue—the tissue that covers surfaces (like the outsides of organs). Most of the cancers found in humans, including breast and lung cancer, are carcinomas. Sarcomas are malignant tumors arising in connective tissue, such as bone or blood. These kinds of cancer are rarer than carcinomas but are more often fatal. No matter the type of cancer, however, progression of the disease is maintained by continued uncontrolled growth of abnormal cells.

The Hallmarks of Cancer

Sustained Cell Growth Signals: In both normal and tumor cells, oncogenes and tumor-suppressor genes are present. In normal cells, these genes are functioning properly. In tumor cells, there is often a mutation that allows for constant activation of oncogenes and inactivation of tumor-suppressor genes. When these genes are not properly regulated, they can drive oncogenesis and tumor progression (i.e., when a normal system would scream "stop," cancer cells keep growing).

Insensitivity to Anti-Growth Signals: Normal cells contain what are known as anti-growth signals, which help regulate cell growth. However, cancer cells have mutated genes that can suppress the expression of anti-growth signals, which can lead to rapid dividing and multiplying of cancer cells.

Resistance to Cell Death: Apoptosis, or programmed cell death, is essentially a self-destruct mechanism in healthy cells. Each cell continuously monitors itself, and when it is no longer needed or becomes altered in a way that can be harmful to the body, apoptosis occurs to prevent the now-abnormal cell from growing, dividing, and producing additional abnormal cells. Think of a zombie movie: there is always one person who, once infected, kills himself in order to avoid harming or infecting anyone else. Similarly, in apoptosis, cells sacrifice themselves in order to keep from passing on any abnormality they may have. Cancer cells have several mechanisms by which they can avoid apoptosis, allowing these abnormal cells to flourish and grow—a zombie apocalypse.

Limitless Replicative Potential: Normal cells possess internal programming that limits the number of times they can divide. Cancer cells, however, have the ability to turn off this replication limit. This allows them to multiply at an accelerated pace with no clear end in sight.

Sustained Angiogenesis: Angiogenesis is the process by which new blood vessels are formed. Blood vessels are feeding tubes for tissues, providing oxygen and nutrients needed for proper cell function, survival, and growth. In healthy tissue, angiogenesis is tightly regulated, but cancer cells are capable of not only inducing but also sustaining angiogenesis, ensuring that the tumor is supplied with adequate nutrients to continue growing and spreading.

Tissue Invasion and Metastasis: In metastasis, cancer cells break away from the site where they first formed, travel through the circulatory or lymph system, and form new tumors in other parts of the body. Metastasis is one of the deadliest characteristics of cancer because as cancer spreads throughout the body, it affects more and more organs and systems and becomes very difficult to eradicate; metastasis is responsible for more than 90 percent of cancer-related deaths (Liotta et al., 1991). In fact, whether or not a tumor has metastasized is often used to determine the severity of the disease. Certain cancers have preferred sites of metastasis, but the liver, bones, and brain are the sites that most commonly receive metastasized cancer cells.

The following are the more recently developed and researched enabling characteristics of cancer, which include novel ways in which cancer cells can develop, grow, thrive, and cause issues within the body (Hanahan and Weinberg, 2011).

Genome Instability and Mutations: As a tumor grows, the genes in the cancer cells that detect DNA damage and activate its repair lose their ability to function. Once this loss of function occurs, these cellular caretakers can no longer prevent mutations in the genome, which allows for further cancer growth. Over time, mutations in DNA occur, and this is exacerbated by a loss of DNA repair, etc.

Tumor-Promoting Inflammation: Inflammation is common in many diseases, including cancer. Cancer-related inflammation was initially thought to be an attempt by the immune system to fight abnormal cells, but it has since been found that inflammation can activate anti-apoptosis factors and pro-angiogenic factors. Inflammatory cells can also induce the release of reactive oxygen species (ROS), which are like little pinballs bouncing around the cells, causing damage that can further mutate cancer cells. Interestingly, ROS can trigger apoptosis if it becomes elevated enough (i.e., hyperbaric oxygen therapy), but cancer cells typically display increased levels of antioxidant proteins that keep ROS within the healthy limits that allow the cancer cells to benefit (Liou et al., 2010). Later we will discuss strategies to increase ROS past the apoptotic threshold to induce cancer cell death.

Altered Energy Metabolism: Because we know that cancer cells grow and divide at an accelerated rate, it's easy to understand why a change in energy metabolism is beneficial for sustained growth. Cancer cells have been found to be in a state of aerobic glycolysis, which means that even in the presence of adequate oxygen, they increase the fermentation of glucose—which typically occurs only when oxygen is limited. This increase can activate many oncogenes, as well as cause mutations in the tumor-suppressor genes that make them less effective. In addition, the increase in glucose metabolism causes an increase in the production of lactate (glucose is broken down into pyruvate, and excess pyruvate is converted to lactate) within the cancer cells. Lactate can then be taken in by neighboring cells, where it fuels growth. Incomplete glucose oxidation through the typical mitochondrial pathways also allows glucose carbons to be used to synthesize the lipids, proteins, and DNA needed to make new tumor cells.

Avoidance of Our Immune System: Normal cells are watched by immune cells that eliminate abnormal or dysfunctional cells. Cancer cells appear to have developed the ability to avoid this detection, allowing them to progress into tumors (i.e., evading the "castle" defense and infiltrating organs and tissues).

These hallmarks and enabling characteristics are what define cancer, regardless of the type. Although they are widely accepted, there is still much debate behind their origin: what makes a normal, healthy cell develop these mutations and become cancerous.

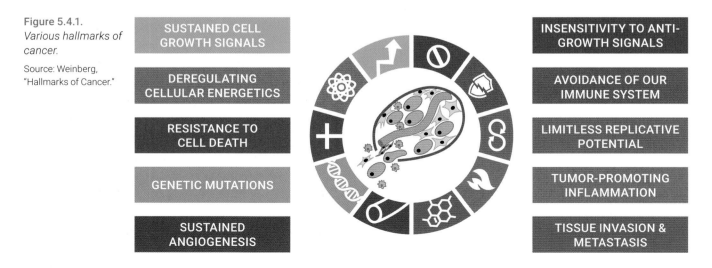

Figure 5.4.1.
Various hallmarks of cancer.

Source: Weinberg, "Hallmarks of Cancer."

SUSTAINED CELL GROWTH SIGNALS

DEREGULATING CELLULAR ENERGETICS

RESISTANCE TO CELL DEATH

GENETIC MUTATIONS

SUSTAINED ANGIOGENESIS

INSENSITIVITY TO ANTI-GROWTH SIGNALS

AVOIDANCE OF OUR IMMUNE SYSTEM

LIMITLESS REPLICATIVE POTENTIAL

TUMOR-PROMOTING INFLAMMATION

TISSUE INVASION & METASTASIS

How Do Cells Become Cancerous?

One of the primary features of a cancer cell is its ability to divide or proliferate rapidly and unchecked. Of course, normal, healthy cells also proliferate—it's necessary for growth and proper function in some adult tissues. So if both healthy and cancerous cells undergo cell growth, what makes a cell become cancerous? When do normal growth and proliferation turn dangerous?

Somatic Mutation Theory

Because many of the characteristics of cancer revolve around genetic mutations, many experts refer to cancer as a genetic disease. The most widely accepted explanation for the origin of cancer is the somatic mutation theory. This theory states that over time, damage to a normal cell's DNA initiates a cascade of events that cause the cell to become cancerous. Some doctors take this theory as the be-all, end-all explanation for why cancer develops. However, this theory has met with several limitations recently. For example, we know that cancer is a disease of great heterogeneity: the genetic mutations in cancer vary from person to person, even within the same type of cancer (Stratton et al., 2009). In an attempt to explain these paradoxes, it's been proposed that cancer is a *metabolic disease* rather than a *genetic disease*.

Metabolic Dysfunction Theory

The idea that cancer springs from dysfunction in energy production was discussed in the 1920s by Dr. Otto Warburg. Under normal circumstances, glucose is taken in by a cell and broken down without the need for oxygen; lactate is a by-product of this process. Dr. Warburg found that cancer cells metabolize glucose at a higher-than-normal rate, resulting in an increased production of lactate—and when there is an abundance of lactate, it can be fermented and used for energy. Healthy cells don't ferment lactate in the presence of oxygen, but cancer cells do, in a process called aerobic glycolysis.

Lactate fermentation is one of cancer cells' main sources of energy for growth, proliferation, and metastasis. However, this is an extremely inefficient way to acquire cellular energy. The fact that cancer cells rely on lactate fermentation raises the question, why do cancer cells favor this inefficient method of producing energy? Could it be that they have an impaired ability to properly use mitochondria for energy production?

Damaged Mitochondria

The understanding of aerobic glycolysis has led researchers to propose that cancer cells are unable to efficiently produce energy due to defective or damaged mitochondria. This has sparked a lot of research into the metabolism of cancer cells and how mitochondrial function relates to the disease.

According to Warburg (1956), "The first phase in cancer development is the irreversible injuring of respiration." "Respiration" in this sense refers to a cell's ability to use oxygen to break down glucose. It is thought that once a cell loses its ability to effectively utilize oxygen, as occurs with mitochondrial dysfunction, it develops other characteristics that define cancer (Seyfried et al., 2012).

Figure 5.4.2. *Normal cell metabolism vs. cancer cell metabolism.*

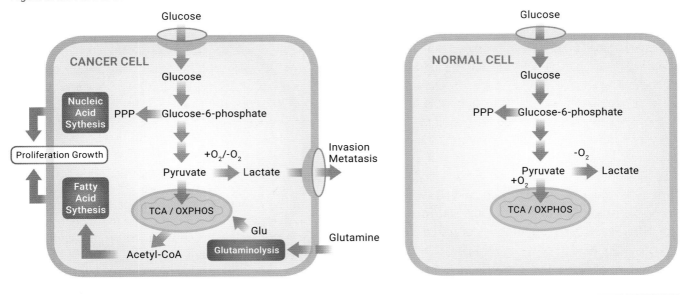

These theories have been validated based on the fascinating findings of mitochondrial swap studies. One study found that when the mitochondria from a normal cell was fused with the mitochondria from a highly metastatic cell, mitochondrial function was fine despite the presence of a cancerous nucleus (Kaipparettu et al., 2013). Similarly, if you take the mitochondria from a tumor cell and put it into a cell with a normal nucleus, the cell becomes cancerous. Additional studies have found that cells with functional mitochondria display increased ATP synthesis and oxygen consumption despite having a mutated nucleus (Cruz-Bermudez et al., 2015). Together, these findings suggest that mitochondrial function (rather than the nucleus itself) may play a large role in determining whether a cell is cancerous or not—or oncogenic regulation.

The chicken-or-the-egg argument often gets brought up. Some argue that genetic mutations cause the problems with the mitochondria rather than the other way around. However, the mitochondria and nuclear transfer experiments discussed above, by scientists like Dr. Thomas Seyfried, indicate that the somatic mutations often cannot entirely explain the origins of cancer because rates of tumor formation in normal mitochondria change when the mitochondria is combined with a nucleus from a tumor (Seyfried, 2012). While this may be a step in the right direction, there is still much struggle to further our understanding of this new principle of cancer. Some research indicates

that not all cancer cells display damaged respiration (Moreno-Sanchez et al., 2007), and even that healthy and cancerous cells have similar mitochondrial function (Cairns et al., 2015; Koppenol et al., 2011). Though there are many limitations to these studies, it's possible that even when mitochondria are not damaged, cancer cells reprogram how they get energy anyway. Therefore, as we hope to get across throughout this section, it is unlikely that this one theory can entirely explain cancer cell abnormalities, although it may play an extremely large part.

Reprogramming of Energy Metabolism
Whether genetic mutations cause mitochondrial dysfunction or mitochondrial dysfunction causes genetic mutations, it's been well established that in cancer cells, there is a shift in metabolism—a metabolic dysfunction. As previously discussed, cancer cells reprogram energy metabolism in order to thrive. Is this a survival method or a preferred mechanism by these cells? When a cancer cell divides, the result is two daughter cells, which means a doubling of the need for biological materials such as proteins, lipids, and nucleic acids. These cells do whatever it takes (in this case, reprogram energy metabolism) to ensure that they get fed and can survive (Bauer et al., 2004).

In order for cancer cells to grow and thrive, they must be properly nourished. If you look at PET scans of a tumor, you will see a drastic increase in glucose uptake (Groves et al., 2007). Cancer cells have remarkably higher rates of glucose uptake than normal cells, resulting in a high cellular glycolytic flux and lactate production. Under normal circumstances, glucose is taken in by a cell and broken down without the need for oxygen, which results in the production of some energy (ATP) and pyruvate. Typically, pyruvate is shuttled into the mitochondria and into the Krebs cycle, where it is used to generate electron carriers that participate in the electron transport chain to fuel ATP production through an oxygen-requiring process called oxidative phosphorylation. When pyruvate is abundant (such as times when there is a large influx of glucose), pyruvate can be converted to lactate if not properly broken down. In cancer, we tend to see a lowering of pyruvate dehydrogenase complex (PDH), which is the complex responsible for breaking down pyrvuate. In turn, this decreases pyruvate entry into the mitochondria and forces lactate fermentation to occur. Lactate fermentation is a fundamental feature that virtually all cancer cells display, and it can be responsible for some progressive mechanisms of the disease. It is important to understand that all cells possess the ability to transition to this method of metabolism (lactate fermentation), but it typically occurs only when oxygen availability is low (hypoxia). While it is true that cancer cells often display a hypoxic (low-oxygen) environment, what makes them unique is their ability to ferment lactate in the presence of oxygen, a process called aerobic glycolysis (Racker et al., 1972). Therefore, if we were able to provide an alternative source of fuel while limiting the production of the cancer cells' preferred fuel source (glucose), it could have a significant impact on the cancer cells' ability to grow and proliferate.

Cancer is complex beyond imagination, and a conclusive understanding of the disease may not be possible. But whether it is of metabolic origin or genetic origin, cancer is a disease of great genetic heterogeneity—that is, in two people with the same kind of cancer, cancer cells may have very different attributes. This means trying to treat the disease solely from a genetic perspective is probably not realistic. Of course, this also poses a challenge in treating the disease metabolically: cancer cells within the body can display metabolic differences (Frezza et

al., 2011; Jeon et al., 2012). However, this shouldn't be discouraging; while we may not fully understand what causes cancerous metabolic features, we do know that they can occur, and targeting these consistent metabolic characteristics may improve our ability to manage the disease through a combination of approaches.

Current Cancer Treatment Options

Traditional nonsurgical treatments for cancer are highly toxic. Imagine you discover one day that the spiders living in your attic have started to crawl throughout your house and are showing up in the bedrooms, the kitchen, the living room … Rather than call an exterminator, you decide to go around spraying every room with Raid. In the process you end up staining and messing up your bed, couch, and other materials that might not have been in the way. This is the basic approach of traditional nonsurgical treatments for cancer, which unfortunately leave the door open to complications, such as muscle wasting and depleted immune function.

Chemotherapy, one of the most common forms of treatment, may be effective to a degree in fighting cancer. What is alarming, though, is that it lacks specificity. Chemotherapy kills healthy cells along with cancer cells, which leads to an array of nasty side effects, including fatigue, nausea, hair loss, anemia, blood-clotting problems, nerve and muscle defects, and infertility.

Cytotoxic chemotherapy is often coupled with radiation, which is used to shrink and hopefully kill cancerous tumors. The side effects of radiation include fibrosis (the thickening or scarring of connective tissue), memory loss, infertility, and potentially even the development of a secondary form of cancer from the radiation.

New treatments, such as immunotherapy and hormone therapy, are attempts to move away from the toxicity of chemotherapy and radiation; however, they are still novel treatment strategies that need more work.

Targeting What Fuels Cancer

When we understand that cancer can be attributed to metabolic dysfunction, it's easy to see that targeting the metabolism of cancer cells could be extremely effective. If we could prevent cancer cells from getting or using the primary energy that they need to survive, multiply, and spread, we'd have an amazing tool for treating the disease.

Evidence suggests that there is a direct relationship between high blood glucose levels and tumor growth (Seyfried et al., 2003; Seyfried et al., 2008; Gnagnarella et al., 2008). For this reason, targeting glucose, the major fuel of cancer, could be beneficial in slowing the progression of tumors.

The following are some additional ways in which glucose can help cancer thrive:

- **Angiogenesis:** Angiogenesis, or the development of blood vessels, is necessary for providing nutrients and oxygen to tumors. The increase in glucose metabolism in cancer cells ultimately creates a more acidic tumor environment by producing lactate, which can help promote angiogenesis and thereby enhance cancer's ability to progress. (Gatenby and Gillies et al., 2004).

- **Providing Fuel for Neighboring Cancer Cells:** One by-product of glucose breakdown, lactate, can be used for fuel itself when there is an abundance of it. Because cancer cells increase the breakdown of glucose, they also increase the amount of lactate produced. It has been found that a cancer cell can release unused lactate into the area around the cell, where it can be taken up by neighboring cancer cells that are in need of energy. Nice neighbors, huh?

- **Growth Substrate:** When a cancer cell increases its glucose consumption, it can use that glucose in different ways. Glucose does not have to be fully broken down. After certain steps of the metabolic pathway have been completed, by-products can be used to synthesize new lipids, proteins, and DNA, all of which are important to continue the uncontrolled growth of the tumor.

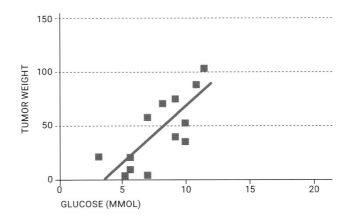

Figure 5.4.3. *Tumor weight is directly proportional to the amount of glucose in the blood.*

Source: Seyfried, "Cancer as a Metabolic Disease."

Given the fact that glucose is cancer's primary fuel source, it's obvious that we should focus on limiting glucose metabolism. If we can limit glucose, then theoretically we can limit the growth of cancer cells. In fact, multiple drugs that target glucose metabolism, such as metformin, have already been developed for use in cancer treatment. However, many people fail to realize that there are dietary measures that also limit glucose and could prove to be helpful for cancer patients. Restricting calories and carbohydrates to the point of achieving ketosis is a simple way to use diet to restrict glucose and thereby starve cancer cells of their primary fuel.

KETO CONCEPT

Cleaning with a Dirty Rag

The fact that soda, chips, pretzels, and candy are offered to patients after chemotherapy and radiation blows our minds. It's been shown that cancer cells thrive on glucose, and cancer patients are being offered the foods that are not only low in quality but also extremely high in sugar! It's almost like trying to dry the dishes you just washed using a towel that's been soaked in mud: it negates a lot of the work you just did. Why would we spend hours trying to clean up the body with chemo and radiation only to immediately hand those cancer cells the tool they need—sugar—to make it dirty again?

Diet-Based Therapies

We will discuss three ways to reduce glucose by changing the way you eat: restricting calories, fasting, and following a ketogenic diet. (There are also drugs and supplements that can lower blood glucose—see page 125.) Let's look at each approach and evaluate its effectiveness in treating cancer.

However, first, it's important to note that these approaches don't necessarily exist in isolation. A combination of calorie restriction, ketogenic dieting, and even periods of fasting can coexist—and allows for more flexibility and accommodation of a patient's needs.

Restricting Calories

Consistently restricting calories has been shown to slow the rate of cancer growth (Hursting et al., 2010; Kritchevsky et al., 2001; Mukherjee et al., 1999; Tannenbaum et al., 1942). While the exact reason is unknown, it's likely due to the following effects of calorie restriction, all of which are related to hallmarks of cancer (see page 117):

- Decreased production of growth factors and anabolic hormones, which can contribute to the growth of cancer cells

- Decreased reactive oxygen species (ROS) production

- Improvement in the body's antioxidant and immune systems

- Decreased inflammation

- Enhanced DNA repair processes

- Increased removal of damaged or abnormal cells through apoptosis

It is likely that many of these benefits occur from the reduction in blood glucose as well as the potential for a minor increase in ketone bodies, which may have anticancer properties themselves—as we'll get to shortly.

3-Bromopyruvate: Miracle Drug?

In one research study, the molecule 3-Bromopyruvate (3-BP) was able to rid all nineteen animals of advanced cancer (Ko, 2004). 3-BP inhibits glycolysis (the breakdown of glucose), thus reducing cellular ATP and starving cancer cells of the energy they need (Ko, 2001).

More recently, researchers used 3-BP to treat a sixteen-year-old boy suffering from a rare form of liver cancer. They found that 3-BP killed more cancer cells than any drug that had been tested. Although the boy died two years later, he survived much longer than was originally expected. There is still a lack of scientific understanding of 3-BP's exact mechanisms, and legal disputes over its patent are preventing further investigation, but the success of this drug clearly stems from its ability to act on the metabolic alteration of cancer cells (Ko et al., 2012).

Studies dating back to 1909 have shown that calorie restriction can inhibit the growth of tumors in mice. One study on rhesus monkeys found that when the monkeys were fed 10 to 20 percent fewer calories than usual, the incidence of developing cancer was reduced by 50 percent (Colman et al., 2009). Similarly, Albanes (1987) found a linear relationship between the degree of calorie restriction and tumor incidence (on average, the rate of tumors was 42 percent lower in the restricted groups). Thus there is strong evidence that reducing total caloric intake plays a role in reducing the occurrence of cancer, but as always, there are considerations to keep in mind.

For instance, the effects of calorie restriction on cancer are not uniform—some types of cancer respond better than others. And the degree of calorie restriction needed to effectively reduce tumor size or possibly even to prevent cancer from developing at all is still not definitively known. Another consideration is that calorie restriction can result in rapid weight loss and potentially muscle wasting. Ideally, individuals should adopt the least restriction needed to yield the best result in order to help preserve muscle mass and prevent wasting.

Fasting

Fasting—abstaining from food for set periods—has been shown to be therapeutic in the treatment and management of various types of cancer. There are several ways in which fasting could provide benefits in the management of cancer that are similar to calorie restriction. Fasting can result in a reduction in blood glucose and insulin and, depending on the length of the fast, can increase ketone levels, which may be beneficial against cancer on its own. (We'll talk more about that below.)

Additionally, fasting may actually sensitize cancer cells to chemotherapy (Lee et al., 2012). This offers a solution to one of the biggest limitations of chemo: it is difficult to get the dose high enough to completely kill the cancer because of how toxic the treatment is to normal cells and tissues. If fasting for, say, sixteen to twenty-four hours before a chemo treatment sensitizes cancer cells to chemo, a lower dose theoretically would be just as effective on cancer cells as a higher dose. That means less damage to healthy cells, more damage to cancer cells, and fewer side effects for patients. Additionally, fasting has shown promise in protecting healthy cells during various toxic cancer treatments in both animals and humans (Lee et al., 2012; Safdie et al., 2009).

However, to our knowledge, no studies have directly investigated how fasting before chemotherapy affects cancer cell growth in humans. However, studies have shown that fasting prior to chemotherapy may allow for a reduction in fatigue, weakness, and gastrointestinal side effects (Safdie et al., 2009). More research is needed, but fasting seems to be a feasible option as an additional cancer treatment aid.

Following a Ketogenic Diet

Unlike restricting calories and fasting, following a ketogenic diet allows for substantial food intake, yet because it dramatically reduces carbohydrate consumption (and therefore glucose), it has the same effects: lower insulin and glucose, decreased ROS, improved immune function, and even HDAC (histone deacetylase) inhibition (which we will discuss on page 173). All of these effects have been shown to slow tumor growth.

Restricting carbohydrate and sugar intake seems to be ideal, whether or not an individual is on a true ketogenic diet. As discussed earlier, there is a direct relationship between plasma glucose levels and tumor growth; therefore, lowering plasma glucose by reducing carbohydrates seems to be beneficial. So what further benefit does a ketogenic diet have compared to just lowering carbohydrates? Is there something unique that comes with the diet that can further assist in battling cancer? Interestingly, research has demonstrated that ketones can have anticancer effects even when glucose is not reduced (Scheck et al., 2012; Poff et al., 2014). Using ketones for fuel can be anti-angiogenic, anti-inflammatory,

---

KETO CONCEPT

Can Some Cancer Cells Use Ketones?

You might be thinking, "Wouldn't ketones feed cancer cells, too?" Some of the current literature demonstrates that cancer cells are unable to utilize ketones, likely due to their mitochondrial abnormalities, but there is still much debate on this topic. Other studies have demonstrated that ketones are toxic to cancer cells, possibly due to the fact that cancer cells are unable to metabolize ketone bodies because of their impaired oxidative machinery or lack of ketolytic enzymes (Chang et al., 2013). However, some cell cultures suggest that ketones can be used as a fuel source by cancer cells (Martinez-Outschoorn et al., 2011). Although a direct comparison to glucose hasn't been made, it is likely that even if ketones could be utilized, ketones would be much less efficient at providing energy to cancer cells than glucose is, still lending credence to the theory that ketones are the better alternative for fuel.

The Dog Days Are Over: KetoPet Sanctuary

We are huge dog lovers, and we're excited to see the work being done at the KetoPet Sanctuary (KPS) in Georgetown, Texas. KPS, by the Epigenix Foundation, helps rescue dogs with terminal cancer. Their goal is not only to provide love and care for these animals but also to offer the dogs groundbreaking cancer therapies. KPS is currently implementing an approach that combines ketogenic diets, exercise, calorie restriction, and a well-rounded standard of care with their animals, with impressive success. We highly recommend that you check out their website, www.ketopetsanctuary.com.

and pro-apoptotic (Seyfried et al., 2003)—in other words, it discourages the development of blood vessels that feed cancer cells, reduces tumor-promoting inflammation, and promotes the necessary death of abnormal and potentially cancerous cells. Essentially, the ketogenic diet could not only fight cancer cells but also protect healthy cells from exposure during other treatment options!

Some studies suggest that cancer cells cannot effectively and efficiently utilize ketones, offering a potential method for starving cancer cells of fuel (Seyfried et al., 2011). Other studies have demonstrated that ketones are actually toxic to cancer cells, possibly because cancer cells are unable to utilize them effectively (Chang et al., 2013); however, these results conflict with some earlier studies.

Additionally, new research has demonstrated that ketosis leads to improved immunity in animals with cancer, which could slow the progression of the disease (Lussier et al., 2016).

It goes without saying that any approach you take for therapeutic purposes should be overseen by your doctor. Some doctors may be resistant at first, but if you're looking to make a dietary change for yourself or a loved one, the research we will discuss shortly highlights some important information that you should understand and then run by your healthcare team. For example, to optimize the benefits of a ketogenic diet, it may be important to restrict calories, even slightly at first. Some animal research suggests that unrestricted feeding on a ketogenic

Metabolic Drugs

While we do feel that drugs may be overused in the treatment of various diseases, not just cancer, certain drugs may beneficially target metabolic pathways. An example is 2-deoxyglucose (2DG), which is a potent inhibitor of glycolysis (the breakdown of glucose) and has even demonstrated the ability to kill prostate cancer cells (Liu, 2001).

Metformin, a drug commonly used to lower blood glucose in individuals suffering from diabetes, has gained some popularity in the cancer world. Metformin exerts its effects by making people more sensitive to insulin, therefore allowing them to use less insulin to take up glucose from the blood. It also limits the amount of sugar produced by the liver (Vallianou, 2013). Studies have found that metformin can also inhibit the growth of prostate, ovarian, and breast cancer cells (Algire, 2010). There is still much debate surrounding these effects, but at the very least, metformin could provide a benefit by reducing blood glucose levels and therefore substrate for cancer cells to use to grow and divide.

More research is required before the use of metabolic drugs to treat cancer becomes a standard practice, but it appears as though some of these drugs could work well in combination with standard treatments such as chemotherapy and radiation. As we will discuss later, there are some readily available supplement options on the market today that may be comparable to these metabolic drugs, with fewer side effects.

diet can lead to insulin resistance and possibly even elevations in blood glucose and insulin (Meidenbauer et al., 2014). This often is the result of eating too many calories and ultimately carbohydrates. Unlike the potential limitations discussed earlier with CR and muscle mass, being in a state of ketosis can actually preserve muscle mass even in the presence of calorie restriction, meaning that cachexia (weight loss and muscle wasting) may not be as big of an issue under these circumstances. This is just one example of how the dynamics change, especially when discussing cancer and ketosis, and should always be tailored to an individual's needs and situation.

Research on the Ketogenic Diet and Cancer

In *The Art of War*, Sun Tzu mentions a strategy called a blockade, in which you cut off the enemy's food supply. Similarly, if we were able to cut off cancer's food supply in our war on the disease, what might happen?

On paper, it sounds simple: cancer feeds on glucose and cannot effectively use ketones for fuel. Thus, after cutting way back on glucose and allowing the body to run on ketones instead, you starve the cancer cells of fuel and they die. Unfortunately, although the general school of thought is on the right track, it's much more complex than that.

Cell Culture Studies

Most research begins with preclinical trials, or trials done in nonhuman subjects, to test various scientific theories. In some cases, these trials start with cell culture studies. In cancer research, this involves growing cancerous cells in a test tube or culture dish and testing different theories to further our understanding of the disease. Early cell culture studies involving ketosis and cancer gave us great insight into potential mechanisms for ketosis as an aid for cancer. One study demonstrated that a cancer cell bathed in ketone bodies not only had decreased glucose utilization and lactate production (which, as described earlier, can fuel cancer) but also demonstrated growth inhibition (Magee et al., 1979). Further, Dr. Eugene Fine, a leading researcher in this area, found that the ketone body acetoacetate upregulated enzymes responsible for inhibiting cancer cell growth (Fine et al., 2009). Lastly, researchers determined that cancer cells were unable to efficiently utilize ketones as an energy source, and therefore their rate of survival decreased when the cells were in dishes containing ketone bodies (Skinner et al., 2009). This cell culture work shows promise for ketones and the use of a ketogenic diet as a helpful therapy for cancer in conjunction with other treatments.

However, one of the biggest limitations of cell culture research is that it bears little resemblance to real life. It's hard to assume that what happens in the controlled setting of a lab, in isolated cells, will also happen in humans with cancer.

Animal Research

Once we begin getting into "in vivo," or live, research on animals, interpreting the results becomes much more challenging. Animal studies on the ketogenic diet and cancer often vary in the type of animal used, the duration of treatment, and the type of diet the animals are fed. However, one benefit of animal research is that they will eat exactly what you feed them, so researchers can be certain of their calorie and nutrient intake and easily control their environment to isolate other factors—unlike with humans, who can sneak a candy bar in spite of the prescribed diet, whose stress and activity levels vary widely, and so on.

In most studies involving the ketogenic diet and cancer in animals, animals are implanted with tumors and then treated. For example, one study implanted adult mice with brain tumors and then put them on either an unrestricted or a restricted ketogenic diet; those two groups were compared to a group on an unrestricted high-carbohydrate diet (Zhou et al., 2007). The researchers found that a restricted ketogenic diet decreased the growth of tumors by about 65 percent and enhanced health and survival compared to the high-carbohydrate group.

Growth of Brain Tumors in Mice on Standard Diet vs Restricted Ketogenic Diet

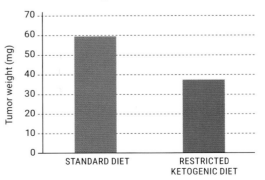

Figure 5.4.4. Mice on a restricted ketogenic diet showed decreased tumor size compared to those on a standard, unrestricted diet.

Source: Zhou et al., 2007.

Doesn't Red Meat Cause Cancer?

To say that red meat is a direct "cause" of cancer is just plain false. However, what most people are likely alluding to is a correlation between red meat intake and cancer incidence. Good news: research has shown that eating beef, pork, and processed meat has no association with colorectal cancer, and neither does total or saturated fat intake (Kimura et al., 2007). Keep in mind that correlation does not equal causation; however, this does remind us that quality, of meat or any other food source, should always be taken into consideration.

Other studies using low- or sometimes even no-carbohydrate ketogenic diets tend to show the same effects. Mice injected with prostate cancer were fed the same number of calories of either a no-carb ketogenic diet (84 percent fat and 16 percent protein), a low-fat diet (12 percent fat, 72 percent carbohydrate, and 16 percent protein), or a typical Western diet (40 percent fat, 44 percent carbohydrate, and 16 percent protein) (Freedland et al., 2008). Fifty-one days later, the tumors in the mice on the no-carb ketogenic diet were 33 percent smaller than those in the mice on the Western diet. The mice on the ketogenic diet also survived longer than the mice in the other two groups.

Of course, the ketogenic diet doesn't have to be and likely shouldn't be a stand-alone treatment. Rather, it can work in conjunction with other treatments. Studies have shown that mice with cancer on a ketogenic diet were more responsive to radiation and ultimately had fewer tumor cells (Abdelwahab et al., 2012). Our good friend and colleague Dr. Angela Poff led much of the work investigating mice with metastatic cancer on a ketogenic diet alone or in combination with hyperbaric oxygen therapy (Poff et al., 2013). Hyperbaric oxygen therapy (HBOT) involves administration of 100 percent oxygen at elevated pressure, which increases ROS—those particles that damage cells—to a level even cancer cells can't handle, ultimately making it toxic for the cells. She found that a ketogenic diet alone slowed tumor growth and increased survival time by 57 percent, but a ketogenic diet in combination with hyperbaric oxygen therapy decreased tumor growth and increased survival by 78 percent!

Treatment	Cohort Size (N)	Mean Survival Time (days)
Control (Standard Diet)	13	31.2
Ketogenic Diet	8	48.9
Standard Diet plus HBOT	8	38.8
Ketogenic Diet plus HBOT	11	55.5

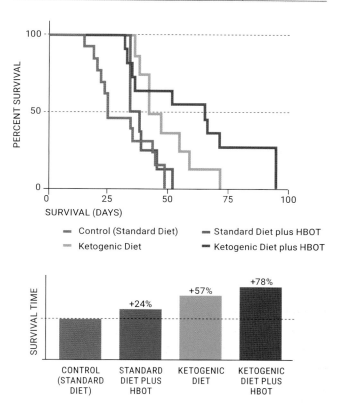

Figure 5.4.5. *A ketogenic diet alone and in combination with HBOT increased survival time significantly more than a standard diet or a standard diet in combination with HBOT.*

Source: Poff et al., 2013.

Tumor size in mice before and after treatment

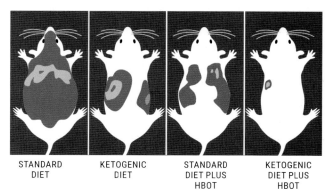

STANDARD DIET   KETOGENIC DIET   STANDARD DIET PLUS HBOT   KETOGENIC DIET PLUS HBOT

Figure 5.4.6. *A ketogenic diet alone and in combination with HBOT decreased tumor size much more than a standard diet or a standard diet in combination with HBOT.*

Source: Poff et al., 2013.

Human Trials

Last but certainly not least are human trials. These are few and far between due to challenges in getting approval for studies this experimental in a population that is vulnerable (i.e., people who have cancer). Nonetheless, the results of the studies we do have, along with anecdotal reports from people across the world, are promising:

1. Two female pediatric patients with advanced-stage malignant brain cancer saw a 21.8 percent decrease in tumor cell glucose uptake after eight weeks on a ketogenic diet. Both saw significant clinical improvements, and one remained on the diet for one year and was free of disease progression, meaning a stable remission (i.e., the tumor had not progressed further) (Nebeling et al., 1995).

2. Ten subjects with advanced, incurable cancer were put on a ketogenic diet. More than half of them achieved a stable or partial remission (where the tumor remains but has shrunk) after just twenty-eight days on the diet. In fact, the greater the level of ketosis, the higher the chance of stable or partial remission (Fine et al., 2012).

3. A sixty-five-year-old woman with brain cancer did a three-day water-only fast followed by four weeks of a 4:1 ketogenic diet at about 600 calories per day (80 percent fat, 20 percent protein and carbs) and radiation and chemotherapy. An MRI done after the four-week period detected no brain tumor tissue. The patient then switched to a low-calorie, non-ketogenic diet for five months, still with no tumor recurrence. However, three months after stopping strict diet therapy, the tumor recurred (Zuccoli et al., 2010).

4. Recently, eleven patients with advanced or metastatic tumors (not on chemotherapy) were put on a modified ketogenic diet (20 to 40 grams of carbohydrates per day). The authors concluded that a ketogenic diet is safe and feasible in advanced cancer patients and slightly improved quality of life scores. At four weeks, 54.5 percent of patients had stable or improved disease, and those who saw the best benefit were patients who lost at least 10 percent of their body weight (Tan-Shalaby et al., 2016).

5. Six patients who underwent radiotherapy and concurrently consumed a self-administered ketogenic diet had no adverse diet-related side effects. These patients all experienced weight loss, which was confirmed to be primarily fat mass, and their quality of life remained stable throughout. Tumor regression occurred in five of six patients with early-stage disease; however, one subject with metastatic small-cell lung cancer experienced slight progression during three cycles of combined chemotherapy plus ketogenic diet, which progressed rapidly after ending the ketogenic diet (Klement et al., 2016).

6. One hurdle that we consistently face in this type of research is compliance. Recently, Zahra et al. (2017) stated that "patients with locally advanced NSCLC and pancreatic cancer receiving concurrent radiotherapy and chemotherapy had suboptimal compliance to the oral ketogenic diet and thus, poor tolerance." Due to these confounding variables, it is hard to make conclusions on what, if any, effect the diet is having. In order to continue down this road of research, better compliance and coaching will be needed for patients and researchers to truly be able to assess the effect of the ketogenic diet on specific outcomes.

7. Recently, an extensive literature review looked at whether cancer-specific survival in rectal cancer patients is affected by medical history and lifestyle factors, conditional on radiation treatment. The authors found that individuals eating a modified ketogenic diet (defined as at least 40 percent calories from fat and less than 100 grams per day glycemic load based on overall distributions) significantly reduced their risk of cancer-specific death. The hazard ratio—the ratio of the hazard/death rates corresponding to the conditions—was significantly lower in the individuals consuming a ketogenic diet compared to other deaths in the irradiated group (Kato et al., 2016).

To improve our understanding of how the ketogenic diet affects cancer, more human research is needed. Physicians and healthcare professionals should be willing to look at this as an alternative strategy as long as proper guidance, support, and oversight are provided. Nutritional intervention in conjunction with current and emerging treatment options could prove to be a very effective tool for fighting cancer. By no means is diet the be-all, end-all approach, but its ability to sensitize the body to other treatments, such as chemotherapy and radiation, may prove valuable. The lower the amount of chemotherapy and radiation we can do while still yielding optimal results, the better off we likely will be.

Dr. Seyfried proposes a "press-pulse" approach that looks at treating cancer like driving in a drag race: the driver presses the gas pedal the entire time, but at certain points during the race will pulse the turbo to give the car an extra boost. In the case of cancer treatment, the "press" could be a calorie-restricted ketogenic diet—maintained consistently to prevent the growth and spread of tumors—while the "pulse" could be things like hyperbaric oxygen therapy, nontoxic drugs, and chemotherapy, which can further shrink tumors and improve health.

Possible Concerns

We have outlined a lot of potential ways in which the ketogenic diet could be beneficial for fighting cancer, slowing tumor growth, or preventing cancer from ever developing. The data presented thus far is compelling, but there are possible limitations to the ketosis and cancer theory that should be addressed.

We discussed earlier how cancer cells do not use ketones as efficiently as they utilize glucose. However, over time, cancer cells adapt and can use a variety of different fuels, including fatty acids, for growth and energy production (Lin et al., 2017). Indeed, the ability of a cancer cell to utilize fatty acids poses a threat to the use of a ketogenic diet as a therapy. There are two possible (and opposing) fears:

- If rates of fatty acid synthesis are elevated in cancer cells and fatty acid uptake is increased, then a high-fat diet could lead to lipid toxicity in cancer cells.

- Increased dietary fat intake could contribute to the progression of the disease by providing more fat for the cancer cells to use.

These are two very different outcomes, and which one is more likely may depend on the cancer type, the stage of the cancer, or even the health of the patient. Cancer cells are going to do whatever they can to get fuel to help them grow and thrive. The

Brain Cancer

In the past several years, we have heard many stories of individuals with brain cancer seeing success with the ketogenic diet. One important thing to note is that fatty acids don't readily cross the blood-brain barrier to enter the brain, which may be a reason why this approach seems to work so well in these individuals. Any concerns one might have about cancer cells using fatty acids would be alleviated by the fact that the brain wouldn't have much access to them, just to ketones that are produced in the body (which do enter the brain). As we have said many times already, we need a lot more information about when the ketogenic diet is applicable and in which cancers/conditions it might not apply. The lack of consistent results may be a result of inconsistent study methods (e.g., some subjects achieving a state of ketosis while others do not, lack of compliance, etc.) as well as cancer heterogeneity. This is why it is important for us to continue to build our understanding of the disease and keep testing various combinations of therapeutic approaches. For more information, check out Dr. Adrienne Scheck's work at the Barrow Neurological Institute, where she is actively investigating these situations.

question ultimately becomes, would you rather offer them a non-preferred, "possible" fuel (i.e., fatty acids and ketones) or pour gasoline on the fire by feeding them their preferred fuel (glucose)? At this time, we feel the data is compelling that targeting glucose metabolism is a much better option.

Besides, with the other benefits of ketosis and a well-formulated ketogenic diet—such as lowered inflammation, decreased oxidative stress, and enhancement of immune function—ketones need to be looked at as more than just a fuel source. And just because cancer cells may be able to take up ketones and utilize fatty acids doesn't mean that they can use them as effectively as glucose. It is possible that even just a lower-carbohydrate, higher-protein (non-ketogenic) diet could slow tumor growth compared to a traditional Western diet (Ho et al., 2011); this indicates that the level of carbohydrate restriction and degree of ketosis can be tailored to the individual and situation (e.g., cancer type, degree of metastasis, etc.).

Exogenous Ketones

Imagine that you and your friends are having a challenge to see who can drive from New York to California the fastest. There are three options: a motorcycle, a Porsche, and a pickup truck. Unfortunately, you draw the short straw and get stuck with the pickup truck. Several hours into the journey, everyone needs to stop for gas. However, the only gas station around provides just diesel fuel. You, driving a pickup truck, are fine since diesel is what your truck uses. However, the two other drivers are at a standstill because their vehicles can't run on the diesel fuel. Needless to say, you make it to California first, while they remain stranded at the gas station.

Now think of cancer cells as the motorcycle and Porsche and ketones as the diesel fuel. Unlike normal tissues and cells, many cancer cells are unable to *effectively* utilize ketone bodies for energy. As discussed earlier, this is why the ketogenic diet holds so much promise for cancer patients, and preliminary case studies in animals and humans have verified its potential effectiveness. On the other hand, the ketogenic diet is thought of as a rather restrictive way of eating that can be difficult to stick to, especially for individuals already suffering the stress of living with cancer. Fortunately, exogenous ketones may provide an alternative way to achieve ketosis and push blood levels to a point where beneficial effects may be seen.

Remember the pilot trial by Dr. Eugene Fine and colleagues (2012), who put eight patients with advanced incurable cancers on a ketogenic diet and found that more than 60 percent of those who were tumor stable or had partial remission had threefold higher levels of ketones at the conclusion of the study than those whose cancers continued to progress. This trial indicates that there may be something unique about an elevation in ketone bodies—not just the reduction of glucose—that is driving the prevention of the disease's progression.

Want to know what's even more interesting, yet disappointing in the sense that it hasn't been talked about until now? The concept of ketones serving as an adjuvant therapy to cancer treatment isn't new. In the early 1970s, researchers looked at the effects of D-BHB on the growth of leukemia cells (Magee, 1979). Cell growth was inhibited, proportional to the concentration of D-BHB—meaning that the greater the level of D-BHB, the lower the cancer cell growth. To build on this work, decades later researchers took cancerous nerve cells and bathed them with either AcAc or BHB; those cells lived 52 percent and 61 percent shorter, respectively, while apoptosis (cell death) was significantly higher (Skinner et al., 2009). As mentioned earlier, our friend and colleague Dr. Angela Poff has since carried on this work in models of metastatic cancer, investigating ketones both alone and in combination with other therapies. First, she found that even in the presence of high glucose, brain cancer cells lived shorter with ketone supplementation. Additionally, mice that had metastatic cancer and were supplemented with ketones saw slowed tumor growth and lived more than 60 percent longer than those in a control group (Poff et al., 2014).

Now, you may be wondering how this is possible. How could ketone supplementation itself be exerting effects directly on cancer cells and potentially slowing tumor growth and increasing survival time? There are several plausible mechanisms:

- Ketone supplementation has been shown to increase antioxidant capacity, thus protecting the cells from damage (Poff et al., 2016).

- Ketone supplementation has been shown to increase levels of carnosine, a potent inhibitor of anaerobic glycolysis (the transformation of glucose to lactate when there are limited amounts of oxygen). Carnosine has been shown to slow tumor growth and metastasis, and in studies, ketone supplementation increased cancer survival rates by four times (Poff et al., 2016).

- Ketone supplementation reduces particles called lysophospholipids, which are elevated in the blood of cancer patients and have been shown to increase the production of new tumors and the spread of those tumors (Poff et al., 2016).

- Referring to Warburg's hypothesis, cancer cells increase lactate production, which promotes the metastasis and spread of tumors. However, as we already know, BHB and lactate use the same monocarboxylic acid (MCT) transporters, so elevating levels of BHB can elevate the levels of these transporters. Through competitive inhibition (i.e., if cancer cells are utilizing the transporters, then lactate may not be able to), ketones themselves may hinder the tumor-promoting aspects of lactate by not allowing it to get into the cells as easily (Bonuccelli et al., 2010).

- Ketones can limit oxidative stress and inflammation, which could have anticancer effects (Youm et al., 2015).

- Ketones may be exerting signaling cascades that can induce apoptosis, reduce ROS production, and even trigger DNA repair through HDAC inhibition (West and Johnstone, 2014).

- Ketones may enhance the formation of new mitochondria and improve mitochondrial function (Veech, 2004; Frey et al., 2016), which, as we discussed earlier, may reduce the likelihood that cells will become cancerous.

In addition to their effects on tumor growth, ketone supplements may reduce the side effects of radiation, such as cachexia (weight loss and muscle wasting). Besides ketones' ability to preserve lean muscle mass, a recent study showed that when a ketone ester was administered, bone marrow damage markers following radiation exposure were attenuated (decreased) by 50 percent. In addition, the production of red blood cells (which can be significantly decreased by both cancer itself and cancer treatments) was significantly rescued by ketone supplementation (Kemper et al., 2016). Therefore, ketone supplementation may serve a synergistic relationship when combined with other current therapies and treatment modalities; however, more research needs to be done in human models using various ketone supplements (esters, salts, isomers, etc.).

Deuterium Depletion? What's That?

If you've never heard of deuterium or deuterium depletion (Dd), don't worry; we hadn't either until we met Que Collins and Laszlo Boros, two doctors actively investigating this area of research, and read the book *Defeating Cancer* by Gabor Somlyai.

In brief, the mitochondria in our cells use oxygen and hydrogen from food to produce ATP and water. Imagine that to create ATP, each mitochondria has a windmill that powers its energy production. Normally, hydrogens can easily bind to the blades of the windmill; however, deuterium, a heavier-than-normal hydrogen, starts slowing down the windmill when it binds due to its weight. Eventually, the deuterium will break the windmill. Everything we consume has different levels of deuterium and contributes to this process.

One theory is that over time, deuterium contributes to dysfunctional mitochondria and ultimately metabolic disease—including cancer. Processed foods, which typically contain high amounts of carbohydrates, contain a lot of deuterium. Several studies show promise for deuterium-depleted water as well as foods that are low in deuterium and their ability to destroy or inhibit tumor cell growth (unlike our normal drinking water). It's possible that with unbroken "windmills," healthy cells are better able to adapt, and this could lead to better-functioning mitochondria that can overwhelm cancer cells. Much more research is needed on this; however, it is especially interesting because ketogenic foods tend to be much lower in deuterium than carbohydrate-rich foods.

Future Directions

Because cancer is extremely complex and varies from person to person, multiple approaches are likely needed to fight it. While targeting metabolism seems advantageous, we likely will have to explore various ways to do so in order to address different aspects of the disease and its progression. While it's clear that ketosis may have unique benefits that might be helpful for individuals with cancer, there are still questions to be answered, such as what level of ketosis is optimal for these individuals and whether/how a ketogenic diet and supplemental ketones affect cancer differently. We may find that a ketogenic diet is beneficial during certain stages of cancer but not during others, or that calorie restriction is required in some cases but not in others. We may find that exogenous ketones are the preferred treatment method for certain types of cancer or that, following remission, using exogenous ketones prevents tumors from recurring and spares lean body mass from cachexia, or muscle wasting. However, we may also find that ketogenic therapies should not be used for some cancers. It's likely, however, that a combination of treatment options administered in a "press-pulse" manner will give patients the best results.

The evidence in favor of exposing cancer cell metabolism is too extensive to ignore. Due to the fact that we have yet to find a cure, it may be time to consider novel approaches. At the end of the day, the goal is to improve both the management of the disease and the quality of life of cancer patients. Keeping in mind the Hippocratic Oath—"First, do no harm"—finding the best approach to target cancer's metabolic pathways in an attempt to win this war on the disease will require a huge effort from many brilliant minds.

In closing, we are often asked, "What would you do if, God forbid, you or a loved one were diagnosed with cancer?" While we are not medical doctors, and what we have to say should in no way be construed as medical advice, we can suggest what our regimen would be and possible steps that we would take to make ketosis part of our cancer treatment plan.

1. Fast for forty-eight to seventy-two hours to initiate ketosis.

2. Adopt a calorie-restricted ketogenic diet with intermittent fasting—for instance, one or two meals per day. (See Chapter 3 for more on how this ketogenic diet might look.)

3. Take medications or supplements that reduce blood glucose, such as metformin, berberine, or, better yet, dihydroberberine.

4. Supplement with exogenous ketones, HMB (a supplement that can prevent muscle protein breakdown), and high-dose probiotics (which can help boost immune function and gut function).

5. Exercise daily, whether that is going on a walk, lifting weights, or a combination of the two.

6. Seek hyperbaric oxygen therapy treatment.

7. Undergo pulsed chemotherapy or radiation based on our doctors' recommendation. (Prior to the actual chemotherapy or radiation, we would supplement with exogenous ketones and fast for at least sixteen hours in an attempt to sensitize cells to the treatment.)

As you can see, cancer is a tricky disease, and likely the most complicated one we have ever come across. By no means is cancer treatment or therapy our area of expertise; rather, we hope to provide you with a brief understanding of the disease and the research behind why ketosis may be a potential treatment option when paired with other standards of care. By no means are we stating that a ketogenic diet or ketone supplementation is a magical cure for cancer, but it may be a logical option for individuals looking to lower blood glucose and insulin levels and overcome defective mitochondria. Nothing stated here should be construed as medical advice; rather, it's meant as a breakdown of information for you to interpret and use as you feel is appropriate. It is likely that a combination of various therapies will be ideal for most individuals, and we hope to continue to see great strides in this area.

References

Abdelwahab, M. G., K. E. Fenton, M. C. Preul, J. M. Rho, A. Lynch, P. Stafford, and A. C. Scheck. "The ketogenic diet is an effective adjuvant to radiation therapy for the treatment of malignant glioma." *PLOS ONE* 7, no. 5 (2012): e36197. doi: 10.1371/journal.pone.0036197.

Albanes, D. "Total calories, body weight, and tumor incidence in mice." *Cancer Research* 47, no. 8 (1987): 1987–92.

Algire, C., L. Amrein, M. Zakikhani, L. Panasci, L., and M. Pollak. "Metformin blocks the stimulative effect of a high-energy diet on colon carcinoma growth in vivo and is associated with reduced expression of fatty acid synthase." *Endocrine-Related Cancer* 17, no. 2 (2010): 351–60. doi: 10.1677/ERC-09-0252.

Allen, B. G., S. K. Bhatia, J. M. Buatti, K. E. Brandt, K. E. Lindholm, A. M. Button, ... and M. A. Fath. "Ketogenic diets enhance oxidative stress and radio-chemo-therapy responses in lung cancer xenografts." *Clinical Cancer Research* 19, no. 14 (2013): 3905–13. doi: 10.1158/1078-0432.CCR-12-0287.

Bauer, D. E., M. H. Harris, D. R. Plas, J. J. Lum, P. S. Hammerman, J. C. Rathmell, ... and C. B. Thompson. "Cytokine stimulation of aerobic glycolysis in hematopoietic cells exceeds proliferative demand." *The FASEB Journal* 18, no. 11 (2004): 1303–5.

Beck, S. A., and M. J. Tisdale. "Nitrogen excretion in cancer cachexia and its modification by a high fat diet in mice." *Cancer Research* 49, no. 14 (1989): 3800–4.

Cairns, R. A., I. S. Harris, and T. W. Mak. "Regulation of cancer cell metabolism." *Nature Reviews Cancer* 11, no. 2 (2011): 85–95. doi: 10.1038/nrc2981.

Chang, H. T., L. K. Olson, and K. A. Schwartz. "Ketolytic and glycolytic enzymatic expression profiles in malignant gliomas: implication for ketogenic diet therapy." *Nutrition & Metabolism* 10, no. 1 (2013): 47.

Chen, X., Y. Qian, and S. Wu. "The Warburg effect: evolving interpretations of an established concept." *Free Radical Biology and Medicine* 79 (2015): 253–63. doi: 10.1016/j.freeradbiomed.2014.08.027.

Colman, R. J., Anderson, R. M., Johnson, S. C., Kastman, E. K., Kosmatka, K. J., Beasley, T. M., ... and R. Weindruch. "Caloric restriction delays disease onset and mortality in rhesus monkeys." *Science* 325, no. 5937 (2009): 201–4. doi: 10.1126/science.1173635.

Cruz-Bermúdez, A., C. G. Vallejo, R. J. Vicente-Blanco, M. E. Gallardo, M. Á. Fernández-Moreno, M. Quintanilla, and R. Garesse. "Enhanced tumorigenicity by mitochondrial DNA mild mutations." *Oncotarget* 6, no. 15 (2015): 13628–43.

DeBerardinis, R. J., et al. "The biology of cancer: metabolic reprogramming fuels cell growth and proliferation." *Cell Metabolism* 7, no. 1 (2008): 11–20. doi: 10.1016/j.cmet.2007.10.002.

Fine, E. J., A. Miller, E. V. Quadros, J. M. Sequeira, and R. D. Feinman. "Acetoacetate reduces growth and ATP concentration in cancer cell lines which over-express uncoupling protein 2." *Cancer Cell International* 9 (2009): 14. doi: 10.1186/1475-2867-9-14.

Fine, E. J., C. J. Segal-Isaacson, R. D. Feinman, S. Herszkopf, M. C. Romano, N. Tomuta, ... and J. A. Sparano. "Targeting insulin inhibition as a metabolic therapy in advanced cancer: a pilot safety and feasibility dietary trial in 10 patients." *Nutrition* 28, no. 10 (2012): 1028–35. doi: 10.1016/j.nut.2012.05.001.

Freedland, S. J., J. Mavropoulos, A. Wang, M. Darshan, W. Demark-Wahnefried, W. J. Aronson, ... and S. V. Pizzo. "Carbohydrate restriction, prostate cancer growth, and the insulin-like growth factor axis." *The Prostate* 68, no. 1 (2008): 11–19. doi: 10.1002/pros.20683.

Frezza, C., L. Zheng, O. Folger, K. N. Rajagopalan, E. D. MacKenzie, L. Jerby, ... and G. Kalna. "Haem oxygenase is synthetically lethal with the tumour suppressor fumarate hydratase." *Nature* 477, no. 7363 (2011): 225–8. doi: 10.1038/nature10363.

Gatenby, R. A., and R. J. Gillies. "Why do cancers have high aerobic glycolysis?" *Nature Reviews Cancer* 4, no. 11 (2004): 891–9. doi: 10.1038/nrc1478.

Gnagnarella, P., S. Gandini, C. La Vecchia, and P. Maisonneuve. "Glycemic index, glycemic load, and cancer risk: a meta-analysis." *American Journal of Clinical Nutrition* 87, no. 6 (2008): 1793–801.

Groves, A. M., et al. "Non-[18 F] FDG PET in clinical oncology." *Lancet Oncology* 8, no. 9 (2007): 822–30. doi: 10.1016/S1470-2045(07)70274-7.

Guppy, M., E. Greiner, and K. Brand. "The role of the Crabtree effect and an endogenous fuel in the energy metabolism of resting and proliferating thymocytes." *European Journal of Biochemistry* 212, no. 1 (1993): 95–9.

Hanahan, D., and R. A. Weinberg ."The hallmarks of cancer." *Cell* 100, no. 1 (2000): 57–70.

Hanahan, D., and R. A. Weinberg. "Hallmarks of cancer: the next generation." *Cell* 144, no. 5 (2011): 646–74. doi: 10.1016/j.cell 2011.02.013.

Ho, V. W., K. Leung, A. Hsu, B. Luk, J. Lai, S. Y. Shen, ... and B. H. Nelson. "A low carbohydrate, high protein diet slows tumor growth and prevents cancer initiation." *Cancer Research* 71, no. 13 (2011): 4484–93.

Hursting, S. D., S. M. Smith, L. M. Lashinger, A. E. Harvey, and S. N. Perkins. "Calories and carcinogenesis: lessons learned from 30 years of calorie restriction research." *Carcinogenesis* 31, no. 1 (2010): 83–89. doi: 10.1093/carcin/bgp280.

Jarrett, S. G., J. B. Milder, L. P. Liang, and M. Patel. "The ketogenic diet increases mitochondrial glutathione levels." *Journal of Neurochemistry* 106, no. 3 (2008): 1044–51.

Jeon, S. M., N. S. Chandel, and N. Hay. "AMPK regulates NADPH homeostasis to promote tumour cell survival during energy stress." *Nature* 485 (2012): 661–5. doi: 10.1038/nature11066.

Jiang, Y. S., and F. R. Wang. "Caloric restriction reduces edema and prolongs survival in a mouse glioma model." *Journal of Neuro-Oncology* 114, no. 1 (2013): 25–32. doi: 10.1007/s11060-013-1154-y.

Kaipparettu, B. A., Y. Ma, J. H. Park, T. L. Lee, Y. Zhang, P. Yotnda, ... and L. J. C. Wong. "Crosstalk from non-cancerous mitochondria can inhibit tumor properties of metastatic cells by suppressing oncogenic pathways." *PLOS ONE* 8, no. 5 (2013): e61747. doi: 10.1371/journal.pone.0061747.

Kato, I., G. Dyson, M. Snyder, H. R. Kim, and R. K. Severson. "Differential effects of patient-related factors on the outcome of radiation therapy for rectal cancer." *Journal of Radiation Oncology* 5, no. 3 (2016): 279–86.

Kemper, M. F., A. Miller, R. J. Pawlosky, and R. Veech. "Administration of a novel β-hydroxybutyrate ester after radiation exposure suppresses in vitro lethality and chromosome damage, attenuates bone marrow suppression in vivo." *FASEB Journal* 30, suppl 1 (2016): 627.3.

Kimura, Y., S. Kono, K. Toyomura, J. Nagano, T. Mizoue, M. A. Moore, ... and T. Okamura. "Meat, fish and fat intake in relation to subsite-specific risk of colorectal cancer: The Fukuoka Colorectal Cancer Study." *Cancer Science* 98, no. 4 (2007): 590–7.

Klement, R. J., and C. E. Champ. "Calories, carbohydrates, and cancer therapy with radiation: exploiting the five R's through dietary manipulation." *Cancer and Metastasis Reviews* 33, no. 1 (2014): 217–29. doi: 10.1007/s10555-014-9495-3.

Klement, R. J., and R. A. Sweeney. "Impact of a ketogenic diet intervention during radiotherapy on body composition: I. Initial clinical experience with six prospectively studied patients." *BMC Research Notes* 9, no. 1 (2016): 143.

Ko, Y. H., P. L. Pedersen, and J. F. Geschwind. "Glucose catabolism in the rabbit VX2 tumor model for liver cancer: characterization and targeting hexokinase." *Cancer Letters* 173, no. 1 (2001): 83–91.

Ko, Y. H., B. L. Smith, Y. Wang, M. G. Pomper, D. A. Rini, M. S. Torbenson, ... and P. L. Pederser. "Advanced cancers: eradication in all cases using 3-bromopyruvate therapy to deplete ATP." *Biochemical and Biophysical Research Communications* 324, no. 1 (2004): 269–75.

Ko, Y. H., H. A. Verhoeven, M. J. Lee, D. J. Corbin, T. J. Vogl, and P. L. Pedersen. "A translationa study 'case report' on the small molecule 'energy blocker' 3-bromopyruvate (3BP) as a potent anticancer agent: from bench side to bedside." *Journal of Bioenergetics and Biomembranes* 44, no. 1 (2012): 163–70.

Koppenol, W. H., P. L. Bounds, and C. V. Dang. "Otto Warburg's contributions to current concepts of cancer metabolism." *Nature Reviews Cancer* 11, no. 5 (2011): 325–37. doi: 10.1038/nrc3038.

Kritchevsky, D. "Caloric restriction and cancer." *Journal of Nutritional Science and Vitaminology* 47, no. 1 (2001): 13–19.

Lee, C., L. Raffaghello, S. Brandhorst, F. M. Safdie, G. Bianchi, A. Martin-Montalvo, ... and L. Emionite. "Fasting cycles retard growth of tumors and sensitize a range of cancer cell types to chemotherapy." *Science Translational Medicine* 4, no. 124 (2012): 124ra27. doi: 10.1126/scitranslmed.3003293.

Lewis, N. E., and A. M. Abdel-Haleem. "The evolution of genome-scale models of cancer metabolism." *Frontiers in Physiology* 4 (2013): 237. doi: 10.3389/fphys.2013.00237.

Lin, H., S. Patel, V. S. Affleck, I. Wilson, D. M. Turnbull, A. R. Joshi, ... and E. A. Stoll. "Fatty acid oxidation is required for the respiration and proliferation of malignant glioma cells." *Neuro-Oncology* 19, no. 1 (2017): 43–54. doi: 10.1093/neuonc/now128.

Liotta, L. A., P. S. Steeg, and W. G. Stetler-Stevenson. "Cancer metastasis and angiogenesis: an imbalance of positive and negative regulation." *Cell* 64, no. 2 (1991): 327–36.

Liou, G. Y., and P. Storz. "Reactive oxygen species in cancer." *Free Radical Research* 44, no. 5 (2010): 479–96. doi: 10.3109/10715761003667554.

Liu, H., Y. P. Hu, N. Savaraj, W. Priebe, and T. J. Lampidis. "Hypersensitization of tumor cells to glycolytic inhibitors." *Biochemistry* 40, no. 18 (2001): 5542–7.

Lussier, D. M., E. C. Woolf, J. L. Johnson, K. S. Brooks, J. N. Blattman, and A. C. Scheck. "Enhanced immunity in a mouse model of malignant glioma is mediated by a therapeutic ketogenic diet." *BMC Cancer* 16 (2016): 310. doi: 10.1186/s12885-016-2337-7.

Magee, B. A., N. Potezny, A. M. Rofe, and R. A. Conyers. "The inhibition of malignant cell growth by ketone bodies." *Australian Journal of Experimental Biology Medical Science* 57, no. 5 (1979): 529–39.

Marsh, J., P. Mukherjee, and T. N. Seyfried. "Drug/diet synergy for managing malignant astrocytoma in mice: 2-deoxy-D-glucose and the restricted ketogenic diet." *Nutrition & Metabolism* 5 (2008): 33. doi: 10.1186/1743-7075-5-33.

Martinez-Outschoorn, U. E., M. Prisco, A. Ertel, A. Tsirigos, Z. Lin, S. Pavlides, ... and R. G. Pestell. "Ketones and lactate increase cancer cell 'stemness,' driving recurrence, metastasis and poor clinical outcome in breast cancer: achieving personalized medicine via Metabolo-Genomics." *Cell Cycle* 10, no. 8 (2011): 1271–86. doi: 10.4161/cc.10.8.15330.

Maurer, G. D., D. P. Brucker, O. Bähr, P. N. Harter, E. Hattingen, S. Walenta, ... and J. Rieger. "Differential utilization of ketone bodies by neurons and glioma cell lines: a rationale for ketogenic diet as experimental glioma therapy." *BMC Cancer* 11 (2011): 315. doi: 10.1186/1471-2407-11-315.

Mavropoulos, J. C., W. C. Buschemeyer, A. K. Tewari, D. Rokhfeld, M. Pollak, Y. Zhao, ... and W. Demark-Wahnefried. "The effects of varying dietary carbohydrate and fat content on survival in a murine LNCaP prostate cancer xenograft model." *Cancer Prevention Research* 2, no. 6 (2009): 557–65. doi: 10.1158/1940-6207.CAPR-08-0188.

Meidenbauer, J. J., N. Ta, and T. N. Seyfried. "Influence of a ketogenic diet, fish-oil, and calorie restriction on plasma metabolites and lipids in C57BL/6J mice." *Nutrition & Metabolism* 11 (2014): 23.

Miller, D. M., S. D. Thomas, A. Islam, D. Muench, and K. Sedoris. "c-Myc and cancer metabolism." *Clinical Cancer Research* 18, no. 20 (2012): 5546–53. doi: 10.1158/1078-0432.CCR-12-0977.

Moreno-Sánchez, R., S. Rodríguez-Enríquez, A. Marín-Hernández, and E. Saavedra. "Energy metabolism in tumor cells." *FEBS Journal* 274, no. 6 (2007): 1393–418.

Morscher, R. J., S. Aminzadeh-Gohari, R. G. Feichtinger, J. A. Mayr, R. Lang, D. Neureiter, ... and B. Kofler. "Inhibition of neuroblastoma tumor growth by ketogenic diet and/or calorie restriction in a CD1-Nu mouse model." *PLOS ONE* 10, no. 6 (2015): e0129802. doi: 10.1371/journal.pone.0129802.

Mukherjee, P., A. V. Sotnikov, H. J. Mangian, J. R. Zhou, W. J. Visek, and S. K. Clinton. "Energy intake and prostate tumor growth, angiogenesis, and vascular endothelial growth factor expression." *Journal of the National Cancer Institute* 91, no. 6 (1999): 512–23. doi: 10.1093/jnci/91.6.512.

Mukherjee, S. *The Emperor of All Maladies: A Biography of Cancer.* New York: Simon and Schuster, 2010.

Mulrooney, T. J., J. Marsh, I. Urits, T. N. Seyfried, and P. Mukherjee. "Influence of caloric restriction on constitutive expression of NF-κB in an experimental mouse astrocytoma." *PLOS ONE* 6, no. 3 (2011): e18085. doi: 10.1371/journal.pone.0018085.

Nebeling, L. C., F. Miraldi, S. B. Shurin, and E. Lerner. "Effects of a ketogenic diet on tumor metabolism and nutritional status in pediatric oncology patients: two case reports." *Journal of the American College of Nutrition* 14, no. 2 (1995): 202–8.

Otto, C., U. Kaemmerer, B. Illert, B. Muehling, N. Pfetzer, R. Wittig, ... and J. F. Coy. "Growth of human gastric cancer cells in nude mice is delayed by a ketogenic diet supplemented with omega-3 fatty acids and medium-chain triglycerides." *BMC Cancer* 8 (2008): 122. doi: 10.1186/1471-2407-8-122.

Pelser, C., A. M. Mondul, A. R. Hollenbeck, and Y. Park. "Dietary fat, fatty acids, and risk of prostate cancer in the NIH-AARP diet and health study." *Cancer Epidemiology and Prevention Biomarkers* 22, no. 4 (2013): 697–707. doi: 10.1158/1055-9965.EPI-12-1196-T.

Poff, A. M., C. Ari, P. Arnold, T. N. Seyfried, and D. P. D'Agostino. "Ketone supplementation decreases tumor cell viability and prolongs survival of mice with metastatic cancer." *International Journal of Cancer* 135, no. 7 (2014): 1711–20. doi: 10.1002/ijc.28809.

Poff, A. M., C. Ari, T. N. Seyfried, and D. P. D'Agostino. "The ketogenic diet and hyperbaric oxygen therapy prolong survival in mice with systemic metastatic cancer." *PLOS ONE* 8, no. 6 (2013): e65522. doi: 10.1371/journal.pone.0065522.

Puzio-Kuter, A. M. "The role of p53 in metabolic regulation." *Genes & Cancer* 2, no. 4 (2011): 385–91. doi: 10.1177/1947601911409738.

Racker, E. "Bioenergetics and the problem of tumor growth: an understanding of the mechanism of the generation and control of biological energy may shed light on the problem of tumor growth." *American Scientist* 60, no. 1 (1972): 56–63.

Safdie, F. M., T. Dorff, D. Quinn, L. Fontana, M. Wei, C. Lee, ... and V. D. Longo. "Fasting and cancer treatment in humans: a case series report." *Aging (Albany, NY)* 1, no. 12 (2009): 988–1007.

Scheck, A. C., M. G. Abdelwahab, K. E. Fenton, and P. Stafford. "The ketogenic diet for the treatment of glioma: insights from genetic profiling." *Epilepsy Research* 100, no. 3 (2012): 327–37. doi: 10.1016/j.eplepsyres.2011.09.022.

Schmidt, M., N. Pfetzer, M. Schwab, I. Strauss, and U. Kämmerer. "Effects of a ketogenic diet on the quality of life in 16 patients with advanced cancer: a pilot trial." *Nutrition & Metabolism* 8, no. 1 (2011): 54. doi: 10.1186/1743-7075-8-54.

Schwartz, K., H. T. Chang, M. Nikolai, J. Pernicone, S. Rhee, K. Olson, ... and M. Noel. "Treatment of glioma patients with ketogenic diets: report of two cases treated with an IRB-approved energy-restricted ketogenic diet protocol and review of the literature." *Cancer & Metabolism* 3 (2015): 3. doi: 10.1186/s40170-015-0129-1.

Seyfried, T. *Cancer as a Metabolic Disease: On the Origin, Management, and Prevention of Cancer.* Hoboken, NJ: John Wiley & Sons, 2012.

Seyfried, T. N., R. E. Flores, A. M. Poff, and D. P. D'Agostino. "Cancer as a metabolic disease: implications for novel therapeutics." *Carcinogenesis* 35, no. 3 (2014): 515–27.

Seyfried, T. N., M. Kiebish, P. Mukherjee, and J. Marsh. "Targeting energy metabolism in brain cancer with calorically restricted ketogenic diets." *Epilepsia* 49, suppl 8 (2008): 114–6. doi: 10.1111/j.1528-1167.2008.01853.x.

Seyfried, T. N., T. M. Sanderson, M. M. El-Abbadi, R. McGowan, and P. Mukherjee. "Role of glucose and ketone bodies in the metabolic control of experimental brain cancer." *British Journal of Cancer* 89, no. 7 (2003): 1375–82. doi: 10.1038/sj.bjc.6601269.

Seyfried, T. N., and L. M. Shelton. "Cancer as a metabolic disease." *Nutrition & Metabolism* 7 (2010): 7.

Shelton, L. M., L. C. Huysentruyt, P. Mukherjee, and T. N. Seyfried. "Calorie restriction as an anti-invasive therapy for malignant brain cancer in the VM mouse." *ASN Neuro* 2, no. 3 (2010): e00038. doi: 10.1042/AN20100002.

Skinner, R., A. Trujillo, X. Ma, and E. A. Beierle. "Ketone bodies inhibit the viability of human neuroblastoma cells." *Journal of Pediatric Surgery* 44, no. 1 (2009): 212−6. doi: 10.1016/j.jpedsurg.2008.10.042.

Stafford, P., M. G. Abdelwahab, M. C. Preul, J. M. Rho, and A. C. Scheck. "The ketogenic diet reverses gene expression patterns and reduces reactive oxygen species levels when used as an adjuvant therapy for glioma." *Nutrition & Metabolism* 7 (2010): 74. doi: 10.1186/1743-7075-7-74.

Stratton, M. R., P. J. Campbell, and P. A. Futreal. "The cancer genome." *Nature* 458 (2009): 719−24. doi: 10.1038/nature07943.

Tan-Shalaby, J., J. Carrick, K. Edinger, D. Genovese, A. D. Liman, V. A. Passero, and R. Shah. "Modified ketogenic diet in advanced malignancies: final results of a safety and feasibility trial within the Veterans Affairs Healthcare System." *Nutrition & Metabolism* 13 (2016): 61.

Tannenbaum, A., and H. Silverstone. "The genesis and growth of tumors." *Cancer Research* 2 (1942): 468−75.

Thompson, H. J., J. N. McGinley, N. S. Spoelstra, W. Jiang, Z. Zhu, and P. Wolfe. "Effect of dietary energy restriction on vascular density during mammary carcinogenesis." *Cancer Research* 64, no. 16 (2004): 5643−50.

Tzu, Sun. *The Art of War.*

Veech, R. L. "The therapeutic implications of ketone bodies: the effects of ketone bodies in pathological conditions: ketosis, ketogenic diet, redox states, insulin resistance, and mitochondrial metabolism." *Prostaglandins, Leukotrienes and Essential Fatty Acids* 70, no. 3 (2004): 309−19.

Warburg, O. "On the origin of cancer cells." *Science* 123, no. 3191 (1956): 309−14.

Woolf, E. C., and A. C. Scheck. "The ketogenic diet for the treatment of malignant glioma." *Journal of Lipid Research* 56, no. 1 (2015): 5−10. doi: 10.1194/jlr.R046797.

Youm, Y. H., K. Y. Nguyen, R. W. Grant, E. L. Goldberg, M. Bodogai, D. Kim, ... and S. Kang. "The ketone metabolite [beta]-hydroxybutyrate blocks NLRP3 inflammasome-mediated inflammatory disease." *Nature Medicine* 21, no. 3 (2015): 263−9. doi: 10.1038/nm.3804.

Zahra, A., M. A. Fath, E. Opat, K. A. Mapuskar, S. K. Bhatia, D. C. Ma, ... and K. L. Bodeker. "Consuming a ketogenic diet while receiving radiation and chemotherapy for locally advanced lung cancer and pancreatic cancer: the University of Iowa experience of two phase 1 clinical trials." *Radiation Research* 187, no. 6 (2017): 743−54. doi: 10.1667/RR14668.

Zhou, W., P. Mukherjee, M. A. Kiebish, W. T. Markis, J. G. Mantis, and T. N. Seyfried. "The calorically restricted ketogenic diet, an effective alternative therapy for malignant brain cancer." *Nutrition & Metabolism* 4 (2007): 5. doi: 10.1186/1743-7075-4-5.

Zhuang, Y., D. K. Chan, A. B. Haugrud, and W. K. Miskimins. "Mechanisms by which low glucose enhances the cytotoxicity of metformin to cancer cells both in vitro and in vivo." *PLOS ONE* 9, no. 9 (2014): e108444. doi: 10.1371/journal.pone.0108444.

Zuccoli, G., N. Marcello, A. Pisanello, F. Servadei, S. Vaccaro, P. Mukherjee, and T. N. Seyfried. "Metabolic management of glioblastoma multiforme using standard therapy together with a restricted ketogenic diet: case report." *Nutrition & Metabolism* 7 (2010): 33. doi: 10.1186/1743-7075-7-33.

Section 5:
Exercise and Performance

"I'm ready to accept the challenge. I'm coming home." LeBron James announced that he would return to Cleveland to play basketball in 2014 after playing several seasons with the Miami Heat. Soon thereafter, he wanted to make another change. LeBron, inspired by several of his talented opponents, decided to take a low-carb approach to shed some pounds over the summer. As LeBron began posting pictures of his slimmed-down physique, there was plenty of media speculation about exactly what he was doing with his diet. A few years earlier, ultramarathon runner Timothy Olson had also decided to switch to a ketogenic diet before competing in the 2011 Western States 100-Mile Endurance Run. What were these two athletes thinking? Isn't it unreasonable to expect to play basketball at an elite level without consuming a carbohydrate-rich diet? Wouldn't it be impossible that someone could run 100 miles without relying on sugary goos and gels?

> "Impossible is just a big word thrown around by small men who find it easier to live in the world they've been given than to explore the power they have to change it. Impossible is not a fact. It's an opinion. Impossible is not a declaration. It's a dare. Impossible is potential. Impossible is temporary. Impossible is nothing."
> —Muhammad Ali

Yet LeBron had an outstanding season that year, averaging more than twenty-five points per game and leading his team all the way to the NBA Finals back on his home turf. And Tim, the ultramarathoner, not only won the race but did so in a record time of 14:46:44, which was more than twenty minutes faster than anyone had ever run the course before.

How low-carb/ketogenic diets impact performance is one of the most controversial topics in the fitness community to date. Many people agree that the ketogenic diet is useful for certain therapeutic or alternative therapy modalities; however, some are adamant that it is physically impossible to maintain physical performance on a ketogenic diet. We used to think along the same lines—until we heard Dr. Jeff Volek's talk on ketogenic dieting and performance at a conference in 2011, which sparked our interest and made us want to investigate further. And when we have a question like "Can an athlete still perform on a ketogenic diet?" we can go into the lab at the Applied Science and Performance Institute and find out for ourselves rather than wait years for other people to research it. In this section, we will review previous research as it relates to ketogenic diets and performance as well as brand-new data from our lab and from colleagues of ours who are researching and exploring these areas.

Finally, we want to note that neither this chapter nor this book as a whole is intended to argue that a ketogenic diet is always better than another nutritional approach. That's not what we are about. Rather, we want to provide context and lay a foundation of understanding for those who may be seeking alternatives to traditional recommendations. Many people believe that the road to peak performance is black or white: you either eat carbohydrates or you don't perform. We are here to provide evidence that performance is far beyond just black or white, and if we become fat-fueled machines, we can certainly still perform at a high level.

Switching the Fuel Tank: Why You Can't Measure the Effects of Keto After Just a Few Days

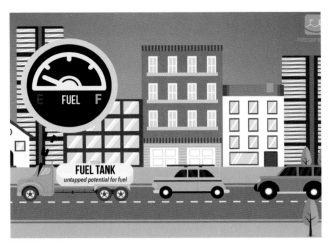

Figure 5.5.1. *"Hitting the wall" is like running out of gas in a fuel truck. You have fuel, you just can't tap into it as well.*

Source: Ketogenic.com.

"Hitting the wall" is a common phrase used among long-distance cyclists, marathon runners, and other endurance athletes to describe the point where it feels as if you can't take even one step farther. Imagine running for hours, more miles than you'd believe possible, and then suddenly your feet feel like they are encased in cement and you literally can't pick them up anymore. "Frustrating" is an understatement.

In the 2016 Olympics, French athlete Yohann Diniz experienced this phenomenon firsthand. Leading the pack about forty-five minutes into a 50k race walk, Yohann collapsed in agony, not only from exhaustion but also from severe stomach pains that literally had him struggling to get up (possibly due to all the goos and gels these athletes typically consume). Whether it is from pure exhaustion or a combination of tiredness and intense GI distress, athletes strive to find ways to avoid this "bonking" in order to run an entire race strong.

Drs. Jeff Volek and Stephen Phinney explain why this happens in their book *The Art and Science of Low Carbohydrate Performance*. Imagine that you are driving on the highway in a fuel tanker truck powered by diesel fuel, and then you realize that the truck's gas gauge is on empty and your truck stalls right there in the middle of the road. The irony is clear: you have a tank filled with hundreds of gallons of gasoline, yet you can't utilize it. The same idea applies to humans. The maximum amount of glycogen—the stored form of glucose—that most humans can store is around 400 to 500 grams, about 1,600 to 2,000 calories' worth. Meanwhile, our fat stores are nearly endless; even the leanest individuals store around 40,000 calories' worth of fat. So the question becomes: which storage tank would you rather tap into? Athletes who rely on carbohydrates as their main fuel source tend to have a difficult time tapping into this nearly limitless supply of fuel during races. Therefore, they consume sugary drinks, goos, and gels in a continuous effort

to refill their glucose tanks, which often leads to "hitting the wall" or, as in Yohann Diniz's case, severe pain and distress.

As discussed earlier in this book, becoming keto-adapted is the process of getting your body to switch from using primarily glucose to using primarily fat and ketones as its main fuel source. To effectively utilize that large reserve tank of fat, we must be adapted to utilizing fat as fuel—and that takes time. We can't emphasize this enough. Many studies looking at performance employ only a short window of just a couple days to three weeks on a high-fat, low-carb diet. From this, some researchers draw the conclusion that this "low-carbohydrate diet" impairs performance. Think about that time frame for a moment. Imagine if Derek Jeter, one of the greatest baseball players of all time, had to switch to batting left-handed midseason. Granted, he might be able to pull it off, but his performance would certainly suffer.

The experience is the same when we make the switch from running on carbs to running on fat. Since most of us have been carbohydrate-adapted and primarily glucose-dependent our entire lives, eating a ketogenic diet for a few weeks likely wouldn't allow us enough time to fully adapt to burning fat instead of carbs, and a decline in performance would be expected.

Once we are fully adapted and can tap into that fat fuel tank, though, is it possible to perform at a competitive level? For many athletes, the answer seems to be yes.

Effects on Endurance Performance

Numerous studies have shown that a carbohydrate-rich diet can be beneficial for endurance athletes. Over the past several decades, researchers have been investigating optimal carbohydrate-dosing strategies that help endurance athletes perform at their best. Why are so many researchers interested in this topic? In the late 1960s, nephrologist Jonas Bergström found a positive association between glycogen levels prior to exercise and exercise capacity (Bergstrom et al., 1967): basically, the more glycogen you start with, the better your performance will be. As a result, researchers spent decades looking at ways for athletes to maximize glycogen stores prior to races by eating absurdly high amounts of carbohydrates. This led to years of studies showing that short-term high-fat diets aren't as beneficial as high-carbohydrate diets for optimal performance. Researchers assumed the reason must be that muscle glycogen—stored glucose that can fuel muscle performance—is lower on a high-fat diet.

On paper, this sounds logical. If you aren't eating carbohydrates to replenish the glycogen you use, how can your muscle glycogen level remain steady? But as you can see in the table on page 140, most of these studies were very short-term—just a couple days in duration—and did not allow for a period of adaptation to a high-fat, low-carbohydrate diet to occur. Therefore, the decline in performance may instead be due to the fact that the athletes were in the process of becoming fat-adapted—a period during which the body doesn't function optimally.

So what really happens to muscle glycogen on a high-fat, low-carb diet? If allowed time to become keto-adapted, can someone who is eating very limited carbohydrates perform as well as someone who is carbohydrate loading? Can the bacon-fueled athlete compete with the bagel-fueled athlete?

Over three decades ago, one of the first studies on this topic investigated whether endurance athletes could perform on a low-carbohydrate ketogenic diet. Five well-trained cyclists were put on a ketogenic diet. Each of them ate the same number of calories, the same amount of protein, and less than 20 grams of carbohydrates per day. After just four weeks, three of the five subjects had not just maintained but actually *improved* their time-to-exhaustion trial, and on average, the subjects' riding times didn't change significantly from those they achieved when they ate a carbohydrate-based diet—147 minutes versus 151 minutes (Phinney et al., 1983). This gave us the first

---

KETO CONCEPT

Gels, Goos, and Poo

Many ultra-marathoners and long-distance runners have experienced the dreaded gastrointestinal distress that comes with the constant glucose gels and goos they have to consume in order to keep their energy up during a long-distance race. In one study of more than 200 endurance athletes, carbohydrate intake was positively correlated to nausea and flatulence (Pfeiffer et al., 2012). Dr. Volek and Dr. Phinney (2012) postulate that these athletes might see relief when competing in a keto-adapted state because they would need to consume fewer calories during the race.

KETO CONCEPT

Do You Need to Carb Load?

One study indicated that a short period of carbohydrate loading following carbohydrate restriction resulted in no increase in performance (Burke et al., 2000). This study divided subjects into two groups: one who ate an average of 709 grams of carbohydrates per day, and the other who ate an average of 177 grams of carbohydrates per day, for five days. On day six, before their performance trial, both groups ate about 730 grams of carbohydrates in an attempt to refill their glycogen tanks. Yet there was no significant difference in performance between the two groups. On top of that, the group whose carbohydrates had been restricted for the first five days had higher rates of fat oxidation, meaning that they were better able to tap into their fat stores than the group eating very large amounts of carbohydrates. This study points to the fact that, irrespective of a ketogenic diet, endurance athletes likely don't need to consume extremely high levels of carbohydrates throughout their training year. It appears that as long as glycogen levels are comparable, there are no differences in performance.

insight that performance may not necessarily decline in high-level athletes, even after just a short transition period (four weeks). Further, this study showed that the rate of fat oxidation for athletes on a ketogenic diet was, on average, three times that of individuals who were not on a ketogenic diet: the cyclists in this study burned an average of 1.5 grams of fat per minute, whereas most non-keto-adapted individuals burn an average of 0.5 gram of fat per minute. This was our first clue that endurance athletes could maintain performance on a ketogenic diet while becoming extraordinary fat burners.

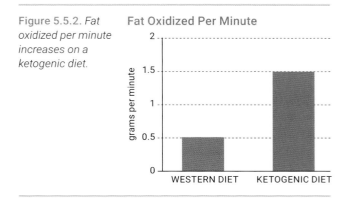

Figure 5.5.2. *Fat oxidized per minute increases on a ketogenic diet.*

Fat Oxidized Per Minute

Though this study has received a great deal of criticism because of its small sample size and the fact that the subjects experienced a range of outcomes (i.e., some significantly improved, some stayed the same, and some got worse), it paved the way for more research into the idea that it is possible to perform well on a diet that isn't predicated on consuming copious amounts of carbohydrates. Over the years, several studies have been done trying to answer the question, "Can endurance athletes perform well on a low-carbohydrate or ketogenic diet?" As you see in the table on page 140, these studies differ drastically in their duration, the type of diet, and what is actually being measured.

Until recently, no studies had looked at the performance of endurance athletes who were truly keto-adapted. In 2016, Dr. Jeff Volek and his team created the FASTER study—Fat-Adapted Substrate Use in Trained Elite Runners—to examine the metabolic characteristics of elite endurance athletes consuming either a low-carbohydrate or a high-carbohydrate diet (Volek et al., 2016). Twenty elite ultra-marathoners and Ironman distance triathletes were involved in this trial. Most of these individuals had more than ten years of competitive running

experience, and some held national and international records in competition. The low-carbohydrate group (ten subjects) had to consume less than 20 percent of calories from carbohydrate and more than 60 percent from fat for at least six months, making this the first study to look at long-term keto adaptation in elite endurance athletes. Based on what most people have been preaching for decades, one would suspect that these athletes wouldn't be able to perform as well due to their limited muscle glycogen. As it turned out, this was *not* the case!

It is a rare privilege to study high-caliber athletes in a research setting, so Dr. Volek and his team collected everything that they could, including blood, muscle tissue, fat tissue, gut bacteria, and even urine and feces. You name it, they got it. One key element that they looked at was muscle glycogen levels both before and after exercise. The keto-adapted athletes drank a high-fat shake prior to exercise, while the high-carbohydrate athletes drank a carb-filled shake. Then both groups ran on a treadmill for three hours at 65 percent of their VO_2 max (an average running pace for an endurance athlete).

Average Habitual Daily Intake	Low-Carbohydrate Athletes	High-Carbohydrate Athletes
Calories (kcal)	2,884	3,174
Fat (g)	226	91
Protein (g)	139	118
Carbs (g)	82	486

Peak fat oxidation—the highest rate of fat oxidation—in the athletes on the low-carbohydrate diet was, on average, 2.3 times higher than in the high-carbohydrate athletes, with the average being 1.5 grams of fat burned per minute. In addition, over the three-hour exercise period, all of the subjects perceived their level of exertion to be about the same: the low-carbohydrate athletes didn't feel that it was any harder than the high-carb athletes did.

The most important and eye-opening finding of this study came in terms of muscle glycogen. The study reported that "there were no significant differences in pre-exercise or post-exercise glycogen concentrations between groups" (Volek et al., 2016). How could that be? Both groups started with about the same amount of muscle glycogen and decreased it by about the same amount during exercise,

HOW DOES A KETOGENIC DIET AFFECT AEROBIC PERFORMANCE?

Study	Number of Subjects	Duration	Composition of Diet	Outcome
Burke et al., 2000	8	5 days (carb load day 6, exercise day 7)	> 65% fat, ~15% protein, <20% carbs	↓ respiratory exchange ratio (RER)* ↑ fat oxidation ↓ carbohydrate oxidation
Burke et al., 2002	8	5 days	70% fat, 12% protein, 18% carbs	↓ RER
Stellingwerff et al., 2006	7	5 days (carb load day 6)	67% fat, 15% protein, 18% carbs	↓ RER ↓ carbohydrate metabolism ↓ breakdown of glycogen ↑ breakdown of fatty acids via hormone-sensitive lipase (HSL)—a key regulatory enzyme in the breakdown of fats
Carey et al., 2001	7	6 days (standard carbs day 1, high-fat days 2–7, carb load day 8, test day 9)	69% fat, 15% protein, 16% carbs	↓ RER ↑ fat oxidation during exercise ↑ carbohydrate oxidation ↓ power output
Lambert et al., 2001	5	10 days (carb load days 11–14)	> 65% fat, 20% protein, < 15% carbs	↑ fat oxidation ↓ carbohydrate oxidation ↓ breakdown of glycogen and lactate ↑ improved time-trial times
Lambert et al., 1994	5	14 days	70% fat, 23% protein, 7% carbs	↑ time to exhaustion ↓ RER ↓ muscle glycogen
Rowlands et al., 2002	7	14 days	65% fat, 20% protein, 15% carbs	↓ cycling distance covered ↑ power output during final 5 kilometers ↑ mean power output ↓ plasma insulin ↑ plasma glucose ↑ breakdown of fatty acids ↑ peak fat oxidation
Goedecke et al., 1999	16	15 days	70% fat, 11% protein, 19% carbs	↑ CPT1 (enzymes responsible for fat breakdown)
Burke et al., 2016	10 in KD group	3 weeks	80% fat, 16% protein, 4% carbs	↑ fat oxidation ↓ oxygen demand ↑ peak aerobic capacity ↓ performance
Phinney et al., 1983	5	4 weeks	85% fat, 13% protein, 2% carbs	↑ time to exhaustion ↑ fat oxidation
Zajac et al., 2014	8	4 weeks	70% fat, 15% protein, 15% carbs	↑ heart rate ↑ maximal oxygen uptake (VO_2 max) ↓ muscle breakdown/damage
Klement et al., 2013	12	5–7 weeks	68% fat, 29% protein, 3% carbs	Body composition improved (↓ fat mass, ↑ muscle mass)
Helge et al., 1996	20	7 weeks	62% fat, 17% protein, 21% carbs	↓ RER ↑ noradrenaline—an important neurotransmitter ↑ heart rate
Helge et al., 2001	13	7 weeks	62% fat, 17% protein, 21% carbs	↓ RER ↑ breakdown of fatty acids ↓ breakdown of glycogen
Volek et al., 2016	20	20 months	71% fat, 19% protein, 10% carbs	↑ fat oxidation (muscle glycogen maintained; no different from carbohydrate group)

*The lower the RER, the greater the reliance on fat as fuel and the higher the fat oxidation.

regardless of carbohydrate consumption. Following the exercise, both groups replenished muscle glycogen to a similar degree as well. For the first time, a long-term study of fat-adapted individuals showed that those on a low-carbohydrate ketogenic diet have muscle glycogen levels similar to individuals eating abundant amounts of carbohydrates.

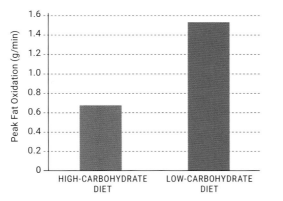

Figure 5.5.3. *Average fat oxidation in the FASTER study.*
Source: Volek et al., 2016.

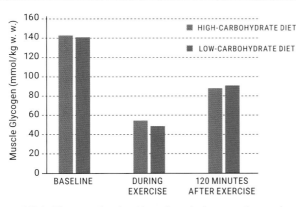

Figure 5.5.4. *Glycogen levels at baseline, during exercise, and 120 minutes after exercise in both the high-carbohydrate and low-carbohydrate groups.*
Source: Volek, 2016.

It's important to understand the implications of Dr. Volek's research on long-term ketogenic diets in endurance athletes. Even though the low-carbohydrate athletes in the study relied less on glucose for fuel, they still burned muscle glycogen (our stored form of carbohydrates) at a high rate. The question most people have asked is, why would a fat-adapted athlete need to break down muscle glycogen in order to maintain performance? It is possible that this muscle glycogen helps keep the Krebs cycle (see page 54) running smoothly and may even help replenish liver glycogen stores (Volek et al., 2016).

Dr. Volek's lab also looked at the rate of glycogen resynthesis: how much glycogen was restored after exercise. Despite receiving only 4 grams of carbohydrates in a post-exercise shake, the low-carbohydrate athletes were able to resynthesize (remake) glycogen to the same degree as the high-carbohydrate athletes who consumed 40-plus grams of carbohydrates post-exercise. How could this be? What is fueling the glycogen resynthesis if not carbohydrates? One possibility is that the lactate and glycerol, which were nearly two times higher in the low-carbohydrate athletes than in the high-carbohydrate athletes following exercise, are converted to glycogen (Volek et al., 2016). Remember that a triglyceride is three fatty acids with a glycerol backbone. Since we are breaking down triglycerides at such a rapid rate and utilizing those fatty acids, the glycerol backbone might be used to help resynthesize glycogen.

> "Even in the absence of food intake, skeletal muscles have the capacity to replenish some of their glycogen."
> —Fournier et al. (2004)

Around the same time that Dr. Volek came to these conclusions, we were finishing up an animal study looking at the very same thing. We fed animals either a Western diet or a low-carbohydrate ketogenic diet for six weeks (keep in mind that animals tend to become keto-adapted a lot faster than humans) while they performed weighted resistance exercise on a running wheel (Roberts et al., 2016). After six weeks, we found no differences in glycogen levels between the ketogenic and the Western diet groups. Again, the results confirm that when we're keto-adapted, our bodies likely are able to upregulate processes to help maintain glycogen levels. However, what we found might have given us more insight into how our bodies are able to resynthesize glycogen under low-carbohydrate conditions, even beyond the lactate and glycerol.

In Chapter 1, we discussed gluconeogenesis, the process by which the body creates glucose from things like amino acids (the building blocks of protein). People often fear that those amino acids are going to come straight from skeletal muscle or branched-chain amino acids (BCAAs), the primary amino acids responsible for muscle growth and

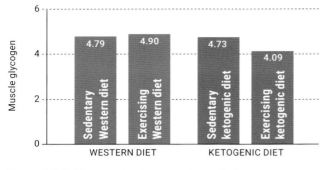

Figure 5.5.5. *Glycogen levels comparing sedentary versus exercising animals on either a traditional Western diet or a ketogenic diet.*

Source: Roberts et al., 2016.

repair. Thus one concern that people have about a low-carbohydrate ketogenic diet is that our bodies are going to break down these essential amino acids that are important for muscle growth, so a ketogenic diet wouldn't allow for muscle building. However, contrary to popular belief, we found that the ketogenic and Western diet groups had the same levels of BCAAs. However, alanine, another amino acid that's used to create glucose (it is very glucogenic), was lower in the ketogenic dieting group. This indicates that in keto-adapted individuals, the important BCAAs may be spared and amino acids that aren't as important for muscle building, such as alanine, are used for glycogen replenishment instead. Regardless of the mechanisms of action, our results, along with Dr. Volek's results, indicate that once keto-adapted, our bodies can regulate muscle glycogen levels to the same degree as those who are consuming a carbohydrate-rich diet.

Should every endurance athlete or ultra-marathoner go on a ketogenic diet? That is absolutely not the takeaway here. In fact, several athletes perform extremely well on a carbohydrate-based diet. Rather, we want to give you the tools to understand how and why it could be beneficial to switch to using primarily fat as fuel, especially during these types of long-distance activities. Remember that individuals and athletes who want to employ a ketogenic diet need to allow time to truly adapt to the diet. A couple days or even a couple weeks likely won't allow you to reap the benefits of being fat-adapted. Additionally, very few studies have examined the effects of supplementing with carbohydrates prior to or during an exercise bout—sometimes known as a targeted ketogenic

Alaskan sled dogs typically consume a high-fat, low-carbohydrate diet and perform several hours of physical activity a day. One study showed that dogs running 160 kilometers per day for five days had very little overall muscle glycogen depletion, even though they were consuming only 15 percent of their calories from carbohydrates (McKenzie et al., 2005). The researchers discovered that the dogs possess a remarkable ability to replenish their muscle glycogen. Here, too, it is possible that glycerol, lactate, or even amino acids like alanine are largely contributing to the sustained glycogen levels in these dogs (Miller et al., 2015). In other words, similar to humans, these dogs, despite running thousands of miles, can perform well despite not eating traditional kibble but rather more high-fat, low-carbohydrate meats.

approach—or how many grams of carbohydrates endurance athletes can consume while staying in ketosis. In Dr. Volek's study, individuals were able to eat 80 grams or more of carbohydrates and stay in ketosis, while studies involving more sedentary individuals show that they may need to stick to 30 to 50 grams per day or less.

If you're an endurance athlete and you want to try a ketogenic diet, Dr. Steve Phinney, an expert in the field, offers three key tips (Phinney, 2004):

1. Allow at least two to four weeks to become keto-adapted (the exact amount of time varies by individual).

2. Maintain appropriate electrolyte balance with 3 to 5 grams of sodium per day and 2 to 3 grams of potassium (see page 48 for more on electrolytes).

3. Personalize protein intake to optimize ketosis and performance for yourself (see page 47 for more on protein consumption on a ketogenic diet).

We have a lot more work to do to figure out how to utilize supplemental carbohydrates and even supplemental ketones to optimize the ketogenic diet for endurance athletes; however, feel free to experiment around yourself. Start small and titrate up. Remember, you are your own scientist!

Effects on Strength, Power, and Anaerobic Performance

With our backgrounds in anaerobic sports (Jacob in hockey and boxing, Ryan in baseball and football), we are fascinated by how changes in diet could affect these type of athletes as well. For example: how would a competitive CrossFit athlete perform on a ketogenic diet? What about bodybuilders and bikini competitors, who often crash-diet on low-fat, low-carb diets to prepare for shows, only to realize that their hormones and metabolism are completely out of whack when the show is over? Or MMA athletes and wrestlers, who need to diet for weight loss in order to make their weight class but also need to preserve as much muscle mass and strength as possible? Or professional football players, who want a healthy way to extend their careers and protect their bodies as much as possible? All of these topics piqued our interest and drove us to find out more about the ability of individuals to maintain performance, strength, and power while on a ketogenic diet.

Even in people who aren't necessarily exercising, body composition has been shown to improve on a ketogenic diet (Volek et al., 2010). Lean body mass (muscle) increases and body fat decreases. Therefore, individuals who aren't "highly trained" certainly could see improvements in strength due to a sheer improvement in muscle mass and relative strength from losing body fat. But the question that most individuals have is, what happens to higher-level athletes or individuals who have been resistance training for a longer period?

The first attempt to crack this code was a study that looked at eight twenty-year-old elite male gymnasts who were put on a thirty-day modified ketogenic diet (22 grams of carbs, 200 grams of protein, and 120 grams of fat per day) consisting of healthy whole foods such as fish, meats, oil, and vegetables (Paoli et al., 2012). After thirty days, they were tested and then switched back to their standard Western diet for thirty days. After that thirty-day period, the gymnasts were tested again. There were no significant differences in any performance measures (including vertical jumps, push-ups, chin-

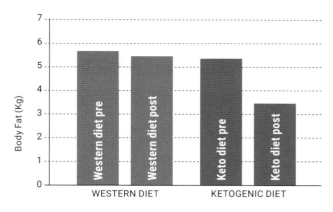

Figure 5.5.6. *Gymnasts on a modified ketogenic diet lost a significant amount of body fat..*
Source: Paoli, 2012.

ups, and dips). However, while on the ketogenic diet, the gymnasts lost significantly more fat mass (nearly 2 kilograms) while their lean body mass increased slightly. The key takeaway is that even though the gymnasts were on the ketogenic diet for just thirty days, they were able to maintain performance and significantly improve body composition. Thus, for athletes in sports in which weight is a concern, a modified ketogenic diet may result in a significant loss of primarily fat mass while muscle mass and performance are maintained.

Like gymnasts, Taekwondo athletes need to be conscious of their weight in order to compete at a high level. These athletes often use unhealthy methods to slim down to extremely low weights to compete in a lighter weight class. This often results in decreased muscle mass and immune system function, and it is a catastrophe for hormones. In one study (Rhyu and Cho, 2014), ten Taekwondo athletes were put on a higher-protein, low-carbohydrate, modified ketogenic diet (55.0 percent fat, 40.7 percent protein, and 4.3 percent carbohydrates) for three weeks while another group of Taekwondo athletes adhered to a non-ketogenic diet (30 percent fat, 30 percent protein, 40 percent carbohydrates). Even though three weeks is a very short period that likely doesn't allow for full adaptation, the ketogenic diet group finished a 2,000-meter sprint faster and felt less fatigued than the non-ketogenic diet group. They also found no significant differences between groups for peak or average Wingate Cycle Ergometer anaerobic power, meaning that a ketogenic diet didn't adversely affect power output, even after adhering to the diet for only a few weeks.

Several recent studies have shown that CrossFit athletes can improve body composition and still perform well on a ketogenic diet. For example, one study found that after six weeks on a ketogenic diet, men and women athletes significantly decreased fat mass (−6.2 pounds), maintained muscle, and improved overall performance (Gregory et al., 2016). In addition, Dr. Mike Roberts and his lab team at Auburn University looked at twelve weeks of a ketogenic diet in well-trained athletes performing cross-training (Roberson et al., in review). During the study, the athletes on the ketogenic diet lost nearly 7.5 pounds more fat mass than the control group. Better yet, there were no significant differences in muscle mass or performance between the two groups. It's more evidence that athletes competing in areas that require great physical fitness, such as CrossFit, can perform well and improve their body composition on a carbohydrate-restricted ketogenic diet.

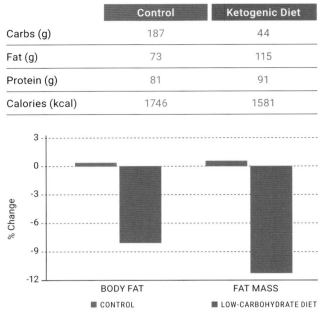

	Control	Ketogenic Diet
Carbs (g)	187	44
Fat (g)	73	115
Protein (g)	81	91
Calories (kcal)	1746	1581

Figure 5.5.7. *Percent change in body fat and fat mass in CrossFit athletes on either their normal diet or a ketogenic diet.*

Source: Adapted from Gregory et al., 2016.

ANAEROBIC SPORTS AND RESEARCH

Study	Number of Subjects	Duration	Composition of Diet	Outcome
Escobar et al., 2016	18	5 days low-carb followed by 3 days with a carb increase (not keto, but "lower" carb)	< 6 g of carbs per kg per day	⬆ number of reps
Havemann et al., 2006	8	1 week	68% fat (protein and carbs not specified)	⬆ improved heart rate variability ⬇ power output
Rhyu et al., 2014	20	3 weeks	55.0% fat, 40.7% protein, 4.3% carbs	⬇ 2000-meter sprint time ⬇ fatigue
Paoli et al., 2012	8	1 month	54.8% fat, 40.7% protein, 4.5% carbs	⬇ body weight and fat mass ⬆ muscle mass
Agee, 2015	27	6 weeks	50% fat, 45% protein, < 7% carbs	⬆ deadlift power ▬ lean body mass
Gregory et al., 2016	27	6 weeks	66% fat, 23% protein, 11% carbs	⬇ fat mass ▬ lean body mass ⬆ improved CrossFit performance times
Wilson et al., 2017	25	11 weeks	75% fat, 20% protein, 5% carbs	⬆ lean body mass ⬇ fat mass ⬆ testosterone
Roberson et al., 2017	18	12 weeks	Ketogenic diet (about 70% fat, 25% protein, 5% carbs)	⬆ blood ketone levels ⬇ fat mass ▬ strength ▬ muscle mass

What About MMA Fighters?

Since MMA is a weight-restricted sport, it is logical that these athletes would want to lose fat rapidly yet preserve muscle mass. In addition, severe blows to the head—which MMA fighters experience often—can leave individuals temporarily insulin resistant and in need of an alternative fuel source. (See page 106 for more on traumatic brain injury and the ketogenic diet.) Our friend and colleague Jordan Joy published a case study looking at two MMA fighters on a ketogenic diet (75 percent fat, 20 percent protein, and 5 percent carbohydrate) for eight weeks. These athletes lost, on average, 6.3 pounds and improved performance in areas like strength, vertical jump, and fatigue resistance. This likely indicates that these athletes, once keto-adapted, can maintain and even improve performance on a ketogenic diet (Joy et al., 2016).

Take a minute and think about how this could apply to other situations. Take sports with weight classes, for instance. When these athletes cut weight, their performance tends to decline as well. Anyone who has dieted down for a competition or an event knows the feeling of "my strength just isn't there anymore" or "I'm not as powerful as I used to be." It is plausible that a ketogenic diet could allow you to cut weight but still maintain those performance metrics—which could lead to an increase in relative power (how much power you have in relation to your weight). Athletes in these types of sports should consider trying a well-formulated ketogenic diet (under proper supervision) to ensure optimal benefits.

Our lab performed the first-ever well-controlled study looking at high-level resistance-training athletes and long-term body composition and performance (Wilson et al., 2017). We divided twenty-five resistance-trained college males into two groups: one group was put on a ketogenic diet (70 percent fat, 25 percent protein, and 5 percent carbohydrate) and the other continued to eat their traditional carbohydrate-based diet. Both groups ate the same number of calories and the same amount of protein—the only differences between the diets were in the fat and carbohydrate content.

Cyclic Ketogenic Dieting

Is it possible to have your cake and eat it, too? Can you stay in ketosis if you eat a ketogenic diet Monday through Friday and then go back to eating a traditional Western diet that is high in carbohydrates on the weekends?

We took highly resistance-trained guys and split them into two groups: one followed this "weekends-off" scenario, and the other stayed on a ketogenic diet consistently, without any cheat days. After several weeks, both groups on average had lost about 3 kilograms of total body weight. So, if we were going by the scale, we'd say that you can eat keto during the week and go back to eating pizza, cake, and cookies on the weekends and get the same results as staying keto all the time. However, when we took a deeper look at body composition, it turned out that among the individuals on the stricter ketogenic diet, almost all of the weight loss came from body fat. Those on a cyclic ketogenic diet, on the other hand, lost 2 kilograms of muscle mass and only 1 kilogram of fat mass. We believe that part of the reason for this was that the cyclic ketogenic diet athletes were never able to become fully keto-adapted. Once they got back into ketosis after the weekend, it was already Thursday or Friday, and they were ready to carb up again (Lowery et al., in review).

Cyclic ketogenic dieting is a wide-open field, and there are some interesting areas to explore, such as how (and if) a less-aggressive cyclical approach, such as carbing up at just one meal, might make a difference; whether the timing of the higher-carb meal (e.g., just on hard workout days) matters; and how supplemental ketones might affect the results.

We then had these individuals perform a hard resistance-training program. In ten weeks on their respective diets, both groups were able to increase muscle mass to the same extent; however, the ketogenic dieting group lost significantly more fat mass (24 percent versus 13 percent). Interestingly enough, both groups increased strength and power to the same extent. Additionally, we saw no adverse effects on blood lipid profiles and a slight increase in testosterone levels in the ketogenic diet group. This was the first study showing that highly resistance-trained athletes working out several times per week can gain muscle, lose fat, and perform well on a ketogenic diet. For more information and a deeper write-up of this study, check out ketogenic.com/uncategorized/ketogenic-dieting-body-composition-beyond-abstract/.

Last but not least, a recent study investigated the effect of a low-carbohydrate, high-fat modified ketogenic diet in sub-elite Olympic power lifters. The typical thinking is that these individuals would need carbohydrates to fuel their bodies and allow them to lift extremely heavy weights. However, these five athletes ate a diet consisting of 1 gram of carbohydrate per kilogram of body weight per day (e.g., someone who weighs 80 kilograms would eat no more than 80 grams of carbohydrates). They could eat as much protein and fat as they wanted. Most of the participants lost from 2.1 to 3.6 kilograms over the eight-week study while increasing strength. Thus these individuals, despite eating a lower-carbohydrate diet, were still able to perform well and improve their body composition (Chatterton, 2015).

Exogenous Ketones and Performance

Though they have numerous other applications, exogenous ketones were created largely to provide an alternative source of energy that ultimately could improve performance.

In the mid-1990s, researchers found that injecting a rat heart with BHB increased the hydraulic efficiency of the heart by 28 percent, decreased its oxygen consumption, and increased ATP (cellular energy) production (Kashiwaya et al., 1994). Let that sink in for a moment. BHB increased the efficiency of one of the most important organs in our bodies while simultaneously decreasing the amount of oxygen needed to generate ATP. For us, as former athletes, the idea of being more efficient and needing less oxygen to create energy at least warrants a deeper look into the potential of ketone supplements.

Dr. Richard Veech and Dr. Kieran Clarke have done a lot of work on ketones and performance. First, they supplemented a small group of athletes with the D-BHB monoester, and the athletes saw a significant improvement in power output during a rowing exercise (Clarke and Cox, 2013). Second, they performed a study in which animals received 30 percent of their calories in the form of the D-BHB monoester. The results were astounding. Animals supplementing with ketones ran 32 percent farther on a treadmill and completed a maze test 38 percent faster than the control rats did: in other words, not only did they see increases in physical performance, but they also performed better on cognitive tests (Murray et al., 2016). Finally, this group performed a series of experiments investigating the effects of the ketone monoester in highly trained cyclists prior to

Ketones and Muscle

A large part of what dictates athletic performance is the quality of muscle tissue—specifically, its ability to grow and repair itself sufficiently when needed. One study showed that during a caloric deficit, individuals on a low-carb diet that wasn't ketogenic lost significantly more muscle mass than individuals on a ketogenic diet (Young et al., 1971). In addition, ketone levels were strongly correlated with muscle mass: the higher the ketone levels, the less muscle was lost. Another study using sodium BHB found that after several weeks of fasting, individuals given supplemental ketones had lower levels of a marker of protein breakdown (Sherwin et al., 1975). Yet another study (Nair et al., 1988) determined that BHB itself promotes muscle protein synthesis and decreases the breakdown of leucine, the primary amino acid responsible for triggering muscle protein synthesis and thus muscle growth—so preventing its breakdown can help preserve and grow muscle mass. We have brand-new data from a project that we collaborated on with Dr. Mike Roberts' lab showing that D-BHB ketone salts can increase muscle protein synthesis even in the presence of a standard diet (Roberts et al., 2017, in review). The newest study showed that adding a ketone ester to a standard post-exercise recovery beverage enhanced the post-exercise activation of mTORC1—a strong indicator of higher muscle protein synthesis (Vandoorne et al., 2017).

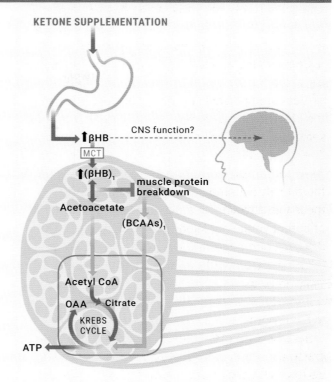

Figure 5.5.8. *Ketone supplementation increases BHB levels, which can positively affect the central nervous system, block muscle protein breakdown, and/or provide an alternative fuel source for cells to use.*

Source: Egan, B., and D. P. D'Agostino. "Fueling performance: ketones enter the mix." *Cell Metabolism* 24, no. 3 (2016): 373–375.

Figure 5.5.9. *Ketone salt supplementation appears to trigger muscle protein synthesis.*

Source: Roberts et al., 2017, in review.

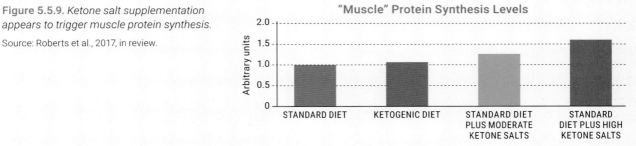

and during exercise (Cox et al., 2016). Some of their findings in these athletes included:

- A great capacity for athletes to both take up and utilize ketones efficiently

- Decreased levels of plasma lactate during exercise, indicating that the athletes were able to clear the lactate easier, which could be important for fatigue

- Steady muscle glycogen levels

- Reduced protein breakdown (i.e., sparing of muscle protein)

- No elevation in insulin levels

- Significant elevation in intramuscular BHB levels, indicating that BHB gets taken up by skeletal muscle

- Consistently lower respiratory exchange ratios during exercise, indicating greater fat oxidation

- Increased performance (on average 411 meters farther) during a 30-minute cycle time trial

This study is one of the first to shed light on the potential performance aspects of supplemental ketones. Its results make it clear that ketone bodies can be taken up and utilized during exercise. Also, the ability of ketones to lower the exercise-induced rise in plasma lactate can be extremely important for endurance athletes by helping prevent fatigue.

This group's most recent study showed that supplemental ketones may also aid in glycogen synthesis in humans, further alluding to some beneficial effects for performance. It has been established that physical endurance can be limited by muscle glycogen stores—when glycogen is depleted, physical work and activity may suffer. Twelve well-trained male athletes completed a study that looked at a glucose drink with or without a ketone monoester following an exercise protocol. The researchers found that the glucose plus ketone ester drink increased glucose uptake and muscle glycogen synthesis, which may be important for athletes looking to optimize performance—"dual fuel."

However, not all studies have found performance increases with exogenous supplementation. In fact, one study found that supplementation with ketone salts resulted in no increases in physical or cognitive performance (Rodger, 2015). However, in stark contrast to other ketone supplementation trials, the ketones used in this study were racemic (DL) ketone salts mixed in a sugar-free liquid solution, and they elevated blood ketones only slightly, from 0.2 to 0.6 mmol over the duration of the trial. There are two possible concerns here: First, the fact that this supplement was already dissolved in a solution could have diluted its effects. Second, the racemic form (DL-BHB) of the ketones could have significantly impacted the results of the trial. To put this in perspective, in most of the work we've done in the lab looking at racemic ketone salts, blood ketone levels have risen to between 0.3 and 0.8 mmol, while D-BHB alone, rather than the mixed isomers, has consistently raised blood ketone levels more than twice as high. (For more on racemic mixes and BHB isomers, see page 60.)

Our lab has seen significant improvements in both cognitive function and physical measures of fatigue in athletes using ketone supplements during high-intensity exercise. There are obvious implications for competition here: you would want your team to have less "perceived fatigue" toward the end of the game so that they feel fresher. With exogenous ketones, we have seen that to be the case in trained individuals.

More pilot studies from our lab have examined the cognitive and physical effects of a wide dosing range of exogenous ketone salts (D-BHB) and found significant improvements in perceived energy and focus, body composition, metabolism, and time-trial performance—in both general populations and well-trained athletes. Though there is limited published research on exogenous ketones and their impact on performance, we suspect that in the coming months or years, as awareness of this alternative source of fuel continues to grow, we will see a lot more studies in this area.

CHAPTER SUMMARY

There is strong evidence that a well-formulated ketogenic diet can serve as a tool for athletes who are looking to optimize body composition and perform exceptionally. However, in order to optimize these benefits, the body needs to become keto-adapted before improvements in body composition and performance are seen. Whether you're an endurance athlete, a CrossFit athlete, an MMA fighter, or an athlete in another sport that has weight classes, the loss of body fat and maintenance of muscle mass that occur on a well-formulated ketogenic diet can benefit your performance. Additionally, the ketogenic diet may help with other aspects of being a competitive athlete, such as inflammation and head trauma, which we discuss more in Section 3. While a limited number of studies have been done using supplemental ketones, those that have indicate that exogenous ketones may improve both physical and cognitive function while exhibiting beneficial effects for muscle mass and power. More research is needed, so it's important to be your own scientist and experiment to find out if or what kind of ketogenic diet or ketone supplementation may work for you.

References

Agee, J. L. "Effects of a low-carbohydrate ketogenic diet on power lifting performance and body composition." Master's Thesis. Retrieved from JMU Scholarly Commons. Paper 36. (2015).

Bergström, J., L. Hermansen, E. Hultman, and B. Saltin. "Diet, muscle glycogen and physical performance." *Acta Physiologica* 71, no. 2–3 (1967): 140–50. doi: 10.1111/j.1748-1716.1967.tb03720.x.

Burke, L. M., D. J. Angus, G. R. Cox, N. K. Cummings, M. A. Febbraio, K. Gawthorn, J. A. Hawley, M. Minehan, D. T. Martin, and M. Hargeaves. "Effect of fat adaptation and carbohydrate restoration on metabolism and performance during prolonged cycling." *Journal of Applied Physiology* 89, no. 9 (2000): 2413–21.

Burke, L. M., J. A. Hawley, D. J. Angus, G. R. Cox, S. A. Clark, N. K. Cummings, B. Desbrow, and M. Hargeaves. "Adaptations to short-term high-fat diet persist despite high carbohydrate availability." *Medicine & Science in Sports & Exercise* 34, no. 1 (2002): 83–91.

Burke, L. M., J. A. Hawley, E. J. Schabort, A. S. C. Gibson, I. Mujika, and T. D. Noakes. "Carbohydrate loading failed to improve 100-km cycling performance in a placebo-controlled trial." *Journal of Applied Physiology* 88, no. 4 (2000): 1284–90.

Burke, L. M., M. L. Ross, L. A. Garvican-Lewis, M. Welvaert, I. A. Heikura, S. G. Forbes, J. G. Mirtschin, L. E. Cato, N. Strobel, A. P. Sharma, and J. A. Hawley. "Low carbohydrate, high fat diet impairs exercise economy and negates the performance benefit from intensified training in elite race walkers." *Journal of Physiology* 23 (2016): 2785–807. doi: 10.1113/JP273230.

Carey, A. L., H. M. Staudacher, N. K. Cummings, N. K. Stept, V. Nikolopoulos, L. M. Burke, and J. A. Hawley. "Effects of fat adaptation and carbohydrate restoration on prolonged endurance exercise." *Journal of Applied Physiology* 91, no. 1 (2001): 115–22.

Chatterton, S. "The effect of an 8-week low carbohydrate high fat diet on maximal strength performance, body composition and diet acceptability in sub-elite Olympic weightlifters and powerlifters." Doctoral dissertation, Auckland University of Technology. (2015).

Clarke, K., and P. Cox. (2013). U.S. Patent Application No. 14/390,495.

Cox, P. J., T. Kirk, T. Ashmore, K. Willerton, R. Evans, A. Smith, ... and M. T. King. "Nutritional ketosis alters fuel preference and thereby endurance performance in athletes." *Cell Metabolism* 24, no. 2 (2016): 256–68. doi: 10.1016/j.cmet.2016.07.010.

Escobar, K. A., J. Morales, and T. A. Vandusseldorp. "The effect of a moderately low and high carbohydrate intake on Crossfit performance." *International Journal of Exercise Science* 9, no. 4 (2016): 460–70.

Fournier, P. A., T. J. Fairchild, L. D. Ferreira, and L. Bräu. "Post-exercise muscle glycogen repletion in the extreme: effect of food absence and active recovery." *Journal of Sports Science & Medicine* 3, no. 3 (2004): 139.

Goedecke, J. H., C. Christie, G. Wilson, S. C. Dennis, T. D. Noakes, W. G. Hopkins, and E. V. Lambert. "Metabolic adaptations to a high-fat diet in endurance cyclists." *Metabolism* 48, no. 12 (1999): 1509–17.

Gregory, R. M. "A low-carbohydrate ketogenic diet combined with 6 weeks of CrossFit training improves body composition and performance." Master's thesis. (2016).

Havemann, L. "Nutritional strategies for endurance and ultra-endurance cycling." Doctoral dissertation, University of Cape Town. (2008).

Havemann, L., S. J. West, J. H. Goedecke, I. A. Macdonald, A. St. Clair Gibson, T. D. Noakes, and E. V. Lambert. "Fat adaptation followed by carbohydrate loading compromises high-intensity sprint performance." *Journal of Applied Physiology* 100, no. 1 (2006): 194–202. doi: 10.1152/japplphysiol.00813.2005.

Helge, J. W., E. A. Richter, and B. Kiens. "Interaction of training and diet on metabolism and endurance during exercise in man." *Journal of Physiology* 492, Pt. 1 (1996): 293–306.

Helge, J. W., P. W. Watt, E. A. Richter, M. J. Rennie, and B. Kiens. "Fat utilization during exercise: adaptation to a fat-rich diet increases utilization of plasma fatty acids and very low density lipoprotein-triacylglycerol in humans." *Journal of Physiology* 537, Pt. 3 (2001): 1009–20. doi: 10.1111/j.1469-7793.2001.01009.x.

Holdsworth, D. A., P. J. Cox, T. Kirk, H. Stradling, S. G. Impey, and K. Clarke. "A ketone ester drink increases postexercise muscle glycogen synthesis in humans." *Medicine and Science in Sports and Exercise* (2017). doi: 10.1249/MSS.0000000000001292.

Joy, J. M., R. M. Vogel, A. C. Tribby, J. C. Preisendorf, P. H. Falcone, M. M. Mosman, ... and J. R. Moon. "A ketogenic diet's effects on athletic performance in two professional mixed-martial-arts athletes: case reports." Texas Woman's University. Denton, TX. 2016.

Kashiwaya, Y., K. Sato, N. Tsuchiya, S. Thomas, D. A. Fell, R. L. Veech, and J. V. Passonneau. "Control of glucose utilization in working perfused rat heart." *Journal of Biological Chemistry* 269, no. 41 (1994): 25502–14.

Klement, R. J., T. Frobel, T. Albers, S. Fikenzer, J. Prinzhausen, and U. Kämmerer. "A pilot study on the impact of a self-prescribed ketogenic diet on biochemical parameters and running performance in healthy physically active indivicuals." *Nutrition and Medicine* 1, no. 1 (2013): 10.

Lambert, E. V., J. H. Goedecke, C. van Zyl, K. Murphy, J. A. Hawley, S. C. Dennis, and T. D. Noakes. "High-fat diet versus habitual diet prior to carbohydrate loading: effects on exercise metabolism and cycling performance." *International Journal of Sport Nutrition and Exercise Metabolism* 11, no. 2 (2001): 209–25.

Lambert, E. V., D. P. Speechly, S. C. Dennis, and T. D. Noakes. "Enhanced endurance in trained cyclists during moderate intensity exercise following 2 weeks adaptation to a high fat diet." *European Journal of Applied Physiology and Occupational Physiology* 69, no. 4 (1994): 287–93.

McKenzie, E., T. Holbrook, K. Williamson, C. Royer, S. Valberg, K. Hinchcliff, ... and M. Davis. "Recovery of muscle glycogen concentrations in sled dogs during prolonged exercise." *Medicine and Science in Sports and Exercise* 37, no. 8 (2005): 1307–12.

Miller, B. F., J. C. Drake, F. F. Peelor, L. M. Biela, R. Geor, K. Hinchcliff, ... and K. L. Hamilton. "Participation in a 1,000-mile race increases the oxidation of carbohydrate in Alaskan sled dogs." *Journal of Applied Physiology* 118, no. 12 (2015): 1502–9. doi: 10.1152/japplphysiol.00588.2014.

Murray, A. J., N. S. Knight, M. A. Cole, L. E. Cochlin, E. Carter, K. Tchabanenko, ... and K. Clarke. "Novel ketone diet enhances physical and cognitive performance." *FASEB Journal* 30, no. 12 (2016): 4021–32. doi: 10.1096/fj.201600773R.

Nair, K. S., S. L. Welle, D. Halliday, and R. G. Campbell. "Effect of beta-hydroxybutyrate on whole-body leucine kinetics and fractional mixed skeletal muscle protein synthesis in humans." *Journal of Clinical Investigation* 82, no. 1 (1988): 198–205. doi: 10.1172/JCI113570.

Paoli, A., K. Grimaldi, D. D'Agostino, L. Cenci, T. Moro, A. Bianco, and A. Palma. "Ketogenic diet does not affect strength performance in elite artistic gymnasts." *Journal of the International Society of Sports Nutrition* 9 (2012): 34. doi: 10.1186/1550-2783-9-34.

Pfeiffer, B., T. Stellingwerff, A. B. Hodgson, R. Randell, K. Pöttgen, P. Res, and A. E. Jeukendrup. "Nutritional intake and gastrointestinal problems during competitive endurance events." *Medicine & Science in Sports & Exercise* 44, no. 2 (2012): 344–51. doi: 10.1249/MSS.0b013e31822dc809.

Phinney, S. D. "Ketogenic diets and physical performance." *Nutrition & Metabolism* 1 (2004): 2. doi: 10.1186/1743-7075-1-2.

Phinney, S. D., B. R. Bistrian, W. J. Evans, E. Gervino, and G. L. Blackburn. "The human metabolic response to chronic ketosis without caloric restriction: preservation of submaximal exercise capability with reduced carbohydrate oxidation." *Metabolism* 32, no. 8 (1983): 769–76.

Phinney, S. D., E. S. Horton, E. A. Sims, J. S. Hanson, E. Danforth Jr.,and B. M. LaGrange. "Capacity for moderate exercise in obese subjects after adaptation to a hypocaloric, ketogenic diet." *Journal of Clinical Investigation* 66, no. 5 (1980): 1152–61.

Rhyu, H., and S. Y. Cho. "The effect of weight loss by ketogenic diet on the body composition, performance-related physical fitness factors and cytokines of Taekwondo athletes." *Journal of Exercise Rehabilitation* 10, no. 5 (2014): 326–31. doi: 10.12965/jer.140160.

Roberson, P. A., W. C. Kephart, C. Pledge, P. W. Mumford, K. W. Huggins, J. S. Martin, K. C. Young, R. P. Lowery, J. M. Wilson, and M. D. Roberts. "The physiological effects of 12 weeks of ketogenic dieting while cross-training." (2016). Abstract.

Rodger, S. "Oral ketone supplementation: effect on cognitive function, physiology and exercise performance." Doctoral dissertation, University of Waikato. (2015).

Rowlands, D. S., and W. G. Hopkins. "Effects of high-fat and high-carbohydrate diets on metabolism and performance in cycling." *Metabolism* 51, no. 6 (2002): 678–90.

Sato, K., Y. Kashiwaya, C. A. Keon, N. Tsuchiya, M. T. King, G. K. Radda, andR. L. Veech. "Insulin, ketone bodies, and mitochondrial energy transduction." *FASEB Journal* 9, no. 8 (1995): 651–8.

Sherwin, R. S., R. G. Hendler, and P. Felig. "Effect of ketone infusions on amino acid and nitrogen metabolism in man." *Journal of Clinical Investigation* 55, no. 6 (1975): 1382–90. doi: 10.1172/JCI108057.

Stellingwerff, T., L. L. Spriet, M. J. Watt, N. E. Kimber, M. Hargreaves, J. A. Hawley, and L. M. Burke. "Decreased PDH activation and glycogenolysis during exercise following fat adaptation with carbohydrate restoration." *American Journal of Physiology—Endocrinology and Metabolism* 290, no. 2 (2006): 380–8. doi: 10.1152/ajpendo.00268.2005.

Vandoorne, T., S. De Smet, M. Ramaekers, R. Van Thienen, K. De Bock, K. Clarke, and P. Hespel. "Intake of a ketone ester drink during recovery from exercise promotes mTORC1 signalling but not glycogen resynthesis in human muscle." *Frontiers in Physiology* 8 (2017): 310.

Veech, R. L., B. Chance, Y. Kashiwaya, H. A. Lardy, and G. F. Cahill Jr. "Ketone bodies, potential therapeutic uses." *IUBMB Life* 51, no. 4 (2001): 241–7. doi: 10.1080/152165401753311780.

Volek, J. S., D. J. Freidenreich, C. Saenz, L. J. Kunces, B. C. Creighton, J. M. Bartley, ... and S. D. Phinney. "Metabolic characteristics of keto-adapted ultra-endurance runners." *Metabolism* 65, no. 3 (2016): 100–10.

Volek, J. S., and S. D. Phinney. *The Art and Science of Low Carbohydrate Performance*. Miami, FL: Beyond Obesity LLC, 2012.

Volek, J. S., E. E. Quann, and C. E. Forsythe. "Low-carbohydrate diets promote a more favorable body composition than low-fat diets." *Strength and Conditioning Journal* 32, no. 1 (2010): 42–47. doi: 10.1519/SSC.0b013e3181c16c41.

Wilson, J. M., R. P. Lowery, M. D. Roberts, M. H. Sharp, J. M. Joy, K. A. Shields, ... and D. D'Agostino. "The effects of ketogenic dieting on body composition, strength, power, and hormonal profiles in resistance training males." *Journal of Strength & Conditioning Research* (2017). doi: 10.1519/JSC.0000000000001935.

Wing, R. R., J. A. Vazquez, and C. M. Ryan. "Cognitive effects of ketogenic weight-reducing diets." *International Journal of Obesity and Related Metabolic Disorders* 19, no. 11 (1995): 811–6.

Young, C. M., S. S. Scanlan, H. S. Im, and L. Lutwak. "Effect on body composition and other parameters in obese young men of carbohydrate level of reduction diet." *American Journal of Clinical Nutrition* 24, no. 3 (1971): 290–6.

Zajac, A., S. Poprzsecki, A. Maszczyk, M. Czuba, M. Michalczyk, and G. Zydek. "The effects of a ketogenic diet on exercise metabolism and physical performance in off-road cyclists." *Nutrients* 6, no. 7 (2014): 2493–508. doi: 10.3390/nu6072493.

Section 6:
New and Emerging Areas of Interest

"Wonder is the beginning of wisdom."
—Socrates

We seem to be discovering new applications of the ketogenic diet every day. Scientists and researchers are hard at work, looking to expand upon the current applications and investigate new areas in which a ketogenic diet and/or an elevation in ketones may be beneficial. Remember, however, that in a lot of these areas we are just beginning to crack open the door to understanding how and why a ketogenic diet may be beneficial. Over the next decade, we expect to see much more data emerging on the effects of a ketogenic diet; to date, however, the horizon is bright for the implementation of the ketogenic diet in a wide variety of therapeutic applications.

Crohn's Disease

Let's start with an area that is near and dear to our hearts. Ryan here: My mom is truly my hero and has been there to support me my entire life. Unfortunately, she has been dealing with Crohn's disease for over a decade, and it takes a toll on her daily life. Thus I completely understand the hardships that people suffering from Crohn's disease face: constant trips to the bathroom, pain, lack of appetite, bloating, sickness/vomiting, inflammation, and overall disruption of life. My mom never lets this disease get her down and continues to fight through each and every day, even without prescription drugs or medical treatment. Due to both the rising costs and the adverse effects she has experienced with prescription medications, she has opted not to take them. My number-one mission is to figure out a way that I can help her mitigate her symptoms and reduce the pain that she experiences on a daily basis.

Crohn's is an autoimmune disease in which the immune system attacks the gastrointestinal (GI) tract, causing inflammation, bleeding, and scarring. Current statistics in the U.S. suggest that 5 out of 100,000 people are diagnosed with this disease, yet the number may even be higher due to underreporting or misdiagnosis (Hanauer and Sandborn, 2001). Crohn's is an inflammatory bowel disease (IBD), which is different from irritable bowel syndrome (IBS) in that IBS does not cause inflammation or ulcers, thereby damaging the bowel. The other main inflammatory bowel disease is ulcerative colitis (UC). UC is typically located in the colon, beginning at the rectum, while Crohn's can affect any part of the gastrointestinal tract. Unlike IBS, neither Crohn's nor UC is thought to be curable.

Many treatment options have been used in an attempt to ease the burden of Crohn's disease, with varying results. Often these strategies target the gut directly. The most common treatments for Crohn's, anti-inflammatory drugs and immunosuppressants, are aimed at reducing inflammation in bowel tissues. From there, surgery is often necessary to remove damaged portions of the small intestine and/or colon.

Other treatment options focus on boosting the good bacteria that live in the gut, such as probiotics, prebiotics, and, more recently, fecal matter transplants (described further below). Boosting the good bacteria in the colon improves the immune system and protects intestinal tissue. However, a study found that patients with Crohn's disease in remission who were treated with a probiotic for one year were nearly twice as likely to have a recurrence of the disease as those who were treated with a placebo (Prantera et al., 2002). These results seem counterintuitive and indicate that even heavy supplementation with certain beneficial probiotic strains did not prevent recurrence at one year or reduce the severity of recurrent lesions in patients dealing with Crohn's. Therefore, these options should be looked at as additional tools rather than standalone therapies.

Since Crohn's disease is primarily the result of severe chronic inflammation, is it possible that a properly formulated diet can decrease inflammatory markers and improve quality of life? Currently, many dietitians and physicians recommend a diet that eliminates FODMAPs—fermentable oligo-, di-, and monosaccharides and polyols, which are gas-producing carbohydrates that are not easily digested by the body. This recommendation is meant to provide foods that lower inflammation and do not trigger bloating, stomach pain, etc. Further, one study showed that a low-carbohydrate, high-fat diet can reduce levels of C-reactive protein (CRP), a marker of inflammation (Rankin and Turpyn, 2007). More recently, a case report involving a fourteen-year-old boy diagnosed with Crohn's disease reported significant improvements with a "Paleolithic ketogenic diet" (Tóth et al., 2016) that consisted of animal fat, meat, organ meat, eggs, and minuscule amounts of honey with a 2:1 fat-to-protein ratio. At-home monitoring confirmed that he was in ketosis. Two weeks after starting the diet, the boy stopped taking all his medications; more than a year later, he was still off them. Symptoms that typically accompany autoimmune diseases, such as night sweats, disrupted sleep, and joint pain, disappeared just weeks after he began the diet. Bloodwork showed that inflammatory markers like C-reactive protein decreased significantly during the first couple of weeks, and thickening of the ileum wall (part of the small intestine that is often affected by Crohn's) as measured by ultrasound significantly went down. Within ten months on the diet, the boy achieved full remission from symptoms as well as normalization of intestinal inflammation (Tóth et al., 2016).

It's interesting to note how important sticking to the diet was: when the boy strayed from the diet and ate a piece of "Paleo" cake (ingredients: coconut oil, flour from oilseeds, and sugar alcohols), his symptoms immediately returned.

Individuals with compromised intestinal issues may not be able to absorb high amounts of fat in the same way that most other people do, and this can lead to bloating, gassiness, and diarrhea. Fats like MCT oil, which are typically recommended on a ketogenic diet, may cause irritation in someone who has Crohn's disease. Individuals looking to adopt a similar approach should be cognizant of this effect and possibly employ a modified ketogenic diet that incorporates periods of intermittent fasting combined with a moderate-protein, moderate-fat, low-carbohydrate diet.

What Is a Fecal Matter Transplant?

Briefly, a fecal matter transplant (FMT) is exactly what it sounds like: doctors take the fecal matter of a healthy individual and transplant it into a patient's ecosystem (e.g., their intestines, etc.). The thinking is that this entirely new "army" of good bacteria that is brought in could populate and flourish in the individual who needs it. This treatment is very promising, but in the U.S. it is only used to treat *C. difficile*—but anecdotal reports from around the world for other conditions are encouraging.

It may even be beneficial for individuals with Crohn's to supplement with ketones without changing their diet. We recently performed a pilot study in which we gave a woman with Crohn's (diagnosed for over twenty-five years) 6 to 8 grams of D-BHB per day (a mix of sodium, calcium, and magnesium) with water. After three months of supplementation, alongside no changes in diet, her white blood cell count and fasting blood glucose improved, and, most importantly, her C-reactive protein (a marker of inflammation) dropped from 62.5 to 4.4 mg/L (normal range is 0 to 4.9 mg/L). She also was able to start walking on a treadmill for twenty minutes a day because she felt better and had significantly more energy.

Lastly, we need to be cognizant that important short-chain fatty acids like butyrate tend to decrease acutely with low carbohydrate (fiber) consumption (Duncan et al., 2007). Specifically, indigestible fiber may be fermented in the colon by the residing bacteria, which then produce short-chain fatty acids, such as butyrate, which serve as a healthy fuel source for the cells that line the colon. It is unknown whether ketones can increase the amount of butyrate directly, but it's plausible that the butyrate component of BHB (beta-hydroxybutyrate) can improve gut bacteria and aid in improving overall health. It may be a good idea to supplement with butyrate-promoting probiotics or sodium butyrate itself at the beginning of the transition to a lower carbohydrate intake. This may help encourage butyrate production, especially if vegetable consumption is cut down significantly, as it was for the boy with Crohn's who found success on a Paleolithic ketogenic diet. However, be extremely careful when introducing fibers with high prebiotic activity (i.e., inulin). Remember, the gut is its own ecosystem, and in some individuals there is a constant battle between bad and good bacteria, where the bad bacteria often win. Dropping food (e.g., fibers, inulin, etc.) into the battlefield could lead to inflammation and bloating if the bad bacteria eat it up first.

KETO CONCEPT

Mom's Keto Case Study

So how is my mom doing? I tried putting her on a typical high-fat, low-carbohydrate ketogenic diet and soon realized that she couldn't handle the fat the way most other people can. I felt really bad about it, but my mom is a trooper and continued to trust me. Over the past several months, she has adhered to a modified ketogenic diet in which she fasts for part of the day and then eats some eggs and cheese and another meat-based meal later in the day. She also does light exercise five times per week and supplements daily with exogenous ketones, vitamins, and occasionally a strong probiotic. We've seen dramatic improvements in inflammatory markers in her bloodwork, while she's continued to lose fat mass and maintain muscle mass (I measure her stats at the lab. Sorry for making you a science project, Mom!), and her quality of life has improved. I'm ecstatic to see her doing so well and look forward to seeing more research in this area.

Multiple Sclerosis

Multiple sclerosis (MS) is another disease that hits home for me (Ryan). My aunt has been dealing with MS for over a decade, and I have seen the impact that it can have on quality of life and motor and cognitive function. I cringe every time I hear my aunt talk about how she stumbled or fell due to the fact that her motor function isn't what it used to be. The first clear description of MS dates back to 1868 in a diary written by neurologist Jean-Martin Charcot, in which he describes a patient with "demyelinating lesions" in the brain. Fast-forward more than 100 years, and the medical community is still unsure about what causes this disease and what types of treatment options help prevent its progression.

MS is traditionally classified as an autoimmune disease characterized by a degeneration of neurons and of the myelin sheath, which covers nerve fibers in the brain and spinal cord. When the myelin sheath is damaged, it can cause nerve impulses to slow or even stop. Symptoms of MS include impaired coordination, fatigue, pain, weakness, and sometimes loss of vision.

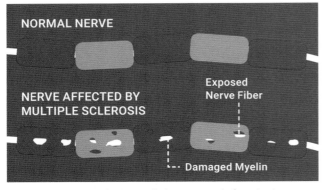

Figure 5.6.1. *Normal nerve cells have properly functioning myelin sheaths, while MS nerve cells do not.*

Source: Ketogenic.com.

The traditional school of thought is that with MS, the immune system attacks the central nervous system, giving rise to inflammatory lesions that can cause a variety of neurological symptoms. Current drug treatments are, therefore, designed to suppress the immune system; however, some scientists have challenged the idea that MS is only the result of inflammation. Rather, these researchers suggest, MS may be the primary result of cellular degeneration, which then initiates and triggers inflammation. This is a chicken-and-egg battle, yet all scientists agree that both degeneration of cells and inflammation likely play a strong role in the disease.

Evidence showing that MS involves both neurodegeneration and neuroinflammation is rapidly emerging (Storoni and Plant, 2015). Studies have discovered that cognitive impairments, such as learning and memory difficulties, occur in 43 to 70 percent of MS patients (Choi et al., 2016). In fact, brain MRIs in patients with MS have shown structural disorders of both the cerebral cortex and the hippocampus, a primary locus of memory consolidation (Hao et al., 2012). The damaged areas of the brain in MS are similar to the damaged areas in Parkinson's and Alzheimer's disease, thus it is possible that a ketogenic diet may also benefit individuals with MS.

Dietary manipulation strategies that target inflammation have been attempted to reduce symptoms of MS and, at a minimum, slow the progression of the disease. In animals, a condition called experimental autoimmune encephalomyelitis (EAE) is commonly employed to mimic MS in humans because it is characterized by inflammation and neurodegeneration in the central nervous system (CNS) and has been shown to result in impairments in spatial learning and memory (Hao et al., 2012). One study found that in mice with EAE, a ketogenic diet suppressed motor and memory dysfunction and reversed structural brain lesions, possibly by reducing inflammation and oxidative stress (Hao et al., 2012).

More recently, a "fasting-mimicking diet," or FMD, has been examined as a possible MS therapy. FMD typically follows this weekly regimen:

- Day 1: Subjects consume 50 percent of normal caloric intake.

- Days 2 and 3: Subjects consume 10 percent of normal caloric intake.

- Days 4 through 7: Subjects consume normal caloric intake.

Studies have shown that FMD induces a state of ketosis and has profound effects on ameliorating EAE symptoms and reversing disease progression. Further, sixty MS patients on FMD or a ketogenic diet for six months saw improved quality of life and decreased fatigue, and researchers found that it was both safe and feasible for MS patients to follow a FMD or ketogenic diet (Choi et al., 2016).

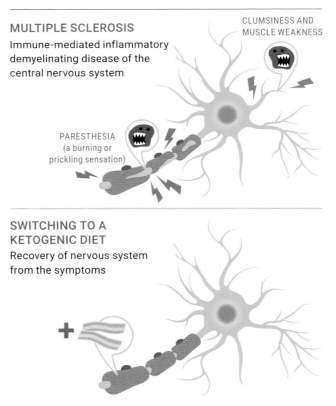

Figure 5.6.2. *Immune system inflammation can drive demyelination, but an anti-inflammatory diet, such as a ketogenic diet, may allow the nervous system to recover from those symptoms.*

Source: Ketogenic.com.

As in Alzheimer's and Parkinson's disease (see pages 101 and 94), impaired mitochondrial function may play an integral role in MS. In animals with EAE, mitochondrial injury precedes inflammation and therefore can trigger neurodegeneration (Storoni and Plant, 2015). Also, similar to what is seen in Alzheimer's patients, MS patients have demonstrated 40 percent lower brain glucose uptake compared to healthy controls, possibly indicating impaired brain energy metabolism—which suggests that the brains of MS patients could benefit from an alternative fuel source, such as ketones.

A pilot study looking at eighty-five patients with MS showed that glucose metabolism correlated with disease progression—as their disease got worse, so did their brain's ability to use glucose. This indicates that impaired mitochondrial function and glucose metabolism play a significant role in the progression of MS (Regenold et al., 2008). There is also evidence that the body recognizes the problem that the brain experiences in taking up and utilizing glucose and therefore increases the number of ketone transporters in an attempt to supply more fuel to the brain (Nijland et al., 2014).

To date, there are limited human studies looking directly at the impact of ketogenic diets or ketone supplementation in MS patients; however, we are hopeful that there will be plenty of studies over the next several years. Due to the fact that the ketogenic diet has been shown to be safe and to increase ATP production, overcome dysfunctional mitochondria, increase antioxidant levels, and reduce oxidative damage, it may offer therapeutic benefits for MS patients.

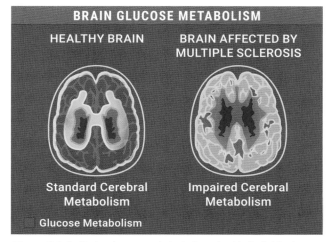

Figure 5.6.3. *Brain glucose uptake is impaired in individuals with MS.*

Source: Ketogenic.com.

Autism

Some reports estimate that 1 in 160 individuals are affected by autism spectrum disorder (ASD), a complex neurodevelopmental condition (Elsabbagh et al., 2012). However, the CDC reports that 1 in 68 children are affected by ASD, and the rate has been steadily increasing over the past several decades. Typically, individuals diagnosed with ASD express three core symptoms: impaired social interactions, repetitive behaviors, and communication difficulties. Additionally, seizures and problems with the gastrointestinal, immune, and endocrine systems are common in children with autism (Spence and Schneider, 2009). The term *spectrum* is used because the types and level of impairment can vary from case to case. To date, despite vast research on the topic, limited scientific discoveries have been made on what causes ASD; however, most researchers agree that a combination of genetic and environmental factors are likely major contributors.

Many researchers feel that, as in other disorders discussed throughout this book, mitochondrial dysfunction and impaired glucose metabolism play a large role in ASD. In fact, markers associated with mitochondrial dysfunction are significantly elevated in individuals with ASD. Additionally, nearly 40 percent of individuals with ASD also experience epilepsy, indicating that there is significant overlap between the two conditions (Frye, 2015). Given that a ketogenic diet has been shown to have substantial success in treating epilepsy and other conditions in which mitochondrial dysfunction is present, it is plausible that the diet could have beneficial effects on ASD-associated symptoms.

Several studies have shown improvements in sociability and behavior in mice when they are put on a ketogenic diet. In addition, studies looking at autistic children on a ketogenic diet recorded improvements in the Childhood Autism Rating Scale (CARS), a rating scale commonly used to diagnose the degree of autism (Evangeliou et al., 2003; Spilioti et al., 2013). Further, a case study involving a twelve-year-old girl with ASD found that her seizures improved within weeks of starting a low-carb, high-fat (MCT-based) diet (Herbert and Buckley, 2013).

After a year, her anticonvulsant medication dosage was reduced by 50 percent, and she had experienced a 60-pound weight loss, improved cognitive and language function, markedly improved social skills, increased calmness, increased intelligence quotient, and a significant improvement in CARS score (from 49 to 17), indicating a change from severe autism to a non-autistic state.

It's not completely clear how the ketogenic diet helps with ASD, but there are some theories.

If, as is believed, autism involves impairment of the mitochondria and how they produce energy from glucose, a ketogenic diet may help by increasing the number of mitochondria and providing an alternate source of fuel to glucose, one that can bypass the problem areas in mitochondria or create new, properly functioning mitochondria (Greco et al., 2015; Hyatt et al., 2016). Also, people with ASD often display increased levels of inflammation and reactive oxygen species (ROS), which can damage tissue and DNA; being in a state of ketosis may reduce these issues (Maalouf et al., 2007; Youm et al., 2015). Finally, the ketogenic diet increases adenosine, which acts on the brain as a sleep modulator—autistic children tend to have reduced adenosine and difficulty sleeping. Increasing adenosine also seems to help reduce anxiety, seizures, and repetitive behaviors (Masino et al., 2009).

Overall, the exact mechanisms for why a ketogenic diet may be beneficial for autism spectrum disorder are still not entirely clear—more research is certainly needed. Anecdotally, many parents have reached out to us who have implemented either the diet, exogenous ketones, or a combination in their children with ASD and have seen remarkable improvements. However, it's important to point out some limitations and considerations to keep in mind when implementing a ketogenic diet in autistic children:

1. A high-fat diet that's *not* ketogenic may worsen symptoms (Zilkha et al., 2016). This could be due to the fact that some people with ASD have difficulty breaking down certain types of long-chain fatty acids (Clark-Taylor and Clark-Taylor, 2004). Therefore, it may be important to seek out more ketogenic fats, such as MCTs or short-chain fatty acids, which they should be able to metabolize more easily. Supplementing with exogenous ketones may be helpful in combination with a well-formulated diet (see Chapters 3 and 4).

2. In children especially, severely limiting protein and other nutrients can lead to a lack of weight gain and growth inhibition. Due to the fact that children with autism tend to be underweight already, they should be closely monitored by a trained physician and dietitian when put on a ketogenic diet. Ensuring that these children get proper nutrients and vitamins along with adequate protein is of the utmost importance for their development, and they should follow a well-formulated ketogenic diet that is customized to their needs (see Chapter 3). In addition, supplementation with thiamine, lipoic acid, and l-carnitine have been shown to help in these situations, as they may help the body break down and utilize dietary macronutrients (Wexler et al., 1997).

KETO CONCEPT

Rett Syndrome

Rett syndrome, first recognized in 1966, is a neurological/neurodevelopmental disorder that primarily affects females. The cause and effects of this disease differ from autism; however, children affected by Rett syndrome often exhibit autistic-like behaviors, such as repetitive hand movements, prolonged toe walking, body rocking, sleep problems, and an overall progressive deterioration of motor, mental, and social functions. One study investigated the effects of a ketogenic diet on seven girls with Rett syndrome who also exhibited anticonvulsant-resistant seizures. Five of the seven girls who tolerated the diet saw behavioral and motor improvements. The authors concluded that "with a possible defect in carbohydrate metabolism and a difficult seizure disorder, use of a ketogenic diet is logical and appears to produce clinical benefit in patients with Rett syndrome" (Haas et al., 1986). Later, a case report was published about a twelve-year-old girl who was diagnosed with refractory seizures and Rett syndrome (identified by a mutation in the MECP2 gene). The researchers found that when this patient was placed on a ketogenic diet, she saw a reduction in seizure frequency and her behavior improved significantly (Liebhaber et al., 2003).

Angelman Syndrome

Angelman syndrome (AS) is a rare neurogenetic disorder that occurs in 1 in 15,000 live births and is often misdiagnosed as cerebral palsy or autism. It is characterized by severe developmental delay, seizures, speech impairment, uncoordinated movements and/or trembling of the limbs, and a unique set of behaviors that includes happy demeanor and excessive laughter (Williams et al., 2010). Typically, antiseizure drugs and physical and speech therapy are used to manage the disorder.

Although Rett and Angelman syndromes occur due to different gene mutations (Rett: MECP2, AS: UBE3A), there is overlap in the clinical presentation (Jedele, 2007). Limited direct data exists with AS; however, in one study involving a five-year-old girl with AS and uncontrollable daily seizures (resistant to anticonvulsant therapy), the girl became seizure free and experienced improved sleep and reduced hyperactivity several months after starting a 4:1 ketogenic diet (Evangeliou et al., 2010). This could be due to an improvement in the impaired glucose metabolism seen in AS, as well as a balancing of GABA (gamma-aminobutyric acid), which is normally dysfunctional in conditions of AS.

More recently, researchers looked at ketone ester supplementation in a mouse model of AS (Ciarlone et al., 2016). AS mice were supplemented with the R,S-1,3-butanediol acetoacetate diester (BD-AcAc2) ad libitum (as much as they wanted) for eight weeks. The ketone ester improved motor coordination, learning and memory, and synaptic plasticity in the AS mice. The ester also exhibited anticonvulsant properties, which indicates that both the ketogenic diet and ketone supplementation show great promise in this population.

Depression/Anxiety

According to the Anxiety and Depression Association of America, depression affects about 6.7 percent of the U.S. population and more than 15 million American adults. Anxiety disorders are the most common mental illness in the U.S., affecting nearly 40 million adults. There is a large overlap between the two: nearly half of those diagnosed with depression are also diagnosed with an anxiety disorder. Some researchers suggest that a ketogenic diet may have mood-stabilizing properties due to its ability to positively change brain energy metabolism, which is typically lowered in depressed/anxious individuals (El-Mallakh and Paskitti, 2001). The ketogenic diet has been shown to raise levels of dopamine and serotonin, neurotransmitters that are often lower in people with depression (Murphy et al., 2004) and anxiety (van der Wee et al., 2008).

In animals, the Porsolt test is used to determine levels of depression: rats are placed in a water-filled chamber with smooth walls, and researchers record the amount of time they spend immobile after they give up trying to escape the chamber. One study put a group of rats on a 4:1 ketogenic diet and another group on a standard carbohydrate-based diet; all variables—protein, vitamins, minerals—were the same, only the amounts of carbohydrate and fat differed. The ketogenic diet group spent less time immobile than the rats in the control group, suggesting that the ketogenic diet may have antidepressant effects

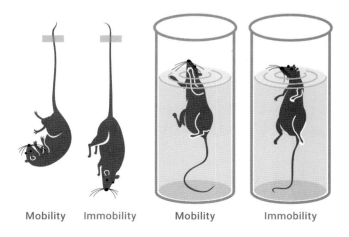

Mobility   Immobility   Mobility   Immobility

Figure 5.6.4. *The Porsolt test is commonly used to test depression in animals.*

(Murphy et al., 2004). In another study, pregnant mice were fed a ketogenic diet, but when their offspring were born, those offspring were fed a traditional carbohydrate-based diet. The offspring showed less susceptibility to depression and anxiety as adults (Sussman et al., 2015). They also had reduced blood glucose levels and were more physically active than their standard diet–fed counterparts.

Research on anxiety and depression in humans on a ketogenic diet is limited. However, studies have shown that many depression disorders, such as unipolar and bipolar disorders, are linked to a reduction in brain glucose utilization and altered chemicals in the brain (Schwartz et al., 1987; Baxter et al., 1989). (See the following section for more on bipolar disorder.) Therefore, because ketones help supply energy when glucose isn't being utilized efficiently, a ketogenic diet or ketone supplementation may improve mood and/or reduce anxiety (Kashiwaya et al., 2013). Also, as noted earlier, the ketogenic diet has been shown to raise serotonin and dopamine levels in the brain, which can also help reduce anxiety and depression. Most antidepressant drugs come with some pretty harsh side effects, so it's important to explore alternative treatments. More research into the effects of a ketogenic diet on depression and anxiety in humans is needed.

KETO CONCEPT

Can Your Diet Change Your Child's Life?

We were excited to see this type of research come out in the area of depression and anxiety. One study we hope to see or complete ourselves is on the disease susceptibility of the offspring of animals fed a ketogenic diet for their entire lives. Based on the study that looked at mice exposed to high levels of ketones in utero, it appears that lifestyle habits (exercise, diet, etc.) can have an impact on our offspring. The authors state that "there may be additional behavior alterations in offspring of animals fed a ketogenic diet including changes in learning and memory, and altered susceptibility to neurodegenerative disease later on in life" (Sussman et al., 2015). This indicates that certain epigenetic changes (modification of gene expression) may have positive long-term benefits on the offspring of animals who were fed a ketogenic diet.

Bipolar Disorder

Bipolar disorder (formerly known as manic-depressive disorder) involves dramatic shifts in mood, energy, and activity levels that affect a person's ability to carry out day-to-day tasks. The first line of treatment is antipsychotic and antidepressant medications. Interestingly enough, many anticonvulsant medications are also widely used as mood stabilizers (Ballenger and Post, 1980).

The mania and depression that characterize bipolar disorder are associated with a reduction in the brain's utilization of glucose for energy (Buchsbaum et al., 1997). Although genetics likely plays a significant role in the susceptibility to this illness, psychological, environmental, and lifestyle factors also appear to be important. It's interesting that people with bipolar disorder tend to consume more total carbohydrates, sugar, and sweetened drinks than others (Elmslie et al., 2001)—possibly unconsciously trying to self-medicate with sweets in an attempt to feel better in the moment. It's possible that the high-sugar diets consumed by bipolar individuals are not fueling their brains sufficiently due to impaired brain glucose utilization, thereby contributing further to the disorder.

Individuals with bipolar disorder have elevated levels of oxidative stress, which is the harmful overproduction of free radicals that may damage cell components such as DNA and protein. Strategies such as caloric restriction and lower-carbohydrate diets have shown to reduce oxidative stress by producing antioxidants, specifically glutathione, which combat damaging free radicals (Lopresti and Jacka, 2015). In addition, insulin resistance is often associated with bipolar disorder and is thought to possibly hamper treatment for the disorder (Calkin et al., 2015). On the surface, the increase in oxidative stress and insulin resistance seen in individuals with bipolar disorder point to the fact that diet may play a significant role in the condition. On top of that, many of the medications that are used to treat bipolar disorder may cause weight gain and ultimately lead to metabolic syndrome, a combination of negative health measures (e.g., excess body fat around the waist) that increase risk for heart disease, stroke, and diabetes. The ketogenic diet has been shown to reduce insulin resistance (Boden et al., 2005), so whether or not the ketogenic diet actually helps bipolar disorder directly, it still can indirectly improve the overall health and quality of life of individuals with bipolar disorder.

Two case reports have been published showing the positive effects that a ketogenic diet may have on bipolar disorder. First, a sixty-nine-year-old woman who had bipolar symptoms since her midtwenties was put on a ketogenic diet for two years; over that period her symptoms improved to the point that she was able to stop taking medication. She stated, "Even on the [medication], I often felt a sense of foreboding, waiting for the other shoe to drop. While it helped a lot with depression, the medication did not do much for my agitation, or my hair-trigger temper. However, I have not lost my temper once since establishing consistent ketosis . . . [I] just simply find myself reacting differently. . . . I believe that being in ketosis has been life changing for me" (Phelps et al., 2013). Second, a twenty-five-year-old woman who had had bipolar disorder since she was thirteen and had been on a multitude of medications, including antidepressants, started a ketogenic diet (70 percent fat, 22 percent protein, 8 percent carbs). She stated that her mood felt "significantly calmer," and she remained stable on the diet for several years (Phelps et al., 2013).

No adverse side effects were reported in either of these cases. In fact, both patients noted a clear association between the extent of ketosis (blood ketone levels) and diminishing bipolar symptoms, potentially opening doors for further studies looking at supplemental ketones as an option as well to help further the process.

Migraines/Headaches

Migraines are the third most prevalent illness in the world; according to the Migraine Research Foundation, nearly 12 percent of the world's population suffers from them, affecting over a billion people. While headaches are uncomfortable, migraines are more severe and, in addition to intense head pain, induce a collection of symptoms, such as nausea/vomiting and visual disturbances. Like seizures, migraines consist of episodes of neurologic dysfunction that lead to these symptoms, and anticonvulsants are often used to treat them.

An interesting article was published in 1924 by G. N. W. Thomas, who stated, "I believe sugar to be a potent factor in migraine. Many persons who now regularly suffer from migraine will find the attacks disappear entirely if sugar be eliminated from the diet." A bold statement from nearly a hundred years ago! The first documented case of a ketogenic diet being used for migraines occurred not much later, in 1928. The study authors said that although some patients had trouble sticking to the diet, "nine out of twenty-three patients did show some improvement and we feel sufficiently encouraged to continue with a diet at least relatively high in fats and low in carbohydrates. . . . It is hoped that others may have an opportunity to try out a series of patients in a similar way" (Schnabel, 1928; Maggioni et al., 2011).

There has been renewed interest in this area. Here are some of the more recent studies that have found that a ketogenic diet benefits migraines:

- A woman in her forties who had reoccurring migraines enrolled in a weight-loss program involving a modified fast with three or four high-protein, low-carbohydrate shakes a day. While this might not be the best ketogenic approach, due to sheer caloric restriction and reduced carbohydrate intake, she still achieved a state of ketosis. Upon inducing a state of ketosis, the woman become completely free of migraines and continued to remain migraine-free for fourteen months (Strahlman, 2006).

- Adolescents ages twelve to nineteen who had chronic daily headaches were given a modified Atkins diet with less than 15 grams of carbohydrates per day (see page 98 for more on MAD). The three subjects who completed the three-month trial saw an improvement in headache severity and quality of life (Kossoff et al., 2010). (Unfortunately, it's not surprising that only three teens were able to stick to the diet: avoiding snacks and treats that aren't keto friendly while all their friends and classmates are eating whatever they want can be a big obstacle for children and teens.)

- In a study done on twins who developed neurological episodes, including migraines, those who were put on a 3:1 ketogenic diet saw complete resolution of migraine attacks during the treatment, and the level of improvement was strongly correlated with the degree of ketosis (DiLorenzo et al., 2013).

- A study of forty-five overweight women who followed a ketogenic diet for just one month demonstrated fewer days with headaches, from about five per month to one (Di Lorenzo et al., 2015).

The direct cause of migraines and headaches is unknown; however, the fact that a ketogenic diet has been found to be beneficial may provide a clue: we don't mean to sound like a broken record, but as in so many other health problems, mitochondrial dysfunction and its accompanying decreased ATP production in the brain may play a significant role (Roos-Araujo et al., 2014). Ketones would alleviate that issue by providing an alternative fuel that bypasses the problem areas of the mitochondria. The ketogenic diet's ability to reduce inflammation may also play a role, as migraines may involve neural inflammation.

Anecdotally, we have received numerous reports of exogenous ketones being extremely helpful for migraines as well. If mitochondrial dysfunction and neural inflammation are indeed causes of migraines, it seems plausible that exogenous ketones would be helpful—however, no studies have been done directly looking at this hypothesis yet.

Before treating migraines with a ketogenic diet or ketones, several factors, such as age, frequency of attacks, accompanying complications, and medication, need to be considered. We recommend that individuals with migraines talk to their doctors before changing their diets.

Post-Traumatic Stress Disorder (PTSD)

Post-traumatic stress disorder (PTSD) is defined as a mental disorder that some people develop after experiencing or witnessing life-threatening events that may cause physical harm, intense fear, feelings of helplessness, and/or horror, such as military combat, a natural disaster, a car accident, or sexual assault. PTSD affects an estimated 8 percent of Americans, or 24.4 million people. It's diagnosed more in women than in men—about 10 percent of women have PTSD compared to 4 percent of men, possibly due to more women seeking medical help for symptoms than men.

PTSD can happen to anyone, but it's often most associated with members of the military because it's particularly common among soldiers who have seen combat. According to the Pentagon, suicide has caused more American veteran casualties than actual combat in Iraq or Afghanistan, regardless of whether the veterans had been deployed to either war zone—an alarming statistic. Between 11 and 20 percent of the military personnel who served in Iraq and Afghanistan have PTSD in any given year (www.ptsd.va.gov). Beyond its physical and emotional impact on individuals and their families, PTSD brings about an annual cost of well over $40 billion. Often, PTSD is misdiagnosed or overlooked due to other symptoms, which can further increase the cost and the amount of time someone is dealing with this condition.

Symptoms of PTSD may include flashbacks, nightmares, heightened reactions to loud noises or similar traumatic stimuli, depression, insomnia, avoidance of similar traumatic situations, and anxiety. PTSD is also characterized by elevated blood glucose, increased triglycerides and LDL cholesterol, and decreased HDL (good) cholesterol (Karlović et al., 2004). Unfortunately, this combination places individuals with PTSD at a high risk for type 2 diabetes and cardiovascular disease (Norman et al., 2006).

Some research indicates that PTSD-related impairments in health may result from a disrupted gut-brain axis (Kharrazian et al., 2015). The gut and the brain are closely connected, as they have many of the same chemical messengers that relay signals back and forth. The gut helps control many body systems, from immune function to cognitive processes. Individuals with PTSD commonly exhibit irritable bowel syndrome, increased intestinal permeability (a condition in which gaps in the lining of the small intestines allow large food particles into the bloodstream, causing an immune response), altered balance of good bacteria in the gut, increased levels of the stress hormone cortisol, and increased systemic inflammation, all of which result in gastrointestinal complications (Bienenstock, 2016). The brain side of the axis is also impaired with PTSD: sufferers have impaired short-term memory, lower attention span, and increased hostility. In addition, they are more likely to be dependent on alcohol and more likely to commit domestic violence (Kharrazian, 2015). Thus, addressing the gut-brain axis holds promise for addressing many of the symptoms of PTSD—a healthier gut may allow for reduced brain-related symptoms, while a healthier brain may allow for reduced gut-related symptoms.

Current treatment options for PTSD include psychotherapy or counseling and various medications, particularly antidepressants. These can be beneficial, but they can come with side effects, such as addiction/dependence.

The ketogenic diet may be another possible therapy. It has been shown to improve cholesterol profiles, lower blood glucose levels, and reduce inflammation (Holland et al., 2016). It may also enhance the health of intestinal walls by supplying them with butyrate, a short-chain fatty acid that is a by-product of the breakdown of the ketone body BHB that supplies fuel to the good bacteria in the intestines. It is also possible that BHB may cause a mild euphoric state that can improve mood and cognitive function (Brown, 2007). Furthermore, a ketogenic diet and ultimately the production of ketones could increase substances associated with improved cognition, better serotonin metabolism, and reduced aging of the brain (Fontán-Lozano, 2008). Therefore, it is possible that through a multitude of mechanisms, elevated ketone levels achieved on a ketogenic diet or with supplementation could lead to improvements in PTSD. However, more direct research needs to be done (and is currently being conducted).

Schizophrenia

Schizophrenia affects about 1 percent of Americans. However, its devastating impact shouldn't be understated, as it is a very costly and burdensome condition. In 2002, the overall U.S. cost of schizophrenia was estimated to be about $62.7 billion. Schizophrenia, a serious neurological brain disorder ranked among the world's top ten causes of long-term disability, is characterized by perceptual, cognitive, and behavioral disturbances. Symptoms may include agitation, social isolation, repetitive movements, delusion, paranoia, and hearing voices. However, the success rate of antipsychotic medications and psychosocial therapies is promisingly high.

People with schizophrenia often experience other health concerns, such as hypertension, cardiovascular disease, poor cholesterol profiles, high amounts of fat around the internal organs, insulin resistance, and type 2 diabetes (Harris et al., 2013). Most antipsychotic drugs have side effects that cause weight gain and contribute to insulin resistance and potentially other complications, such as type 2 diabetes. A ketogenic diet is known to improve these health concerns and/or limit the drug-related side effects.

It's also possible that a ketogenic diet may generate improvements in the symptoms of schizophrenia itself. A seventy-year-old female diagnosed with schizophrenia at age seventeen reported severe hallucinations on a daily basis and had attempted suicide multiple times (Kraft and Westman, 2009). She was then put on a ketogenic diet of unlimited meat and eggs, 4 ounces of cheese, and vegetables, with total carbohydrate restricted to less than 20 grams per day. After just nineteen days on the diet, she reported no longer experiencing auditory or visual hallucinations. There was no change in her medication during this time; the only thing that differed was her diet. Over the course of a year, she continued the diet without any recurrence of hallucinations and with continuing improvements in both energy and body composition.

Research has hinted at potential ways in which a ketogenic diet may work for this condition. Schizophrenics tend to have increased activity in the hippocampus, the part of the brain responsible for emotion and memory (Tregellas et al., 2015). Studies have shown that in mice, a ketogenic diet can improve hippocampal function, which may reduce the hyperactivity that is seen in schizophrenic patients (Tregellas et al., 2015). Though the exact mechanisms are still not clear, over fifty years ago, correlational research reports came out stating that individuals with high consumption of cereals and wheat were more likely to have schizophrenia (Pacheco et al., 1965). Though more research is needed, implementing a well-formulated ketogenic diet may be a viable option for someone with schizophrenia as a nutritional rather than a pharmacological approach.

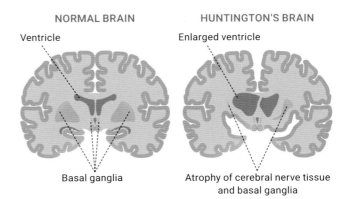

NORMAL BRAIN   **HUNTINGTON'S BRAIN**

Ventricle   Enlarged ventricle

Basal ganglia   Atrophy of cerebral nerve tissue and basal ganglia

Figure 5.6.5. Huntington's disease directly affects the brain by enlarging some areas and decreasing others. It can have debilitating side effects.

Source: www.shutterstock.com/image-vector/ normal-brain-huntingtons-disease-showing-enlarged-311615132.

Huntington's Disease

Huntington's disease is an inherited neurodegenerative disease typically characterized by uncontrolled movements, emotional problems, and impairments in cognitive function. This disease is caused by an inherited mutation in a single gene. The gene mutation causes tangles of amyloid plaques like those present in Alzheimer's, Parkinson's, and ALS. Over time, symptoms and complications possibly resulting from these plaques become significantly worse, eventually leading to death.

Though it's not necessarily a mitochondrial disorder, studies have shown that individuals with Huntington's have impaired energy metabolism in the brain and skeletal muscle (Koroshetz et al., 1997). In addition, studies have shown that individuals with this condition have decreased ATP (energy) production in muscle, reduced activity of the electron transport chain (which is a primary pathway that produces ATP), and increased oxidative stress, all of which may be improved by a ketogenic diet. In addition to motor and cognitive problems, progressive weight loss (including muscle tissue) is a striking symptom of Huntington's and can itself cause serious complications. One study found that the ketogenic diet preserved weight in individuals with Huntington's; however, no significant effect was

seen on coordination or working memory (Ruskin et al., 2011).

Drug treatments for type 2 diabetes that control blood glucose have been shown to increase survival rates and reduce symptoms in Huntington's disease (Ma et al., 2007), which suggests that the reduction and stabilization of blood glucose provided by a ketogenic diet may also be beneficial. In addition, evidence suggests that adenosine, one of the four nucleoside units of ribonucleic acid (RNA; carriers of instructions from DNA), can improve symptoms of Huntington's due to its ability to increase dopamine levels (Masino et al., 2009); therefore, instituting a ketogenic diet, which can improve both glucose/ insulin control and adenosine levels, may have an impact on HD.

Polycystic Ovary Syndrome (PCOS)

PCOS is the result of an imbalance of reproductive hormones in women; in fact, it is the most common cause of infertility in women. According to the PCOS Foundation, about 10 percent of women of childbearing age are affected by PCOS. Over half of the women who are diagnosed with PCOS are overweight or obese (Liepa et al., 2008). In addition,

PCOS is often associated with insulin resistance, metabolic syndrome, elevated blood glucose, decreased short-term memory, and impaired glucose uptake in the brain (Castellano et al., 2015). Women diagnosed with PCOS are more likely to see early cognitive decline than their healthy counterparts.

Currently, there is no cure for PCOS, although diabetes medications seem to improve many of its accompanying conditions. Because so many of its associated problems are related to impaired glucose uptake and metabolism, implementing a proper nutritional strategy to improve brain energy metabolism and decrease insulin resistance seems logical for women with PCOS. Furthermore, PCOS is known as being extremely inflammatory in nature, which is confirmed by high levels of C-reactive protein (a marker of inflammation). Thus, logically, a ketogenic diet may aid by both improving glucose metabolism and decreasing inflammation.

In a six-month study, five women diagnosed with PCOS were instructed to keep carbohydrates below 20 grams per day and to eat animal foods and low-carbohydrate vegetables, which led to a state of ketosis (Mavropoulos et al., 2005). Over the course of the study, the subjects lost, on average, more than 12 percent of their body weight and saw a significant improvement in reproductive hormone and insulin levels. As if that wasn't promising enough, two women became pregnant during the study despite previous fertility complications! It is unknown whether these effects are the result of the weight loss or of being in ketosis; however, this study provides strong evidence that a ketogenic diet may be beneficial for women suffering with PCOS.

We have seen and heard stories from many women who suffer from PCOS implementing a low-carbohydrate ketogenic diet (and even supplementing with ketones in some cases) with significant improvements in various aspects of their health and quality of life. Therefore, interventions that improve insulin sensitivity and reduce body weight (for instance, blood glucose–lowering supplements and exercise) may also be effective at decreasing high levels of androgens and testosterone, regulating ovulation, and reducing the various symptoms associated with PCOS.

Amyotrophic Lateral Sclerosis (ALS) / Lou Gehrig's Disease

As huge baseball fans, we are familiar with ALS from baseball legend Lou Gehrig being diagnosed with it. This brutal and extremely debilitating disorder affects the nerves and functions of the muscles. According to the ALS Association, about fifteen new cases of ALS are diagnosed every day. At any given time, 20,000 Americans have the disease, primarily Caucasian males between forty and seventy years old; however, ALS is seen throughout the world. The average survival time after diagnosis is about three years, and once the disease starts, it almost always progresses, eventually taking away the ability to walk, dress, write, speak, swallow, and breathe.

From a scientific perspective, ALS is a neurodegenerative disorder in which nerve cells in the brain and spinal cord die, causing a weakening and wasting away of the muscles in the body. Though the exact mechanisms underlying ALS are not clearly understood, some scientists suggest that its primary instigators are oxidative damage, inflammation, mitochondrial dysfunction, and excessive stimulation of the neurotransmitter glutamate, which causes cells to become damaged or die (Vucic et al., 2014). While a drug called Riluzole has been shown to slow the progress of ALS due to its anti-glutamate properties, it's expensive and its effectiveness may be limited to its effect on glutamate—it doesn't improve the other factors involved in ALS. By reducing oxidative damage and inflammation and providing an alternative source of energy, the ketogenic diet and/or exogenous ketones may help improve symptoms and ultimately outcomes for ALS patients.

In about 10 percent of ALS patients, the disease is inherited, possibly as a result of a mutation in a gene that affects the mitochondria (Zhao et al., 2006). We're sure you can guess where this is going. Studies in ALS patients have noted decreased mitochondrial function (Wiedemann et al., 2002). One study found that when animals with ALS-like symptoms were fed a ketogenic diet, they maintained motor function longer than a control group. Even more interesting was that when researchers took mitochondria from these mice and added pure D-BHB to them, ATP synthesis increased dramatically within just twelve minutes. In addition, the researchers found that D-BHB actually slowed the rate of cell death in the motor neurons of the spinal cord (Zhao et al., 2006).

Other research has found that C8 MCT, a medium-chain triglyceride that can be metabolized into ketone bodies (see page 56 for more on the different kinds of MCTs), protects against neuron loss in the spinal cord, improves motor function, and decreases muscle weakness, likely because of some conversion to ketones such as BHB (Zhao et al., 2012; Pasinetti, 2013). In addition, a study looking at the ketogenic diet in conjunction with the Deanna Protocol (DP)—a system of supplementation designed to aid in energy production—found that in mice with ALS-like symptoms, those fed the ketogenic diet plus the DP improved motor function and extended survival time/lifespan (Ari et al., 2014).

This evidence clearly indicates that higher ketone levels, whether induced by diet or supplementation, can improve mitochondrial function and ATP production and may protect motor neurons from dying.

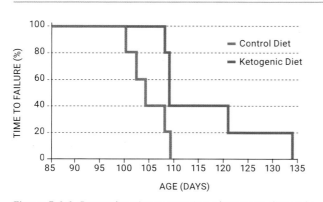

Figure 5.6.6. *Rotarod testing comparing a ketogenic diet and a standard diet on the loss of motor function in animals. Mice on the ketogenic diet maintained motor function longer than mice fed a standard diet.*

Source: Zhao et al., 2006.

Attention-Deficit Hyperactivity Disorder (ADHD)

ADHD is a worldwide problem that affects both kids and adults. It is characterized by inattention (lack of focus, being easily distracted), hyperactivity (difficulty sitting still, excessive talking), and impulsivity (interrupting others during conversation, acting without considering the consequences). Brain activity may be affected in individuals with ADHD, as circuits that connect different areas of the brain may be altered and the volume of various regions of the brain may be reduced—leading to many of the noted symptomatic characteristics.

Currently, there is debate about whether this disorder is "real" or if the symptoms associated with ADHD stem from other issues. The challenge comes from the fact that there is no specific lab test to identify ADHD and even complex scans such as an MRI can't diagnose someone with it. Nevertheless, according to the Centers for Disease Control, as of 2011, 11 percent of children ages four to seventeen (6.4 million) have been diagnosed with ADHD. As you can see in Figure 5.6.7, these numbers have continued to rise each year since 2003. Perhaps the most alarming statistic is that in 2011, 6.1 percent of children in America were taking ADHD medication, and the total yearly cost to Americans for this disorder alone is over $42 billion.

Recently, more discussion has occurred about potential dietary interventions that can help with ADHD, especially in kids and youth (Millichap and Yee, 2012). Several reports point to sugar intake being a primary culprit for a lot of the symptoms seen in kids with ADHD. For instance, some reports indicate that inattention is proportional to sugar intake (Arnold and Lofthouse, 2013). In addition, when looking at the electro-activity in the brains of kids consuming excess sugar, we see that the low blood sugar levels that occur after consuming a lot of sugar (and therefore releasing insulin) are associated with an impairment of the normal electrical activity of the cerebral cortex in the brain (Millichap and Yee, 2012). It's interesting to note

How Much Sugar Do Kids Really Eat?

Recently, several researchers have made a push to lower the acceptable rate for children's sugar intake. In 2015, the World Health Organization recommended that children ages two to eighteen should eat or drink less than 6 teaspoons (about 25 grams) of added sugars a day (Vos et al., 2016). Some reports state that kids today consume an average of 19 teaspoons (over 80 grams) of added sugar per day!

Sugar is added to nearly all of our food products, especially prepackaged foods; it's often listed under names like "high-fructose corn syrup," "maltodextrin," and "dextrose." To put this in perspective, one serving of BBQ sauce can easily contain 13 grams of added sugar (over half of the allotted amount for children). Fruit juice boxes that some parents perceive as healthy can contain over 20 grams of added sugar, and just one can of soda can blow past the suggested limit with over 40 grams of sugar. Take a second to think about how often we let kids and teens chow down on pizza, french fries, and soda and then follow it up with a candy bar dessert. This kind of eating was typical in our school cafeterias growing up. (The tomato sauce on the pizza was counted as a "vegetable.") This is absurd: meals like these can easily quadruple a kid's daily intake of sugar.

children's alertness, cognitive functioning, and behavior improved, alluding to the fact that the diet may be beneficial in improving focus and attention in children who need it the most (Pulsifer et al., 2001). Additionally, parents had less stress, which eases the burden on both them and the children. These improvements may stem from the possibility that the mitochondria in the brain cells are abnormal, as noted in previous studies, and therefore require an alternate energy source, such as ketones (Marazziti, 2012). More research needs to be done looking directly at improvements in ADHD symptoms with the ketogenic diet, but its potential therapeutic use in these individuals is promising.

Anecdotally, supplemental ketones may also benefit ADHD. We have received numerous reports of parents whose children are hyperactive but may not have been officially diagnosed with ADHD who are seeing substantial improvements in many aspects of cognitive function with supplemental ketones. Children coming off their typical ADHD medication isn't unheard of and makes sense when an alternative fuel source is introduced to the brain.

that children with epilepsy often exhibit symptoms of ADHD, and children with ADHD often have brain electrical activity similar to children with epilepsy (Millichap et al., 2010). The benefits of a ketogenic diet for reducing sugar consumption are obvious, and that alone may help improve symptoms of ADHD.

Limited studies have looked directly at the ketogenic diet for ADHD. One study found that children on a ketogenic diet saw steady improvements in brain activity (Kessler et al., 2011). Animal studies using a 4:1 ketogenic diet in models of ADHD have seen normalized brain activity levels, which "suggests that the diet may be useful in the treatment of ADHD" (Murphy and Burnham, 2006). Lastly, one human study looked at the effects of the ketogenic diet on development and behavior in children diagnosed with ADHD. The researchers found that after twenty months on the diet, the

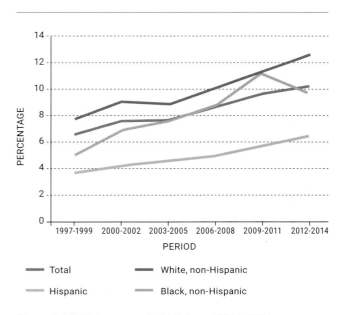

Figure 5.6.7. *Rising rates of ADHD from 1997 to 2014.*

Source: www.chadd.org/understanding-adhd/about-adhd/data-and-statistics/general-prevalence.aspx.

Glut1 Deficiency Syndrome

Glucose transporter type 1 deficiency syndrome is a genetic brain disorder that again involves impaired brain energy metabolism. In this case, the main transporter that takes glucose into the brain, Glut1, isn't functioning properly. Some reports indicate that in a resting state, the adult brain utilizes 25 percent of what the body as a whole uses; in infants and children, that number can rise to 80 percent (Klepper, 2008). Since the brain relies heavily on glucose for energy, when the transporters used to move glucose into the brain aren't functioning as they should, brain energy metabolism and overall health and function are seriously compromised. The majority of individuals with Glut1 deficiency display early-onset seizures, developmental delays, and a complex movement disorder.

The ketogenic diet is by far the most recommended treatment for Glut1 deficiency because it provides an alternative source of fuel for the brain: ketones. However, one thing to keep in mind is that this syndrome is often misdiagnosed as epilepsy. Proper diagnosis and strategic implementation is key in order to provide patients with the best care (Lee and Hur, 2016).

Most studies implementing a ketogenic diet for Glut1 deficiency use a 4:1 or 3:1 ratio with much success. However, alternatives such as the MCT diet (2:1) and the modified Atkins diet (MAD; see page 98) have also been used successfully (Klepper, 2008). One seven-year-old boy with Glut1 deficiency was put on a modified Atkins diet (less than 10 grams of carbs per day, 2:1 fat to protein) with unrestricted calories (Ito et al., 2008). Within three days, his blood BHB levels were over 5 mmol/L, and many of his symptoms, including tremors and movement coordination, had drastically improved. He also was able to walk faster and longer.

While there is some concern that the ketogenic diet is unsustainable for children or adolescents, one study found that thirteen of fifteen children with epilepsy continued the diet over several years, with ten of those thirteen remaining seizure-free. When asked how they felt about the diet, 75 percent of parents ranked it as very effective, while 25 percent said it was moderately effective. All reported improved alertness, demeanor, and physical and mental endurance while on the diet (Klepper et al., 2005). Satisfaction with the daily practicality of the diet was ranked high by 29 percent of parents, moderate by 54 percent, and poor by 17 percent. However, the diet used in this study was a 3:1 ketogenic diet. Therefore, a modified ketogenic diet, along with more keto-friendly snacks, products, and aids like supplemental ketones, may help improve long-term satisfaction for both parents and children.

Supplemental ketones also may be effective on their own. One study administered triheptanoin (a C7 fatty acid, which gets broken down into C5 ketones, which are similar to but slightly different than BHB) to fourteen children and adults with Glut1 deficiency who were not on a ketogenic diet. This resulted in an improvement in seizure rate and spike-and-wave activity (brain wave pattern typical of an epileptic seizure), and most patients also experienced an improvement in neuropsychological performance and cerebral metabolic rate (Pascual et al., 2014).

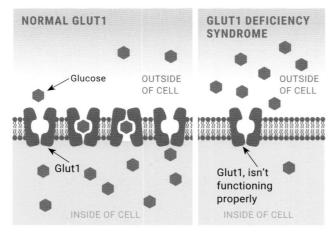

Figure 5.6.8. *Illustration of Glut1 deficiency compared to a normal functioning cell.*

Can the Ketogenic Diet Be Modified?

Most studies of the ketogenic diet implement strict strategies, such as 4:1 or sometimes even higher, in order to facilitate a deeper level of ketosis. For conditions like epilepsy, this degree of ketosis may be necessary to be effective, but in other cases, like Glut1 deficiency, a modified approach could work. In the future, a combination of a ketogenic diet, ketone supplements, and agents that replenish metabolic pathways, such as triheptanoin (C7 MCT oil) or C5 ketones, may create a perfect cocktail for individuals with inherited metabolic disorders such as Glut1 deficiency. An effective ketogenic diet may not need to be as restrictive as previously thought.

Glycogen Storage Disease (GSD)

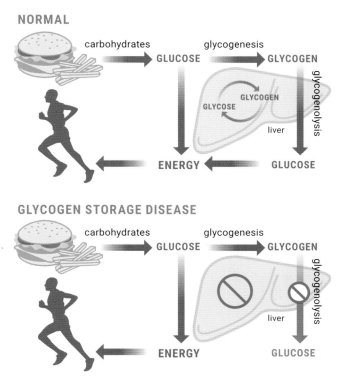

Figure 5.6.9. *An inability to properly break down glucose is the hallmark of GSD.*

As the name implies, glycogen storage disease is the result of inherited dysfunction in glycogen metabolism. Throughout the day or during exercise, the body normally taps into glycogen (the stored form of glucose), which it breaks down into glucose for fuel. However, in the case of GSD, certain enzymes that control the change of glucose into glycogen and glycogen into glucose are missing. Thus, people with GSD may be able to store glycogen in various tissues yet are unable to break it down. If they don't get a constant supply of glucose from the diet, their blood sugar can drop dangerously low and have serious adverse effects.

The traditional treatment of choice for GSD is a steady diet of carbohydrates and avoidance of fasting periods. Makes sense, right? Our bodies need a consistent amount of fuel, and if we can't get it from what is stored as glycogen, we need to get it consistently from our diet. Imagine that you are seventy years old and you have worked your entire life to put away money in your savings and retirement accounts. However, when you go to buy something, you can't access that money; the bank won't let you use what you have put away. In that case, you need to continue to work every day in order to pay bills and buy the items you need. In people with GSD,

carbohydrates are like the money in this analogy, and thus people feel that their only option is to "work" every day, or supply their bodies with a constant stream of carbohydrates to keep themselves going, often unaware that there are alternatives. But as you can see, it is difficult to maintain a constant supply of glucose over an entire lifetime. In addition, chronically elevated glucose (and thus insulin levels), caused by a high-carbohydrate diet, can lead to a host of other issues.

Because the ketogenic diet shifts the body from relying on glucose to relying on fat as its primary fuel, it frees those with GSD from having to constantly monitor their blood glucose and eat a high-carbohydrate diet. In ketosis, the body easily taps into fat stores whenever fuel is needed, so the difficulty in tapping into glycogen is no longer as significant.

There are a several types of glycogen storage disease, but we will primarily focus on type III (also known as debranching enzyme deficiency, or Forbes or Cori disease) and type V (also known as muscle glycogen phosphorylase deficiency, or McArdle's disease).

In GSD III, the deficiency in a particular enzyme not only causes difficulty tapping into glycogen but also leads to a buildup of glycogen in the liver, heart, and skeletal muscles, which can cause serious complications. The implementation of a ketogenic diet has demonstrated benefits in this case. First, two siblings (a seven-year-old girl and a five-year-old boy) who had GSD III were put on a diet consisting of 60 percent fat, 25 percent protein, and 15 percent carbohydrate. After just one year on the diet, their blood tests, cardiac enzymes, and congestive heart failure markers all had significantly improved (Brambilla et al., 2014). Second, two boys (ages nine and eleven) diagnosed with GSD III were treated with a modified Atkins diet in which they ate less than 10 grams of carbohydrates per day but had no restriction on protein and fats. Both boys saw improvements in cardiac function (markers of muscle damage) and exercise tolerance when following the diet over several months (Mayorandan et al., 2014).

Is it possible that supplemental ketones could be beneficial in conjunction with the diet? Another study looked at a two-month-old boy with GSD III and used a combination of BHB ketone supplementation plus a higher-protein 2:1 ketogenic diet (Valayannopoulos et al., 2011). After twenty-four months on this protocol, echocardiography showed an improvement of cardiomyopathy (disease of the heart muscle), blood glucose levels were stable, and no side effects were observed. Thus, it is possible that a combination of a ketogenic diet plus supplemental ketones could be beneficial.

Similar work has been done with GSD V (McArdle's disease). GSD V is caused by a defect of a different enzyme, which results in exercise intolerance, premature fatigue, and exercise-induced muscle pain. A fifty-five-year-old man who had had McArdle's disease since the age of four was put on a ketogenic diet (80 percent fat, 14 percent protein, 6 percent carbohydrate). At the end of the study, his exercise tolerance and strength were over three times as high for higher-intensity activities and up to sixty times as high for low- to moderate-intensity activities, such as walking (Busch et al., 2005).

Each of these studies shows promising results for the use of a ketogenic diet for GSD. Since it can lower insulin and lower blood glucose, yet provides an alternative energy source for the body, the ketogenic diet may be a more viable, sustainable option than traditional therapies that involve a constant supply of glucose/carbohydrates.

Other Inherited Metabolic Disorders

GSD VII (Tarui's disease): Impairment of the enzyme affected in this type of GSD can lead to a disturbance in ATP production and the inability to properly break down glucose into usable energy. Therefore, people with this deficiency often have exercise intolerance, muscle weakness, and fatigue. One study showed that a baby boy with GSD VII who was put on a 3:1 ketogenic diet at four months of age saw significant improvements in motor skills and strength by age two (Swoboda et al., 1997).

Pyruvate dehydrogenase complex deficiency (PDCD): Deficiency in the enzyme PDC results in an energy deficit, especially for the brain, which can lead to brain malformation early on if not treated appropriately. One case study showed that in two brothers (ages two and eleven), a mild ketogenic diet (65 percent fat plus MCTs) resulted in a decrease in neurological deterioration, a significant increase in growth and developmental maturation, and an increase in strength and endurance (Falk et al., 1976).

Lastly, studies utilizing ketogenic diets have also been shown to be beneficial for other conditions, such as complex I deficiency, complex II deficiency, and complex IV deficiency (Kang et al., 2007); argininosuccinate lyase (ASL) deficiency (Peuscher et al., 2011); and adenylosuccinate lyase (ADSL) deficiency (Jurecka et al., 2014).

Inflammation and Wounds

When you take a deeper look at diseases and conditions ranging from diabetes, kidney disease, Crohn's disease, and multiple sclerosis (MS) to Alzheimer's disease and cancer, one key attribute seen across the board is chronic low-grade inflammation/neuroinflammation. A compromised immune system can trigger or provoke further inflammatory markers, which leads to a cascade of unpleasant events. In 2015 alone, for example, more than 3 million people were diagnosed with irritable bowel syndrome (IBS). This number represents a small fraction of disease states and conditions that tie back to inflammation (Dahlhamer, 2016).

Nonsteroidal anti-inflammatory drugs (NSAIDs) are the Pop Rocks of the twenty-first century. Athletes and individuals with chronic pain continually pop NSAIDs such as aspirin in order to alleviate symptoms and problems. Some become reliant on the masking of pain that these drugs provide and consistently take more than is ever "recommended." However, people often fail to realize that the consistent use of NSAIDs has been associated with potentially serious dose-dependent gastrointestinal (GI) complications, such as upper GI bleeding. In fact, GI complications resulting from NSAID use are among the most common drug side effects in the United States, due to widespread use. Think about that for a second. The most common drug side effects are caused by something that anyone can buy at any convenience store and ingest in excessive amounts to numb or mask their pain. Recent reports have shed light on individuals who have even experienced gastric ulcers following chronic NSAID use (Goldstein and Cryer, 2015).

Fortunately, we are here to bring attention to a potential way in which ketones themselves, specifically BHB, can play a role in inflammatory-mediated conditions. First, we need to briefly go over some of the things that drive inflammation from a mechanistic standpoint. One key factor is something known as the "NLRP3 inflammasome," which is really the control center for pro-inflammatory cytokines. Think of the NLRP3 inflammasome as a sensor. If you've ever watched a movie in which a criminal is trying to steal money from a vault, he or she often finds that the vault that has several lasers running across it and one slight misstep could set off all the alarms. Similarly, our inflammasome sensor is very sensitive to such things as toxins, excess glucose, amyloids, and cholesterol, and alterations in these can trigger inflammatory markers. Nevertheless, if you were to completely remove the NLRP3 inflammasome from someone, you could theoretically rid them of type 2 diabetes, atherosclerosis, MS, Alzheimer's, age-related functional decline, bone loss, and gout (Youm et al., 2015). However, since removing the NLRP3 inflammasome is currently not possible, identifying mechanisms that can help control and regulate the NLRP3 inflammasome deactivation may provide insights into the control of several chronic diseases.

The anti-inflammatory properties of a ketogenic diet are well known and established in both animals and humans. The question, then, is what aspect of being in a physiological state of ketosis is driving this anti-inflammatory response? One thought is that BHB itself could be the driving force behind all these effects seen on inflammation. After testing this theory, researchers discovered that BHB inhibited the NLRP3 inflammasome (AcAc wasn't effective here) (Youm et al., 2015). They went on to test this further in mice by providing a ketone ester that, when administered, protected the mice from hyperglycemia. This led the authors to conclude that ketone supplementation holds promise in reducing the severity of multiple NLRP3 mediated chronic inflammatory diseases. More recently, Dr. Angela Poff and her colleagues looked at numerous pro-inflammatory markers in mice supplementing with ketone salts and ketone esters and found significant decreases with exogenous ketone supplementation (Poff et al., 2017). These studies pave the way for looking at inflammation and various related conditions through a new lens.

Wound Healing, Too?!

Recently, Dr. Dominic D'Agostino's lab examined the effects of oral ketone supplementation in animals without dietary restriction on wound healing. Most people don't realize how big an issue chronic wounds are, but in fact, reports indicate that over 1.8 million patients report chronic wounds each year, costing the U.S. healthcare system $25 billion. That should be enough to wake people up to this often-overlooked epidemic. Exogenous ketone supplementation in animals promoted wound healing/closure via enhancement of physiological factors, such as increasing cell growth, advancing cell migration, reducing reactive oxygen species (ROS) production, and resolving inflammation (Kesl et al., 2016). These are brand-new and very interesting findings that we hope will be carried over into more human research.

Aging and Longevity

> "Today is the oldest you've been and the youngest you'll ever be again."
> —Eleanor Roosevelt

Why do we age? How come some people start getting gray hair in their thirties while others still get carded at the bar in their fifties? Superman is one of our favorite superheroes for a multitude of reasons, but we especially love that he is still flying around saving the world in his eighties (the character was created in 1933)—it gives us hope that age is "just a number."

All kidding aside, even though Superman may be fictional, the money and energy being spent on research into antiaging and extending human life is certainly real. According to the U.S. Department of Health and Human Services, the elderly population in the United States, defined as sixty-five-plus years of age, is around 44.7 million, and that number is expected to more than double by 2060 (Moreno and Mobbs, 2016). Along with this rising number comes an increase in costly diseases. What potential impact do diet and lifestyle have on living not only a long life but also a fulfilling life?

"Blue Zones" are areas of the world where people live measurably longer. Unfortunately, Blue Zones have caused a major rift among experts and nutrition enthusiasts, who disagree about what type of diet these people are eating and how diet may affect their longevity. First, it's challenging enough for scientists to track what subjects eat over a ten-week study, let alone identify what people eat over their entire lives. To then try to correlate that data to longevity is rather difficult. But people in Blue Zones share some key characteristics that we think are important irrespective of diet:

- Most people living in these zones typically are physically active throughout the day, usually outdoors, so they get ample amounts of vitamin D.

- They have strong family and community relationships, which give them a sense of purpose.

- They have lower levels of stress and anxiety.

- They eat whole foods (that is, not processed foods).

Whether or not you're on a ketogenic diet, all of these are likely important factors for living a long and healthy life.

> "In the end, it's not the years in your life that count. It's the life in your years."

With that out of the way, let's dig into some theories surrounding aging and possible ways in which a ketogenic lifestyle may help. Keep in mind that there are numerous theories, but we will touch on a few major biological ones.

Theory	Description
Programmed Longevity	Aging is the result of a sequential switching on and off of certain genes.
Endocrine Theory	Hormones regulate the aging process (specifically the insulin/IGF-1 signaling pathway).
Immunological Theory	The immune system is programmed to weaken over time and thus make the elderly more susceptible to infections and diseases.
Free Radical Theory	Free radicals cause damage to cells over time and eventually cause them to stop functioning properly.
Wear and Tear Theory	Due to repeated use over a lifetime, our cells and tissues experience "wear and tear" that eventually causes them to break down and die.
Somatic Damage / Mutation Theory	DNA damage occurs in cells throughout our lives. In addition, each time a cell divides, there is a chance that some of the genes will be copied incorrectly. These mutated cells can malfunction and cause problems in the body's functioning.
Telomere Theory	Telomeres, which cap the ends of chromosomes, have been shown to shorten with each successive cell division; this leads to fraying of our chromosomes.
Glycation Theory/Advanced Glycation End Products (AGEs)	Over time, glucose reacts with fat and protein to create AGEs through a process known as glycation. The more AGEs we have, the faster we age.

We won't go into too much detail on each theory, but we hope you get the gist of some processes that can lead to aging and to cells becoming dysfunctional and/or dying.

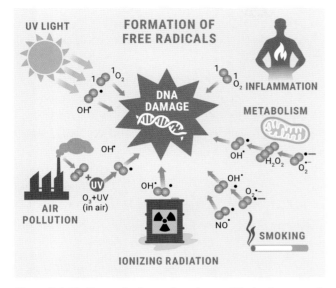

Figure 5.6.10. *Free radicals can form in a multitude of ways and ultimately attack DNA, causing damage.*

Source: www.dreamstime.com/stock-illustration-formation-free-radicals-concept-editable-clip-art-jpg-attacking-dna-image56580573.

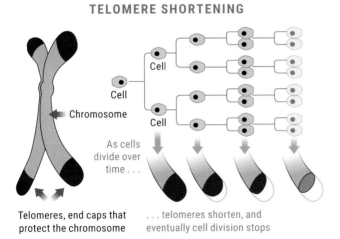

Figure 5.6.11. *Over time, telomeres shorten, which signals the cells to stop dividing. Shorter telemores are associated with earlier risk of heart attacks and death.*

Source: www.wholehealthinsider.com/newsletter/2012/a-genetic-solution-to-slowing-aging-and-preventing-disease/.

Protecting the Aging Brain

Our body's and brain's ability to effectively use glucose declines as we age. Being in a state of ketosis not only provides an energy source that we may be able to utilize more efficiently later in life, but it also may have some unique properties that may help the aging process.

If we haven't gotten this message across yet, we will emphasize it again right now: properly functioning and healthy mitochondria are essential for wellness and longevity. Under conditions where oxidative stress is high (for instance, following a heart attack or traumatic brain injury), there is a clear mismatch between the high energy demand of the brain and the supply of energy from glucose. Under these conditions, there is a deficit in glucose metabolism, leading to build up of lactate and other by-products that further contribute to oxidative stress and prevent mitochondria from functioning properly. Several studies have shown that a ketogenic diet can stimulate the formation of new mitochondria as well as provide a more efficient energy source—essentially cleaning out the dirty tank and providing it with a clean-burning fuel to utilize (Bough et al., 2006; Hyatt et al., 2016).

Another way to protect the brain as we age is to enhance our antioxidant capacity. Over a lifetime we tend to build up free radicals and reactive oxygen species (ROS), a substance created by mitochondria, both of which can bind to our cells, cause damage, and increase inflammation in cellular DNA and other proteins. Free radicals float around the body stealing electrons from other molecules, like robbers on a crime spree trying to steal jewelry and money from as many stores as possible. Referred to as "oxidation," this process basically results in a chainlike process. Once the robber (that is, free radical) steals an electron from a neighboring molecule, that molecule is now short an electron, so it joins in the mischief to replace its electron, creating further damage. As you can imagine, the damage to cells over time can significantly accelerate the aging process. There is a solution, however: antioxidants. Antioxidants contain extra electrons that they can donate to free radicals to make them stable. Thus the solution for decreasing free radical damage and slowing the aging process could be to increase

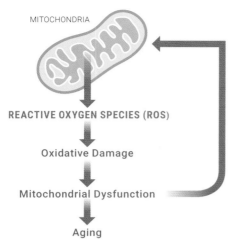

MITOCHONDRIA

REACTIVE OXYGEN SPECIES (ROS)

Oxidative Damage

Mitochondrial Dysfunction

Aging

Figure 5.6.12. Feedback loop between reactive oxygen species (ROS) and mitochondrial dysfunction and their overall effect on aging.

Source: http://sphweb.bumc.bu.edu/otlt/mph-modules/ph/aging/aging3.html.

the body's production of antioxidants—and give the jewelry stores back their merchandise and money.

There are three main areas in which the ketogenic diet may offer an antioxidant benefit:

1. Ketone body breakdown has been shown to improve the amount of coenzyme Q potential, which is an antioxidant, thereby decreasing free radical production (Veech et al., 2004).

2. Certain enzymes that prevent free radicals from forming have been shown to quadruple on a ketogenic diet (Ziegler et al., 2003).

3. Mitochondrial uncoupling proteins (UCPs) are proteins that embed themselves in the mitochondria and help release energy in the form of heat. These proteins, which can help protect against formation of ROS, have been shown to increase on a ketogenic diet (Sullivan et al., 2004).

In addition, in high school athletes, lower oxidative stress has been seen after just three weeks on the ketogenic diet (Rhyu et al., 2014).

Apoptosis is the process by which old or damaged cells self-destruct (i.e., programmed cell death) in order to maintain balance and prevent unhealthy cells from accumulating. However, in disorders such as epilepsy, apoptosis of neurons occurs in response to brain damage. Several studies have shown that a ketogenic diet may have a neuroprotective effect by reducing markers of apoptosis in parts of the brain (Noh et al., 2003), which may reduce cell death directly (Noh et al., 2005).

In addition, inflammation may play a large role in neurodegeneration and impaired cognitive functioning, as is seen in neurodegenerative diseases like Alzheimer's. Ketogenic diets, when properly formulated and implemented, have been shown to be anti-inflammatory (Ruskin et al., 2009).

Finally, ketogenic diets stabilize a substance known as HIF1 alpha, which has been shown to prevent tissue damage in the brain, improve blood flow to the brain, and activate certain growth factors to improve brain metabolism under conditions like aging where those factors may be lacking (Bergeron et al., 2000).

Improving Longevity

Our bodies are extremely complex machines with a host of signals and processes going on all the time. We'd like to share with you some key considerations for why the ketogenic diet may be beneficial for long-term health:

1. Ketogenic diets have been shown to enhance immunity (Woolf et al., 2015; Wright and Simone, 2016). This is helpful for aging because the immune system gradually deteriorates with age, which reduces the capacity to fight infection.

2. One of the most well-researched areas for aging is caloric restriction and fasting, and these have been shown to increase longevity. Ketogenic diets often involve some type of innate caloric restriction compared to traditional diets due to a reduced appetite from more stable blood sugar levels. A diet low in carbohydrates mimics the physiological alterations seen with fasting (Klement, 2014).

3. Some scientists theorize that a substance known as AMPK, which maintains our cells' energy at optimal levels, controls the aging process by regulating stress resistance, the recycling of cell parts, and energy metabolism (Salminen and Kaarniranta, 2012). Ketogenic diets have been shown to increase AMPK in mice (Kennedy et al., 2007). AMPK activity declines with age, hence a diet that can increase this activity should slow cell aging.

4. Glycation is the process by which sugar molecules bond to proteins and fats, and it results in the formation of particles called advanced glycation end products (AGEs), which disrupt the proper functioning of cells. AGEs accumulate in tissues in age-related chronic diseases. Fructose has been shown to accelerate glycation in the body ten times faster than even traditional glucose (McPherson et al., 1988); even after just one meal, having higher blood glucose has been shown to accelerate the formation of AGE precursors (Beisswenger et al., 2001). By reducing the consumption of carbohydrates, which are broken down into sugar, the ketogenic diet also reduces the production of AGEs.

5. In 1953, Denham Harman, an accomplished chemist, proposed a new theory called the "free radical theory of aging," which declared that aging is caused by reactive oxygen species (ROS) accumulating within cells (Harman, 1955). As we've discussed, mitochondria are the energy factories within our cells. Like brain cells, body tissues are exposed to free radicals, and the damage they cause accumulates over time. Antioxidants can help protect against free radicals—and, as discussed above, the ketogenic diet offers several antioxidant effects, from reducing coenzyme Q to increasing the activity of an enzyme that prevents free radicals from forming (Sullivan, 2004).

6. Ketogenic diets have been shown to significantly extend life in rats with cancer (Poff et al., 2013) and epilepsy (Simeone et al., 2016), as well as other diseases.

7. Mice fed a ketogenic diet their entire lives had less body fat, higher energy levels, and higher expression of things like FGF21, which is very important for fat oxidation and has been shown to extend lifespan in mice. In addition, a ketogenic diet prevents amino acids from being broken down, which can be important for body composition and preventing age-related muscle loss (Douris et al., 2015).

Ketones and Longevity

By now, we hope it is clear that ketones themselves should be looked at as far more than a simple alternative fuel source. In fact, ketones have numerous other properties, including acting as signaling molecules. When it comes to longevity, one of BHB's properties is particularly relevant: it acts as an inhibitor of histone deacetylases (HDACs).

Histones are proteins that play a role in how DNA is copied and its instructions are carried out. DNA is wrapped around histones, and any modifications in the histones can control the expression of DNA. HDAC interacts with the surface of the histone, and high levels of HDAC (like we see in cancer cells) can suppress gene expression. The DNA becomes so tightly wrapped around the histone (similar to a boa constrictor wrapping itself around something and squeezing) that it is no longer readable. In the human body, this may affect a variety of signaling pathways, mitochondrial function, and various markers that are important for health and longevity.

BHB, even in moderate amounts of 1.0 to 2.0 mmol, inhibits HDACs from doing what they do and preserves the expression of DNA. Ketones act as a releaser by not allowing the boa constrictor (HDAC) to wrap around the DNA and suppress its activity. Thus ketone bodies may regulate cellular physiology and ultimately alter gene expression (Xie et al., 2016).

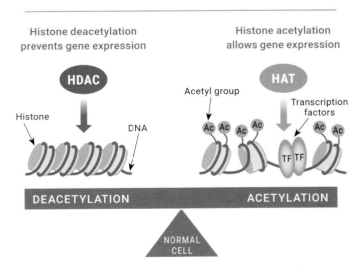

Figure 5.6.13. *Over time, as people age, high amounts of HDACs cause a silencing of genes. However, ketones act as HDAC inhibitors and prevent that silencing from occurring.*

Source: https://biology441.wordpress.com/2015/09/07/histone-deacetylase-and-cancer-cancers-best-friend-is-your-worst-enemy-by-bradley-lasseigne/.

HDAC inhibition by BHB may be what's behind many of the positive effects of a ketogenic diet. For instance, HDAC inhibition has been shown to improve metabolic disease, lower fasting glucose and insulin levels, prevent weight gain, increase the number of new mitochondria, and increase metabolic rate—the rate at which the body burns fuel when at rest (Newman and Verdin, 2014). Clearly, the ability to prevent HDACs from overexpressing themselves and acting like boa constrictors should offer metabolic benefits for individuals dealing with various disease states and even aging.

Another important aspect of BHB's unique functioning lies in cellular NAD balance. (NAD, or nicotinamide adenine dinucleotide, is a coenzyme found in all living cells involved in metabolism; oxidized and reduced forms are abbreviated as NAD+ and NADH, respectively.) The NAD/NADH ratio is a measurement that reflects both the metabolic activities and the health of cells (when NAD is higher than NADH, cells are healthier), and it is rapidly becoming one of the most researched aspects of aging and disease. NAD plays a key role in energy metabolism, and as we age, NAD levels significantly decrease (Chini et al., 2016). This leads to a decrease in the activity of SIRT, an important protein signaler associated with metabolic health, as well as a decrease in mitochondrial and metabolic function. SIRT is one of the targets of resveratrol (found in wine) and is behind the notion that drinking wine improves longevity. You can see why scientists are interested in this pathway for aging and disease. Low-carb wine for the win! Compared to glucose, BHB metabolism uses less NAD to produce energy, therefore potentially increasing the NAD pool inside the body—if you are using/burning less, you have more hanging around. The more NAD there is in cells, the more SIRT is activated, leading to the formation of new mitochondria as well as the cleaning and maintenance of current mitochondria, which helps them run smoothly. Thus, sparing this breakdown of NAD could have important implications in aging by improving energy metabolism.

Now it's time to put all these theories to the test. A recent study found that supplementing with D-BHB increased the average lifespan of worms by 26 percent (Edwards et al., 2014). In addition, these researchers found that BHB supplementation delayed amyloid plaques from degenerating neurons

in Alzheimer's and decreased certain proteins associated with Parkinson's.

Lastly, one key component of cognitive function as we age is brain-derived neurotrophic factor (BDNF). BDNF helps to protect neurons from damage caused by infection or injury. As we age, BDNF levels start to decline, and this has been shown to negatively affect not only the size of the hippocampus in the brain but also memory (Erickson et al., 2010). A recent study found that BHB itself may actually increase BDNF gene expression (Marosi et al., 2016). Since BDNF plays an important role in synaptic plasticity and neuronal stress resistance, ketones may positively impact this cognitive aspect of aging.

It is important to remember that this was done in a specific sample, and the practical applications for humans are still to be determined. That said, we were particularly interested in this area of research, so we personally funded a study looking at ketone supplementation (D-BHB) and its effects on a multitude of health markers and longevity over the course of an animal's life. Though the study is still ongoing, we are comparing three different conditions: a ketogenic diet versus a low-fat diet versus a low-fat diet with exogenous ketone supplementation. To date, 30 percent more of the ketone supplementation group is still alive than the low-fat diet group. Granted, these are just initial results, but it is interesting that this study is confirming the findings regarding ketone supplementation and lifespan. One thing that is evident from all this research is that HDAC inhibition and the ability to regulate mitochondrial function are at the core of health and human lifespan.

The Latest Research on the Ketogenic Diet and Longevity

The effects of the ketogenic diet on aging and longevity have sparked our interest over the last several years for many reasons. For one, we want our families and friends (including you reading this book!) to be able to live longer. Second, the mere fact that a diet or a unique metabolic state may actually help someone live longer blows our minds, especially in light of the fact that this diet is contrary to what most nutritionists and guidelines recommend. Thus, in an attempt to learn more, we have teamed up with some of the most brilliant scientists in the world to search for answers and key insights into what is really going on with the ketogenic diet and how can it affect long-term outcomes.

One of our first studies looked at the effects of a ketogenic diet on adipose (fat) tissue as well as several other markers of health in non-exercising and exercising animals (Holland et al., 2016). All animals ate the same number of calories; the only difference in their diets was the percentage of fat and carbohydrates. We divided the animals into three groups: The Western diet group ate a diet high in carbohydrates (43 percent) and fat (42 percent) and relatively low in protein (15 percent). The standard diet group ate a diet higher in protein (24 percent) and carbohydrates (58 percent) and lower in fat (18 percent). The ketogenic diet group ate 70 percent fat, 20 percent protein, and 10 percent carbohydrates. After just six weeks, body mass, body fat, liver triglycerides, insulin, glucose, and total cholesterol were lowest in the ketogenic diet group. This was one of the first studies that actually matched protein levels and calories. In fact, the ketogenic diet group had slightly less protein than the standard diet group yet saw greater benefits, leading to a possible unique, healthful metabolic state induced by ketosis in which liver, adipose tissue, and blood parameters all benefited.

CHAPTER SUMMARY

In this chapter, we touched on a variety of emerging areas, from autoimmune diseases to brain disorders to aging and longevity. A common theme throughout is impaired mitochondrial function combined with impaired glucose metabolism. You've learned that ketones themselves are far more than just a fuel source; they're signaling metabolites that can have a host of other functions as well. Keep in mind that these are all emerging areas in which new research is coming out every day. For all the conditions mentioned, the ketogenic diet, ketone supplementation, or a combination at least holds some promise for future research and investigations.

Next, we set out to discover what effect a ketogenic diet may have on mitochondria compared to a Western diet. Two groups of mice were fed the same number of calories, but one group was fed a ketogenic diet and the other was fed a Western diet. The macronutrients for each diet were the same as described above. After six weeks, we looked at mitochondria in the mice's skeletal muscle. Our results showed that mice fed a ketogenic diet saw improved mitochondrial function and respiration compared to their Western diet counterparts (Hyatt et al., 2016).

With those two experiments completed, we knew that a ketogenic diet resulted in significant improvements in several biomarkers and enhanced mitochondrial adaptations. However, the ultimate question we want to answer is, what is the effect of a ketogenic diet on longevity? Knowing that this project would take years to design and complete, we set out with our great friends and collaborators at Auburn University to investigate. As of this writing, this research project is still ongoing, but the preliminary findings are nothing short of promising. Currently, twice as many animals being fed a ketogenic diet are alive than those being fed a Western diet. These results are the first to track animals fed a consistent diet over a large majority of their lives. The data gathered throughout this project will be nothing short of groundbreaking.

One last thing we would like to point out is that incredible advancements are being made in this area. Companies like Human Longevity Inc. and Epigenix are making exponential strides every day using the latest scientific technology to help lengthen lifespan while improving quality of life. Whether through a ketogenic diet, supplemental ketones, stem cell therapy, genetic recoding, or some combination thereof, we will soon be able to live longer, healthier, and more fulfilling lives, and we believe nutrition and exercise will be at the core of these solutions.

"Bad men live that they may eat and drink, whereas good men eat and drink that they may live."
—Socrates

References

Ari, C., A. M. Poff, H. E. Held, C. S. Landon, C. R. Goldhagen, N. Mavromates, and D. P. D'Agostino. "Metabolic therapy with Deanna protocol supplementation delays disease progression and extends survival in amyotrophic lateral sclerosis (ALS) mouse model." *PLOS ONE* 9, no. 7 (2014): e103526. doi: 10.1371/journal.pone.0103526.

Arnold, L. E., E. Hurt, and N. Lofthouse. "Attention-deficit/hyperactivity disorder: dietary and nutritional treatments." *Child and Adolescent Psychiatric Clinics of North America* 22, no. 3 (2013): 381–402.

Ballenger, J. C., and R. M. Post. "Carbamazepine in manic-depressive illness: a new treatment." *American Journal of Psychiatry* 137, no. 7 (1980): 782–90. doi: 10.1176/ajp.137.7.782.

Baxter, L. R., J. M. Schwartz, M. E. Phelps, J. C. Mazziotta, B. H. Guze, C. E. Selin, ... and R. M. Sumida. "Reduction of prefrontal cortex glucose metabolism common to three types of depression." *Archives of General Psychiatry* 46, no. 3 (1989): 243–50.

Beisswenger, P. J., S. K. Howell, R. M. O'Dell, M. E. Wood, A. D. Touchette, and B. S. Szwergold. "α-Dicarbonyls increase in the postprandial period and reflect the degree of hyperglycemia." *Diabetes Care* 24, no. 4 (2001): 726–32.

Bergeron, M., J. M. Gidday, A. Y. Yu, G. L. Semenza, D. M. Ferriero, and F. R. Sharp. "Role of hypoxia-inducible factor-1 in hypoxia-induced ischemic tolerance in neonatal rat brain." *Annals of Neurology* 48, no. 3 (2000): 285–96.

Boden, G., K. Sargrad, C. Homko, M. Mozzoli, and T. P. Stein. "Effect of a low-carbohydrate diet on appetite, blood glucose levels, and insulin resistance in obese patients with type 2 diabetes." *Annals of Internal Medicine* 142, no. 6 (2005): 403–11.

Bottini, N., D. De Luca, P. Saccucci, A. Fiumara, M. Elia, M. C. Porfirio, ... and P. Curatolo. "Autism: evidence of association with adenosine deaminase genetic polymorphism." *Neurogenetics* 3, no. 2 (2001): 111–3.

Bough, K. J., J. Wetherington, B. Hassel, J. F. Pare, J. W. Gawryluk, J. G. Greene, ... and R. J. Dingledine. "Mitochondrial biogenesis in the anticonvulsant mechanism of the ketogenic diet." *Annals of Neurology* 60, no. 2 (2006): 223–35. doi: 10.1002/ana.20899.

Brambilla, A., S. Mannarino, R. Pretese, S. Gasperini, C. Galimberti, and R. Parini. "Improvement of cardiomyopathy after high-fat diet in two siblings with glycogen storage disease type III." *JIMD Reports* 17 (2014): 91–95. doi: 10.1007/8904_2014_343.

Brown, A. J. "Low-carb diets, fasting and euphoria: Is there a link between ketosis and γhydroxybutyrate (GHB)?" *Medical Hypotheses* 68, no. 2 (2007): 268–71.

Buchsbaum, M. S., T. Someya, J. C. Wu, C. Y. Tang, and W. E. Bunney. "Neuroimaging bipolar illness with positron emission tomography and magnetic resonance imaging." *Psychiatric Annals* 27, no. 7 (1997): 489–95. doi: 10.3928/0048-5713-19970701-10.

Busch, V., K. Gempel, A. Hack, K. Müller, M. Vorgerd, H. Lochmüller, and F. A. Baumeister. "Treatment of glycogenosis type V with ketogenic diet." *Annals of Neurology* 58, no. 2 (2005): 341. doi: 10.1002/ana.20565.

Calkin, C. V., M. Ruzickova, R. Uher, T. Hajek, C. M. Slaney, J. S. Garnham, ... and M. Alda. "Insulin resistance and outcome in bipolar disorder." *British Journal of Psychiatry* 206, no. 1 (2015): 52–57. doi: 10.1192/bjp.bp.114.152850.

Castellano, C. A., J. P. Baillargeon, S. Nugent, S. Tremblay, M. Fortier, H. Imbeault, ... and S. C. Cunnane. "Regional brain glucose hypometabolism in young women with polycystic ovary syndrome: possible link to mild insulin resistance." *PLOS ONE* 10, no. 12 (2015): e0144116. doi: 10.137/journal.pone.0144116.

Chini, C. C., M. G. Tarragó, and E. N. Chini. "NAD and the aging process: role in life, death and everything in between." *Molecular and Cellular Endocrinology* (2016; epub ahead of print). doi: 10.1016/j.mce.2016.11.003.

Choi, I. Y., L. Piccio, P. Childress, B. Bollman, A. Ghosh, S. Brandhorst, ... and M. Wei. "Diet mimicking fasting promotes regeneration and reduces autoimmunity and multiple sclerosis symptoms." *Cell Reports* 15, no. 10 (2016): 2136–46. doi: 10.1016/j.celrep.2016.05.009.

Clark-Taylor, T., and B. E. Clark-Taylor. "Is autism a disorder of fatty acid metabolism? Possible dysfunction of mitochondrial β-oxidation by long chain acyl-CoA dehydrogenase." *Medical Hypotheses* 62, no. 6 (2004): 970–5. doi: 10.1016/j.mehy.2004.01.011.

Coppola, G., A. Verrotti, E. Ammendola, F. F. Operto, R. della Corte, G. Signoriello, and A. Pascotto. "Ketogenic diet for the treatment of catastrophic epileptic encephalopathies in childhood." *European Journal of Paediatric Neurology* 14, no. 3 (2010): 229–34. doi: 10.1016/j.ejpn.2009.06.006.

de Graaf, R., R. C. Kessler, J. Fayyad, M. ten Have, J. Alonso, M. Angermeyer, ... and J. M. Haro. "The prevalence and effects of adult attention-deficit/hyperactivity disorder (ADHD) on the performance of workers: results from the WHO World Mental Health Survey Initiative." *Occupational and Environmental Medicine* 65, no. 12 (2008): 835–42. doi: 10.1136/oem.2007.038448.

Deutsch, S. I., M. R. Urbano, S. A. Neumann, J. A. Burket, and E. Katz. "Cholinergic abnormalities in autism: is there a rationale for selective nicotinic agonist interventions?" *Clinical Neuropharmacology* 33, no. 3 (2010): 114–20. doi: 10.1097/WNF.0b013e3181d6f7ad.

Di Lorenzo, C., G. Coppola, G. Sirianni, G. Di Lorenzo, M. Bracaglia, D. Di Lenola, ... and F. Pierelli. "Migraine improvement during short lasting ketogenesis: a proof-of-concept study." *European Journal of Neurology* 22, no. 1 (2015): 170–7. doi: 10.1111/ene.12550.

Di Lorenzo, C., A. Currà, G. Sirianni, G. Coppola, M. Bracaglia, A. Cardillo, ... and F. Pierelli. "Diet transiently improves migraine in two twin sisters: possible role of ketogenesis?" *Functional Neurology* 28, no. 4 (2013): 305–8.

Douris, N., T. Melman, J. M. Pecherer, P. Pissios, J. S. Flier, L. C. Cantley, ... and E. Maratos-Flier. "Adaptive changes in amino acid metabolism permit normal longevity in mice consuming a low-carbohydrate ketogenic diet." *Biochimica et Biophysica Acta (BBA)-Molecular Basis of Disease* 1852, no. 10 Pt A (2015): 2056–65. doi: 10.1016/j.bbadis.2015.07.009.

Duncan, S. H., A. Belenguer, G. Holtrop, A. M. Johnstone, H. J. Flint, and G. E. Lobley. "Reduced dietary intake of carbohydrates by obese subjects results in decreased concentrations of butyrate and butyrate-producing bacteria in feces." *Applied and Environmental Microbiology* 73, no. 4 (2007): 1073–8. doi: 10.1128/AEM.02340-06.

Edwards, C., J. Canfield, N. Copes, M. Rehan, D. Lipps, and P. C. Bradshaw. "D-beta-hydroxybutyrate extends lifespan in C. elegans." *Aging* (Albany, NY) 6, no. 8 (2014): 621–44.

El-Gharbawy, A. H., A. Boney, S. P. Young, and P. S. Kishnani. "Follow-up of a child with pyruvate dehydrogenase deficiency on a less restrictive ketogenic diet." *Molecular Genetics and Metabolism* 102, no. 2 (2011): 214–5. doi: 10.1016/j.ymgme.2010.11.001.

El-Mallakh, R. S., and M. E. Paskitti. "The ketogenic diet may have mood-stabilizing properties." *Medical Hypotheses* 57, no. 6 (2001): 724–6. doi: 10.1054/mehy.2001.1446.

Elmslie, J. L., J. I. Mann, J. T. Silverstone, and S. E. Romans. "Determinants of overweight and obesity in patients with bipolar disorder." *Journal of Clinical Psychiatry* 62, no. 6 (2001): 486–91.

Elsabbagh, M., G. Divan, Y. J. Koh, Y. S. Kim, S. Kauchali, C. Marcín, ... and M. T. Yasamy. "Global prevalence of autism and other pervasive developmental disorders." *Autism Research* 5, no. 3 (2012): 160–79. doi: 10.1002/aur.239.

Erickson, K. I., R. S. Prakash, M. W. Voss, L. Chaddock, S. Heo, M. McLaren, ... and E. McAuley. "Brain-derived neurotrophic factor is associated with age-related decline in hippocampal volume." *Journal of Neuroscience* 30, no. 15 (2010): 5368–75.

Evangeliou, A., I. Vlachonikolis, H. Mihailidou, M. Spilioti, A. Skarpalezou, N. Makaronas, ... and S. Sbyrakis. "Application of a ketogenic diet in children with autistic behavior: pilot study." *Journal of Child Neurology* 18, no. 2 (2003): 113–8. doi: 10.1177/08830738030180020501.

Falk, R. E., S. D. Cederbaum, J. P. Blass, G. E. Gibson, R. P. Kark, and R. E. Carrel. "Ketonic diet in the management of pyruvate dehydrogenase deficiency." *Pediatrics* 58, no. 5 (1976): 713–21.

Fontán-Lozano, Á., G. López-Lluch, J. M. Delgado-García, P. Navas, and Á. M. Carrión. "Molecular bases of caloric restriction regulation of neuronal synaptic plasticity." *Molecular Neurobiology* 38, no. 2 (2008): 167–77.

Frye, R. E. "Metabolic and mitochondrial disorders associated with epilepsy in children with autism spectrum disorder." *Epilepsy & Behavior* 47 (2015): 147–157. doi: 10.1016/j.yebeh.2014.08.134.

Giulivi, C., Y. F. Zhang, A. Omanska-Klusek, C. Ross-Inta, S. Wong, I. Hertz-Picciotto, ... and I. N. Pessah. "Mitochondrial Dysfunction in Autism." *JAMA: The Journal of the American Medical Association* 304, no. 21 (2010): 2389–96. doi: 10.1001/jama.2010.1706.

Greco, T., T. C. Glenn, D. A. Hovda, and M. L. Prins. "Ketogenic diet decreases oxidative stress and improves mitochondrial respiratory complex activity." *Journal of Cerebral Blood Flow & Metabolism* 36, no. 9 (2016): 1603–13. doi: 10.1177/0271678X15610584.

Haas, R. H., M. A. Rice, D. A. Trauner, T. A. Merritt, J. M. Opitz, and J. F. Reynolds. "Therapeutic effects of a ketogenic diet in Rett syndrome." *American Journal of Medical Genetics* 25, suppl 1 (1986): 225–46.

Hanauer, S. B., and W. Sandborn. "Management of Crohn's disease in adults." *American Journal of Gastroenterology* 96, no. 3 (2001): 635–43. doi: 10.1111/j.1572-0241.2001.3671_c.x.

Harman, D. "Aging: a theory based on free radical and radiation chemistry." *Journal of Gerontology* 11, no. 3 (1956): 298–300.

Harris, L. W., P. C. Guest, M. T. Wayland, Y. Umrania, D. Krishnamurthy, H. Rahmoune, and S. Bahn. "Schizophrenia: metabolic aspects of aetiology, diagnosis and future treatment strategies." *Psychoneuroendocrinology* 38, no. 6 (2013): 752–66. doi: 10.1016/j.psyneuen.2012.09.009.

Herbert, M. R., and J. A. Buckley. "Autism and dietary therapy: case report and review of the literature." *Journal of Child Neurology* 28, no. 8 (2013): 975–82. doi: 10.1177/0883073813488668.

Hoge, C. W., D. McGurk, J. L. Thomas, A. L. Cox, C. C. Engel, and C. A. Castro. "Mild traumatic brain injury in US soldiers returning from Iraq." *New England Journal of Medicine* 358, no. 5 (2008): 453–63. doi: 10.1056/NEJMoa072972.

Holland, A. M., W. C. Kephart, P. W. Mumford, C. B. Mobley, R. P. Lowery, J. J. Shake, ... and M. D. Roberts. "Effects of a ketogenic diet on adipose tissue, liver and serum biomarkers in sedentary rats and rats that exercised via resisted voluntary wheel running." *American Journal of Physiology: Regulatory, Integrative and Comparative Physiology* 311, no. 2 (2016): R337–51. doi: 10.1152/ajpregu.00156.2016.

Hyatt, H. W., W. C. Kephart, A. M. Holland, P. Mumford, C. B. Mobley, R. P. Lowery, ... and A. N. Kavazis. "A ketogenic diet in rodents elicits improved mitochondrial adaptations in response to resistance exercise training compared to an isocaloric Western diet." *Frontiers in Physiology* 7 (2016): 533. doi: 10.3389/fphys.2016.00533.

Ito, S., H. Oguni, Y. Ito, K. Ishigaki, J. Ohinata, and M. Osawa. "Modified Atkins diet therapy for a case with glucose transporter type 1 deficiency syndrome." *Brain and Development* 30, no. 3 (2008): 226–8.

Jedele, K. B. "The overlapping spectrum of Rett and Angelman syndromes: A clinical review." *Seminars in Pediatric Neurology* 14, no. 3 (2007): 108–17. doi: 10.1016/j.spen.2007.07.002.

Jurecka, A., M. Zikanova, E. Jurkiewicz, and A. Tylki-Szymańska. "Attenuated adenylosuccinate lyase deficiency: a report of one case and a review of the literature." *Neuropediatrics* 45, no. 01 (2014): 50–55. doi: 10.1055/s-0033-1337335.

Kang, H. C., Y. M. Lee, H. D. Kim, J. S. Lee, and A. Slama. "Safe and effective use of the ketogenic diet in children with epilepsy and mitochondrial respiratory chain complex defects." *Epilepsia* 48, no. 1 (2007): 82–88. doi: 10.1111/j.1528-1167.2006.00906.x.

Karlović, D., D. Buljan, M. Martinac, and D. Marčinko. "Serum lipid concentrations in Croatian veterans with post-traumatic stress disorder, post-traumatic stress disorder comorbid with major depressive disorder, or major depressive disorder." *Journal of Korean Medical Science* 19, no. 3 (2004): 431–6. doi: 10.3346/jkms.2004.19.3.431.

Kennedy, A. R., P. Pissios, H. Otu, R. Roberson, B. Xue, K. Asakura, N. Furukawa, ... and E. Maratos-Flier. "A high-fat, ketogenic diet induces a unique metabolic state in mice." *American Journal of Physiology Endocrinology and Metabolism* 292, no. 6 (2007): E1724–39. doi: 10.1152/ajpendo.00717.2006.

Kessler, S. K., P. R. Gallagher, R. A. Shellhaas, R. R. Clancy, and A. C. Bergqvist. "Early EEG improvement after ketogenic diet initiation." *Epilepsy Research* 94, nos. 1–2 (2011): 94–101. doi: 10.1016/j.eplepsyres.2011.01.012.

Kharrazian, D. "Traumatic brain injury and the effect on the brain-gut axis." *Alternative Therapies in Health Medicine* 21, suppl 3 (2015): 28–32.

Kim, D. Y., J. Hao, R. Liu, G. Turner, F. D. Shi, and J. M. Rho. "Inflammation-mediated memory dysfunction and effects of a ketogenic diet in a murine model of multiple sclerosis." *PLoS One* 7, no. 5 (2012): e35476. doi: 10.1371/journal.pone.0035476.

Kindred, J. H., J. J. Tuulari, M. Bucci, K. K. Kalliokoski, and T. Rudroff. "Walking speed and brain glucose uptake are uncoupled in patients with multiple sclerosis." *Frontiers in Human Neuroscience* 9 (2015): 84. doi: 10.3389/fnhum.2015.00084.

Klement, R. J. "Mimicking caloric restriction: what about macronutrient manipulation? A response to Meynet and Ricci." *Trends in Molecular Medicine* 20, no. 9 (2014): 471–2. doi: 10.1016/j.molmed.2014.07.001.

Klepper, J. "Glucose transporter deficiency syndrome (GLUT1 DS) and the ketogenic diet." *Epilepsia* 49, suppl 8 (2008): 46–49. doi: 10.1111/j.1528-1167.2008.01833.x.

Klepper, J., H. Scheffer, B. Leiendecker, E. Gertsen, S. Binder, M. Leferink, ... and M. A. Willemsen. "Seizure control and acceptance of the ketogenic diet in GLUT1 deficiency syndrome: a 2-to 5-year follow-up of 15 children enrolled prospectively." *Neuropediatrics* 36, no. 05 (2005): 302–8. doi: 10.1055/s-2005-872843.

Koroshetz, W. J., B. G. Jenkins, B. R. Rosen, and M. F. Beal. "Energy metabolism defects in Huntington's disease and effects of coenzyme Q10." *Annals of Neurology* 41, no. 2 (1997): 160–165. doi: 10.1002/ana.410410206.

Kossoff, E. H., J. Huffman, Z. Turner, and J. Gladstein. "Use of the modified Atkins diet for adolescents with chronic daily headache." *Cephalalgia* 30, no. 8 (2010): 1014–6. doi: 10.1111/j.1468-2982.2009.02016.x.

Kraft, B. D., and E. C. Westman. "Schizophrenia, gluten, and low-carbohydrate, ketogenic diets: a case report and review of the literature." *Nutrition & Metabolism* 6 (2009): 10. doi: 10.1186/1743-7075-6-10.

Leclercq, S., P. Forsythe, and J. Bienenstock. "Posttraumatic stress disorder: does the gut microbiome hold the key?" *Canadian Journal of Psychiatry* 61, no. 4 (2016): 204. doi: 10.1177/0706743716635535.

Lee, H. H., and Y. J. Hur. "Glucose transport 1 deficiency presenting as infantile spasms with a mutation identified in exon 9 of SLC2A1." *Korean Journal of Pediatrics* 59, suppl 1 (2016): S29–31. doi: 10.3345/kjp.2016.59.11.S29.

Liebhaber, G. M., E. Riemann, and F. A. M. Baumeister. "Ketogenic diet in Rett syndrome." *Journal of Child Neurology* 18, no. 1 (2003): 74–75. doi: 10.1177/08830738030180011001.

Liepa, G. U., A. Sengupta, and D. Karsies. "Polycystic ovary syndrome (PCOS) and other androgen excess–related conditions: can changes in dietary intake make a difference?" *Nutrition in Clinical Practice* 23, no. 1 (2008): 63–71.

Lopresti, A. L., and F. N. Jacka. "Diet and bipolar disorder: a review of its relationship and potential therapeutic mechanisms of action." *Journal of Alternative and Complementary Medicine* 21, no. 12 (2015): 733–9. doi: 10.1089/acm.2015.0125.

Ma, T. C., J. L. Buescher, B. Oatis, J. A. Funk, A. J. Nash, R. L. Carrier, and K. R. Hoyt. "Metformin therapy in a transgenic mouse model of Huntington's disease." *Neuroscience Letters* 411, no. 2 (2007): 98–103. doi: 10.1016/j.neulet.2006.10.039.

Maalouf, M., P. G. Sullivan, L. Davis, D. Y. Kim, and J. M. Rho. "Ketones inhibit mitochondrial production of reactive oxygen species production following glutamate excitotoxicity by increasing NADH oxidation." *Neuroscience* 145, no. 1 (2007): 256–64. doi: 10.1016/j.neuroscience.2006.11.065.

Maggioni, F., M. Margoni, and G. Zanchin. "Ketogenic diet in migraine treatment: a brief but ancient history." *Cephalalgia* 31, no. 10 (2011): 1150–1. doi: 10.1177/0333102411412089.

Marazziti, D., S. Baroni, M. Picchetti, P. Landi, S. Silvestri, E. Vatteroni, and M. Catena Dell'Osso. "Psychiatric disorders and mitochondrial dysfunctions." *European Review for Medical and Pharmacological Sciences* 16, no. 2 (2012): 270–5.

Marosi, K., S. W. Kim, K. Moehl, M. Scheibye-Knudsen, A. Cheng, R. Cutler, ... and M. P. Mattson. "3-hydroxybutyrate regulates energy metabolism and induces BDNF expression in cerebral cortical neurons." *Journal of Neurochemistry* 139, no. 5 (2016): 769–81.

Masino, S. A., M. Kawamura Jr., C. A. Wasser, L. T. Pomeroy, and D. N. Ruskin. "Adenosine, ketogenic diet and epilepsy: the emerging therapeutic relationship between metabolism and brain activity." *Current Neuropharmacology* 7, no. 3 (2009): 257–68.

Mavropoulos, J. C., W. S. Yancy, J. Hepburn, and E. C. Westman. "The effects of a low-carbohydrate, ketogenic diet on the polycystic ovary syndrome: a pilot study." *Nutrition & Metabolism* 2 (2005): 35.

Mayorandan, S., U. Meyer, H. Hartmann, and A. M. Das. "Glycogen storage disease type III: modified Atkins diet improves myopathy." *Orphanet Journal of Rare Diseases* 9 (2014): 196. doi: 10.1186/s13023-014-0196-3.

McPherson, J. D., B. H. Shilton, and D. J. Walton. "Role of fructose in glycation and cross-linking of proteins." *Biochemistry* 27, no. 6 (1988): 1901–7. doi: 10.1021/bi00406a016.

Millichap, J. G.,and M. M. Yee. "The diet factor in attention-deficit/hyperactivity disorder." *Pediatrics* 129, no. 2 (2012): 330–7.

Millichap, J. J., C. V. Stack, and J. G. Millichap. "Frequency of epileptiform discharges in the sleep-deprived electroencephalogram in children evaluated for attention-deficit disorders." *Journal of Child Neurology* 26, no. 1 (2010): 6–11. doi: 10.1177/0883073810371228.

Moreno, C. L., and C. V. Mobbs. "Epigenetic mechanisms underlying lifespan and age-related effects of dietary restriction and the ketogenic diet." *Molecular and Cellular Endocrinology* (2016). doi: 10.1016/j.mce.2016.11.013.

Murphy, P., S. Likhodii, K. Nylen, and W. M. Burnham. "The antidepressant properties of the ketogenic diet." *Biological Psychiatry* 56, no. 12 (2004): 981–3. doi: 10.1016/j.biopsych.2004.09.019.

Murphy, P., and W. M. Burnham. "The ketogenic diet causes a reversible decrease in activity level in Long–Evans rats." *Experimental Neurology* 201, no. 1 (2006): 84–89. doi: 10.1016/j.expneurol.2006.03.024.

Mychasiuk, R.,and J. M. Rho. "Genetic modifications associated with ketogenic diet treatment in the BTBRT+ Tf/J mouse model of autism spectrum disorder." *Autism Research* 10, no. 3 (2016): 456–71.

Napoli, E., N. Dueñas, and C. Giulivi. "Potential therapeutic use of the ketogenic diet in autism spectrum disorders." *Frontiers in Pediatrics* 2 (2014): 69.

Newell, C., M. R. Bomhof, R. A. Reimer, D. S. Hittel, J. M. Rho, and J. Shearer. "Ketogenic diet modifies the gut microbiota in a murine model of autism spectrum disorder." *Molecular Autism* 7 (2016): 37.

Newman, J. C., and E. Verdin. "Ketone bodies as signaling metabolites." *Trends in Endocrinology and Metabolism* 25, no. 1 (2014): 42–52.

Nijland, P. G., I. Michailidou, M. E. Witte, M. R. Mizee, S. Pol, A. Reijerkerk, ... and J. van Horssen. "Cellular distribution of glucose and monocarboxylate transporters in human brain white matter and multiple sclerosis lesions." *Glia* 62, no. 7 (2014): 1125–41. doi: 10.1002/glia.22667.

Noh, H. S., S. S. Kang, D. W. Kim, Y. H. Kim, C. H. Park, J. Y. Han, ... and W. S. Choi. "Ketogenic diet increases calbindin-D28k in the hippocampi of male ICR mice with kainic acid seizures." *Epilepsy Research* 65, no. 3 (2005): 153–9.

Noh, H. S., Y. S. Kim, H. P. Lee, K. M. Chung, D. W. Kim, S. S. Kang, ... and W. S. Choi. "The protective effect of a ketogenic diet on kainic acid-induced hippocampal cell death in the male ICR mice." *Epilepsy Research* 53, nos. 1–2 (2003): 119–28.

Norman, S. B., A. J. Means-Christensen, M. G. Craske, C. D. Sherbourne, P. P. Roy-Byrne,and M. B. Stein. "Associations between psychological trauma and physical illness in primary care." *Journal of Traumatic Stress* 19, no. 4 (2006): 461–70. doi: 10.1002/jts.20129.

Pacheco, A., W. S. Easterling,and M. W. Pryer. "A pilot study of the ketogenic diet in schizophrenia." *American Journal of Psychiatry* 121, no. 11 (1965): 1110–1. doi: 10.1176/ajp.121.11.1110.

Pascual, J. M., P. Liu, D. Mao, D. I. Kelly, A. Hernandez, M. Sheng, ... and J. Y. Park. "Triheptanoin for glucose transporter type i deficiency (g1d): modulation of human ictogenesis, cerebral metabolic rate, and cognitive indices by a food supplement." *JAMA Neurology* 71, no. 10 (2014): 1255–65. doi: 10.1001/jamaneurol.2014.1584.

Pearce, J. M. "Historical descriptions of multiple sclerosis." *European Neurology* 54, no. 1 (2005): 49–53. doi: 10.1159/000087387.

Peuscher, R., M. E. Dijsselhof, N. G. Abeling, M. Van Rijn, F. J. Van Spronsen, and A. M. Bosch. "The ketogenic diet is well tolerated and can be effective in patients with argininosuccinate lyase deficiency and refractory epilepsy." *JIMD Reports* 5 (2012): 127–30. doi: 10.1007/8904_2011_115.

Phelps, J. R., S. V. Siemers, and R. S. El-Mallakh. "The ketogenic diet for type II bipolar disorder." *Neurocase* 19, no. 5 (2013): 423–6. doi: 10.1080/13554794.2012.690421.

Poff, A. M., C. Ari, T. N. Seyfried, and D. P. D'Agostino. "The ketogenic diet and hyperbaric oxygen therapy prolong survival in mice with systemic metastatic cancer." *PLOS ONE* 8, no. 6 (2013): e65522. doi: 10.1371/journal.pone.0065522.

Poff, A., S. Kesl, A. Koutnik, N. Ward, C. Ari, J. Deblasi, and D. D'Agostino. "Characterizing the metabolic effects of exogenous ketone supplementation–an alternative or adjuvant to the ketogenic diet." *The FASEB Journal* 31, suppl 1 (2017): 970–7.

Prantera, C., M. L. Scribano, G. Falasco, A. Andreoli, and C. Luzi. "Ineffectiveness of probiotics in preventing recurrence after curative resection for Crohn's disease: a randomised controlled trial with Lactobacillus GG." *Gut* 51, no. 3 (2002): 405–9.

Pulsifer, M. B., J. M. Gordon, J. Brandt, E. P. Vining, andJ. M. Freeman. "Effects of ketogenic diet on development and behavior: preliminary report of a prospective study." *Developmental Medicine & Child Neurology* 43, no. 05 (2001): 301–6. doi: 10.1111/j.1469-8749.2001.tb00209.x.

Rankin, J. W., and A. D. Turpyn. "Low carbohydrate, high fat diet increases C-reactive protein during weight loss." *Journal of the American College of Nutrition* 26, no. 2 (2007): 163–9.

Regenold, W. T., P. Phatak, M. J. Makley, R. D. Stone, and M. A. Kling. "Cerebrospinal fluid evidence of increased extra-mitochondrial glucose metabolism implicates mitochondrial dysfunction in multiple sclerosis disease progression." *Journal of the Neurological Sciences* 275, nos. 1–2 (2008): 106–112. doi: 10.1016/j.jns.2008.07.032.

Rhyu, H. S., S. Y. Cho, and H. T. Roh. "The effects of ketogenic diet on oxidative stress and antioxidative capacity markers of Taekwondo athletes." *Journal of Exercise Rehabilitation* 10, no. 6 (2014): 362–6. doi: 10.12965/jer.140178.

Robinson, R. J., T. Krzywicki, L. Almond, F.al-Azzawi, K. Abrams, S. J. Iqbal, and J. F. Mayberry. "Effect of a low-impact exercise program on bone mineral density in Crohn's disease: a randomized controlled trial." *Gastroenterology* 115, no. 1 (1998): 36–41.

Roos-Araujo, D., S. Stuart, R. A. Lea, L. M. Haupt, and L. R. Griffiths. "Epigenetics and migraine; complex mitochondrial interactions contributing to disease susceptibility." *Gene* 543, no. 1 (2014): 1–7. doi: 10.1016/j.gene.2014.04.001.

Ruskin, D. N., J. A. Fortin, S. N. Bisnauth, and S. A. Masino. "Ketogenic diets improve behaviors associated with autism spectrum disorder in a sex-specific manner in the EL mouse." *Physiology & Behavior* 168 (2017): 138–45. doi: 10.1016/j.physbeh.2016.10.023.

Ruskin, D. N., M. Kawamura Jr., and S. A. Masino. "Reduced pain and inflammation in juvenile and adult rats fed a ketogenic diet." *PLoS One* 4, no. 12 (2009): e8349. doi: 10.1371/journal.pone.0008349.

Ruskin, D. N., J. L. Ross, M. Kawamura Jr., T. L. Ruiz, J. D. Geiger, and S. A. Masino. "A ketogenic diet delays weight loss and does not impair working memory or motor function in the R6/2 1J mouse model of Huntington's disease." *Physiology & Behavior* 103, no. 5 (2011): 501–7. doi: 10.1016/j.physbeh.2011.04.001.

Ruskin, D. N., J. Svedova, J. L. Cote, U. Sandau, J. M. Rho, M. Kawamura Jr., ... and S. A. Masino. "Ketogenic diet improves core symptoms of autism in BTBR mice." *PLoS One* 8, no. 6 (2013): e65021. doi: 10.1371/journal.pone.0065021.

Salminen, A., and K. Kaarniranta. "AMP-activated protein kinase (AMPK) controls the aging process via an integrated signaling network." *Ageing Research Reviews* 11, no. 2 (2012): 230–41. doi: 10.1016/j.arr.2011.12.005.

Scheibye-Knudsen, M., S. J. Mitchell, E. F. Fang, T. Iyama, T. Ward, J. Wang, ... and A. Mangerich. "A high-fat diet and NAD+ activate Sirt1 to rescue premature aging in cockayne syndrome." *Cell Metabolism* 20, no. 5 (2014): 840–55. doi: 10.1016/j.cmet.2014.10.005.

Schnabel, T. G. "An experience with a ketogenic dietary in migraine." *Annals of Internal Medicine* 2, no. 4 (1928): 341–7. doi: 10.7326/0003-4819-2-4-341.

Scholl-Bürgi, S., A. Höller, K. Pichler, M. Michel, E. Haberlandt, and D. Karall. "Ketogenic diets in patients with inherited metabolic disorders." *Journal of Inherited Metabolic Disease* 38, no. 4 (2015): 765–73.

Schwartz, J. M., L. R. Baxter, J. C. Mazziotta, R. H. Gerner, and M. E. Phelps. "The differential diagnosis of depression: relevance of positron emission tomography studies of cerebral glucose metabolism to the bipolar-unipolar dichotomy." *JAMA* 258, no. 10 (1987): 1368–74.

Shanahan, F. "Crohn's disease." *The Lancet* 359, no. 9300 (2002): 62–69. doi: 10.1016/S0140-6736(02)07284-7.

Simeone, K. A., S. A. Matthews, J. M. Rho, and T. A. Simeone. "Ketogenic diet treatment increases longevity in Kcna1-null mice, a model of sudden unexpected death in epilepsy." *Epilepsia* 57, no. 8 (2016): e178–82. doi: 10.1111/epi.13444.

Slade, S. L. "Effect of the ketogenic diet on behavioral symptoms of autism in the poly (IC) mouse model." Senior thesis, Trinity College (2015).

Spence, S. J., and M. T. Schneider. "The role of epilepsy and epileptiform EEGs in autism spectrum disorders." *Pediatric Research* 65, no. 6 (2009): 599–606. doi: 10.1203/01.pdr.0000352115.41382.65.

Spilioti, M., A. Evangeliou, D. Tramma, Z. Theodoridou, S. Metaxas, E. Michailidi, ... and K. M. Gibson. "Evidence for treatable inborn errors of metabolism in a cohort of 187 Greek patients with autism spectrum disorder (ASD)." *Frontiers in Human Neuroscience* 7 (2013): 858. doi: 10.3389/fnhum.2013.00858.

Stafstrom, C. E., and J. M. Rho. "The ketogenic diet as a treatment paradigm for diverse neurological disorders." *Frontiers in Pharmacology* 3 (2012): 59. doi: 10.3389/fphar.2012.00059.

Storoni, M., and G. T. Plant. "The therapeutic potential of the ketogenic diet in treating progressive multiple sclerosis." *Multiple Sclerosis International* (2015). doi: 10.1155/2015/681229.

Strahlman, R. S. "Can ketosis help migraine sufferers? A case report." *Headache: The Journal of Head and Face Pain* 46, no. 1 (2006): 182. doi: 10.1111/j.1526-4610.2006.00321_5.x.

Sullivan, P. G., N. A. Rippy, K. Dorenbos, R. C. Concepcion, A. K. Agarwal, and J. M. Rho. "The ketogenic diet increases mitochondrial uncoupling protein levels and activity." *Annals of Neurology* 55, no. 4 (2004): 576–80. doi: 10.1002/ana.20062.

Sussman, D., J. Germann, and M. Henkelman. "Gestational ketogenic diet programs brain structure and susceptibility to depression & anxiety in the adult mouse offspring." *Brain and Behavior* 5, no. 2 (2015): e00300. doi: 10.1002/brb3.300.

Swoboda, K. J., L. Specht, H. R. Jones, F. Shapiro, S. DiMauro, and M. Korson. "Infantile phosphofructokinase deficiency with arthrogryposis: clinical benefit of a ketogenic diet." *Journal of Pediatrics* 131, no. 6 (1997): 932–4.

Tóth, C., A. Dabóczi, M. Howard, N. J. Miller, and Z. Clemens. "Crohn's disease successfully treated with the paleolithic ketogenic diet." *International Journal of Case Reports and Images (IJCRI)* 7, no. 10 (2016): 570–8. doi: 10.5348/ijcri-2016102-CR-10690.

Tregellas, J. R., J. Smucny, K. T. Legget, and K. E. Stevens. "Effects of a ketogenic diet on auditory gating in DBA/2 mice: a proof-of-concept study." *Schizophrenia Research* 169, no. 1–3 (2015): 351–4. doi: 10.1016/j.schres.2015.09.022.

Urbizu, A., E. Cuenca-León, M. Raspall-Chaure, M. Gratacòs, J. Conill, S. Redecillas, ... and A. Macaya. "Paroxysmal exercise-induced dyskinesia, writer's cramp, migraine with aura and absence epilepsy in twin brothers with a novel SLC2A1 missense mutation." *Journal of the Neurological Sciences* 295, no. 1–2 (2010): 110–3. doi: 10.1016/j.jns.2010.05.017.

Valayannopoulos, V., F. Bajolle, J. B. Arnoux, S. Dubois, N. Sannier, C. Baussan, ... and P. de Lonlay. "Successful treatment of severe cardiomyopathy in glycogen storage disease type III With D, L-3-hydroxybutyrate, ketogenic and high-protein diet." *Pediatric Research* 70, no. 6 (2011): 638–41. doi: 10.1203/PDR.0b013e318232154f.

van der Wee, N. J., J. F. van Veen, H. Stevens, I. M. van Vliet, P. P. van Rijk, and H. G. Westenberg. "Increased serotonin and dopamine transporter binding in psychotropic medication–näive patients with generalized social anxiety disorder shown by 123I-β-(4-Iodophenyl)-tropane SPECT." *Journal of Nuclear Medicine* 49, no. 5 (2008): 757–63. doi: 10.2967/jnumed.107.045518.

Veech, R. L. "The therapeutic implications of ketone bodies: the effects of ketone bodies in pathological conditions: ketosis, ketogenic diet, redox states, insulin resistance, and mitochondrial metabolism." *Prostaglandins, Leukotrienes and Essential Fatty Acids* 70, no. 3 (2004): 309–19. doi: 10.1016/j.plefa.2003.09.007.

Vorgerd, M., and J. Zange. "Treatment of glycogenosys type V (McArdle disease) with creatine and ketogenic diet with clinical scores and with 31P-MRS on working leg muscle." *Acta Myologica* 26, no. 1 (2007): 61–63.

Vos, M. B., J. L. Kaar, J. A. Welsh, L. V. Van Horn, D. I. Feig, C. A. Anderson, ... and R. K. Johnson. "Added sugars and cardiovascular disease risk in children." *Circulation* 135, no. 15 (2016). doi: 10.1161/CIR.0000000000000439.

Vucic, S., J. D. Rothstein, and M. C. Kiernan. "Advances in treating amyotrophic lateral sclerosis: insights from pathophysiological studies." *Trends in Neurosciences* 37, no. 8 (2014): 433–42. doi: 10.1016/j.tins.2014.05.006.

Weber, T. A., M. R. Antognetti, and P. W. Stacpoole. "Caveats when considering ketogenic diets for the treatment of pyruvate dehydrogenase complex deficiency." *Journal of Pediatrics* 138, no. 3 (2001): 390–5. doi: 10.1067/mpd.2001.111817.

Wexler, I. D., S. G. Hemalatha, J. McConnell, N. R. Buist, H. H. Dahl, S. A. Berry, ... and D. S. Kerr. "Outcome of pyruvate dehydrogenase deficiency treated with ketogenic diets: studies in patients with identical mutations." *Neurology* 49, no. 6 (1997): 1655–61.

Wiedemann, F. R., G. Manfredi, C. Mawrin, M. F. Beal, and E. A. Schon. "Mitochondrial DNA and respiratory chain function in spinal cords of ALS patients." *Journal of Neurochemistry* 80, no. 4 (2002): 616–25. doi: 10.1046/j.0022-3042.2001.00731.x.

Williams, C. A., D. J. Driscoll, and A. I. Dagli. "Clinical and genetic aspects of Angelman syndrome." *Genetics in Medicine* 12, no. 7 (2010): 385–95. doi: 10.1097/GIM.0b013e3181def138.

Woolf, E. C., J. L. Johnson, D. M. Lussier, K. S. Brooks, J. N. Blattman, and A. C. Scheck. "The ketogenic diet enhances immunity in a mouse model of malignant glioma." *Cancer Research* 75, suppl 5 (2015): 1344. doi: 10.1158/1538-7445.AM2015-1344.

Wright, C., and N. L. Simone. "Obesity and tumor growth: inflammation, immunity, and the role of a ketogenic diet." *Current Opinion in Clinical Nutrition & Metabolic Care* 19, no. 4 (2016): 294–9. doi: 10.1097/MCO.0000000000000286.

Xie, Z., D. Zhang, D. Chung, Z. Tang, H. Huang, L. Dai, ... and Y. Zhao. "Metabolic Regulation of Gene Expression by Histone Lysine β-Hydroxybutyrylation." *Molecular Cell* 62, no. 2 (2016): 194–206. doi: 10.1016/j.molcel.2016.03.036.

Youm, Y. H., K. Y. Nguyen, R. W. Grant, E. L. Goldberg, M. Bodogai, D. Kim, ...and V. D. Dixit. "The ketone metabolite β-hydroxybutyrate blocks NLRP3 inflammasome-mediated inflammatory disease." *Nature Medicine* 21, no. 3 (2015): 263–9. doi: 10.1038/nm.3804.

Zhao, W., M. Varghese, P. Vempati, A. Dzhun, A. Cheng, J. Wang, ... and G. M. Pasinetti. "Caprylic triglyceride as a novel therapeutic approach to effectively improve the performance and attenuate the symptoms due to the motor neuron loss in ALS disease." *PLoS One* 7, no. 11 (2012): e49191. doi: 10.1371/journal.pone.0049191.

Zhao, Z., D. J. Lange, A. Voustianiouk, D. MacGrogan, L. Ho, J. Suh, ... and G. M. Pasinetti. "A ketogenic diet as a potential novel therapeutic intervention in amyotrophic lateral sclerosis." *BMC Neuroscience* 7 (2006): 29. doi: 10.1136/1471-2202-7-29.

Ziegler, D. R., L. C. Ribeiro, M. Hagenn, I. R. Siqueira, E. Araújo, I. L. Torres, C. Gottfried, ... and C. A. Gonçalves. "Ketogenic diet increases glutathione peroxidase activity in rat hippocampus." *Neurochemical Research* 28, no. 12 (2003): 1793–7. doi: 10.1023/A:1026107405399.

Zilkha, N., Y. Kuperman, and T. Kimchi. "High-fat diet exacerbates cognitive rigidity and social deficiency in the BTBR mouse model of autism." *Neuroscience* 345 (2016): 142–54. doi: 10.1016/j.neuroscience.2016.01.070.

https://migraineresearchfoundation.org/about-migraine/migraine-facts/
www.adaa.org/about-adaa/press-room/facts-statistics
www.alsa.org/about-als/facts-you-should-know.html
www.angelman.org/what-is-as/
www.nia.nih.gov/research/publication/global-health-and-aging/living-longer
www.ptsd.va.gov/index.asp

Chapter 6

KETO KICKSTART:
A PRACTICAL GUIDE
TO GETTING STARTED

In this book, we have presented you with a large amount of information. We have extensively discussed what the ketogenic diet is, its history, the health implications associated with the diet, potential therapeutic uses, and even the science behind exogenous ketones. We hope that you have learned a lot along the way and taken away some key information to help implement the diet yourself and/or help others! In an attempt to do so, we want to equip you with some quick and easy practical tools and tips that you can take away and apply to your life.

The goal of this chapter is to provide you with not only the knowledge to begin your ketogenic lifestyle but also the necessary skills to adjust, optimize, and adhere to the diet.

Keto for You

As you continue to educate yourself on the ketogenic lifestyle, you may find yourself eager to jump in and get started. This is great! We recommend diving in as opposed to straddling the fence, but proper planning is key! For this reason, it is important to tailor the ketogenic diet specifically to you. KETO makes a good acronym for how to make the diet work for you.

Step 1: **K**eep Calories in Mind

Step 2: **E**volve Your Macronutrients

Step 3: **T**ake It Meal by Meal

Step 4: **O**pen Yourself to Change

Step 1: Keep Calories in Mind

Proper planning starts with determining your caloric need. The most accurate method of doing so involves equipment that the general population does not have access to, such as a metabolic cart, which we use in our lab to look directly at a person's metabolism. However, there are a few other ways to figure out a calorie intake that would be pretty close to what you need. For instance, online calorie calculators can be relatively accurate in determining your needs based on your age, body type, and activity level.

We recommend two options:

1) Find an online calorie calculator (check out the one on Ketogenic.com) and enter your information to determine the calories you need according to their algorithm. If you input all your information (age, height, weight, activity level, workout regimen, etc.), it will give you a rough estimate of your caloric needs for maintaining your current weight. From there, you can easily adjust your total calories by adding or subtracting if your goal is to gain or lose weight.

For example, a five-foot-four-inch, forty-year-old female who weighs 150 pounds, is moderately active, and wants to lose weight might be given an output like this:

BMR = 2,070	Deficit
Calories	1,570
Fat	122 g
Protein	98 g
Carbohydrates	20 g

2) Track your food intake using an app like Cronometer or MyFitnessPal and monitor whether you are maintaining, gaining, or losing weight. If you aren't already tracking your food, use the app to enter three full days of normal eating. If your weight has been stable for a couple of weeks, this gives you a good starting point so that you can adjust as needed. A safe bet is to start by adding or subtracting 250 calories. For instance, say you determined that your baseline average intake is 2,250 calories. If you want to gain weight, aim for 2,500 calories a day. If you want to lose weight, aim for 2,000 calories a day.

In the beginning, it is good to monitor your calories to prevent overeating or even undereating and to make sure that you are getting the nutrients you need. However, over time, and as you feel more comfortable with the diet, you can eat to satisfaction and satiety. People tend to eat fewer calories on a ketogenic diet because they aren't as hungry as they were when eating a low-fat, high-carbohydrate diet. Don't get caught up in the numbers, but rather use them as a guiding tool along the way.

Step 2: Evolve Your Macronutrients

Once you have calculated your caloric intake, it is time to tailor the diet more specifically to you. This process will always be evolving based on your goals and activity level and should not be set in stone in most cases. For example, some people are adamant that you must eat exactly 80 percent fat, 15 percent protein, and 5 percent carbohydrates. We do not feel that this is necessary or sustainable. Traditionally, we suggest 60 to 80 percent fat, 15 to 30 percent protein, and 5 to 10 percent carbs. However, these numbers can easily change depending on your goal and the context. For instance, those using the ketogenic diet for certain therapeutic approaches (such as to treat epilepsy, Alzheimer's disease, Parkinson's, or cancer) may want to consume a higher percentage of fat and a slightly lower percentage of protein and carbohydrates in an attempt to drive blood ketone concentration up further, which can be extremely important in those situations. On the other hand, those concerned with increasing muscle mass may find it more beneficial to have a slightly higher protein intake (25 to 30 percent) and scale back on fat (60 to 70 percent). More active people (such as those who lift weights or do CrossFit) may be able to tolerate a slightly higher protein intake than those who are more sedentary.

Once you determine your macronutrient percentages, you will want to calculate the total number of grams of each nutrient to consume daily. You do this by multiplying your daily caloric intake by each macronutrient's respective percentage.

Start by calculating 5 percent and 10 percent of your calorie intake. For example, if your daily calorie intake target is 2,000 calories, 5 percent is 100 calories and 10 percent is 200 calories. This represents the range of calories (not grams) of carbohydrates you may want to start with. To determine grams, take that number of calories and divide it by 4 (the number of calories in a gram of carbohydrate). This gives you a range of 25 to 50 grams of carbohydrates per day.

Next, calculate 20 percent and 30 percent of your calorie intake. Continuing with the example of 2,000 calories per day, 20 percent is 400 calories and 30 percent is 600 calories. This represents the range of calories (not grams) of protein you may want to start with. To determine grams, take that number of calories and divide it by 4 (the number of calories in a gram of protein). This gives you a range of 100 to 150 grams of protein per day.

Finally, fill in the rest with fat, to satiety. What we mean is that now that you know how much carbohydrate and protein to eat, you can fill in the rest of your day's calories with fat, until you're full. For example, athletes tend to err on the side of extra protein. Say you are an athlete aiming for 10 percent carbohydrates and 25 percent protein. On 2,000 calories a day, that would mean 50 grams of carbs (200 calories) and 125 grams of protein (500 calories) per day. If you are trying to maintain your weight—so you want calories to stay stable—then you would need to eat 1,300 calories of fat. Fat has 9 calories per gram, so dividing 1,300 by 9 gives you about 144 grams of fat per day.

Now, that does not mean that you have to put butter and heavy cream in your morning coffee or eat fat bombs at night to hit this number. Eat to satiety. If you are at 100 grams of fat at the end of the day, that is fine—no need to guzzle down some MCT or butter before bed just to "hit your macros." Remember, not everyone is the same. This is Keto for You. When it comes to nutrition, you are the master of your own destiny; don't eat just because you feel like you have to.

Step 3: Take It Meal by Meal

If you are new to tracking macronutrients or percentages, then sticking to calculated numbers each day may seem like quite a headache. For this reason, we suggest taking it one meal at a time. An approach that has been successful with many individuals we have worked with is the following:

First, determine how frequently you plan to eat throughout the day. For example, if you plan on skipping breakfast, that's fine—plan for two meals per day. If you want to start your day with some coffee with butter or heavy cream, that's fine, too. Be realistic about what works with your lifestyle. Many people prefer to have only coffee in the morning and not eat until lunch or even dinnertime. Don't force yourself to eat breakfast just because someone on TV or the internet said you should. However, we do suggest consuming fewer, bigger meals as opposed to five to six small meals per day. (See page 49 for more on meal frequency.)

Once you have determined your number of meals per day, divide the total number of grams of each macronutrient by the number of meals you plan to consume. This will give you a rough idea of how much fat, protein, and carbs you can eat at each meal. For example, say you are eating three meals a day and are using the macronutrient amounts from the earlier example: 25 to 50 grams of carbohydrates, 100 to 150 grams of protein, and 144 grams of fat. That means that at each meal, you would aim for about 8 to 17 grams of carbohydrates, 33 to 50 grams of protein, and 48 grams of fat.

Granted, not everyone eats the same amount of food at each meal. You may have a small breakfast, a medium-sized lunch, and a larger dinner. That is completely okay. However, we recommend eating your biggest meals earlier in the day rather than late at night (i.e., big breakfast, moderate lunch, small to moderate dinner) since we know from studies that movement after meals can help improve digestion and insulin sensitivity, which can be important for long-term fat loss. However, these are just examples. You also may want to incorporate some snacks (pork rinds are a great crunchy snack, for example). Just plan for that and know how much you want to eat at each meal until you get the hang of the diet.

Unless you have a rather extensive background in nutrition, these numbers likely will not do much to help you decide what to actually eat. Remember, take it one meal at a time. For each meal, choose a protein source, whether it be eggs and bacon at breakfast or some type of fatty meat, such as steak, at lunch. (Try to stick with fatty cuts instead of leaner meats—see page 47 for more.) Use a calorie-tracking app like Cronometer or MyFitnessPal or the nutrition facts label to determine how much of that protein source will meet your protein requirement for the meal.

Next, check how much fat that amount of your protein source contains. From there you can adjust your fat intake for the meal by using fatty additions like dressings, butter, oils, seeds, and nuts to help get you closer to your goal.

Now fill in the rest of your meal with the nonstarchy vegetable of your choice to meet your carbohydrate requirement. We recommend this approach because some of our clients tend to take the macronutrient content of these recommendations at face value. For example, we have seen people use an "if it fits your macros" approach and consume 144 grams of fat in the form of butter and/or MCT oil in their coffee, drink 100 to 150 grams of protein in the form of pure protein shakes, and then finish the night off with 25 to 50 grams of carbohydrates from a package of M&Ms. This approach isn't ideal for optimizing ketosis and likely isn't sustainable long term.

Here's what a typical day looks like for each of us.

Jacob: 1,800 calories, 70% fat, 20% protein, 10% carbs	
BREAKFAST	N/A
LUNCH	4 hard-boiled eggs, butter, light spinach salad with crushed nuts and oil-based dressing
SNACK	Pork rinds and handful of nuts
DINNER	Light salad, 4 to 6 ounces of fatty meat, vegetables
DESSERT	Slice of keto cheesecake (page 318) or keto cookies (pages 306 to 310)
ESTIMATED DAILY TOTALS	
140 grams fat, 90 grams protein, 45 grams carbs	

Ryan: 2,300 calories, 65% fat, 25% protein, 10% carbs	
BREAKFAST	Eggs and bacon or keto pancakes (page 220)
LUNCH	Cobb salad with bacon, egg, and blue cheese
SNACK	N/A
DINNER	Light salad, 4 to 6 ounces of fatty meat, vegetables
DESSERT	Keto cookies (pages 306 to 310) or keto milkshake

ESTIMATED DAILY TOTALS
166 grams fat, 144 grams protein, 58 grams carbs

This is a perfect example of why it's not as simple as 75 percent fat, 20 percent protein, and 5 percent carbs, or whatever combination of percentages might be recommended. Jacob eats 70 percent of his calories as fat, while Ryan eats only 65 percent of his calories as fat, yet Ryan still eats more total grams of fat than Jacob. Calorie and macro goals need to be customized for you. Blanket recommendations are a good starting point, but they are just that: a starting point.

Step 4: Open Yourself to Change

When adopting the ketogenic lifestyle, it is important to understand and be open to change. Foods that you may have been told were "bad" (bacon, oils, etc.) are now staples in your diet. Others that you may have loved, such as brownies and cookies, aren't necessarily off the list, but it will take some creativity to "keto-tize" them and make them keto-friendly (see Chapter 8 for keto-tized recipes). Always remember that in order to make the ketogenic approach work, you have to make eating keto work for your lifestyle. What works for someone you know might not be the best approach for you. If you eat twice a day, that's fine. If you have four meals a day, that's fine as well. Look at it as a lifestyle, not a diet. Traditional diets aren't sustainable over time and often lead to a crash and rebound. Don't feel like you are restricted in your food choices. Rather, think of ways to be creative and come up with alternative options for foods that you feel you are missing out on. We want you to be in this for the long haul, not just try it out for a couple of weeks. Once you've learned the tricks of the trade,

PLANNING YOUR MEALS

EXAMPLE Total macros	How many meals do you want to eat per day?	Divide total macros by number of meals
Protein 100g		Protein: 100g/4 → 25g
Carbs 25g	**4**	Carbs: 25g/4 → 6g
Fat 160g		Fat: 160g/4 → 40g

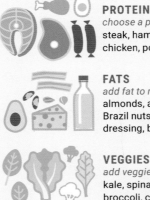

PROTEIN
choose a protein source
steak, hamburger, salmon, flounder, chicken, pork, sausage, eggs

FATS
add fat to meet macro requirements
almonds, avocados, ranch dressing, Brazil nuts, macadamia nuts, Greek dressing, bacon, coconut oil, cheese

VEGGIES
add veggies to meet carb total
kale, spinach, romaine lettuce, broccoli, cauliflower

WATER
Remember to drink ample amounts of water!

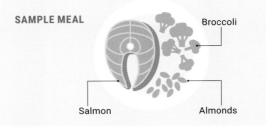

SAMPLE MEAL — Broccoli — Salmon — Almonds

Figure 6.1. *Plan your meals to meet your macros.*
Source: Ketogenic.com.

you may be able to ditch the approach of tracking every meal you eat and stick to eating what you know is keto-friendly.

As a brief recap:

Step 1: Keep calories in mind. Find a starting point that is right for you.

Step 2: Evolve your macronutrients. Customize your macros to fit the ketogenic lifestyle you want.

Step 3: Take it meal by meal. Balance your meals accordingly. (Don't save all your carbs for M&Ms at night!)

Step 4: Open yourself to change. Make it enjoyable. Find ways to keto-tize your favorite recipes and food preferences.

Ketogenic Dieting for Beginners: Dos and Don'ts

Low-carbohydrate dieting is by no means a novel approach to weight loss and improved general health. Many diet fads associated with carbohydrate restriction have come and gone over the years, some remaining more relevant than others. From Atkins to Zone to Paleo, the idea that limiting carbohydrates is a plausible strategy for reaching certain health goals is accepted by many people worldwide. However, society has been a bit resistant to the idea that consuming a low-carbohydrate diet that is also high in fat, such as a ketogenic diet, may be beneficial for long-term health. For this reason, there seems to be a gap between the research involving the ketogenic diet and its practical applications. To combat this gap, we have put together a list of dos and don'ts for successfully following a low-carb/high-fat lifestyle.

> "There are two ways to see the world. Some people see the thing that they want, and some people see the thing that prevents them from getting the thing that they want."
> —Simon Sinek

Dos

Plan your diet according to your goals.
Having a game plan before starting a ketogenic diet may be crucial to the success of the diet. Before beginning your journey into ketosis, you should prepare and plan according to your goal. Are you looking to lose some weight and lean out? Are you looking to implement the diet as a therapy for mild cognitive impairments that you are seeing as you get older? Ultimately, your specific goal will determine how many calories you plan to consume as well as the specific foods you plan to eat. Set out your vision and don't let anything get in the way of achieving those goals.

Remove temptations from your home.
One of the defining features of being in ketosis is the reduction of hunger and food cravings. However, these reductions do not occur immediately; in fact, it may take time to fully experience these benefits. Several studies have looked at something called "willpower depletion," which basically means that we all have a certain amount of willpower that can be depleted after numerous temptations, eventually leading us to break. You don't want to challenge your willpower by staring at soda, chips, donuts, cookies, and candy day in and day out. Facing too many sugary temptations during the initial stages of the diet could lead you to want to cheat, thus preventing you from fully reaching a state of keto adaptation. To combat this threat, remove the non-keto-friendly food options from your pantry. Even better, get your family or housemates on board as well, and you can bond by creating delicious keto-friendly recipes together.

Find recipes to replace your favorite meals.
Everyone's initial thought when implementing a ketogenic diet is, "So you're telling me I have to give up cookies and cheesecake and my favorite Sunday breakfast, pancakes?" Actually, no, you don't. For any food you enjoy that has carbohydrates, there are almost always ketogenic alternatives that are just as delicious, and sometimes even better (mmm, butter). Cookbooks, websites, blogs, and social media accounts dedicated to ketogenic recipes are in no shortage. Is your favorite meal spaghetti and meatballs? Don't worry, because with the proper

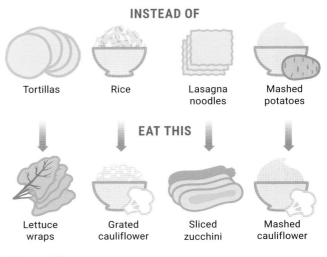

INSTEAD OF

Tortillas · Rice · Lasagna noodles · Mashed potatoes

EAT THIS

Lettuce wraps · Grated cauliflower · Sliced zucchini · Mashed cauliflower

Figure 6.2. *Keto swaps.*

equipment, you can make zucchini noodles and a creamy low-carb spaghetti sauce. Craving a slice of pizza? Cauliflower- or meat-crust pizza can quell that craving! Even ketogenic dessert recipes are becoming more popular, from fat bombs to cheesecake to cookies. We have provided several ketogenic recipes in this book, and if you are looking for "keto swaps" such as alternatives to potato chips, check out our recommended sites at Ketogenic.com/KetoSwap.

Mix it up!

It's a common mistake to think that a ketogenic diet includes only boring, bland food options. The reality is quite the opposite. You can incorporate endless food options into your daily ketogenic meal plan, so mix it up and have fun with it! Eating the same thing every day not only becomes monotonous (regardless of your diet protocol) but also can lead to an excessive intake of certain nutrients and an inadequate intake of others. Try to buy a variety of meats, veggies, and other ingredients to make delicious recipes and desserts!

Stay hydrated.

When you are on a ketogenic diet, your insulin levels tend to be lower. When insulin in the body is low, the kidneys excrete more water and sodium. This can lead to frequent urination and possibly dehydration. For this reason, it is important to focus on your water consumption and make sure you stay hydrated. Remember, when you go to the bathroom, it should be light in color, like lemonade. Darker urine may indicate dehydration.

Supplement with electrolytes.

The side effects we just mentioned in regard to water and insulin make supplementing with electrolytes equally important as drinking enough water. Increased water excretion can lead to deficiencies in certain electrolytes, which can have a rather large impact on factors such as mental clarity, exercise performance, and overall feeling of wellness. These electrolytes include (but are not limited to) calcium, potassium, magnesium, and sodium. Certain electrolytes can be replenished through your diet, while others may require supplementation.

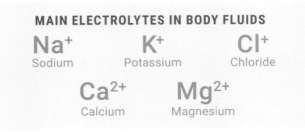

Figure 6.3. *The main electrolytes in our bodies.*

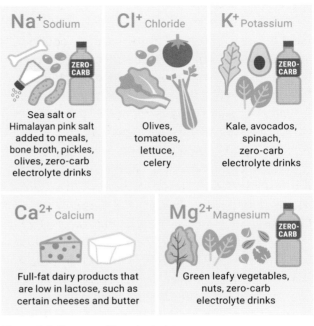

Figure 6.4. *Sources of key electrolytes.*

Sodium and potassium are the most commonly depleted electrolytes; therefore, paying close attention to those levels is important, especially during the adaptation phase. To replenish sodium, we suggest salting your food or adding bone broth to your daily regimen. To replenish potassium, you can focus on consuming foods that are high in potassium, such as avocados and green leafy vegetables, like spinach. Other options include taking an electrolyte supplement like Nuun; if you are taking exogenous ketones, many of those supplements have an adequate electrolyte content.

Experiment with intermittent fasting.

Fasting is a practice often used by ketogenic dieters. Because reduced hunger commonly accompanies a ketogenic diet, fasting is a plausible option that can have a variety of health and body composition benefits. Even incorporating small intermittent fasts can lead to an increased production of ketone bodies. Options include something as simple as skipping breakfast and eating your first meal at lunchtime all the way to eighteen-hour fasts or practicing alternate-day fasting. If you want to experiment with fasting techniques, we recommend that you start with lighter methods and work your way up to the more intense versions of intermittent eating. For more on intermittent eating, see page 49.

Try MCTs and coconut oil.

MCTs, or medium-chain triglycerides, are fats that can be rapidly converted to energy in the body. MCTs are found in a variety of foods, such as coconut, coconut oil, and heavy cream, and in supplement form (for example, MCT oil and MCT powder). The powder seems to be better for cooking and baking, while the oil is better for adding to coffee or shakes. Additionally, the powder doesn't seem to pose the same gastrointestinal challenges as the oil. If you are looking to increase your healthy fat intake and reap such benefits as the antimicrobial properties of lauric acid, then options like coconut oil (also high in MCTs) may be advantageous. Some of our favorite meals can be cooked in coconut oil, which adds a great flavor to most dishes. Just be careful not to overdo it on the MCTs, or you might find yourself spending more time in the bathroom than ever before. See page 55 for more on MCTs.

Eat a variety of healthy fats.

Make sure to mix up your fat choices just as you do your general food choices. Different fats have different health benefits, so exposing your body to a variety of healthy fats can be of great benefit! See page 45 for more on healthy fats.

Be aware of condiment ingredients.

Individuals often fail to look at the nutrition labels for certain condiments. Salads are a great option, but be aware that most salad dressings, despite being high in fat, contain sugar and other carbohydrates as well. Some condiments, like ketchup, are available in reduced-sugar versions; definitely don't fall for the "fat-free" versions of most dressings, which tend to replace fat with added sugars.

Be careful with dairy.

There are plenty of dairy options that are high in fat and may seem like great ketogenic choices. However, many dairy products are also high in lactose (milk sugar). Make sure to check the labels on all dairy items before consuming them, because the lactose content can add up fast!

Experiment with exogenous ketones.

Exogenous or supplemental ketones are synthesized versions of the ketones that our body produces naturally. The use of exogenous ketones can be particularly beneficial while your body is transitioning from relying solely on glucose for fuel to using ketones as its primary fuel source. Not only do ketone salts elevate ketones, but they also can provide additional sodium, magnesium, and calcium. It is plausible that ketone supplementation has the potential to speed up the adaptation period; at the very least, supplements could provide you with more energy during the transition. For more on exogenous ketones, see Chapter 4.

Train hard.

While your motivation to get in the gym and exercise may waver at the beginning of the adaptation period, we recommend that you push through and continue to train hard. Intense training can increase your rate of fat oxidation and therefore your rate of ketone body production. A study conducted in our lab found that those who did high-intensity interval training (HIIT) saw a greater increase in plasma ketones than those doing steady-state training. Therefore, continuing to train hard and exercise might enable you to adapt faster.

Monitor your ketone and glucose levels periodically.

At the beginning of the transition period, testing your ketone levels is a good way to monitor how your body is responding to the diet. Simple testers such as urine strips or breath acetone meters are affordable ways to monitor ketones. Those looking to go the extra mile may want to invest in a blood ketone meter to help during this period. Always test in the morning or right before sleep, as exercise and food intake can cause ketone levels to fluctuate. It also could be beneficial to track your fasting blood glucose to see how your body is handling the

HOW TO TEST KETONES

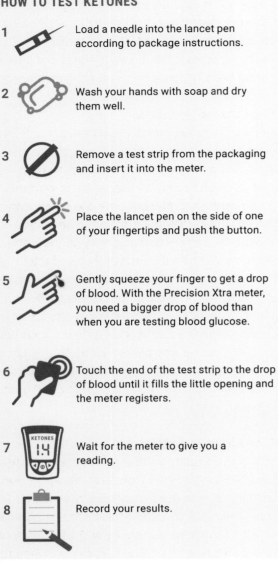

1. Load a needle into the lancet pen according to package instructions.

2. Wash your hands with soap and dry them well.

3. Remove a test strip from the packaging and insert it into the meter.

4. Place the lancet pen on the side of one of your fingertips and push the button.

5. Gently squeeze your finger to get a drop of blood. With the Precision Xtra meter, you need a bigger drop of blood than when you are testing blood glucose.

6. Touch the end of the test strip to the drop of blood until it fills the little opening and the meter registers.

7. Wait for the meter to give you a reading.

8. Record your results.

Figure 6.5. *The process of testing for blood ketones.*
Source: Ketogenic.com.

changes in diet. After you get the hang of the diet, testing isn't necessary, so don't stress out about turning the urine stick purple.

Keep fiber in mind.

Certain fibers have the ability to feed the good bacteria in the gut. Getting enough fiber can also help ensure proper digestion. Therefore, the main carbohydrate sources we recommend are green leafy vegetables that are higher in fiber. Be wary of high-fiber protein bars, which may actually cause an increase in blood glucose—see page 44.

Don'ts

Don't let carbs creep up too high.

One of the biggest reasons for a lack of success on a ketogenic diet is letting carbohydrates creep up too high. Snacks like nuts and nut butters are common culprits in this mistake. While nuts can safely be incorporated into a ketogenic lifestyle, overconsumption can lead to insufficient carbohydrate restriction, thus preventing ketosis. The same is true for nut butters, such as peanut butter or almond butter; in fact, nut butters may be even more problematic because they are usually slightly higher in sugar and lower in fiber than the nuts themselves.

In the initial stages of a ketogenic diet, you may have a bit of a sweet tooth. When cravings strike, peanut butter can really hit the spot, and putting the spoon away may be more difficult than you think! It's easy to overdo it. If you don't want to challenge your willpower, choose higher-fat, lower-carb snack alternatives, like macadamia nuts or pork rinds.

Don't overconsume artificial sweeteners / sugar alcohols.

Natural sweeteners and sugar alcohols can be a great way to liven up a ketogenic diet, but beware of overconsuming them or consuming the wrong ones! (See Chapter 7 for more on natural sweeteners and sugar alcohols.) Overconsumption of certain sugar alcohols can cause digestive issues like gastric distress—even just a handful of sugar-free gummy bears at the movie theater could have you spending the entire movie in the bathroom. Be on the lookout for artificial sweeteners (e.g., Equal, Splenda, etc.) that are combined with maltodextrin, a very non-keto-friendly sweetener. A little bit here and there won't hurt, but when baking or using larger amounts, get straight sucralose or aspartame powder instead. Ideally, we prefer that you use natural sweeteners that are keto-friendly, such as erythritol, stevia, inulin, monk fruit, and even a brand-new one called allulose.

Don't go crazy with high-fiber protein bars.

Many nutrition companies are coming out with low-sugar, high-fiber protein bars. These bars can be a great way to satisfy your sweet tooth, but be aware

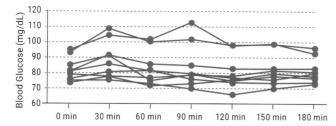

Individual Glucose Response to SCF

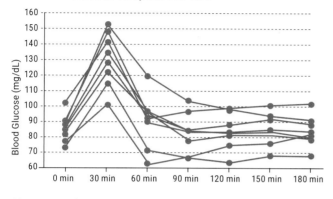

Individual Glucose Response to IMO

Figure 6.6. *Blood glucose responses from soluble corn fiber (SCF) compared to isomaltooligosaccharides (IMOs).*
Source: Lowery et al., 2017.

that not all low-sugar protein bars are actually low-carb! Bars using isomaltooligosaccharides (IMOs) as their fiber source may not be the most keto-friendly. Our lab found that this type of fiber can cause a rise in blood glucose and insulin, which could be harmful to your state of ketosis. Instead, look for protein bars that use soluble corn fiber (SCF) as their main fiber source. We found that this fiber source does not increase blood glucose or insulin and actually serves its purpose of feeding the good bacteria in the gut to a greater extent than IMOs.

Don't live on fast food.
An occasional stop at a fast-food joint to get a lettuce-wrapped burger or a chopped salad is absolutely fine. However, don't let the bunless burger from your favorite fast-food place become a staple of your diet. Remember that *quality is key*—the meat from a lot of fast-food restaurants is not the highest quality, and sometimes those "healthy" salads are loaded with hidden carbohydrates. It's better to consume a small amount of a high-quality food than a lot of a poor-quality food.

Don't fall for low-fat foods.
This may seem obvious since the ketogenic diet is high-fat, but there's another reason to avoid low-fat foods: they tend to replace fat with carbohydrates/sugar. You may find that lower-fat dressings and cheeses have a higher carb count than you thought!

Don't go chasing ketones.
Previously we recommended testing your ketone levels at the beginning of the diet to gain an understanding of how your body is reacting to your ketogenic strategy. However, it's important not to go overboard and become obsessed with testing multiple times per day just to see if you are in ketosis. Ketone levels vary throughout the day as a result of food intake and other factors, such as stress and movement. Additionally, it's not clear what optimal levels of ketones actually are; in fact, the longer you are on the diet, the lower your plasma levels might become due to your body taking them up into the cells much more rapidly. Once you are in ketosis, you tend to be able to tell when you are in or out. Don't stress about it; just stick to your plan.

Don't be afraid of protein.
Far too often, people fear eating too much protein on a ketogenic diet. While this fear has some merit for individuals who need to adhere to a lower protein intake in order to maintain ketosis (such as those with conditions like epilepsy), others may not need to be so strict. For example, people who are training hard can likely get away with the higher end of the range for protein intake. Remember that the most important part of maintaining ketosis is minimizing carbohydrate intake. If you are doing this, then there is likely no need to worry about enjoying a steak smothered in butter from your favorite restaurant.

Don't overconsume MCTs.
MCT oil can be hard on the stomach, leading to gastric distress and even leaving you spending more time in the bathroom if taken in excessive amounts. For this reason, we recommend building up your MCT consumption slowly and listening to your body!

Don't overconsume fruits and vegetables.

Eating fruits and vegetables can be a great way to get fiber and fill up on a ketogenic diet. However, some vegetables and especially fruits have a high carbohydrate content. As one of our colleagues once said, "An apple a day will keep ketosis away." Monitor the sugar content of fruits and vegetables and try to stick to green leafy vegetables.

Don't consider all salad dressings to be keto-friendly.

Drizzling your salad with dressing can be a great way to ensure that you are getting enough fat in your meal when dining out, but beware! Certain vinaigrettes contain enough sugar to make your body say goodbye to ketosis. Low-fat dressings commonly replace fat with carbohydrates, so avoiding those may be beneficial. Stick to oils and dressings like ranch, Caesar, and blue cheese, and use them in moderation. To be safe, when eating out you may want to ask your server to double-check if the dressing was made with added sugar or carbohydrates.

Don't consume too much alcohol.

We understand that people like to have a glass of wine every now and then or go out for a drink. Heck, we do, too. But be especially cautious with flavored liquors and traditional beers, which can be sugar-heavy. Dry red wines, like the ones made by our good friends at Dry Farm Wines, are a solid option, as are low-carb beers and spirits, as long as you consume them in moderation. No strawberry daiquiris or Bahama Mamas!

Don't dine out unprepared.

Eating out on a ketogenic diet may seem intimidating, but it doesn't have to be! Most restaurants display their menus online, and many even make nutrition facts available to view. Don't be afraid to ask your server how a dish is prepared or what types of sauces are used. Quite honestly, we feel that it's a lot easier to dine out keto than it is to eat low-fat. Just ask for a side salad and vegetables and a choice of fatty meat or fish. Beware of sauces, and when in doubt, get the sauce on the side.

Don't stop training.

Even if it is light exercise, keep your body moving: go on walks, play sports, or get in the gym. Trust us, your body will thank you.

Don't give up.

Most importantly, do not give up! You may want to cave in at the beginning or completely stop the diet when you start to feel a little tired. You may want to have that slice of pizza or that cookie. But stay strong! We hear people say all the time, "Yeah, I tried keto. It didn't work for me." When we ask how long they tried it, we commonly hear, "Maybe two weeks?" This is not enough time to fully adapt to the diet. Stick to your plan, and soon you will be feeling great and reaping the benefits of ketosis! See page 191 for more tips on weathering the transition to becoming keto-adapted.

Figure 6.7. *Beer can contain a lot of carbohydrates, so choose wisely.*

Source: Ketogenic.com.

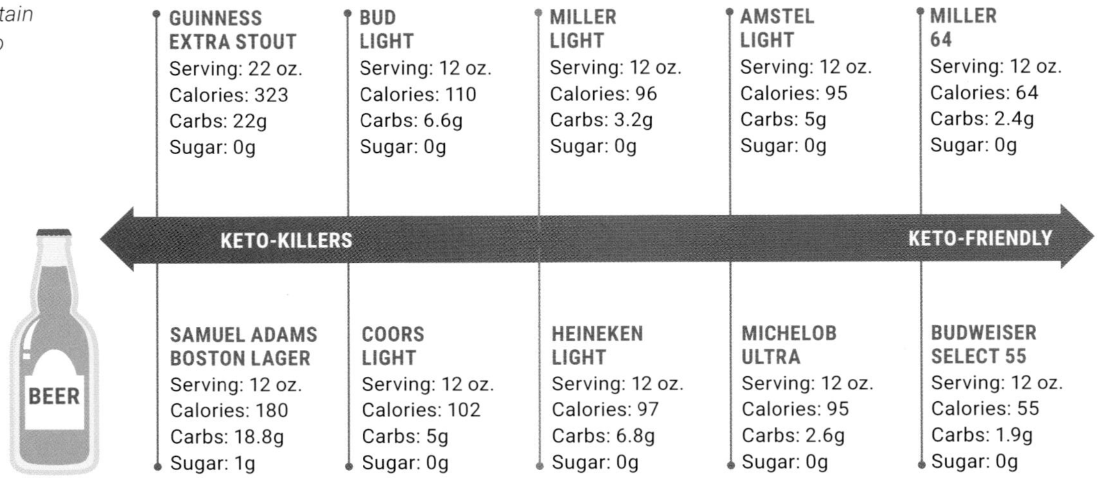

GUINNESS EXTRA STOUT	BUD LIGHT	MILLER LIGHT	AMSTEL LIGHT	MILLER 64
Serving: 22 oz.	Serving: 12 oz.	Serving: 12 oz.	Serving: 12 oz.	Serving: 12 oz.
Calories: 323	Calories: 110	Calories: 96	Calories: 95	Calories: 64
Carbs: 22g	Carbs: 6.6g	Carbs: 3.2g	Carbs: 5g	Carbs: 2.4g
Sugar: 0g	Sugar: 0g	Sugar: 0g	Sugar: 0g	Sugar: 0g

KETO-KILLERS ⟵ ⟶ KETO-FRIENDLY

SAMUEL ADAMS BOSTON LAGER	COORS LIGHT	HEINEKEN LIGHT	MICHELOB ULTRA	BUDWEISER SELECT 55
Serving: 12 oz.	Serving: 12 oz.	Serving: 12 oz.	Serving: 12 oz.	Serving: 12 oz.
Calories: 180	Calories: 102	Calories: 97	Calories: 95	Calories: 55
Carbs: 18.8g	Carbs: 5g	Carbs: 6.8g	Carbs: 2.6g	Carbs: 1.9g
Sugar: 1g	Sugar: 0g	Sugar: 0g	Sugar: 0g	Sugar: 0g

BEER

Adjusting to the Ketogenic Diet

Adapting to the ketogenic diet and switching from primarily utilizing carbohydrates as fuel to using fat and ketones as fuel takes some time. The length of the adaptation period varies from individual to individual, and we see that the longer someone is on the diet, the more adapted they become over time. Most people start to adapt in as little as two weeks, and realistically by the four- to six-week mark. During this time is when most people experience the "keto flu"—symptoms that can accompany the switch from being a glucose-burner to being a fat-burner.

Here are some tips and strategies that can help alleviate symptoms or speed the transition:

- **Fast intermittently** to help with ketone production and lower blood glucose levels. (See page 49 for more on intermittent fasting.)

- **Fat fast** (drink high-fat coffee, fat shakes, etc.) to give your body material to make ketones.

- **Exercise** to increase fat oxidation and ketone production.

- **Replenish electrolytes** (sodium, calcium, magnesium, and potassium) to prevent symptoms associated with electrolyte depletion. (See page 48 for more on electrolytes.)

- **Drink plenty of water,** because beginning a ketogenic diet causes a drop in insulin that triggers the kidneys to release more water. While your body is adjusting, it's important to drink plenty of water to counter this release of fluid and prevent dehydration, which can cause some symptoms of keto flu.

- **Experiment with exogenous ketones** to provide you with energy and possibly to upregulate ketogenic pathways. Supplementing with ketones will boost your ketone levels in the short term, which can help provide more fuel as your body ramps up its own ketone production. The extra fuel can mean more energy during the transition period. (See Chapter 4 for more on exogenous ketones.)

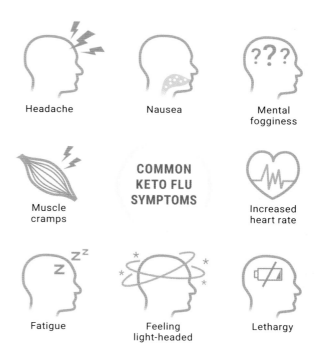

Figure 6.8. *Common symptoms experienced during keto adaptation, also known as the keto flu.*

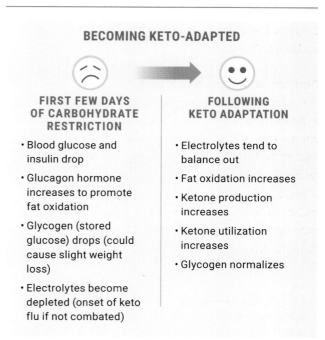

Figure 6.9. *Once keto-adapted, our bodies tend to balance out and regulate biological processes.*

Dining Out Keto

Eating out on a ketogenic diet isn't as hard as you may think. To be honest, it's way easier than eating out on a low-fat diet. Most veggies are cooked in oils and butter anyway, and it's easy to get a fatty cut of meat or a simple salad. Be creative and don't be afraid to ask questions about ingredients. Enjoy yourself!

Be prepared.
Many restaurants offer their menus and even nutrition facts on their websites. If you know where you'll be dining, use this to your advantage by determining which meals are keto-friendly and which are not prior to your visit. When in doubt, picture the Keto Plate (below), which gives you a general idea of what your plate should look like when you dine out. For example, opt for a side salad or green vegetables along with a steak and added butter.

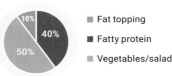

Figure 6.10. *This is what your keto plate should look like.*

10%
40%
50%
■ Fat topping
■ Fatty protein
■ Vegetables/salad

Ask questions.
To the naked eye, some meals may seem more keto-friendly than they are. Some restaurants love to sneak carbs into meals through the use of sauces and glazes. Ask your server about how the food is prepared and what kind of dressings, seasonings, and sauces are used.

Avoid the bread basket.
One of the best ways to do this is to keep it off the table in the first place. If you are out with friends or family who *really* want some bread and you find yourself yearning to dive in, ask for a low-carb appetizer or salad (hold the croutons) instead.

Replace those carb-heavy sides.
Rice and potatoes are among the most common sides. Ask if these can be replaced with keto-friendly vegetables or even a side salad. Some restaurants have even started offering cauliflower rice or mashed cauliflower. WIN!

Get fatty.
When in doubt, order that fatty cut of meat or fish. Even a large salad with added fats from oils and avocados is an excellent option. This, with the addition of a fatty dressing or some butter on your veggies, makes for a great ketogenic meal!

Avoid beer and mixed drinks.
Some people love to have a drink with dinner, but be aware of the options. Try to avoid beers and mixed drinks that are high in sugar; instead, opt for a nice red wine or low-carb beer, which have a lower sugar content.

Drink plenty of water.
Believe it or not, our stomachs have a "full" sensor. While everyone else is filling up on bread or tortilla chips, drink a large glass of water to help fill you up before you even get your low-carb starter or salad. Trust us: the only downside might be having to excuse yourself for a quick restroom break.

Pass on dessert.
Forget the bread basket; skipping dessert may be the hardest part of dining out. When your companions are indulging in after-dinner treats, you may find yourself ready to cave in. Stay strong! Opt for a coffee with heavy cream or even a bowl of sugar-free Jell-O topped with whipped cream. No need for pie or cookies, as you'll likely be full from the nice salad and buttered steak you just ate. If you still find yourself craving sweets, check out the recipe section of this book and wait until you get home to enjoy a keto-friendly dessert.

What to Do If You Hit a Plateau

Upon starting a ketogenic diet, individuals may experience rapid results, including fluctuations in weight, early on. However, people often get frustrated when they hit a plateau after they have been on the diet for some time and are no longer losing weight. Keep in mind that just because your ketone levels aren't registering as high doesn't mean that you have hit a plateau. Here are some quick tips for overcoming a plateau:

• **Track your carbohydrate intake.** People tend to let carbohydrates creep up after they stop tracking. Overcoming a stall in your progress toward your goal could be as simple as cutting out a snack and replacing it with something less "carby."

• **Increase your protein.** Often, people are afraid to bump up their protein intake. Unless you have certain restrictions and absolutely must limit protein for therapeutic reasons, don't be afraid to play around with the protein content of your diet. Granted, you don't want to be eating amounts that are typical of "bros" in the gym or bodybuilders slamming down protein shakes. However, you'd be amazed at the difference adding 15 to 30 grams of protein a day can make for your body composition goals. Though it sounds counterintuitive, slightly bumping up calories from protein or even fat could help get you back on the right track. Less isn't always more.

• **Change your exercise patterns.** Nutrition and exercise are the most important factors in your body composition. If you have hit a plateau and are exercising hard three times a week for an hour each time, try switching it up. Try working out five days a week for 30 to 45 minutes. Providing your body with variation can be the key to seeing results. You'd be amazed at how altering the frequency, duration, and intensity of training can make a difference in body composition.

• **Incorporate mini fasts.** If you aren't incorporating intermittent fasting, experiment with different types of fasting to start. For example, try skipping breakfast and eating only lunch or eating breakfast, skipping lunch, and having only dinner. Then experiment with different fasting styles, such as eighteen-hour, twenty-four-hour, or even longer fasts to see how your body responds.

• **Strategically add carbs around your workouts.** With high-level athletes and people who work out hard, we have found that supplementing with additional carbohydrates around workouts can certainly be beneficial. Now, we aren't saying to load up on candy, but eating a light load (10 to 25 grams) of carbs fifteen to thirty minutes prior to your hardest workouts may help. The adrenaline response you get from a workout can blunt the typical insulin response that would occur. If you are worried about getting kicked out of ketosis, you could use a carbohydrate mouth rinse on your harder training days. Research shows that even just swishing carbohydrates around in your mouth and then spitting them out could have performance benefits.

• **Do a ketogenic cycle.** You may have heard of a practiced called calorie cycling. What we are referring to here is something known as "keto cycling." Dr. Antonio Paoli found that doing a ketogenic diet for a period of time and then transitioning to a lower-carbohydrate diet was beneficial for maintaining progress and then jump-starting further progress after going keto again. Please note: we are not suggesting that you stop eating keto completely and hit a sushi buffet the next day. Rather, a couple days of low- to moderate-carb, higher-protein eating could be a good reset before returning to a ketogenic diet for an extended period. Choosing lower-glycemic carbohydrates is key here. An example protocol might be to go on a ketogenic diet for twelve weeks, then follow a low-carb, higher-protein, moderate-fat diet for one to two weeks, and then repeat the cycle.

Evaluate these suggestions and see where you can play around to optimize the ketogenic diet for *you*. Keep in mind that lowering calories is the last resort we recommend. You can go only so low before it becomes unsustainable, and it can actually slow your metabolism over time, which is definitely not what you want! Our objective is to allow people to eat as much food as possible while continuing to achieve their goal, whether it be to lose fat, gain muscle, or a combination of the two.

Personally, we are fans of keto cycling. We use a slightly modified approach where we typically follow a ketogenic diet for eight to twelve weeks, then go low-carb, high-protein for one to two weeks, and then start going back into ketosis. Remember, everyone is different, and every body reacts and adapts differently. Find what's best for *you*.

Working Out on a Ketogenic Diet

Physical activity is an important part of any lifestyle. Whether it is going for an evening stroll or doing heavy squats, exercise is highly recommended for anyone beginning a ketogenic diet. Given that you are embarking on a complete lifestyle change with the diet, one small addition, such as taking a ten-minute walk at lunch or getting in a workout before or after work, shouldn't be too much to ask. Exercise increases fat metabolism, which can aid in both ketone production and ketone utilization. Our lab has shown that training at higher intensities can increase ketone levels more rapidly compared to training at low intensities or not training at all.

Below we have laid out options for a beginner workout and an advanced workout. Keep in mind that these are just examples, and you can modify them as you see fit—whatever works best with your lifestyle. If you do push-ups, sit-ups, and burpees at home, that's excellent. If you don't want to work out, that's fine, too; try to hit a minimum of 10,000 steps a day (you can track your steps with a fitness watch or even an app on your phone) and stay active in other ways. For more on these workouts, check out www.ketogenic.com/ketogenicbibleworkouts.

Beginner Workout

MONDAY	TUESDAY	WEDNESDAY	THURSDAY	FRIDAY	SATURDAY	SUNDAY
Dumbbell bench press 3x10 Cable chest fly 3x10 Dumbbell shoulder press 3x10 Dumbbell lateral raise 3x10 Cable rope tricep pushdown 3x10	Hit 10,000 steps for daily total	Barbell or Smith machine squat 3x10 Machine leg press 3x10 Bodyweight walking lunge 3x10 Machine leg extension 3x10 Machine leg curl 3x10	Hit 10,000 steps for daily total	One-arm dumbbell row 3x10 Cable lat pulldown 3x10 Seated cable row 3x10 Cable rope face pull 3x10 EZ bar curl 3x10	HIIT 5 rounds: 10 seconds on, 50 seconds off or 1 hour on treadmill	Hit 10,000 steps for daily total

Advanced Workout

MONDAY	TUESDAY	WEDNESDAY	THURSDAY	FRIDAY	SATURDAY	SUNDAY
Barbell bench press 4x12 Barbell row 4x12 Dumbbell chest fly 4x12 Straight-arm pulldown 4x12 Incline dumbbell press 4x12 Single-arm dumbbell row 4x12 Weighted push-up 4xAMRAP* Weighted pull-up 4xAMRAP*	HIIT 5x10 seconds Hanging leg raise 5x25	Barbell squat 4x12 Barbell deadlift 4x12 Barbell walking lunge 4x12 Bulgarian split squat 4x12 Barbell RDL 4x12 Seated leg extension 4x12 Seated leg curl 4x12 Seated leg press 4x12	HIIT 5x15 seconds	Barbell shoulder press 4x12 Dumbbell side lateral raise 4x12 Cable rear delt fly 4x12 Dumbbell Arnold press 4x12 Cable front raise 4x12 EZ bar skull crusher 4x12 EZ bar curl 4x12 Cable rope overhead extension 4x12 Cable rope hammer curl 4x12	5 rounds of 30 seconds each: Mountain climbers Burpees Medicine ball crunches Push-ups	Rest and hit 10,000 steps for daily total

*AMRAP: as many rounds as possible.

Quick-Start Guide

Our best tips, tricks, and strategies for starting out on the ketogenic diet are found in the previous pages, but if you want a quick overview to refer to, this is the page for you.

Educate Yourself

Understand that a ketogenic diet differs from a traditional low-carbohydrate or Paleo diet but encompasses aspects of both. The goal is to become a fat-burner instead of a sugar-burner. (See Chapter 1 for more on the basics.) Look at the recipe section of this book or online (www.ketogenic.com/ketoswap) for keto-friendly alternatives to your favorite dishes and new keto-friendly recipes—there's no reason to feel restricted.

Calculate Your Calories and Macros

Determine your target daily calorie intake and then how much fat, protein, and carbohydrates you plan to eat each day. As a rough estimate, 5 to 10 percent of your daily calorie intake will come from carbohydrates, 20 to 30 percent from protein, and the rest from fat. See page 181 for detailed instructions on calculating calories and macros. In the beginning, it's helpful to use an app like MyFitnessPal to track your meals and ensure that you are staying close to your plan. However, over time the goal is to help you learn how to eat intuitively. Soon enough you will be able to look at certain foods and portions and make your "Keto Plate."

Remove Temptations and Prepare Keto-Friendly Foods

There's no need to test your willpower by having a package of cookies or a batch of cupcakes in the house. Rather, prepare some delicious low-carb alternatives—family members and friends who aren't keto will enjoy them, too. Have fun with it! Also, plan ahead and have on hand keto-friendly snack options, such as string cheese, pork rinds, hard-boiled eggs, beef jerky, and nuts.

Get Moving!

If you are already a gym-goer, continue pushing through. If you don't routinely go to the gym, now is a good time to start. Exercise helps speed the transition to becoming keto-adapted and reduces symptoms of the keto flu.

Push Through the Keto Flu

Becoming keto-adapted can take anywhere from one to three weeks, and during that time you may experience symptoms of the keto flu. Push through and don't give up! Some people adapt a lot faster than others, so give it time. Remember, you have been primarily utilizing glucose your entire life! A few weeks to completely switch your primary fuel source isn't bad. The tips on page 191 can help alleviate the symptoms of keto flu and speed the transition.

Overcome Obstacles

There will always be obstacles, whether plateaus or times when you slip and eat something that's not keto-friendly. Remind yourself why you started a ketogenic diet in the first place. When properly implemented, a ketogenic lifestyle can have numerous benefits. Keep in mind the long-term outcome you are looking for and don't let challenges get in your way.

Enjoy It, Have Fun with It, and Make It a Lifestyle!

Chapter 7:

THE SCIENCE
OF COOKING

After all that information about the science behind the ketogenic diet, you must be eager to start eating this way, if you weren't already. We are scientists, though, so we like to take a scientific approach to everything relating to the ketogenic lifestyle, including cooking. This chapter covers the general functions of macronutrients (fat, protein, and carbohydrate) in cooking and baking. Fiber in itself is not technically a macronutrient; however, it is discussed in this chapter because it falls under a subclassification of carbohydrates. You will also find information about specific ingredient types, such as leaveners, emulsifiers, and cooking fats, in regard to what they do during the cooking process, how they alter a recipe, and how to manipulate them to achieve a desired outcome.

Macronutrients

The three main macronutrients are fat, protein, and carbohydrate. All diets feature some combination of these macronutrients. In Chapter 3, we looked at how fat, protein, and carbohydrate act in the body; here, we'll examine their roles in food and cooking.

Fat

Cooking fats are derived from many different animal and plant sources, including butter from milk fat, lard from pork, coconut oil from coconut, olive oil from olives, nut oils from various nuts, and vegetable oils from grains. These can be further divided into saturated and unsaturated fats; unsaturated fats can be further separated into monounsaturated and polyunsaturated fats (see page 44).

Saturated fats are found primarily in animal foods but are also found in some plant sources, such as coconut and palm oil. At room temperature, saturated fats are solid. Unsaturated fats are found primarily in plant foods, such as grains, nuts, and seeds, but are also present in fatty fish, such as salmon. While different fats are used for different purposes in cooking, as we will discuss later in this chapter, in general fat provides taste, texture, and tenderness.

Protein

Protein comes from both animal and plant sources. Proteins are found in the musculature of animals; in plants, protein is found primarily in the germ of the grain. Amino acids, which are the building blocks of protein, can be categorized as essential and nonessential: there are nine essential amino acids that you need to get from your diet and eleven nonessential amino acids that your body can make on its own. In cooking, protein provides structure, texture, and thickness and acts as an aggregate, binding foods together.

Carbohydrate

Carbohydrates come from plant sources, such as fruits, vegetables, and grains. These can be broken down into many categories, including starch or polysaccharides, fiber, oligosaccharides, disaccharides, and monosaccharides (see page 40). The structure of a grain is the bran, germ, and endosperm. The bran is the outer layer and contains fiber, minerals, and antioxidants. The next layer, the germ, contains fats, vitamins, and phytonutrients. Finally, the endosperm contains primarily carbohydrates and protein. The general functions of carbohydrates in cooking include providing structure/stability, tenderizing (i.e., softening), delaying coagulation/crystallization (i.e., hardening), and adding sweetness.

Fiber

Dietary fiber, found in plants, cannot be digested. Fiber is divided into two categories: soluble and insoluble. Soluble fiber dissolves when added to water, while insoluble fiber does not, but both can be fermented by gut bacteria. The function of fiber in cooking is to add bulk, absorb water, bind ingredients together, and improve the overall nutrient density of a food.

Ingredients and Their Functions

Before going over the various keto-friendly ingredients that are used to make the recipes in this book, it's important to understand the palate: the ultimate judge of your efforts in the kitchen! The palate has five different taste sensors: salty, sweet, sour, bitter, and umami. These five aspects of taste should be taken into consideration when cooking savory or sweet foods. Other things that affect the palate include ingredients such as herbs, spices, flavorings, extracts, fats and oils, and sweeteners, along with cooking times and methods.

Fats and Oils

As mentioned previously, the function of fats and oils in cooking is to provide taste, texture, and tenderness to foods. Different fats have different effects, and using the correct fat for the task at hand is important for achieving the desired outcome. Simply put, ingredients that are higher in saturated fat are solid at room temperature, and ingredients that are higher in polyunsaturated and monounsaturated fats are liquid at room temperature. Some of the most common fats and oils used in cooking are listed below.

Butter
Butter is composed primarily of saturated fat, which is why it is solid at room temperature. Depending on the source (i.e., higher milk fat or lower milk fat), the fat content will range from 70 to 80 percent, with the other 20 to 30 percent being whey protein, lactose, and various milk solids. Butter provides flakiness and crispness to doughs such as puff pastries and pie crusts: as butter is heated, it emits steam, which becomes trapped in the dough and acts as a natural leavener. Butter also adds flavor, particularly to baked goods, by interacting with the lecithin found in eggs. Lecithin is an emulsifier, which means that it binds together compounds that would normally not be attracted. When the fat in butter is attracted to the lecithin in eggs, it emulsifies the fat with the liquids and other compounds to create a more homogenous or evenly distributed flavor. Butter is a friend, not a foe!

Clarified Butter and Ghee
Clarified butter and ghee are essentially butter with the milk solids removed. (See page 348 to learn how to make clarified butter and ghee.) With the milk solids removed, the smoke point of the resulting fat is higher (for a discussion of smoke points, see page 199).

Lard
Lard is a solid fat that has been rendered from pork fat. Lard functions similarly to butter, providing flavor, crispness, flakiness, and tenderness to baked goods, but it has a much stronger flavor. This is because as lard is rendered from pork fat, some connective tissue and muscle in the fat may impart

a "porky" flavor to the lard. After being rendered, the fat is strained to clarify it. Leaf lard, which is made from the fat around the kidneys, is considered to be the very best lard. Lard can be substituted for butter in recipes; just use one-quarter less than the amount of butter called for.

Nut, Seed, and Vegetable Oils

Nut, seed, and vegetable oils are derived from many plants, including peanut, hazelnut, grapeseed, sunflower, sesame, soybean, corn, olive, and safflower plants, to name a few. These oils are liquid at room temperature because they have more unsaturated fat than saturated fat. They are used for cooking over an open flame because they tend to have higher smoke points, which enables them to be used at higher temperatures without burning. In baking they provide not only tenderness but also taste, a more desirable mouthfeel, and lubrication. One of the main advantages of liquid fats is that many of them (especially vegetable oils) are shelf-stable and thus have a longer shelf life. Due to their mild taste, they are generally used to produce dressings, vinaigrettes, and sauces.

Coconut Oil

Coconut oil, unlike nut oils, is solid at room temperature due to its high concentration of saturated fat, but it acts more like a nut oil when added to baked goods. It does not provide good flake or crispness to pastries, but it does provide tenderness and a subtle flavor. Coconut oil is about 50 percent MCTs, making it advantageous on a ketogenic diet (see page 47). Furthermore, coconut oil can be substituted in equal amounts for any liquid nut, seed, or vegetable oil. When substituting coconut oil for a solid fat, such as butter or lard, however, use 25 percent less coconut oil than what's called for in the recipe.

MCT Oil

Medium-chain triglycerides (MCTs) are fatty acids that are quickly and easily burned to produce ketones (see page 55). MCT oil, which is 100 percent MCTs, is liquid at room temperature. Therefore, in cooking, it functions as a liquid oil, not a solid fat. Because it has a relatively low smoke point, it should not be used for high-heat cooking, such as pan-searing, grilling, or sautéing. However, it can be used

Smoke Points

An oil's smoke point is the point at which it begins to give off a bluish smoke and an altered smell. At that point, the fats in the oil are beginning to change, which will affect the smell and taste of the food, sometimes producing an undesirable flavor. The smoke point of an oil depends on various factors, such as the type of fat (saturated or unsaturated), the amount of oil used, and whether the oil has been exposed to light, moisture, higher temperatures, or oxygen. This exposure increases the amount of free fatty acids in the oil, causing them to oxidize, or begin to breakdown.

In addition, highly refined fats and oils have a higher smoke point. Below are the smoke points of common cooking fats and oils that are commonly used on a ketogenic diet.

COOKING FATS AND OILS	SMOKE POINT
Flaxseed oil	225°F
Sunflower oil	225°F–440°F
Extra-virgin olive oil	320°F
MCT oil	320°F
Peanut oil	320°F–450°F
Butter	350°F
Coconut oil	350°F
Lard	370°F
Macadamia nut oil	390°F
Canola oil	400°F
Walnut oil	400°F
Sesame oil	410°F–450°F
Virgin olive oil	420°F
Extra-light olive oil	468°F
Safflower oil	510°F
Avocado oil	520°F

in salad dressings and in relatively low-temperature baking. Because it has a mild flavor, it can be paired with a wide range of ingredients and flavors. Please note, however, that large quantities of MCT oil may cause gastrointestinal complications, so it should be used sparingly when being introduced to a diet to assess tolerance. (See page 56 for more.) If you are new to MCT oil, start with 5 to 7 grams a day and build up from there.

Flours and Binding Agents

The grain-based flours used in traditional baking provide structure and, when mixed with water, form gluten, the elastic and structural component associated with traditional baked goods. When baked goods rise and expand, gluten traps the air that is produced, retaining the expansion. Gluten also provides the chewy, spongy texture found in many breads, such as French bread and English muffins. The mechanical action of kneading helps develop the gluten. Depending on the end product, different doughs are kneaded for varying amounts of time to develop the gluten. For example, a French bread dough is kneaded for longer than the dough used to make soft hamburger buns. In some baked goods, however, the gluten is avoided as much as possible: the ingredients for muffins, which are meant to have a tender, not chewy, crumb, are quickly whisked together, not kneaded.

Flours with high amounts of gluten tend to have high amounts of carbohydrates; therefore, they cannot be used on a ketogenic diet. On a ketogenic diet, a variety of nut and seed flours and meals are used in place of wheat flour to provide chewiness without carbohydrates. These include coconut flour, almond flour, hazelnut flour/meal, peanut flour, flaxseed meal, hempseed meal, and psyllium husk. Emulsification agents such as xanthan gum, guar gum, and cellulose gum are often used in ketogenic baking to bind together these flours and retain moisture in the end product.

Nut butters, ground seeds such as flax, chia seeds, and psyllium husk also act as binding agents with gluten-free flours due to their ability to absorb water. When making baked goods with low-carbohydrate, gluten-free flours, you will have the best chance of achieving a consistency similar to their high-carbohydrate, high-gluten counterparts if you mix these alternative flours with binding agents. In this book, the recipes for zucchini bread (page 226), chocolate chip cookies (page 306), and carrot cake (page 334) all use binding agents.

Another binding agent that works very well in baked goods is whey protein powder. Depending on the type of protein powder and alternative flours being used, it's possible to produce a final product that is very similar to the "real" thing. A blend of whey protein isolate and casein protein, similar to that found in Quest Protein Multi-Purpose Mix, is optimal for baking. Not only is the Quest mix great for replicating the mouthfeel, texture, and consistency of wheat flour, but it also includes xanthan gum and cellulose gum to bind baked goods together.

Leaveners

Leavening gives lift and rise to baked goods and lightens their texture. Leavening can be achieved by mechanical means or by using leavening agents, such as baking soda or baking powder (chemical agents) or yeast (a biological agent). In ketogenic baking, mechanical and chemical leavening is used, but biological leavening is not, for reasons explained below.

Examples of mechanical leavening include creaming butter and sweetener or whipping egg whites to form a meringue. When air is incorporated into a baked good, as it is in these methods, it expands when heated to make the baked good rise.

Leavening agents work by producing carbon dioxide gas bubbles that are trapped in the baked good to make it rise. Examples of chemical leaveners are baking soda and baking powder. Carbon dioxide is created when the sodium bicarbonate in these leaveners (a base) comes into contact with an acidic component, such as lemon juice or vinegar, and water. Baking soda is purely sodium bicarbonate and reacts with the acidic compounds in baked goods. For example, in the blueberry cake recipe on page 328, baking soda is mixed with lemon juice to produce carbon dioxide, which helps the cobbler rise. However, in a recipe that does not use an acidic ingredient like lemon juice, it is advantageous to use baking powder, which is baking soda combined with acidic compounds, typically sodium aluminum sulfate and monocalcium phosphate. When mixed with water, baking powder causes a chemical reaction that produces carbon dioxide, increasing the volume of a baked good. An example is the carrot cake recipe on page 334; baking powder is used in this recipe because the batter does not include an acidic component.

Yeast is a biological leavening agent. Like chemical leaveners, it creates carbon dioxide, but it does so through the natural process of fermentation. A microscopic, single-cell living organism, yeast transforms its food (carbohydrates) into carbon dioxide and ethyl alcohol, which are then trapped in the baked good via the mechanism of gluten and cause the product to rise. Yeast is rarely used in ketogenic baking because there is little to no carbohydrate present for the yeast to ferment.

Sweeteners

Sugar is the standard ingredient for sweetening any food product, but other sweeteners include honey, maple syrup, agave nectar, coconut palm sugar, corn syrup, and fruits. All of these sweeteners are carbohydrate-heavy and therefore are not included in a ketogenic diet. In place of caloric sweeteners, non-caloric sweeteners can be used. Two categories of non-caloric sweeteners are artificial sweeteners and sugar alcohols.

Artificial sweeteners can be made from plants or even sugar. Because they are exponentially sweeter than sugar, they are generally combined with maltodextrin or dextrose—sugars—as a carrying agent for commercial use. If you want to avoid the carrying agent (the maltodextrin or dextrose), opt for the "raw" versions of these sweeteners, which are simply the artificial sweetener with no additive. These raw sweeteners should be used very sparingly because they are so sweet. For example, the chocolate peanut butter fudge recipe on page 326

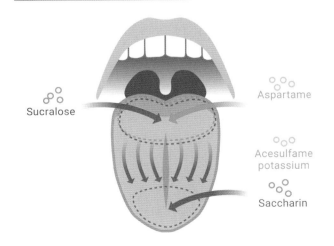

Figure 7.1. *How different artificial sweeteners hit the palate.*

calls for a very small amount of raw sucralose, which is about 600 times as sweet as sugar. Other non-caloric artificial sweeteners include acesulfame potassium, aspartame, neotame, and saccharin.

Artificial sweeteners tend to attack the palate differently, which is why they're usually used in combination. For example, sucralose is tasted on the back of the tongue at first, then slowly makes its way toward the front of the tongue. Aspartame and acesulfame potassium give a stronger sweetness on the back of the tongue, with less on the front. Saccharin gives a stronger sweetness on the front of the tongue, with less on the back. However, as we will discuss, we really don't encourage the use of saccharin.

A relatively new sweetener that has emerged in recent years is monk fruit, or luo han guo, a fruit native to southern China. Monk fruit has been used for centuries in traditional Chinese medicine, but the FDA didn't approve its use as a sweetener until 2010. This fruit is used to create a sweetener that is about 400 times sweeter than cane sugar. Monk fruit is virtually calorie-free; therefore, it can be used on a ketogenic diet.

Another sweetener that falls into the category of natural sweeteners is stevia. Stevia is derived from the *Stevia rebaudiana* plant and contains a compound called steviol glycosides, which are extracted and made into the common sweetener stevia. Stevia is approximately 300 times sweeter than sugar; therefore, it can be used in very small amounts to add sweetness to foods. Research shows that stevia is very safe and has many health benefits, such as acting as an antimicrobial, lowering blood sugar by decreasing glucose production in the liver, improving insulin sensitivity, having anti-inflammatory properties, and protecting the liver.

Sugar alcohols are naturally occurring in plants and are not calorie-free like artificial sweeteners. They range from 1.5 to 3 calories per gram, whereas regular sugar has 4 calories per gram. Sugar alcohols include erythritol, maltitol, mannitol, sorbitol, xylitol, lactitol, and isomalt. Sugar alcohols range in their degree of sweetness, although most of them are less sweet than sugar. Note that they may cause gastrointestinal distress, such as gas, bloating, constipation, and diarrhea. As you can see in Figure 7.3, some of the sugar alcohols typically found in "sugar-free" candy, like maltitol

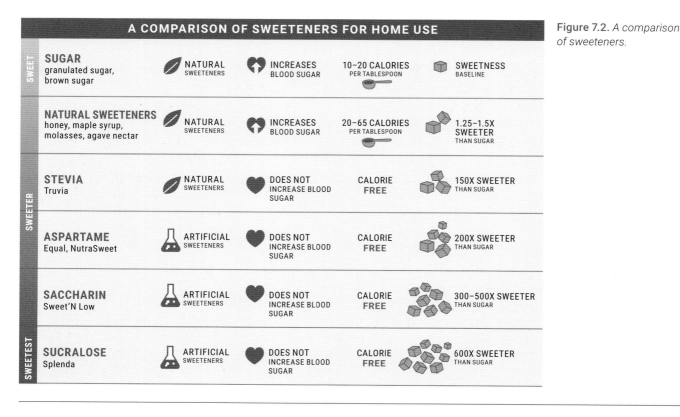

Figure 7.2. *A comparison of sweeteners.*

A COMPARISON OF SWEETENERS FOR HOME USE

SWEET — **SUGAR** granulated sugar, brown sugar	NATURAL SWEETENERS	INCREASES BLOOD SUGAR	10–20 CALORIES PER TABLESPOON	SWEETNESS BASELINE
NATURAL SWEETENERS honey, maple syrup, molasses, agave nectar	NATURAL SWEETENERS	INCREASES BLOOD SUGAR	20–65 CALORIES PER TABLESPOON	1.25–1.5X SWEETER THAN SUGAR
SWEETER — **STEVIA** Truvia	NATURAL SWEETENERS	DOES NOT INCREASE BLOOD SUGAR	CALORIE FREE	150X SWEETER THAN SUGAR
ASPARTAME Equal, NutraSweet	ARTIFICIAL SWEETENERS	DOES NOT INCREASE BLOOD SUGAR	CALORIE FREE	200X SWEETER THAN SUGAR
SACCHARIN Sweet'N Low	ARTIFICIAL SWEETENERS	DOES NOT INCREASE BLOOD SUGAR	CALORIE FREE	300–500X SWEETER THAN SUGAR
SWEETEST — **SUCRALOSE** Splenda	ARTIFICIAL SWEETENERS	DOES NOT INCREASE BLOOD SUGAR	CALORIE FREE	600X SWEETER THAN SUGAR

and polyglycitol, have a robust glycemic index and therefore aren't recommended for consumption in large amounts.

Two new groups of ingredients have surfaced in recent years: functional fibers and rare sugars.

Functional fibers, which occur naturally in small amounts in plants, are added to foods to boost sweetness and increase nutrient density. These fibers are made up of a mixture of short-chain carbohydrates and tend to be very sweet but relatively indigestible by our gut enzymes. Examples include isomaltooligosaccharides (IMOs), inulin, and soluble corn fiber.

Unlike other types of fiber, IMOs raise blood insulin and glucose levels, as shown in Figures 7.4 and 7.5. IMOs are about half as sweet as sugar, can be found in liquid form, and can easily be added to any recipe; simply substitute the IMO for 25 to 50 percent of the indicated sweetener. IMOs have an elevation of blood glucose and insulin similar to slow-digesting oatmeal.

Inulin is also a functional fiber, but unlike IMOs, it doesn't affect blood glucose or insulin. However, in relatively small quantities (5 to 10 grams), inulin has been shown to cause extreme gastrointestinal distress in first-time users, although the gastrointestinal issues tend to diminish over time

as people incorporate the fiber into their diet. Inulin comes in a powdered form that is water-soluble and slightly sweet; when using it in recipes, opt for smaller amounts—3 to 5 grams for single-serving recipes or 8 to 11 grams for bulk recipes.

Soluble corn fiber (SCF) is a versatile fiber similar to IMOs in appearance and sweetness. The benefit of this ingredient is that it produces almost no increase in blood glucose or insulin. The sugar molecules in soluble corn fiber are indigestible by the enzymes in the digestive system, and current research shows that it is minimally digested. Soluble

Glycemic Index

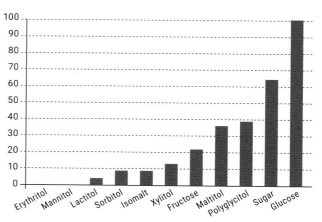

Figure 7.3. *The glycemic index of various sweeteners.*

corn fiber also has a beneficial impact on the gut bacteria. In relatively low doses, SCF has been shown to have the same gastrointestinal benefits as inulin, without the distress. Soluble corn fiber aids in the secretion of hormones PYY and GLP-1, which help increase satiety and decrease hunger. This makes it a good option for a ketogenic diet because it confers the same gut health benefits of fiber as foods containing carbohydrates, decreases hunger, and has little to no effect on blood glucose, with relatively the same sweetness as high-fructose corn syrup.

Allulose is a new ingredient known as a rare sugar, meaning that it is found in small quantities in nature. The benefit of allulose is that it has a syrupy consistency and is almost 95 percent excreted, meaning that the body does not break it down. It can be used very similarly to a liquid sugar in cooking, but it may cause gastrointestinal distress; therefore, it should not be used in significant amounts (more than 10 grams).

Understanding the differences among artificial sweeteners, sugar alcohols, functional fibers, and rare sugars is key in optimizing a ketogenic diet. Although some products claim to be "sugar-free," it's important to do your due diligence and understand the definition of "sugar" in order to avoid foods that could kick you out of ketosis.

Seasonings, Flavorings, Extracts, and Spices

Seasoning, flavorings, extracts, and spices all serve to enhance the flavor of food, but each functions in a different way. For example, salt interacts with the molecules in a food, making them more volatile on the tongue. Salt enhances savory flavors, increases sweetness, decreases bitterness, and stabilizes sour flavors, depending on the concentration of these flavors in the food and the amount of salt used. Many recipes direct you to add salt "to taste" because many factors go into the final taste of a food; therefore, calling for an exact amount of salt will not always yield the best-tasting result. This same rule applies to black pepper, which is added to food not to make it spicy but to open up the taste buds on the tongue to allow more and stronger flavors to come across the palate. This is why tasting food while cooking is encouraged: it helps you understand not only the flavor profile of the dish but also what needs to be added to improve the dining experience.

Flavorings and extracts are concentrated sources of one specific essence. A flavorful substance is steeped or dissolved in a strong alcohol (normally white rum) because the alcohol readily absorbs the flavor. The flavoring in the alcohol is so concentrated that only a very small amount is required in a recipe. Flavorings and extracts are great for ketogenic cooking because they expand the range of flavors available for use. For example, the chocolate peanut butter banana truffle recipe on page 336 uses banana extract to give the truffles a banana flavor because bananas are too high in carbohydrates to be part of a ketogenic diet.

Blood Insulin Response

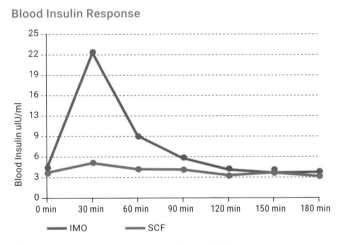

Figure 7.4. *Insulin responses to IMO and SCF.*

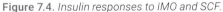

Blood Glucose Response

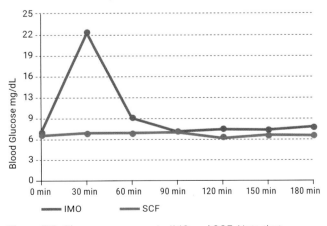

Figure 7.5. *Glucose responses to IMO and SCF. Note that IMO increases glucose while SCF does not.*

Spices are extremely versatile ingredients in any kitchen. Not only do they provide particular flavor compounds and tastes, but they also can improve the experience of eating a dish. For example, in the cardamom snickerdoodles with maple bourbon caramel recipe on page 310, the cardamom, cinnamon, toasted butter, maple extract, and bourbon not only improve the overall taste of the cookie but also offer a layered experience of flavor.

Glossary of Cooking Terms

Al dente. Derived from Italian, it translates as "to the tooth." Generally used to describe when pasta is cooked until firm to the bite, not soft or mushy, but not undercooked. However, since pasta is omitted from a ketogenic diet, in this book *al dente* is used for cooking vegetables. When vegetables are cooked al dente, they have lost their raw, earthy, starchy taste but are not soft or mushy. The cooking time will vary depending on the size, cut, and variety of the vegetable; therefore, tasting the vegetables throughout the cooking process is crucial to avoid undercooking or overcooking.

Blanch. Vegetables are blanched as a par-cooking technique. When blanching a vegetable, the goal is to cook it thoroughly so that it can be quickly sautéed. To blanch vegetables, you fill a large saucepan or stockpot three-quarters full of water and place it over high heat. The water should then be brought to a boil, with the pot covered. Salt, if using, should be added to the water after it has come to a boil. The food is submerged in the boiling water in a colander, strainer, or freely for the amount of time the recipe calls for or until al dente.

Brine. To submerge a meat, normally poultry, in a water and sodium chloride (salt) solution. This is done to increase the moistness of the meat, once cooked. When meat is brined, it undergoes the following two key processes, both of which help to prevent meat from drying out during cooking: first, the water is absorbed into the cells of the meat to increase hydration; second, the salt denatures the protein in the meat, which allows water to be trapped. A standard ratio for a brine is 1 tablespoon of salt per 1 cup of water, but the amount of salt may increase depending on the size of the protein being brined. Depending on the size and weight of the protein being brined, the process can take anywhere from 30 minutes to a few days. Brines can contain many flavoring agents such as herbs, spices, and extracts to impart more flavor into the meat.

Caramelization. The process by which the sugar in flours, syrups, and vegetables begins to brown due to its interaction with heat. Caramelization alters the flavor and texture of a food.

Deglaze. When sautéing or pan-searing meat, the Maillard reaction occurs, which causes the meat to brown. It also leaves a brown residue on the bottom of the pan, which has great flavor for a sauce or glaze. To deglaze the pan, you add hot stock, wine, or liquid to the pan over heat to remove this brown, flavorful residue. After adding the deglazing liquid, you scrape the bottom of the pan with a spatula or other cooking tool to release the flavorful residue.

Depouillage. Derived from French, it translates as "to skim fat." This term refers to the action of removing the fat that may develop when cooking a soup, stock, or sauce. This can be done by offsetting the saucepan or stockpot over the burner so that only half of it is touching the heat. Then bring the liquid to a boil and allow the fat to float to one side. Next, using a spoon or ladle, skim the top of the liquid to remove the excess fat.

Disgorge. To remove excess water from vegetables. Some vegetables, such as eggplant, squash, and zucchini, have a very high water content, which is not optimal when cooking over high heat with oil because caramelization may not occur if the water content is high. Furthermore, vegetables such as eggplant have a very bitter taste due to the phenolic compounds they contain. Along with removing water from eggplant, disgorging it removes any bitter taste. Therefore, if you plan to pan-fry vegetables with a high water content or plan to use a dry heat method, such as grilling or roasting, it is best to disgorge the vegetables first. (If you plan to cook the vegetables in water or to steam them, disgorging isn't necessary.) To disgorge a vegetable, place the sliced vegetable in a colander over a container or sink, generously coat the vegetable with kosher salt, and allow it to sit for 30 to 60 minutes. This will remove excess water from the vegetable, ensuring that it cooks properly.

Fold. To homogenously combine ingredients while preserving volume. Most often, this term is used to describe the action of incorporating a lighter ingredient, such as whipped egg whites or whipped cream, into a heavier ingredient, such as a batter. Due to the fact the whipped ingredient(s) have had air incorporated into them, gently folding it into another ingredient preserves volume so that the final product may rise and maintain volume after cooking.

Homogenous. To make ingredients homogenous is to combine them so that the flavors, textures, and colors are evenly distributed.

Maillard reaction (Maillard browning). The Maillard reaction is the browning of meat. It is caused by the reaction between the sugars and the protein in that meat. When introduced to heat, the proteins break down, which causes the change in flavor, texture, and smell of the meat.

Pickle. Pickling is a method that was used before refrigeration to preserve food, but is still used today. The most common form is to submerge a vegetable, fruit, or meat in a water, vinegar, and sodium chloride (salt) solution. The goal with pickling is to reduce the pH of the food to or below 4.6 so that bacteria cannot grow. This process is normally done at room temperature (70°F to 75°F). Pickled foods can be shelf-stable if the proper recipe is followed.

Pulse. To blend ingredients in a food processor or blender in increments of 1 to 2 seconds. This ensures that the ingredients blend properly and do not simply spin in the vortex of the blender or food processor, and it allows you to have greater control over the consistency of the blended food.

Sear. To cook food over very high heat with a little oil. Searing meats results in a crisp, browned outside, known as Maillard browning. This technique is great for adding flavor to steaks, roasts, and poultry to add another layer of flavor to a dish.

Shock. To stop the cooking process by submerging a cooked food in very cold water. The step of shocking vegetables normally follows the process of blanching. To shock a vegetable, you fill a bowl or container with ice and water, then submerge the blanched vegetable in the cold water to stop the cooking.

Sweat. To cook a vegetable over low heat with a little oil. The goal is to partially cook or soften vegetables to develop their flavor before other ingredients are added. When sweating vegetables, excess moisture is cooked off (during this process, beads of moisture will appear on the surface of the vegetables—thus the term "sweating"). The result is cooked vegetables that can be used in soups, sauces, stews, or any dish where one would want to highlight the presence of that vegetable.

Whip. Whipping is used to make a meringue or whipped cream. It is done by vigorously whisking egg whites or heavy cream for 1 to 3 minutes to create a voluminous mixture that has trapped air.

Chapter 8:

RECIPES

CLASSIC POWDERED CAKE DOUGHNUTS

Macronutrients per serving: Calories 465 | Fat 35.8g | Carbohydrate 5.3g | Fiber 1.8g | Protein 30.5g

Makes: 12 doughnuts (2 per serving) | Prep time: 10 minutes, plus 20 minutes to cool | Cook time: 9 to 11 minutes

1 cup Dymatize Protein Powder Birthday Cake

½ cup Quest Protein Powder Vanilla Milkshake

⅔ cup blanched almond flour

½ teaspoon baking powder

¼ teaspoon ground cinnamon

⅛ teaspoon kosher salt

3 eggs

1 teaspoon vanilla extract

¾ cup (1½ sticks) unsalted butter, softened

1 tablespoon granulated erythritol

⅛ teaspoon raw sucralose

3 tablespoons chopped macadamia nuts

¼ cup powdered erythritol

SPECIAL EQUIPMENT:

2 (6-cavity) nonstick doughnut pans

01 Preheat the oven to 350°F.

02 Sift the protein powders, almond flour, baking powder, cinnamon, and salt into a large bowl.

03 In another bowl, whisk together the eggs and vanilla extract until well combined.

04 In a separate large bowl with a hand mixer, or in the bowl of a tabletop mixer, cream the butter, granulated erythritol, and sucralose. With the mixer running, slowly add the egg mixture and beat until smooth. With the mixer still running, slowly add the dry ingredients and beat until smooth and homogeneous, then fold in the macadamia nuts.

05 Pour the batter into the doughnut pans, filling the cavities three-quarters full. Bake for 9 to 11 minutes, until a toothpick inserted into a doughnut comes out clean.

06 Remove the doughnuts from the pan, place on a cooling rack, and allow to cool for about 20 minutes. Once cool, put the powdered erythritol in a medium-sized bowl and toss the doughnuts one at a time in the sweetener until fully coated.

07 Store in an airtight container in the refrigerator for up to 4 days.

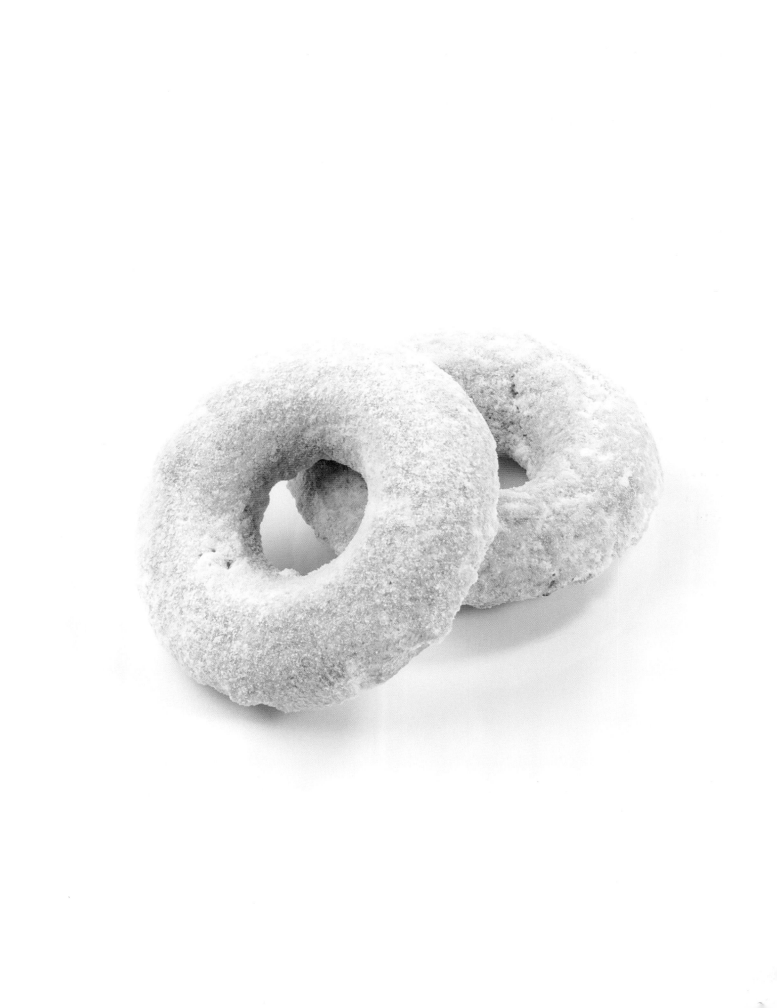

CAULIFLOWER OVERNIGHT "OATS"

Macronutrients per serving: Calories 258 | Fat 18g | Carbohydrate 13.2g | Fiber 8.2g | Protein 10.8g

Makes: 4 servings | Prep time: 20 minutes, plus overnight to thicken | Cook time: —

1 quart water

1 medium head cauliflower (5 to 6 inches in diameter), cored and florets grated

1 cup unsweetened almond milk

¼ cup Quest Protein Powder Vanilla Milkshake

¼ cup ground flax seeds

3 tablespoons coconut oil powder or MCT oil powder

2 tablespoons coconut oil or MCT oil

2 tablespoons chia seeds

2 tablespoons unsweetened coconut flakes

1 tablespoon psyllium husk powder

1 tablespoon ground cinnamon

1 teaspoon vanilla extract

¼ teaspoon ground allspice

¼ teaspoon ground cardamom

¼ teaspoon ground cloves

¼ teaspoon ginger powder

¼ teaspoon ground nutmeg

¼ teaspoon raw stevia powder, or 1 to 2 tablespoons granulated erythritol

01 Bring the water to a boil in a saucepan over high heat. While the water is heating, line a fine-mesh sieve with cheesecloth. Blanch the cauliflower in the boiling water for 3 to 4 minutes. Remove from the water and place in the sieve to drain for 5 to 10 minutes.

02 Place all the ingredients in a large bowl and mix until well incorporated. Divide among four 12-ounce (or larger) containers or jars and refrigerate overnight.

03 Serve chilled. Store leftovers in the refrigerator for up to 5 days.

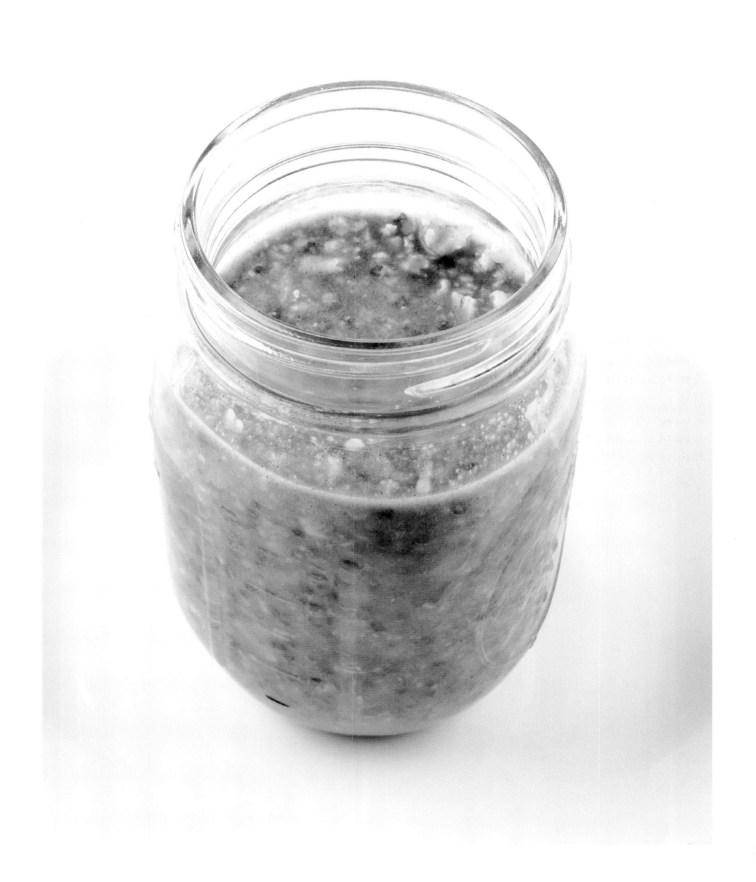

COCONUT CHOCOLATE CHIP MUFFINS

Macronutrients per serving: **Calories 394 | Fat 30g | Carbohydrate 14.9g | Fiber 7.3g | Protein 15.9g**

Makes: **12 muffins (2 per serving)** | Prep time: **20 minutes** | Cook time: **20 to 23 minutes**

⅔ cup high-fiber coconut flour

¼ cup Quest Protein Powder Banana Cream

1½ tablespoons Quest Protein Powder Vanilla Milkshake

¼ cup granulated erythritol

1 teaspoon baking powder

¼ teaspoon kosher salt

6 ounces (¾ cup) cream cheese, softened

⅔ cup plain 2% fat Greek yogurt

3 tablespoons unsalted butter, softened

4 eggs

¼ cup Lily's 55% Cocoa Premium Baking Chips

FOR THE CHOCOLATE COATING:

2 ounces unsweetened chocolate (100% cacao), roughly chopped

1 tablespoon unsalted butter, softened

½ teaspoon raw sucralose

3 tablespoons unsweetened shredded coconut, for garnish

01 Preheat the oven to 350°F and line a 12-well muffin tin with paper liners.

02 Sift the coconut flour, protein powders, erythritol, baking powder, and salt into a large bowl; set aside.

03 In another large bowl or the bowl of a tabletop mixer, using a hand mixer or the whisk attachment for the tabletop mixer, cream the cream cheese, yogurt, and butter until smooth, 2 to 3 minutes. Add the eggs, one at a time, continuing to beat until the wet ingredients are fully combined.

04 Pour the wet ingredients into the dry ingredients and combine with the mixer until smooth. Fold in the chocolate chips.

05 Pour the batter into a pastry bag, then pipe it into the muffin cups, filling them about three-quarters full. Bake for 20 to 23 minutes, until a toothpick inserted in the center of a muffin comes out clean.

06 Remove the muffins from the pan and place on a cooling rack to cool.

07 While the muffins are cooling, prepare the chocolate coating: Place the chopped chocolate in a microwave-safe bowl. Microwave on high for 2 to 3 minutes, stirring every 30 seconds, until smooth. Add the butter and sucralose to the melted chocolate and mix to incorporate.

08 Once the muffins are cool, dip the tops in the melted chocolate (you may need to rewarm the chocolate in the microwave for 15 to 30 seconds if it begins to solidify), then sprinkle the tops with shredded coconut. Store in an airtight container at room temperature for up to 3 days, or freeze for up to 1 month.

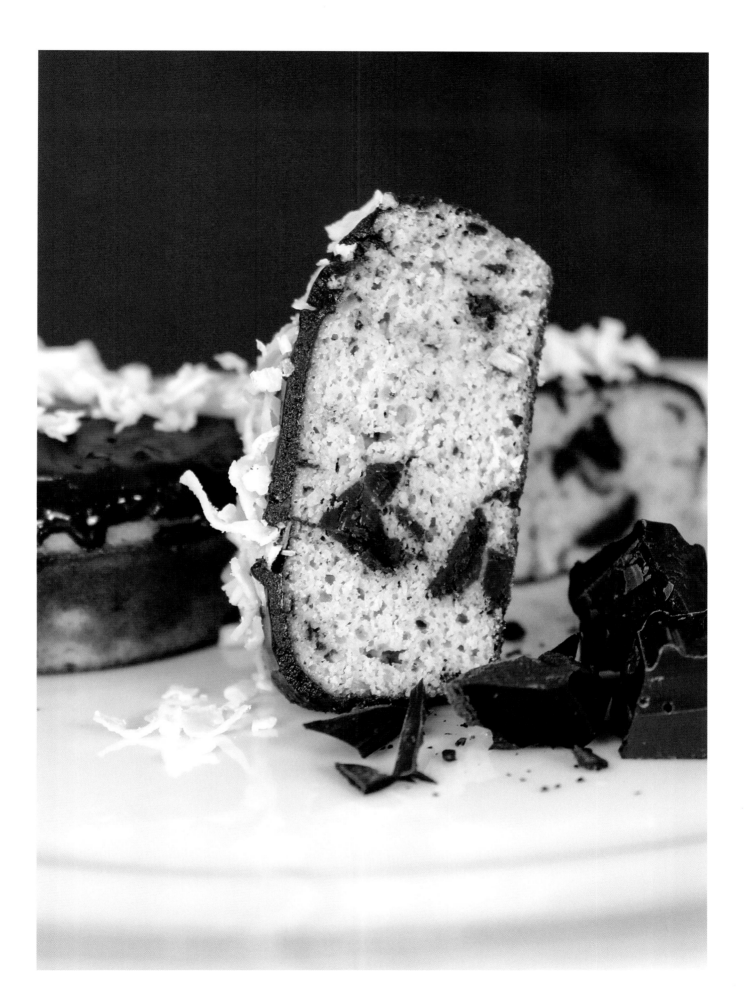

BREAKFAST LASAGNA

Macronutrients per serving: **Calories 434** | **Fat 32.1g** | **Carbohydrate 10.1g** | **Fiber 1.6g** | **Protein 27.4g**

Makes: **4 servings** | Prep time: **20 minutes** | Cook time: **About 50 minutes**

½ (14½-ounce) can crushed tomatoes

½ bunch fresh basil, chopped

1 teaspoon garlic powder

1 tablespoon plus ½ teaspoon kosher salt, divided

6 slices bacon

1 medium yellow squash (about 5 ounces), thinly sliced into half-moons

1 medium zucchini (about 5 ounces), thinly sliced into half-moons

4 ounces ricotta cheese

½ cup shredded mozzarella cheese (about 2 ounces)

2 ounces Serrano ham or other cured ham of choice (optional)

½ small onion, thinly sliced

6 eggs

⅓ cup heavy cream

¼ cup grated Parmesan cheese (about 1 ounce)

01 Preheat the oven to 350°F. Place a cooling rack inside a sheet pan and set aside.

02 Make the sauce: In a large saucepan, simmer the crushed tomatoes, basil, garlic powder, and ½ teaspoon of the salt over medium heat for 20 minutes.

03 Place the bacon on the rack in the sheet pan. Bake for 10 to 15 minutes, until crisp. When the bacon is done, cut the slices in half crosswise.

04 While the sauce and bacon are cooking, place the yellow squash and zucchini slices on a sheet pan and salt evenly with the remaining tablespoon of salt; this will draw out the moisture. Allow to sit for 10 to 15 minutes, then rinse in a colander to remove the majority of the salt.

05 To assemble the lasagna, coat the bottom of a 9 by 5-inch loaf pan or 8-inch square baking dish with 2 to 3 tablespoons of the sauce. Cover the sauce with half of the ricotta, mozzarella, cooked bacon, ham (if using), squash slices, and onion slices. Add the remaining sauce, then repeat with the remaining cheeses, meat, and vegetables.

06 In a large bowl, whisk together the eggs and heavy cream, then pour the mixture over the layered ingredients.

07 Bake the lasagna for 30 to 33 minutes, rotating the pan halfway through, until the eggs have set (the lasagna will have very little visible liquid remaining) and the edges have begun to brown. Remove from the oven, top with the Parmesan cheese, and place back in the oven until the Parmesan has browned, about 2 minutes.

08 Slice into 4 equal portions and serve hot. Store leftovers in an airtight container in the refrigerator for up to 4 days.

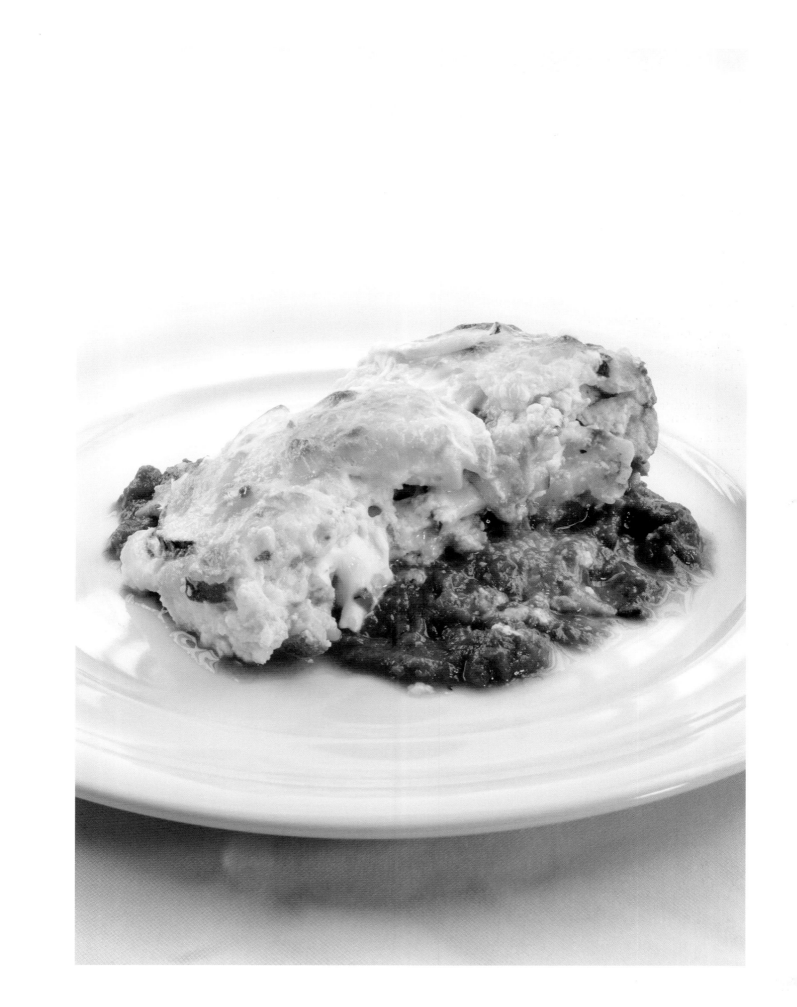

MEAT LOVER'S QUICHE

Macronutrients per serving: **Calories 348** | **Fat 27.5g** | **Carbohydrate 5.3g** | **Fiber 2.2g** | **Protein 18.8g**

Makes: **8 servings** | Prep time: **15 minutes** | Cook time: **About 40 minutes**

FOR THE CRUST:

1 egg

½ cup blanched almond flour

¼ cup (½ stick) unsalted butter, cut into small dice, softened

¼ cup shredded cheddar cheese (about 1 ounce)

2 tablespoons ground flax seed

2 tablespoons high-fiber coconut flour

FOR THE FILLING:

4 slices bacon, chopped

4 ounces Mexican-style fresh (raw) chorizo, chopped

1 medium bell pepper (any color), chopped

1 small tomato, chopped

½ small onion, chopped

1 teaspoon garlic powder

2 ounces prosciutto, chopped (optional)

4 eggs

¼ cup heavy cream

¾ cup shredded Gruyère cheese (about 3 ounces)

⅓ cup grated Parmesan cheese (about 1 ounce; optional)

01 Preheat the oven to 400°F and grease a 9-inch pie pan.

02 In a mixing bowl, combine the ingredients for the crust and mix together to form a dough. Place the dough in the greased pie pan and, using your fingers, press it evenly across the bottom and up the sides of the pan. Par-bake the crust for 5 to 7 minutes. Remove the crust from the oven and lower the temperature to 350°F.

03 While the crust is par-baking, make the filling: Cook the bacon and chorizo in a skillet over medium heat for 3 to 4 minutes, then add the bell pepper, tomato, onion, and garlic powder and sauté for 2 to 3 minutes, until softened. Slide the pan off the heat. If using prosciutto, add it to the pan and stir to combine. Transfer the meat and vegetable mixture to the par-baked crust, spreading it evenly across the bottom.

04 Whisk together the eggs and heavy cream and pour the mixture over the crust and filling. Top with the cheese(s).

05 Bake the quiche for 33 to 37 minutes, rotating the pan halfway through, until the eggs are set and the edges of the crust begin to brown. Cut into 8 equal portions and serve hot. Store leftovers in the refrigerator for up to 4 days.

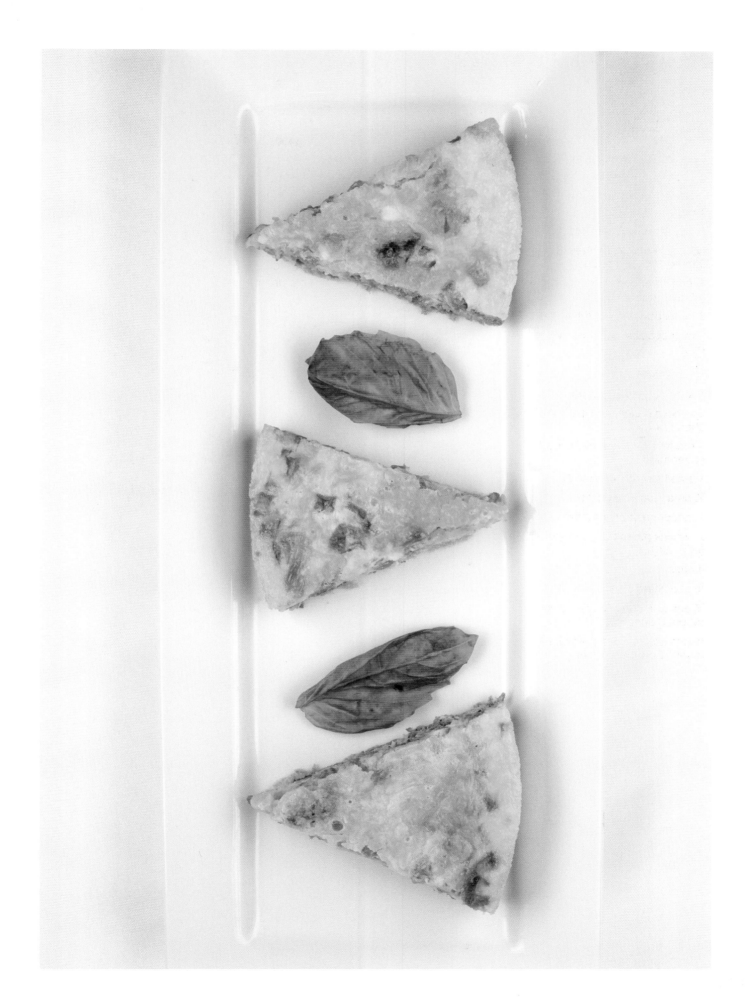

EGGS BENEDICT

Macronutrients per serving: **Calories 521** | **Fat 41.3g** | **Carbohydrate 8.4g** | **Fiber 5.3g** | **Protein 28.9g**

Makes: **4 servings** | Prep time: **15 minutes** | Cook time: **15 minutes**

Poaching is a method in which a vegetable, meat, fruit, or egg is cooked in a simmering liquid such as stock, fruit juice, or water. The temperature of the liquid should be 160°F to 180°F so that liquid is evaporating (i.e., creating steam) but is not at a rolling boil.

FOR THE TOPPINGS:

1 quart water

2 tablespoons white vinegar

8 eggs

8 slices Canadian bacon

1 large tomato, cut into 8 slices

½ cup Hollandaise (page 347)

FOR THE ENGLISH MUFFINS:

½ cup blanched almond flour

⅓ cup high-fiber coconut flour

1 teaspoon baking powder

¼ teaspoon garlic powder

¼ teaspoon onion powder

¼ teaspoon kosher salt

4 eggs

¼ cup (½ stick) unsalted butter, melted, plus at least 1 tablespoon for the pan

01 Bring the water and vinegar to a simmer in a saucepan over medium heat. Set a colander over a large bowl and line a sheet pan with parchment paper. Preheat the oven to 350°F.

02 To make the muffins, place the almond flour, coconut flour, baking powder, garlic powder, onion powder, and salt in a bowl and whisk to combine. In a separate bowl, whisk together the eggs and melted butter until thoroughly blended. Pour the egg mixture into the flour mixture and mix until a batter forms. Set aside until Step 5.

03 To make the toppings, crack an egg into a small bowl, swirl the simmering water to create a vortex, and then gently pour the egg into the water so that the yolk doesn't crack. Cook for 3 minutes for a soft-cooked yolk or 4 to 5 minutes for a harder yolk. Gently remove the egg from the water with a slotted spoon and place in the colander. Once completely drained, transfer to a flat surface and set aside. Repeat with the remaining eggs. *Note:* You can poach more than one egg at a time, but given the amount of liquid used, do not poach more than 3 eggs at once.

04 Spread the Canadian bacon evenly on the prepared sheet pan and place in the oven to warm for 8 to 10 minutes.

05 While the eggs are poaching, make the English muffins: Heat 1 tablespoon of butter in a large sauté pan over medium heat. Using a ¼-cup measure filled two-thirds full, portion out the batter into the pan. Cook for 2 to 3 minutes, until browned, then flip and cook for 1 to 2 minutes on the other side. Remove from the pan, transfer to a plate, and repeat with the remaining batter to make a total of 8 muffins, adding more butter to the pan if needed.

06 To assemble, place 2 English muffins on a plate and top each with 1 slice of Canadian bacon, 1 slice of tomato, and 1 poached egg. Drizzle with hollandaise and serve immediately. This recipe does not store well, so it should be consumed when made.

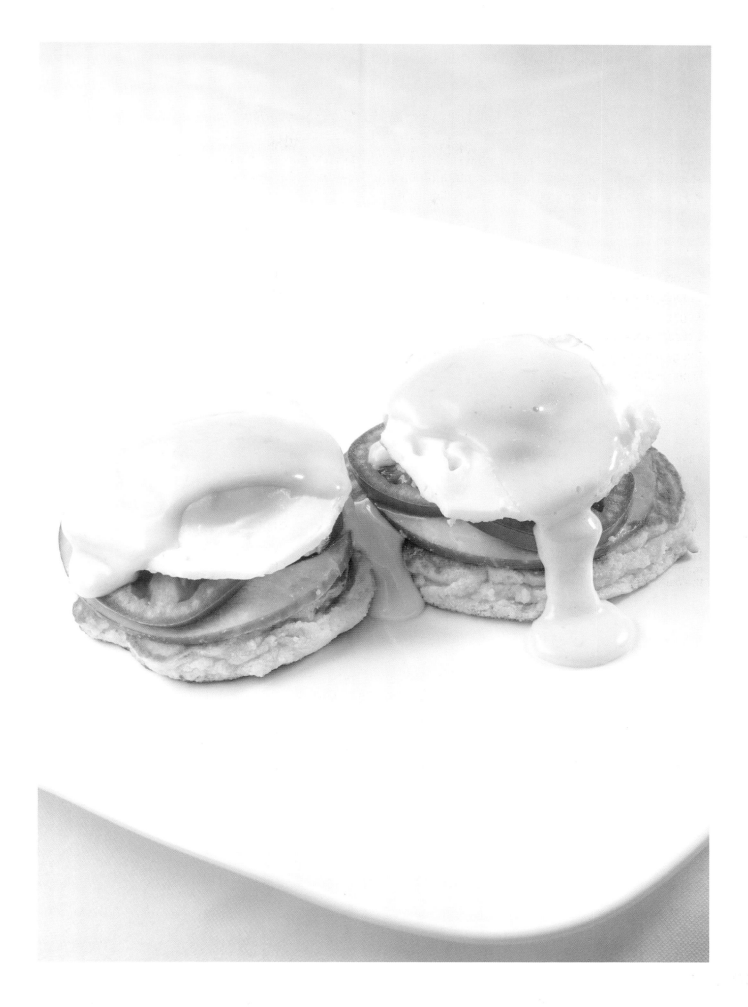

MAPLE BANANA PANCAKES

Macronutrients per serving: Calories 476 | Fat 40.2g | Carbohydrate 6.8g | Fiber 3.9g | Protein 21.8g

Makes: 24 pancakes (4 per serving) | **Prep time:** 10 minutes | **Cook time:** 10 minutes

12 eggs, separated

1 teaspoon cream of tartar

1 (8-ounce) package cream cheese, softened, divided

½ cup high-fiber coconut flour

½ cup plus 3 tablespoons unsweetened almond milk, divided

½ cup plus 2 tablespoons heavy cream, divided

¼ cup blanched almond flour

¼ cup Quest Protein Powder Banana Cream

4 teaspoons ground cinnamon, divided

2 teaspoons vanilla extract

2 teaspoons maple extract, divided

½ teaspoon baking powder

½ teaspoon plus ⅛ teaspoon raw sucralose, divided

¼ cup finely chopped raw pecans

¼ cup roughly chopped raw pecans, for garnish

01 Make the pancakes: In a large bowl, whisk the egg whites until frothy, then add the cream of tartar. Whip until stiff peaks form, about 3 minutes.

02 In a separate bowl, beat together the egg yolks, half of the cream cheese, the coconut flour, ½ cup of the almond milk, ½ cup of the heavy cream, the almond flour, the protein powder, 2 teaspoons of the cinnamon, the vanilla extract, 1 teaspoon of the maple extract, the baking powder, and ½ teaspoon of the sucralose.

03 Gently fold the egg yolk mixture and the finely chopped pecans into the whipped egg whites until evenly blended.

04 Heat a large sauté pan over medium heat, then coat it with cooking spray. Using a ¼-cup measure, spoon the batter into the pan to form pancakes and cook for 2 minutes on each side. Repeat with the remaining batter, recoating the pan with cooking spray between batches.

05 Make the sauce: Beat together the remaining half of the cream cheese with the remaining 3 tablespoons of almond milk, 2 tablespoons of heavy cream, 2 teaspoons of cinnamon, 1 teaspoon of maple extract, and ⅛ teaspoon of sucralose until the sauce is smooth.

06 To serve, drizzle the sauce over the pancakes and garnish with the roughly chopped pecans. Store leftover pancakes and sauce in separate containers in the refrigerator for up to 4 days.

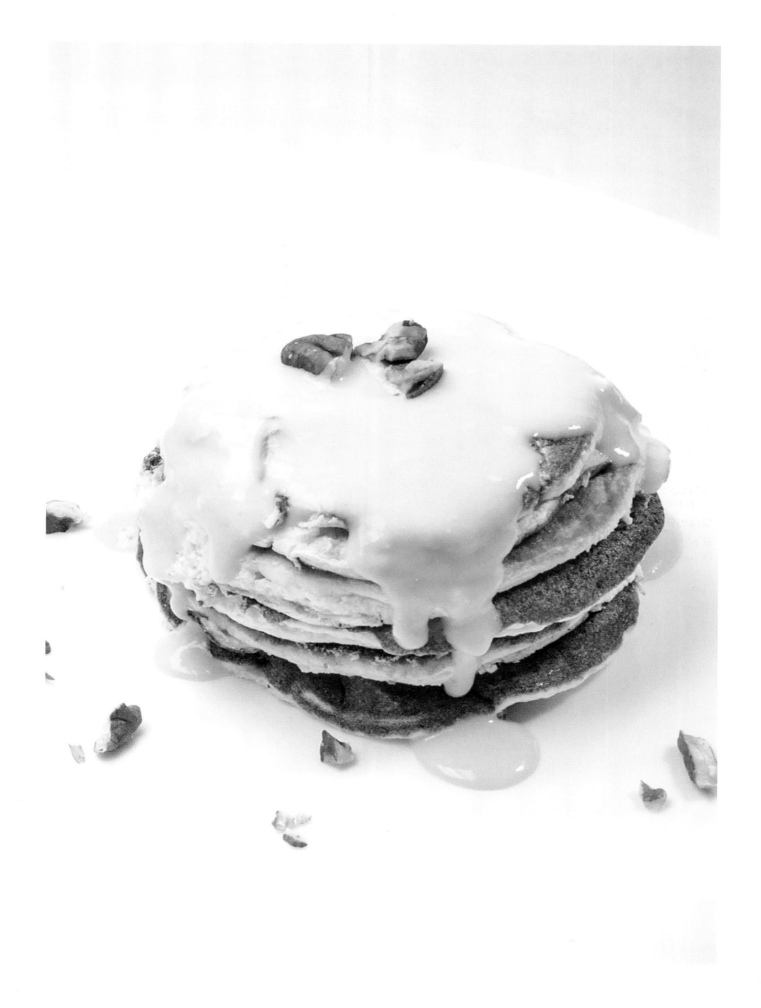

BACON, EGG, AND CHEESE SANDWICH

Macronutrients per serving: Calories 668 | Fat 52g | Carbohydrate 8.6g | Fiber 0.8g | Protein 41.4g

Makes: 2 sandwiches (1 per serving) | Prep time: 10 minutes | Cook time: About 25 minutes

FOR THE FILLINGS:

3 slices bacon

½ small red onion, sliced

½ small tomato, sliced

1 tablespoon coconut oil or MCT oil

4 eggs

2 tablespoons heavy cream

Dash of hot sauce

2 slices cheddar cheese

FOR THE "BREAD":

2 eggs, separated

2 ounces cream cheese (¼ cup), softened

½ teaspoon kosher salt

½ teaspoon smoked paprika

¼ teaspoon garlic powder

¼ teaspoon ground black pepper

¼ teaspoon baking powder

Dash of Worcestershire sauce

¼ teaspoon cream of tartar

⅓ cup grated Parmesan cheese (about 1 ounce)

¼ cup shredded smoked Gouda cheese (about 1 ounce)

01 Preheat the oven to 400°F. Line a sheet pan with parchment paper, then line an 8-inch square baking pan with parchment paper and coat it with cooking spray.

02 Start to prepare the filling: Place the bacon, onion slices, and tomato slices in the lined sheet pan and bake for 10 to 12 minutes, until the bacon is crisp and the vegetables are browned. After removing the pan from the oven, lower the temperature to 350°F. Cut the bacon slices in half crosswise.

03 While the bacon and vegetables are cooking, make the "bread" batter: Mix together the 2 egg yolks, cream cheese, salt, paprika, garlic powder, pepper, baking powder, and Worcestershire sauce. In a separate bowl, whip the egg whites until frothy, then add the cream of tartar and whip until stiff peaks form, about 3 minutes. Fold the yolk mixture into the whites until completely combined, then pour the batter into the prepared baking pan. Sprinkle evenly with the Parmesan and Gouda.

04 Bake the "bread" for 12 to 15 minutes, until the edges begin to brown. Remove from the pan, place on a cooling rack, and let cool for 3 to 4 minutes, then cut into 4 equal portions and set aside.

05 Finish making the filling: Heat the coconut oil in a sauté pan over medium heat, then whisk together the 4 eggs, heavy cream, and hot sauce. Pour into the pan and cook until the eggs are set. Divide the filling into 2 equal portions.

06 To assemble the sandwiches, place 2 pieces of bread on a plate, place 1 slice of cheddar cheese on each piece, and top evenly with the eggs, tomato, onion, and 3 pieces of bacon. Top each with another piece of bread and serve immediately. Store leftovers in an airtight container in the refrigerator for up to 3 days.

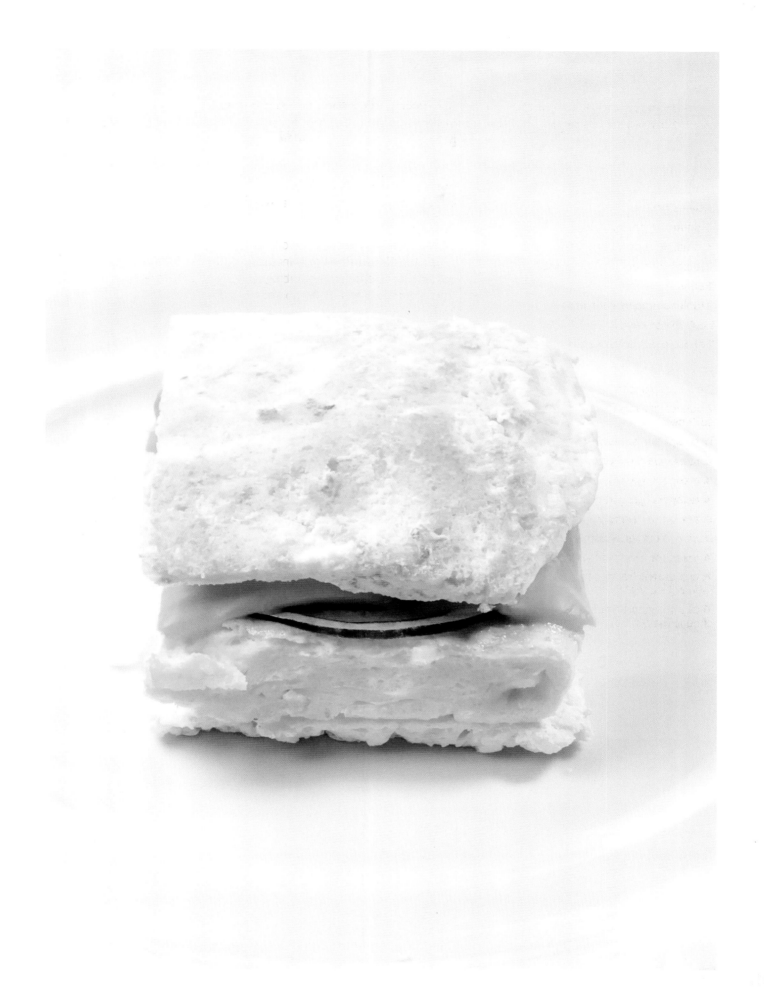

BREAKFAST WRAPS WITH PICO DE GALLO

Macronutrients per serving: Calories 397 | Fat 31g | Carbohydrate 9.5g | Fiber 5.8g | Protein 22g

Makes: 4 servings | Prep time: 15 minutes, plus 1 hour to chill dough | Cook time: 35 minutes

FOR THE WRAPS:

2 cups fresh spinach

¼ ounce pork rinds (about ½ cup)

¼ cup blanched almond flour

3 tablespoons high-fiber coconut flour

1½ teaspoons chia seeds

1 teaspoon psyllium husk powder

½ teaspoon kosher salt

½ teaspoon garlic powder

½ teaspoon onion powder

⅛ teaspoon xanthan gum

Pinch of cayenne pepper

½ cup water, warmed

2 tablespoons coconut oil or MCT oil, divided, for the pan

FOR THE PICO DE GALLO:

2 Roma tomatoes, diced

¼ small red onion, diced

1 teaspoon lime juice

¼ teaspoon kosher salt

FOR THE FILLING:

3 quarts water

¼ cup distilled white vinegar

1 tablespoon kosher salt

8 eggs, room temperature

1 tablespoon coconut oil or MCT oil

2 cups fresh spinach

4 slices cheddar cheese

FOR GARNISH:

4 cherry tomatoes

1 lime, quartered

SPECIAL EQUIPMENT:

Toothpicks

01 Make the dough for the wraps: In a food processor, combine the spinach, pork rinds, almond flour, coconut flour, chia seeds, psyllium husk powder, salt, garlic powder, onion powder, xanthan gum, and cayenne pepper. While pulsing, slowly add the water until a dough forms. Remove the dough from the food processor and knead on a greased flat surface for 1 to 2 minutes, until a smooth dough ball forms. Coat the inside of a bowl with cooking spray, then place the dough in the bowl, cover with plastic wrap, and place in the refrigerator for 1 hour to chill.

02 To prepare the pico de gallo: Combine the tomatoes, red onion, lime juice, and salt; refrigerate until serving time.

03 To hard-boil the eggs for the filling, bring the water to a boil in a 5-quart saucepan over high heat. Add the vinegar and salt and stir until the salt dissolves. Add the eggs one at a time, then set a timer for 10 minutes. When the timer goes off, remove the eggs from the water and place in an ice bath for 3 to 4 minutes. Remove the shells, then roughly chop the eggs; refrigerate the chopped eggs until Step 6.

04 After the dough has chilled, coat a flat surface with cooking spray and place the dough ball on the greased surface. Press down to flatten, cover with parchment paper, and roll out with a rolling pin until it is ¼ inch thick. Remove the parchment and cut out four 9-inch circles using a 9-inch sauté pan or cake pan as a guide.

05 Heat 1 tablespoon of the coconut oil in a 10-inch or larger skillet over medium-high heat. Place a wrap in the skillet and cook for 2 to 3 minutes on each side, until it begins to brown; repeat three more times, adding 1 teaspoon of coconut oil to the pan each time a new wrap is cooked. Set the wraps aside and preheat the oven to 450°F.

06 Finish making the filling: Heat the 1 tablespoon of coconut oil in a 10-inch or larger sauté pan over medium heat for 1 to 2 minutes. Add the spinach and sauté for 2 minutes. Add the hard-boiled eggs to the pan and stir to combine; leave over the heat just long enough to warm them up, then set aside.

07 To assemble, lay a wrap on a flat surface and fill with 1 slice cheddar cheese and ¼ to ⅓ cup of the egg and spinach mixture. Fold the sides of the wrap over the filling, overlapping the ends, and spear with a toothpick to secure; repeat 3 more times with remaining wraps, then place all 4 wraps on a sheet pan and bake for 3 to 4 minutes to melt the cheese.

08 To serve, place a wrap on a plate, garnish with a cherry tomato, 2 tablespoons of pico de gallo, and 1 lime quarter. Store leftover wraps and pico de gallo in separate airtight containers in the refrigerator for up to 4 days.

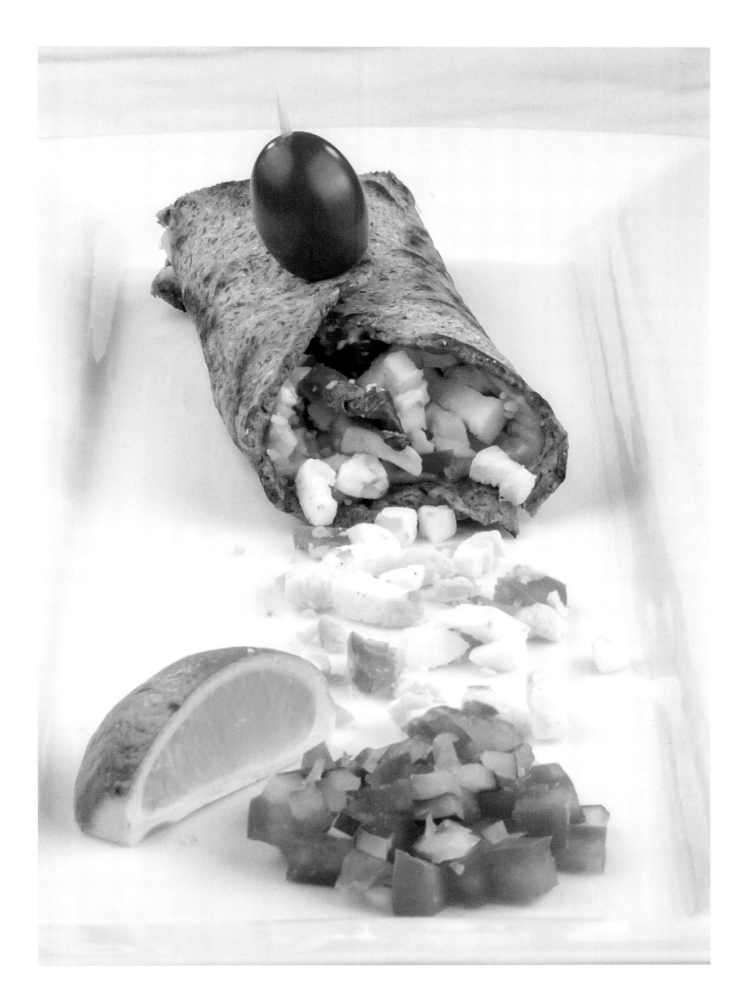

BLACK WALNUT ZUCCHINI BREAD WITH MAPLE BUTTER

Macronutrients per serving: **Calories 399** | **Fat 32.6g** | **Carbohydrate 7.2g** | **Fiber 5.1g** | **Protein 11.1g**

Makes: **One 9 by 5-inch loaf (6 servings)** | Prep time: **15 minutes** | Cook time: **40 minutes**

FOR THE BREAD:

½ cup blanched almond flour

½ cup high-fiber coconut flour

¼ cup hazelnut flour

¼ cup Quest Protein Powder Multi-Purpose Mix

1 tablespoon psyllium husk powder

1 teaspoon baking soda

½ teaspoon baking powder

2 teaspoons ground cinnamon

¼ teaspoon ground nutmeg

¼ teaspoon ground cloves

½ teaspoon xanthan gum, divided

4 eggs

½ cup (1 stick) unsalted butter, softened

3 tablespoons coconut oil or MCT oil

2 tablespoons heavy cream

2 teaspoons vanilla extract

1 teaspoon Splenda Brown Sugar Blend

⅛ to ¼ teaspoon raw sucralose (depending on sweetness preference)

¼ cup black walnuts, chopped

1 zucchini (about 7 ounces), shredded

FOR THE MAPLE BUTTER:

½ cup (1 stick) unsalted butter, softened

1 teaspoon maple extract

1 teaspoon ground cinnamon

¼ teaspoon kosher salt

⅛ teaspoon raw sucralose

01 Preheat the oven to 325°F and coat a 9 by 5-inch loaf pan with cooking spray or oil.

02 Sift the almond flour, coconut flour, hazelnut flour, protein powder, psyllium husk powder, baking soda, baking powder, spices, and ¼ teaspoon of the xanthan gum into a mixing bowl; set aside.

03 Separate the eggs into 2 large bowls. Add the butter and coconut oil to the bowl with the yolks and, using a whisk, mix until the ingredients are smooth and emulsified (with no separation). Add the heavy cream, vanilla extract, Splenda baking blend, and sucralose, and mix until combined; set aside.

04 Whisk the egg whites until frothy. Add the remaining ¼ teaspoon of xanthan gum and whip until stiff peaks form, about 3 minutes.

05 Fold the egg yolk mixture into the egg whites until combined, then add the dry ingredients, walnuts, and shredded zucchini and mix until a thick batter forms.

06 Transfer the batter to the prepared pan, cover with aluminum foil, and bake for 40 minutes, rotating the pan halfway through.

07 While the bread is baking, make the maple butter: Whisk together the butter, maple extract, cinnamon, salt, and sucralose until the mixture is smooth and spreadable.

08 Remove the bread from the oven and turn out onto a cooling rack. When the bread is cool, slice it into 6 equal portions. Serve warm or cool with 1 to 2 tablespoons of the maple butter. Store in an airtight container in the refrigerator for up to 1 week.

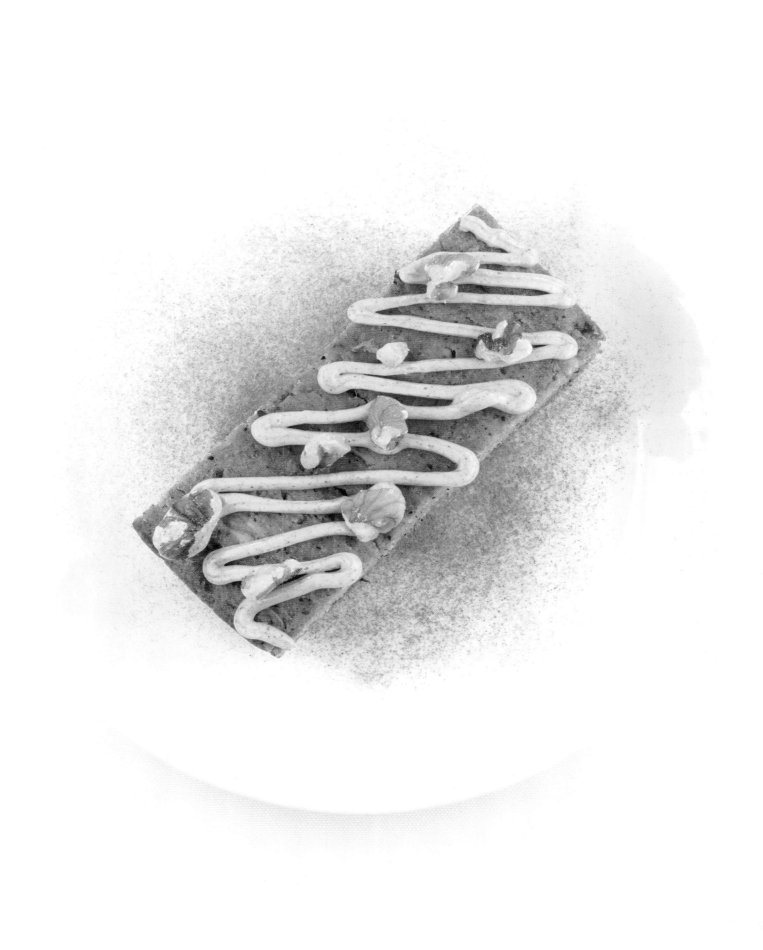

EGGS IN A BASKET

Macronutrients per serving: Calories 393 | Fat 32g | Carbohydrate 12.7g | Fiber 10g | Protein 12.6g

Makes: 4 servings | Prep time: 5 minutes | Cook time: 22 to 25 minutes

4 avocados, halved and pitted

½ teaspoon kosher salt

½ teaspoon garlic powder

½ teaspoon onion powder

1 tablespoon hot sauce, such as Tabasco

8 eggs

01 Preheat the oven to 400°F and line a sheet pan with parchment paper.

02 Place the halved avocados on the sheet pan and season with the salt, garlic powder, onion powder, and hot sauce. Par-bake for 10 minutes.

03 Remove the par-baked avocados from the oven and crack an egg into each half. Bake for 12 to 15 minutes for solid whites and medium-cooked yolks, or longer if you prefer yolks that are set.

04 Remove from the oven and allow to cool. Serve with additional hot sauce, if desired. Store in an airtight container in the refrigerator for up to 3 days.

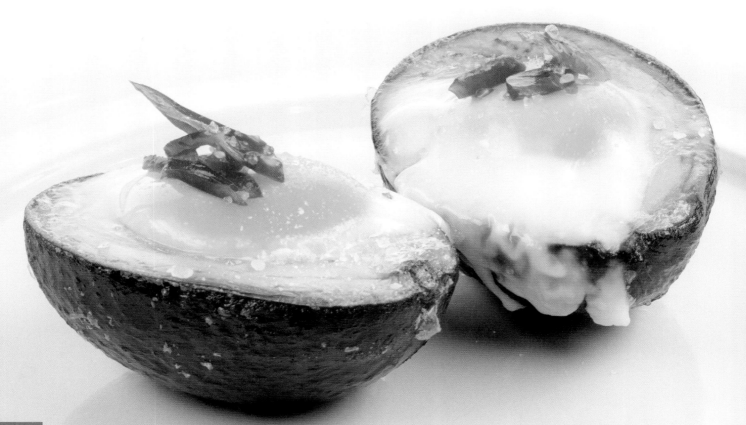

CHORIZO HASH BROWNS AND FRIED EGGS

Macronutrients per serving: Calories 449 | Fat 36.2g | Carbohydrate 11.5g | Fiber 3.6g | Protein 19.2g

Makes: 4 servings | Prep time: 10 minutes | Cook time: About 15 minutes

4 tablespoons (½ stick) unsalted butter, divided

8 ounces Mexican-style fresh (raw) chorizo

½ green bell pepper, chopped

½ red bell pepper, chopped

¼ yellow bell pepper, chopped

¼ onion, chopped

1 teaspoon chopped garlic

1 medium head cauliflower (5 to 6 inches in diameter), cored and florets grated

8 eggs

¼ cup shredded cheddar cheese (about 1 ounce)

1 teaspoon hot sauce

½ teaspoon kosher salt

½ teaspoon ground black pepper

01 Melt 2 tablespoons of the butter in a sauté pan over medium heat. When the butter has begun to brown slightly, add the chorizo, bell peppers, onion, and garlic and cook for 3 to 4 minutes, until the vegetables begin to brown. Turn the heat up to medium-high and add the grated cauliflower; cook for 4 to 5 minutes, until the cauliflower begins to brown.

02 In a separate skillet, melt the remaining 2 tablespoons of butter and fry the eggs until done to your liking.

03 Finish the hash browns with the cheddar cheese, hot sauce, salt, and pepper.

04 Remove the hash browns from the pan and divide them evenly among 4 plates. Serve immediately with the fried eggs, 2 per serving. Store leftover hash browns in the refrigerator for up to 3 days.

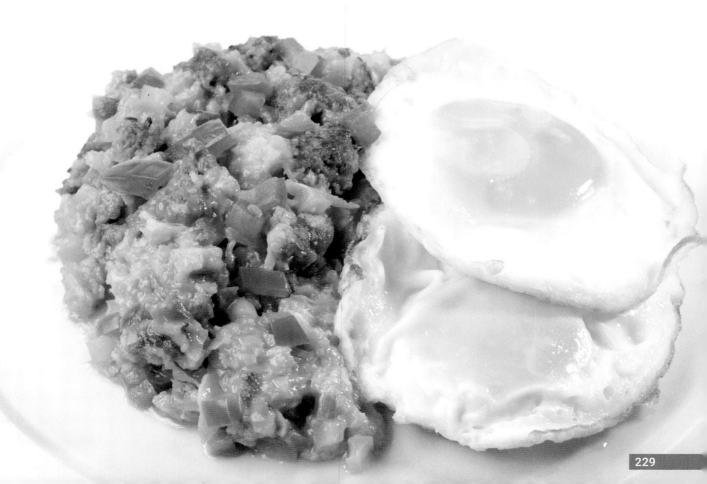

FRITTATA MUFFINS

Macronutrients per serving: Calories 469 | Fat 36.3g | Carbohydrate 7.7g | Fiber 1.3g | Protein 30.3g

Makes: **12 muffins (3 per serving)** | Prep time: **10 minutes** | Cook time: **About 30 minutes**

2 slices thick-cut bacon, chopped

1 tablespoon coconut oil or MCT oil

1 red bell pepper, chopped

1 green bell pepper, chopped

1 small tomato, chopped

1 teaspoon dried basil

1 teaspoon onion powder

½ teaspoon garlic powder

9 eggs

½ cup half-and-half

1 teaspoon hot sauce

½ teaspoon kosher salt

1½ cups shredded smoked Gouda cheese (about 6 ounces)

01 Preheat the oven to 350°F and grease a 12-well muffin tin.

02 Cook the bacon in a skillet over medium heat for 4 to 5 minutes, until it has begun to render its fat and crisp up. Add the coconut oil, bell peppers, and tomato to the pan and sauté for 2 to 3 minutes. Mix in the basil, onion powder, and garlic powder and sauté for 1 more minute, then remove from the heat.

03 In a large bowl, whisk together the eggs, half-and-half, hot sauce, and salt.

04 Divide the bell pepper mixture evenly among the muffin cups. Pour the egg mixture over the pepper mixture, filling the cups about two-thirds full. Sprinkle the top of each muffin with 2 tablespoons of the Gouda.

05 Bake for 20 to 23 minutes, until the egg has set and the tops begin to brown slightly. Remove from the oven and serve hot. Store in an airtight container in the refrigerator for up to 4 days or in the freezer for up to 2 weeks.

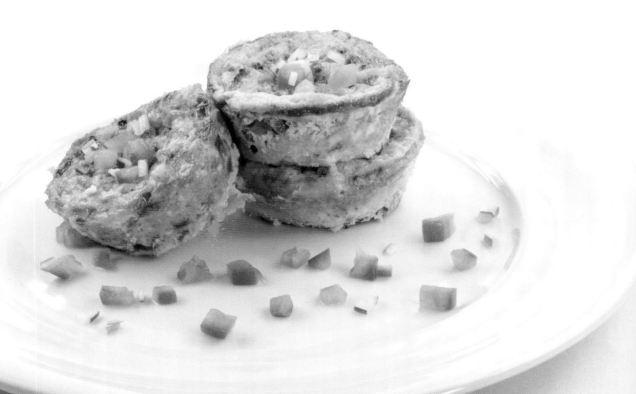

GREEN GOBLIN BREAKFAST SHAKE

Macronutrients per serving: **Calories 376** | **Fat 29.9g** | **Carbohydrate 13.6g** | **Fiber 7.1g** | **Protein 16g**

Makes: **2 servings** | Prep time: **5 minutes** | Cook time: —

12 ounces unsweetened almond milk

1 avocado, peeled, halved, and pitted

1 cup ice cubes

1 cup fresh spinach

¼ cup whey protein powder, flavor of choice

¼ cup heavy cream

¼ cup unsalted cashews

Place all the ingredients in a high-powered blender. Blend for 1 to 2 minutes, until smooth. Divide between 2 glasses and serve immediately.

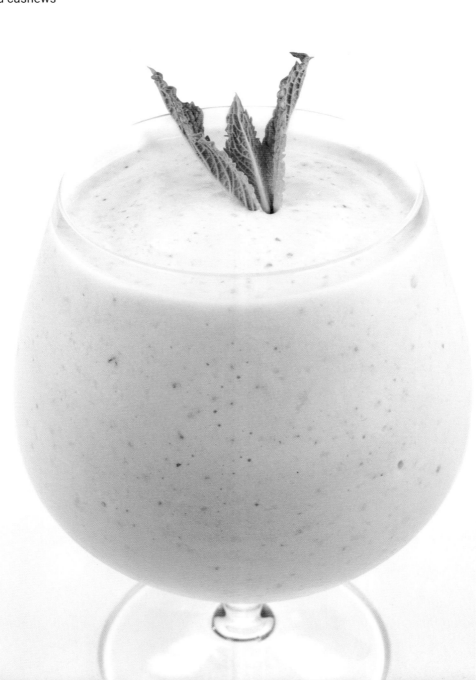

APPETIZERS &
SMALL PLATES

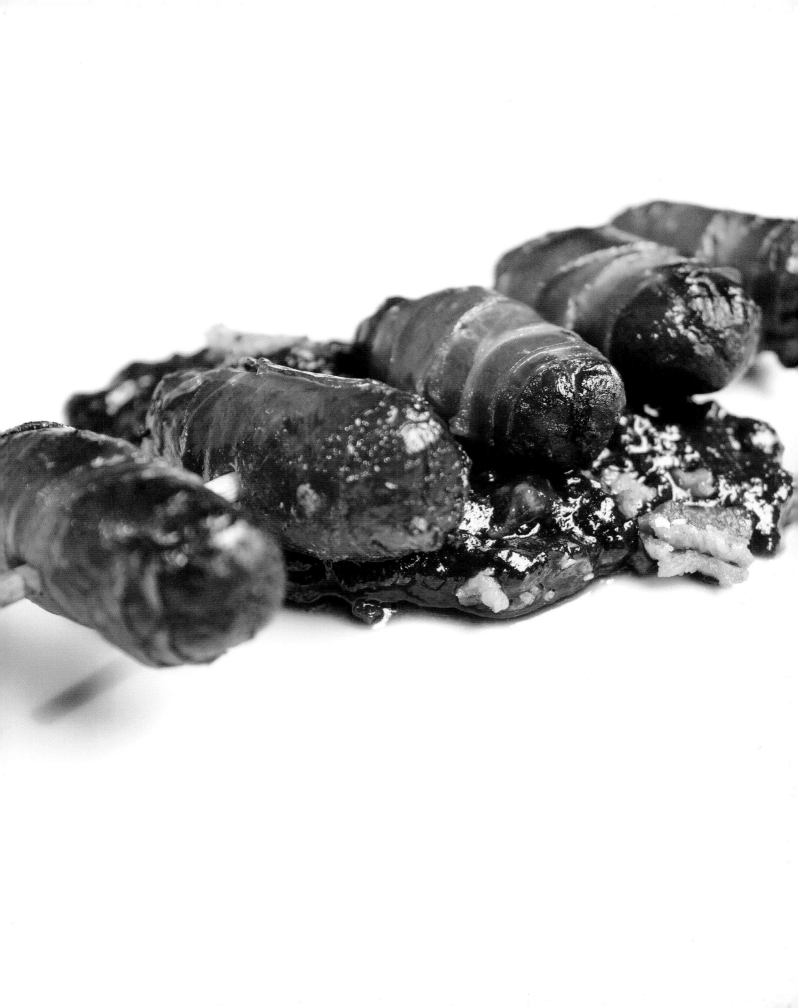

SPINACH DIP

Macronutrients per serving: Calories 208 | Fat 17.5g | Carbohydrate 5.2g | Fiber 1g | Protein 7.5g

Makes: **8 servings** | Prep time: **10 minutes** | Cook time: **About 12 minutes**

1 tablespoon coconut oil

¼ small onion, chopped

8 ounces fresh spinach, chopped

½ small tomato, chopped

1 teaspoon dried or fresh thyme leaves, chopped

½ cup chicken stock (page 345)

1 (8-ounce) package cream cheese, cubed, softened

½ cup shredded cheddar cheese (about 2 ounces)

⅓ cup freshly grated Parmesan cheese (about 1 ounce)

⅓ cup freshly grated Pecorino Romano cheese (about 1 ounce; optional)

½ cup sour cream

1 teaspoon garlic powder

Kosher salt

Pork rinds and/or assorted crudités, for serving

01 In a 5-quart saucepan, heat the coconut oil over medium heat for 1 to 2 minutes, then add the onion and sauté for 2 minutes or until translucent.

02 Add the spinach, tomato, and thyme to the saucepan and sauté for 2 to 3 minutes. Add the chicken stock and simmer for 2 minutes.

03 Whisk in the cheeses, sour cream, and garlic powder until the mixture is smooth and warmed through. Season with salt to taste and transfer to a serving container.

04 Serve warm with pork rinds and/or crudités for dipping. Store in an airtight container in the refrigerator for up to 6 days.

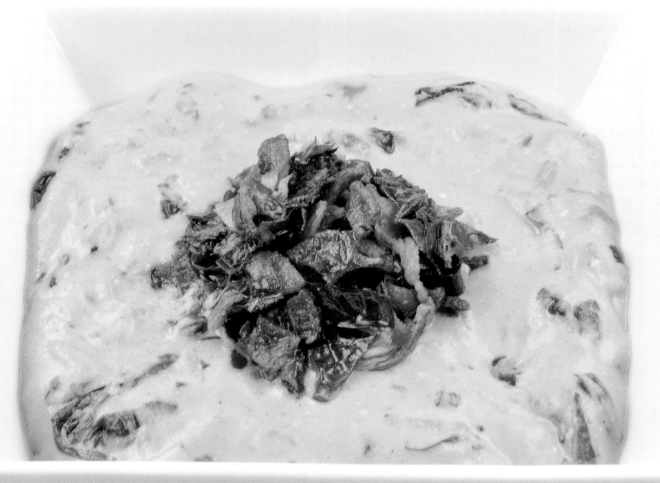

STUFFED MUSHROOM CAPS

Macronutrients per serving: **Calories 176** | **Fat 11.5g** | **Carbohydrate 8.9g** | **Fiber 2.4g** | **Protein 9.3g**

Makes: **10 caps (5 per serving)** | Prep time: **10 minutes** | Cook time: **20 minutes**

10 white mushrooms, about 1½ inches in diameter

1 tablespoon olive oil

¼ cup chopped yellow onions

1 green bell pepper, roughly chopped

1 Roma tomato, roughly chopped

2 cloves garlic, chopped

½ teaspoon kosher salt

¼ teaspoon freshly cracked black pepper

⅓ cup freshly grated Parmesan cheese (about 1 ounce)

01 Preheat the oven to 400°F and set a cooling rack inside a sheet pan.

02 Remove the stems from the mushrooms, then roughly chop the stems and set aside. Place the mushroom caps on the rack in the sheet pan, stem side up.

03 Heat the olive oil in a sauté pan over medium-high heat, then add the chopped mushroom stems, onions, bell pepper, tomato, and garlic and sauté for 4 to 5 minutes, stirring frequently.

04 Season the mushroom mixture with the salt and pepper, then divide the stuffing evenly among the caps.

05 Bake the stuffed mushrooms for 10 minutes. Remove from the oven, top with the Parmesan, then place back in the oven for an additional 5 minutes, until the cheese is slightly browned. Serve immediately.

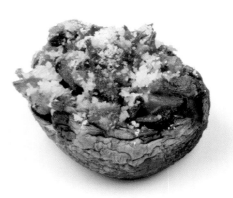
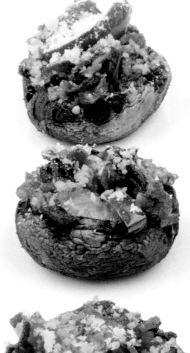
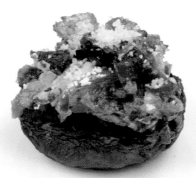
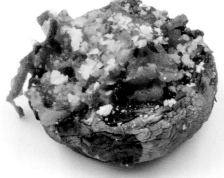

BACON-WRAPPED ASPARAGUS

Macronutrients per serving: **Calories 113** | **Fat 5.2g** | **Carbohydrate 8.2g** | **Fiber 4.5g** | **Protein 8.2g**

Makes: **6 bundles (3 per serving)** | Prep time: **5 minutes** | Cook time: **15 minutes**

30 pencil-thin spears asparagus

3 slices bacon, cut in half crosswise

01 Preheat the oven to 400°F and set a cooling rack inside a sheet pan.

02 Cut the tough ends off the asparagus (approximately the bottom inch of each spear).

03 Wrap a piece of bacon around 5 spears of asparagus and place on the rack in the sheet pan, tucking the loose bacon ends underneath the bundle of asparagus. Repeat until all the asparagus and bacon are used, making a total of 6 bundles.

04 Bake for 20 to 22 minutes, until the bacon is crispy on all sides, turning the bundles over halfway through cooking. Serve immediately. Store leftovers in an airtight container in the refrigerator for 3 to 4 days.

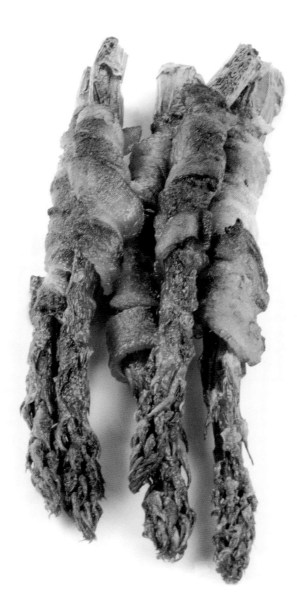

JALAPEÑO POPPERS
WITH CARAMELIZED ONION CHUTNEY

Macronutrients per serving: **Calories 453** | **Fat 35.2g** | **Carbohydrate 5.8g** | **Fiber 2.7g** | **Protein 28.3g**

Makes: **30 poppers (5 per serving)** | Prep time: **30 minutes** | Cook time: **About 30 minutes**

FOR THE POPPERS:

6 ounces 85/15 ground bison

¾ cup crumbled blue cheese (about 3 ounces)

¼ cup chopped red onions

½ bunch fresh cilantro, chopped

1 teaspoon ground cumin

1 teaspoon kosher salt

¼ teaspoon red pepper flakes

15 large jalapeño peppers, halved lengthwise and seeded

15 slices thick-cut bacon, halved crosswise

FOR THE CHUTNEY:

2 tablespoons coconut oil

½ medium red onion, chopped

½ small white onion, chopped

3 radishes, chopped

4 cloves garlic, chopped

2 tablespoons heavy cream

½ teaspoon kosher salt

SPECIAL EQUIPMENT:

Toothpicks

01 Set a cooling rack inside a sheet pan.

02 Place the ground bison, blue cheese, onions, cilantro, cumin, salt, and red pepper flakes in a large bowl. Using your hands, mix the ingredients together thoroughly.

03 Fill each jalapeño half with 1 tablespoon of the bison mixture, then wrap each stuffed pepper with a piece of bacon, securing the ends with a toothpick. Place the wrapped peppers, stuffing side up, on the rack in the sheet pan. Place the pan in the refrigerator and preheat the oven to 400°F.

04 Meanwhile, begin making the chutney: In a large sauté pan, heat the coconut oil over medium-low heat for 1 to 2 minutes. Add the onions, radishes, and garlic and cook for about 20 minutes, stirring occasionally, until the onions are very soft and starting to caramelize.

05 When the onion mixture is about halfway done cooking, remove the stuffed peppers from the refrigerator and place the pan in the oven. Bake for 8 minutes, then flip them over and continue to bake for another 7 to 10 minutes, until the peppers are softened and the temperature of the filling reaches 155°F.

06 When the onion mixture is done, transfer it to a blender or food processor, add the heavy cream and salt, and puree until smooth.

07 Serve the poppers hot with the onion chutney.

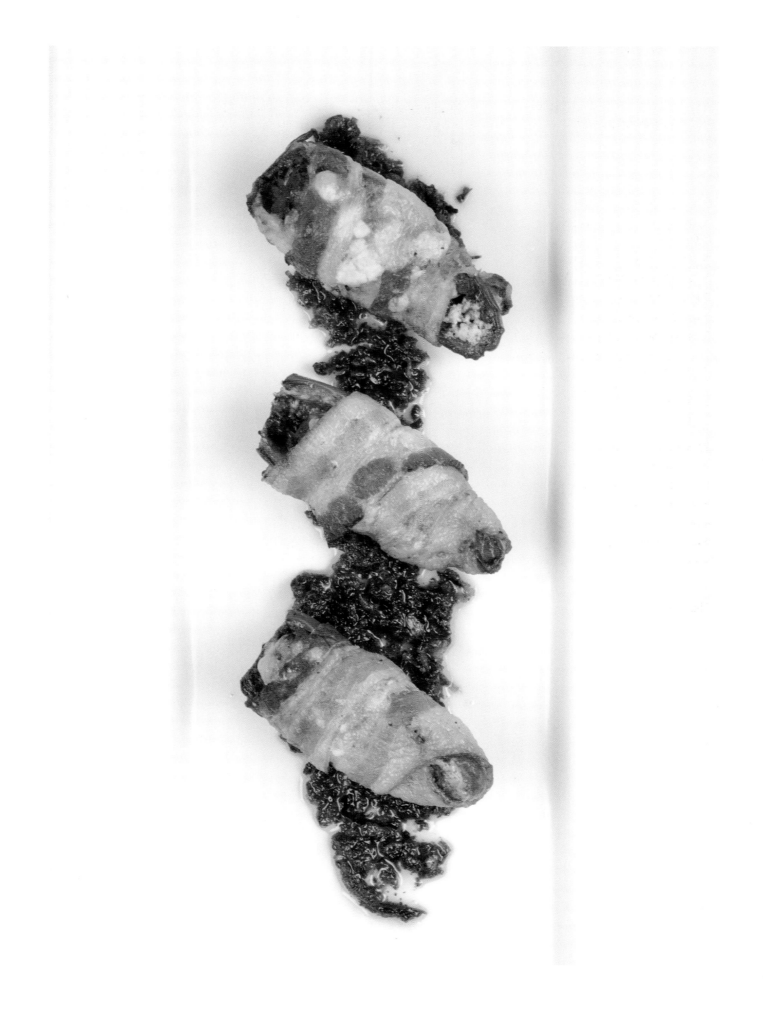

STUFFED ZUCCHINI BOATS WITH SPICY RANCH

Macronutrients per serving: Calories 328 | Fat 27.7g | Carbohydrate 4.8g | Fiber 1.4g | Protein 14.9g

Makes: 8 boats (2 per serving) | Prep time: 15 minutes | Cook time: About 25 minutes

4 medium zucchinis (about 6 ounces each), halved lengthwise

1 tablespoon unsalted butter

¼ cup chopped mushrooms

8 ounces 80/20 ground sirloin

¼ cup crumbled blue cheese (about 1 ounce)

¼ cup chopped fresh cilantro

1 teaspoon dried ground oregano

1 teaspoon ground cumin

⅛ teaspoon cayenne pepper

1 teaspoon kosher salt

2 slices thick-cut bacon

FOR THE SPICY RANCH:

¼ cup ranch dressing

2 teaspoons Sriracha sauce

½ cup cherry tomatoes, for garnish (optional)

01 Preheat the oven to 400°F and set a cooling rack in a sheet pan.

02 Scoop out the cores of the zucchinis to create boats; set the cores aside. Place the boats in a colander, liberally salt, and allow to sit for 5 to 10 minutes to remove the excess moisture. Rinse and pat dry.

03 Place the hollowed-out zucchinis cut side up on the cooling rack in the sheet pan and par-bake for 10 minutes.

04 While the zucchinis are par-baking, make the filling: Roughly chop the cores and place them in a mixing bowl.

05 Preheat a sauté pan over medium-high heat. Add the butter, allow to come to temperature for 1 to 2 minutes, then add the chopped zucchini cores and mushrooms and sauté for 2 to 3 minutes. Remove from the pan and place in a medium-sized mixing bowl.

06 To the bowl with the chopped zucchini cores, add the ground sirloin, blue cheese, cilantro, oregano, cumin, cayenne pepper, and salt. Using your hands, mix the ingredients together thoroughly, then place the filling in the refrigerator until needed.

07 Remove the zucchini boats from the oven. Fill the boats with the sirloin mixture and place back in the oven for 15 to 18 minutes.

08 While the zucchini boats are baking, cook the bacon in a sauté pan over medium heat until crisp, then chop it into small pieces. Mix together the ranch and Sriracha until smooth.

09 When the zucchini boats are done, remove them from the oven and sprinkle the bacon over them; serve immediately with the spicy ranch sauce. Garnish with cherry tomatoes if desired.

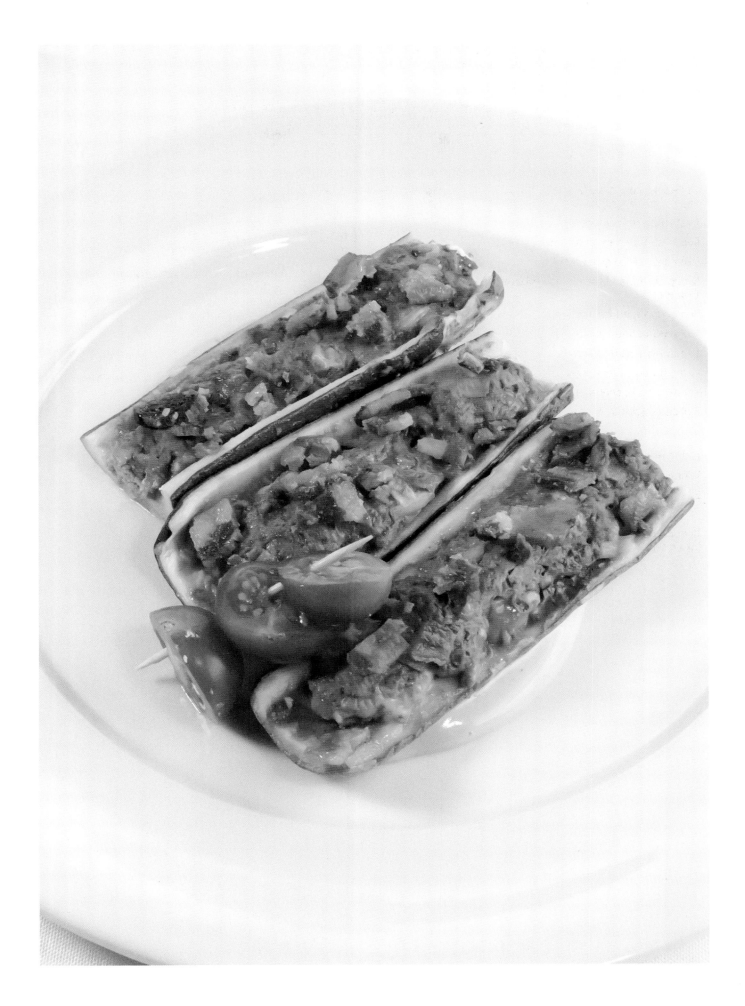

BROCCOLI BITES
WITH SPICY MUSTARD

Macronutrients per serving: Calories 239 | Fat 20.3g | Carbohydrate 6g | Fiber 2.5g | Protein 8.9g

Makes: 6 servings | Prep time: 10 minutes | Cook time: 15 to 20 minutes

Some oils are better than others for deep-frying; reference the oils and smoke points information on page 199 for details. For this recipe, use an oil such as sunflower, safflower, or peanut oil that can withstand high temperatures.

1 quart vegetable oil, for deep-frying

1 pound fresh broccoli florets

Kosher salt

FOR THE BATTER:

½ cup half-and-half

2 eggs

1 teaspoon Worcestershire sauce

¼ cup blanched almond flour

¼ cup Quest Protein Powder Multi-Purpose Mix

1 tablespoon ground flax seeds

1 teaspoon garlic powder

1 teaspoon onion powder

1 teaspoon turmeric powder (optional)

¼ teaspoon smoked paprika (optional)

¼ teaspoon ground black pepper

½ teaspoon kosher salt

FOR THE MUSTARD SAUCE:

¼ cup Dijon mustard

¼ cup mayonnaise

2 teaspoons hot sauce, such as Tabasco

Pinch of cayenne pepper

Kosher salt

01 Preheat the oil in a deep-fryer or 2½-quart saucepan over medium heat until the temperature reaches 350°F. (As you work, monitor the temperature and lower or increase the heat under the pot to maintain a consistent 350°F.) Line a sheet pan with paper towels.

02 While the oil heats up, prepare the batter: In a mixing bowl, whisk together the half-and-half, eggs, and Worcestershire sauce until fully combined. In another bowl, sift together the almond flour, protein powder, ground flax seeds, spices, and salt. Pour the wet ingredients into the dry ingredients and whisk until a thick, homogenous batter forms.

03 Using one hand, dip a broccoli floret into the batter to coat evenly, then place it directly into the hot oil to fry. Fry for 1 to 2 minutes, then flip to fry the other side for 30 to 60 seconds, until all sides are golden brown. You can fry the dipped florets in batches of 3 or 4 at a time; don't overcrowd the pot or the temperature of the oil will drop.

04 Using a slotted spoon, remove the bites from the oil, place on the paper towel–lined sheet pan, and pat dry with paper towels. Sprinkle with salt. Repeat with the remaining broccoli florets.

05 To make the mustard sauce, whisk together the mustard, mayonnaise, hot sauce, cayenne pepper, and salt to taste. Serve the bites immediately, with the sauce on the side for dipping. Store leftover bites and mustard sauce in separate airtight containers in the refrigerator; the bites will keep for 1 day, and the mustard sauce for up to 1 week.

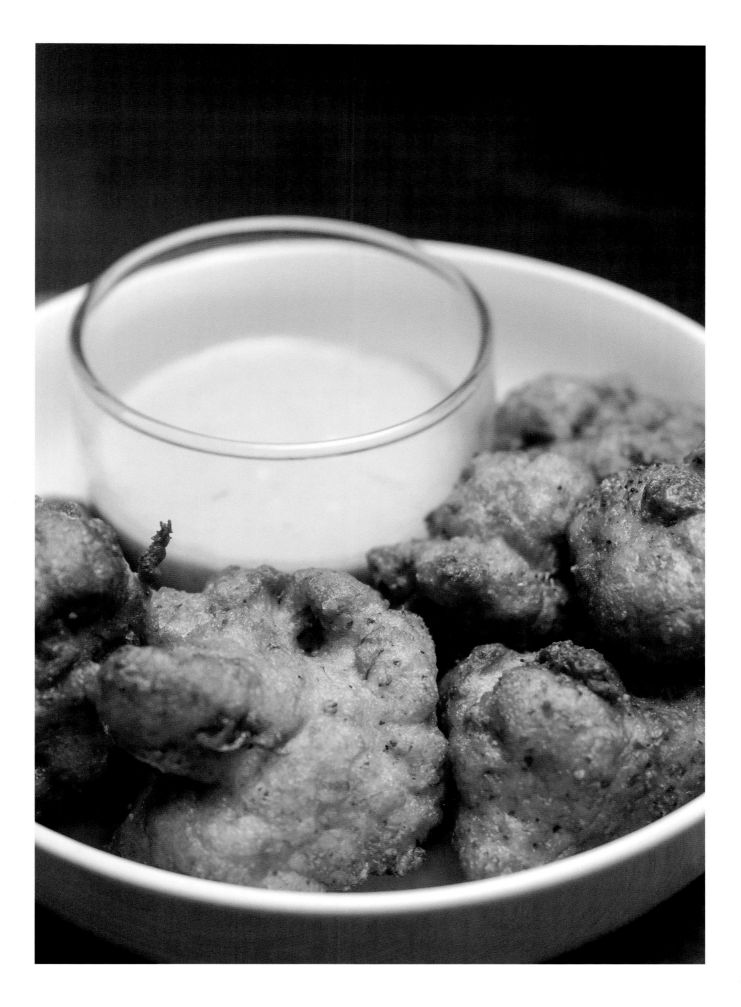

BARBECUE BACON-WRAPPED SHRIMP

Macronutrients per serving: Calories 131 | Fat 6.4g | Carbohydrate 3.1g | Fiber 0.4g | Protein 15.9g

Makes: 4 servings | Prep time: 10 minutes, plus 20 minutes to soak skewers and marinate shrimp | Cook time: About 10 minutes

FOR THE MARINADE AND BARBECUE SAUCE:

¼ cup fish stock (page 346) or water

2 tablespoons tomato paste

1 tablespoon prepared yellow mustard

1 teaspoon hot sauce, such as Tabasco

½ teaspoon Worcestershire sauce

½ teaspoon chili powder

½ teaspoon garlic powder

½ teaspoon onion powder

¼ teaspoon cayenne pepper (optional)

12 peeled and deveined frozen large shrimp (21/25 count), thawed

6 slices bacon

Kosher salt and ground black pepper

SPECIAL EQUIPMENT:

4 (12-inch) wooden skewers

01 Place the skewers in a container and cover with water; allow to soak for 20 to 30 minutes.

02 Marinate the shrimp: In a bowl or shallow dish, whisk together the fish stock, tomato paste, mustard, hot sauce, Worcestershire sauce, chili powder, garlic powder, onion powder, and cayenne pepper, if using. Add the shrimp and marinate for 20 minutes.

03 Preheat a grill to medium heat, or preheat the oven to 350°F.

04 Remove the shrimp from the marinade and set the shrimp aside. Pour the marinade into a small saucepan and bring to a simmer over medium heat. Continue to simmer for 5 minutes, or until the sauce has reduced by one-quarter. Season with salt and pepper to taste, then transfer to a serving bowl. This is your barbecue sauce.

05 Cut the bacon slices in half crosswise and wrap each piece around a shrimp. Place 3 shrimp on each skewer.

06 Grill the shrimp for 3 to 4 minutes on each side, or bake for 7 to 10 minutes, flipping halfway through. When the shrimp is slightly opaque, it is done.

07 Serve the shrimp with the barbecue sauce. Store leftover shrimp and sauce in separate airtight containers in the refrigerator for up to 4 days.

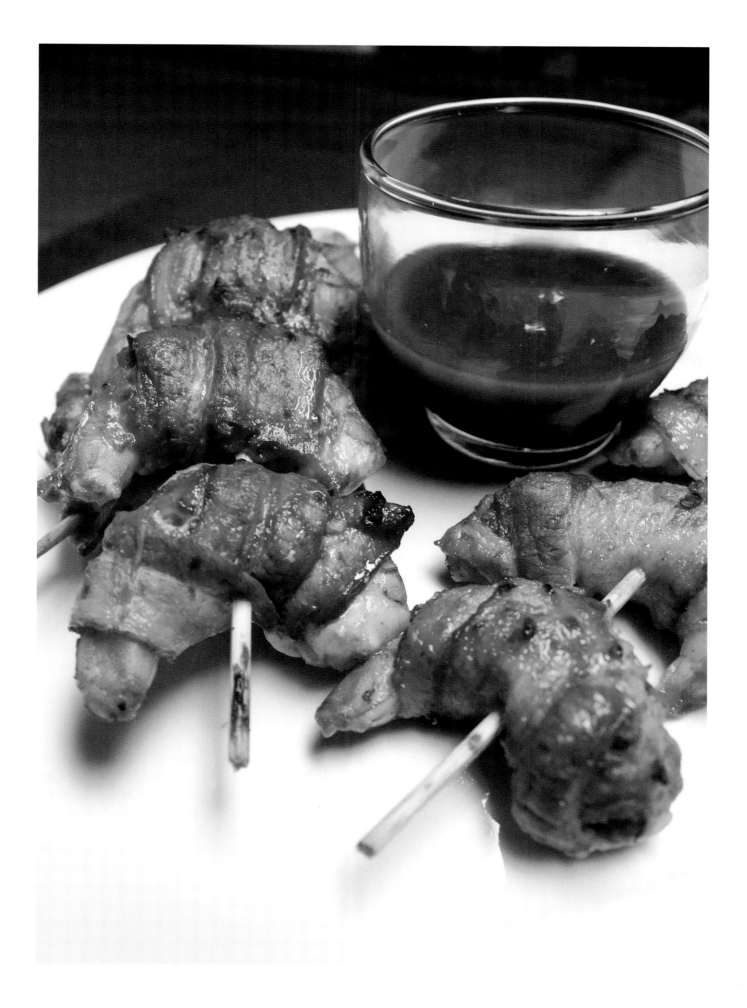

PROSCIUTTO-WRAPPED COCKTAIL SAUSAGES WITH RASPBERRY MAPLE BACON JAM

Macronutrients per serving: **Calories 174** | **Fat 13.7g** | **Carbohydrate 8.2g** | **Fiber 5.2g** | **Protein 7.9g**

Makes: **36 pieces (7 pieces per serving)** | Prep time: **20 minutes** | Cook time: **About 20 minutes**

FOR THE JAM:

4 slices maple bacon, chopped

½ small onion, chopped

½ (12¾-ounce) jar sugar-free raspberry jam

1 teaspoon hot sauce, such as Tabasco

½ teaspoon garlic powder

¼ teaspoon kosher salt

FOR THE SAUSAGES:

12 slices prosciutto (about 3 ounces)

36 smoked cocktail sausages (about 14 ounces)

SPECIAL EQUIPMENT:

7 (12-inch) wooden skewers

01 Place the skewers in a container and cover with water; allow to soak for 20 to 30 minutes.

02 Preheat the oven to 400°F and set a cooling rack inside a sheet pan.

03 Make the jam: Cook the bacon in a sauté pan over medium heat for 4 to 5 minutes to render the fat. Add the onion and sauté for 3 to 4 minutes, until it begins to brown. Add the raspberry jam, hot sauce, garlic powder, and salt and stir to combine. Cook for 2 minutes, stirring occasionally. Transfer the jam to a serving container, let cool slightly, then refrigerate for 15 minutes. It will thicken slightly as it cools.

04 Lay the prosciutto on a flat surface with the short ends facing you. Cut each slice lengthwise into 3 equal strips; you should have 36 thin strips of prosciutto.

05 Roll each sausage in a slice of prosciutto. Place the wrapped sausages on the skewers, 5 to a skewer (one will have 6).

06 Place the skewers on the rack in the sheet pan and bake for 10 minutes or until the outsides begin to crisp, flipping them over halfway through cooking.

07 Serve immediately with the jam. Store leftover sausages and jam in separate airtight containers in the refrigerator for up to 1 week.

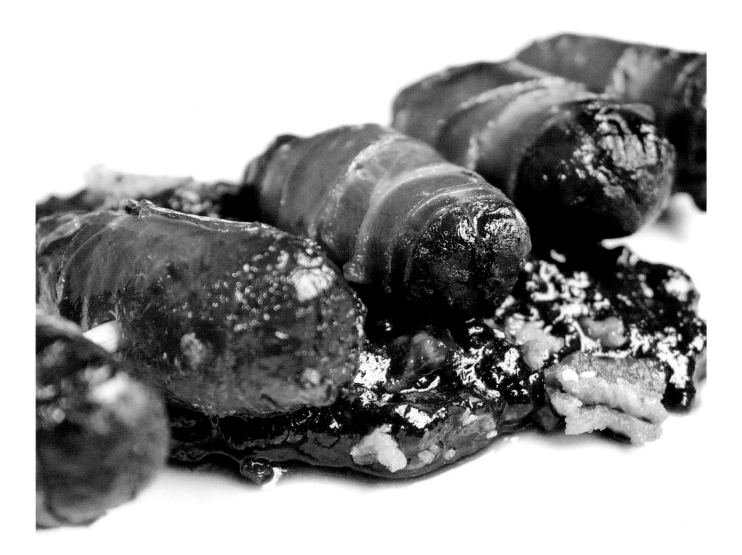

BRUSCHETTA
WITH BASIL OIL

Macronutrients per serving: **Calories 144** | **Fat 12.3g** | **Carbohydrate 2.7g** | **Fiber 0g** | **Protein 4.3g**

Makes: **24 crostini (3 per serving)** | Prep time: **15 minutes** | Cook time: **About 8 minutes**

FOR THE CROSTINI:

4 eggs

½ teaspoon baking soda

½ teaspoon kosher salt

¼ teaspoon cream of tartar

2 tablespoons freshly grated Parmesan cheese

1 teaspoon Italian seasoning

1 teaspoon smoked paprika

½ teaspoon garlic powder

½ teaspoon onion powder

FOR THE BRUSCHETTA:

2 Roma tomatoes, chopped

¼ small red onion, chopped

1 clove garlic, chopped

4 fresh basil leaves, chiffonaded

Salt and pepper to taste

FOR THE BASIL OIL:

Leaves from ½ bunch fresh basil

⅓ cup extra-virgin olive oil

01 Preheat the oven to 400°F. Coat two 12-well muffin tins with olive oil or cooking spray.

02 Separate the eggs, putting the whites in a large bowl and the yolks in a medium-sized bowl.

03 Whisk the egg whites until frothy, then add the baking soda, salt, and cream of tartar and whip until stiff peaks form, about 3 minutes.

04 To the egg yolks, add the Parmesan cheese, Italian seasoning, paprika, garlic powder, and onion powder and beat until smooth. Using a rubber spatula, gently fold the yolk mixture into the egg whites until fully incorporated.

05 Pour the egg mixture into the greased muffin cups, filling them one-quarter full. Bake for 6 to 8 minutes, until lightly browned. Remove from the oven, transfer the crostini to a cooling rack, and let cool.

06 In a small bowl, mix together the ingredients for the bruschetta; set aside.

07 Make the basil oil: In a food processor, blend the basil and olive oil until smooth. Add one-quarter of the basil oil to the bruschetta mixture and stir to combine. Reserve the rest of the basil oil for use as a topping.

08 Once the crostini have cooled, top each with 1 tablespoon of the bruschetta mixture and about 1 teaspoon of the basil oil. Serve immediately. Place leftover crostini, bruschetta, and basil oil in separate containers; store the crostini at room temperature for 1 to 2 days and the bruschetta and basil oil in the refrigerator for up to 4 days.

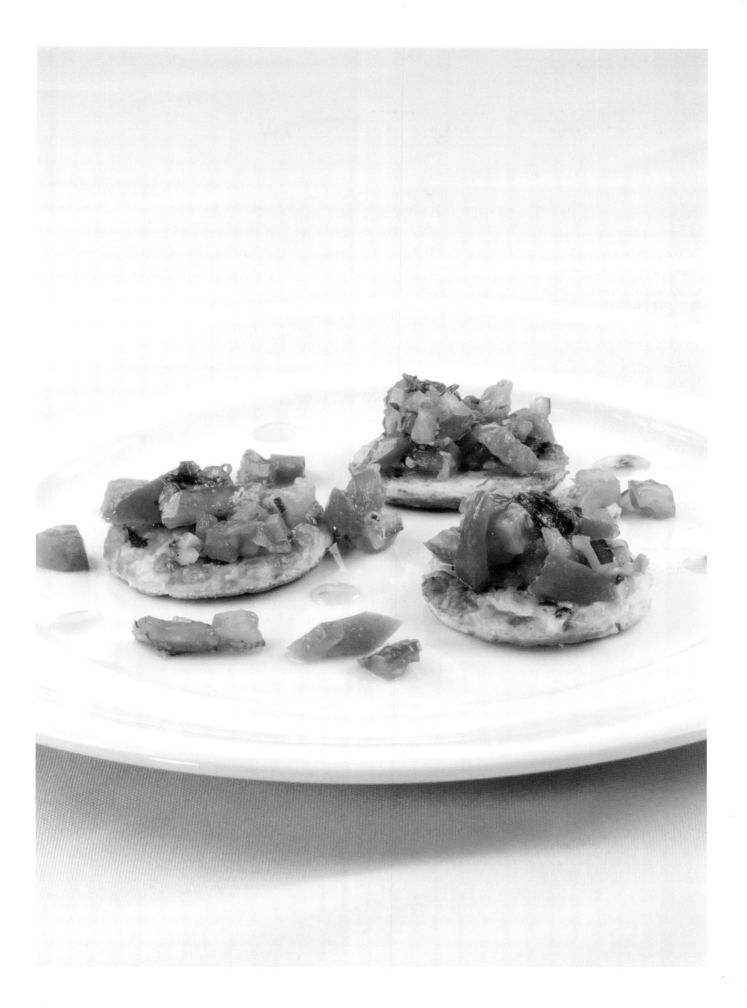

JALAPEÑO PICKLED DEVILED EGGS

Macronutrients per serving: **Calories 265** | **Fat 22.9g** | **Carbohydrate 1.2g** | **Fiber 0g** | **Protein 12.6g**

Makes: **12 deviled eggs (2 per serving)** | Prep time: **10 minutes, plus 1 to 2 days to pickle eggs** | Cook time: **10 minutes**

Serve these eggs with braised purple cabbage and grilled jalapeños for added color and flavor.

2 quarts water

¼ cup white vinegar

2 tablespoons kosher salt

12 eggs, room temperature

2 tablespoons pickling spice

2 jalapeño peppers, sliced

FOR THE DEVILED EGGS:

12 jalapeño-pickled eggs (from above)

¼ cup mayonnaise

1 teaspoon garlic powder

1 teaspoon onion powder

1 teaspoon smoked paprika

1 teaspoon kosher salt

1 teaspoon Worcestershire sauce

⅛ teaspoon cayenne pepper

FOR GARNISH (OPTIONAL):

1 jalapeño pepper, seeded and finely diced

2 tablespoons finely diced red onions

01 To make the pickled eggs: Bring the water to a boil, then mix in the vinegar and salt. Place the eggs in the boiling water and cook for 10 minutes. Remove the eggs from the water with a slotted spoon (reserve the water) and place in a large bowl of ice water to shock the eggs (stop the cooking and cool them).

02 To make the pickling brine: Transfer the egg-cooking water to a heat-proof container, then stir in the pickling spice and sliced jalapeños. Allow the brine to cool to room temperature, then place in the refrigerator to chill.

03 Remove the shells from the hard-boiled eggs.

04 Once the brine is chilled, place the hard-boiled eggs in the brine and return the container to the refrigerator to pickle the eggs for 1 to 2 days.

05 Remove the eggs from the pickling water and cut them in half lengthwise. Transfer the yolks to a bowl and place the whites, cut side up, on a sheet pan.

06 To the bowl with the yolks, add the mayonnaise, garlic powder, onion powder, paprika, salt, Worcestershire sauce, and cayenne pepper; whisk until smooth.

07 Place the egg yolk mixture in a large plastic bag with a corner snipped off or in a pastry bag fitted with a piping tip. Fill each pickled egg white with about 1 tablespoon of the yolk mixture. If desired, garnish with the diced jalapeño and red onions before serving. Store in an airtight container in the refrigerator for up to 5 days.

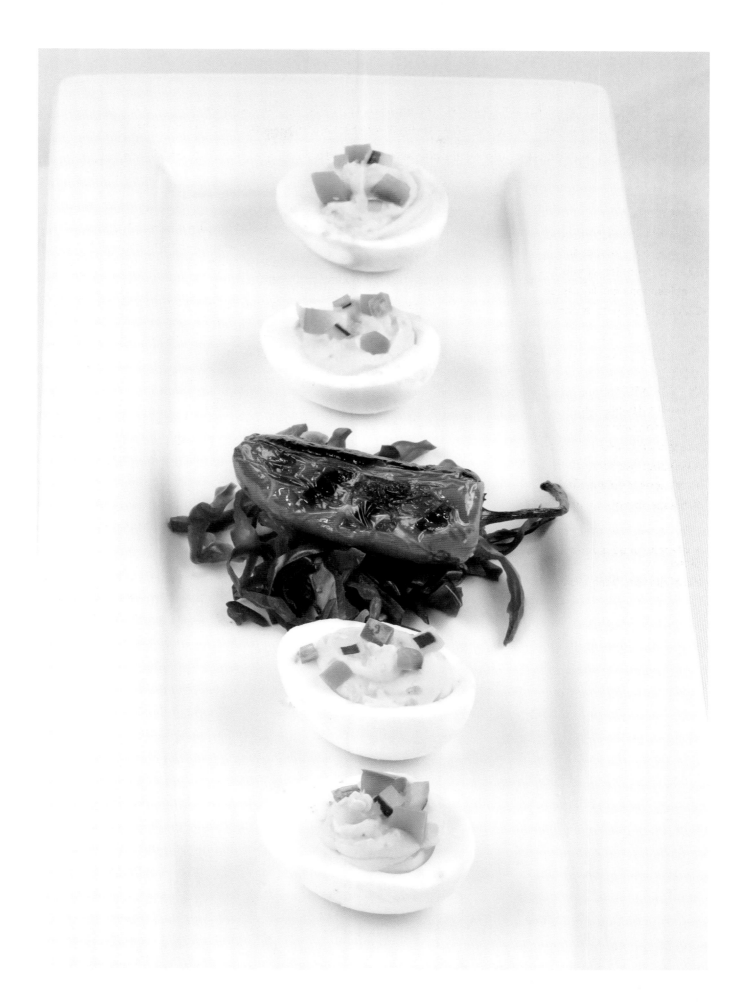

BATTERED BUFFALO BITES

Macronutrients per serving: **Calories 223** | **Fat 18.3g** | **Carbohydrate 9.6g** | **Fiber 3.2g** | **Protein 6.5g**

Makes: **4 servings** | Prep time: **10 minutes, plus 20 minutes to marinate** | Cook time: **About 20 minutes**

¼ cup buttermilk

¼ cup heavy cream

½ cup Buffalo wing sauce, divided

¼ cup plus 2 tablespoons grated Parmesan cheese (about 1¼ ounces), divided

1 tablespoon blanched almond flour

1 tablespoon apple cider vinegar

1 teaspoon smoked paprika

1 teaspoon onion powder

½ teaspoon garlic powder

¼ teaspoon cayenne pepper

¼ teaspoon xanthan gum

1 medium head cauliflower (5 to 6 inches in diameter), cored and cut into 1-inch florets

¼ cup blue cheese dressing

Assorted crudités, for serving (optional)

01 In a large bowl, whisk together the buttermilk, heavy cream, ¼ cup of the Buffalo wing sauce, 2 tablespoons of the Parmesan, almond flour, vinegar, paprika, onion powder, garlic powder, cayenne pepper, and xanthan gum until fully combined. Add the cauliflower florets and toss to coat. Allow to marinate for 20 minutes.

02 Preheat the oven to 450°F and line a sheet pan with parchment paper.

03 Remove the cauliflower florets from the marinade and lay them on the lined sheet pan; reserve the marinade. Roast the cauliflower for 15 to 18 minutes, flipping it over halfway through.

04 While the cauliflower is roasting, transfer the marinade to a small saucepan and bring to a simmer over medium heat. Continue to simmer for 4 to 5 minutes, until reduced by one-quarter. Add the blue cheese dressing and whisk until smooth to make a dipping sauce. Hold over low heat until the cauliflower is done.

05 Remove the cauliflower from the oven and set the broiler to high. Toss the florets in a large bowl with the remaining ¼ cup of Buffalo wing sauce, then return them to the sheet pan and broil for 2 to 3 minutes, until the outsides begin to crisp and turn brown.

06 Remove the cauliflower from the oven and sprinkle with the remaining ¼ cup of Parmesan cheese. Serve hot with the dipping sauce and with crudités, if desired.

07 Store leftover cauliflower and dipping sauce in separate containers in the refrigerator for up to 3 days.

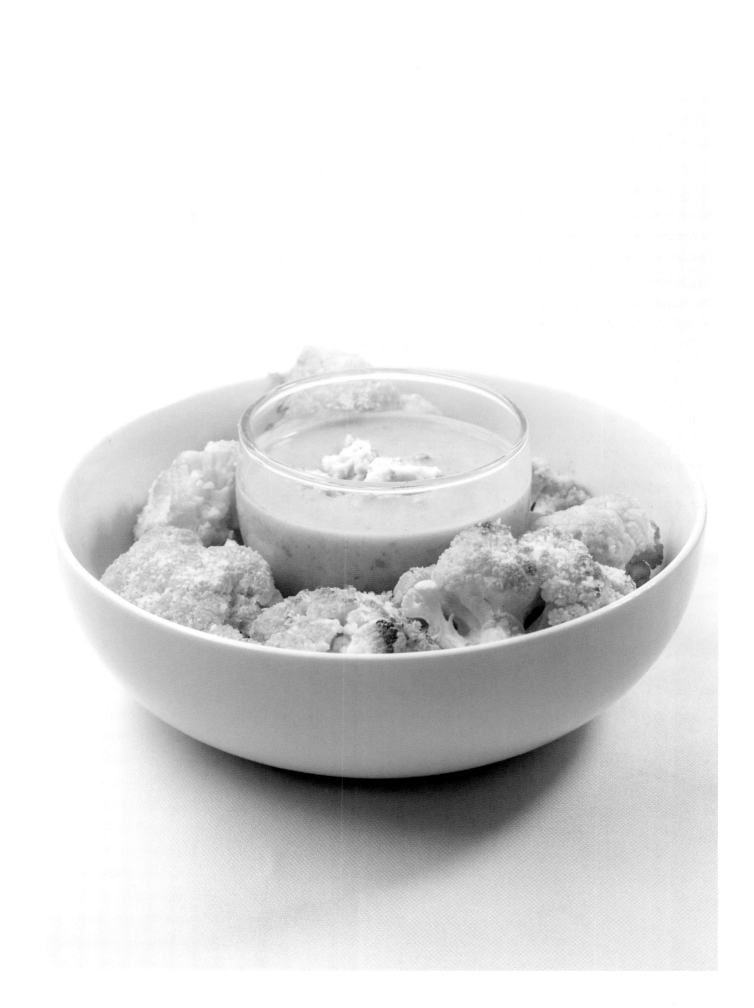

PISTACHIO-COATED GOAT CHEESE WITH RASPBERRY COULIS

Macronutrients per serving: **Calories 262** | **Fat 19.9g** | **Carbohydrate 9.6g** | **Fiber 4g** | **Protein 12.1g**

Makes: **6 servings** | Prep time: **10 minutes** | Cook time: **1 minute**

¼ cup sugar-free raspberry jelly

8 ounces fresh goat cheese

½ cup chopped pistachios

01 Place the raspberry jelly in a microwave-safe bowl, microwave on high for 1 minute, stir until smooth, then set aside until step 4.

02 Form the goat cheese into a log 6 to 8 inches long and place on a flat surface lined with parchment paper.

03 Arrange the chopped pistachios on the parchment paper in a 6 by 4-inch rectangle. Place the goat cheese horizontally along the pistachios. Roll the goat cheese through the pistachios until the cheese is evenly coated.

04 Place the cheese in the refrigerator for 5 minutes to chill. Cut into six equal portions and serve with the raspberry coulis. Store the cheese and coulis in separate airtight containers in the refrigerator for up to 1 week.

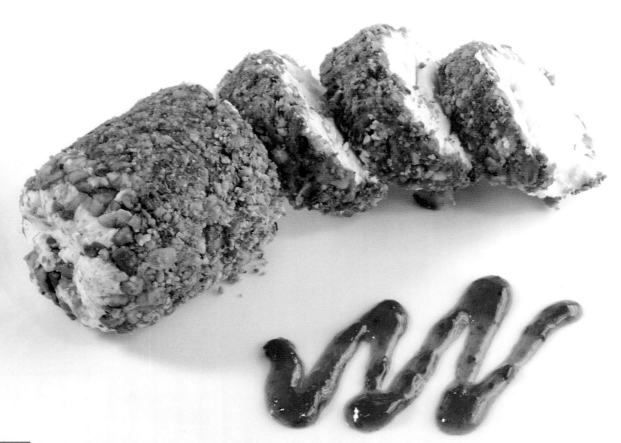

BASIL–CRACKED PEPPER PARMESAN CHIPS

Macronutrients per serving: Calories 204 | Fat 14.3g | Carbohydrate 1.8g | Fiber 0g | Protein 16.8g

Makes: 8 servings | Prep time: 10 minutes | Cook time: 10 minutes

3½ cups freshly grated Parmesan cheese (about 10 ounces)

2 tablespoons chopped fresh basil

Fresh cracked black pepper

1 tablespoon extra-virgin olive oil

01 Preheat the oven to 425°F and line a sheet pan with a silicone baking mat or parchment paper.

02 Place the Parmesan cheese on the sheet pan in tablespoon-sized mounds. Bake for 8 to 10 minutes, until the cheese begins to brown.

03 Remove from the oven, then sprinkle the chips with the basil and some fresh cracked pepper and drizzle with the olive oil. Allow to cool on the pan, then serve. Store in an airtight container for up to 1 week.

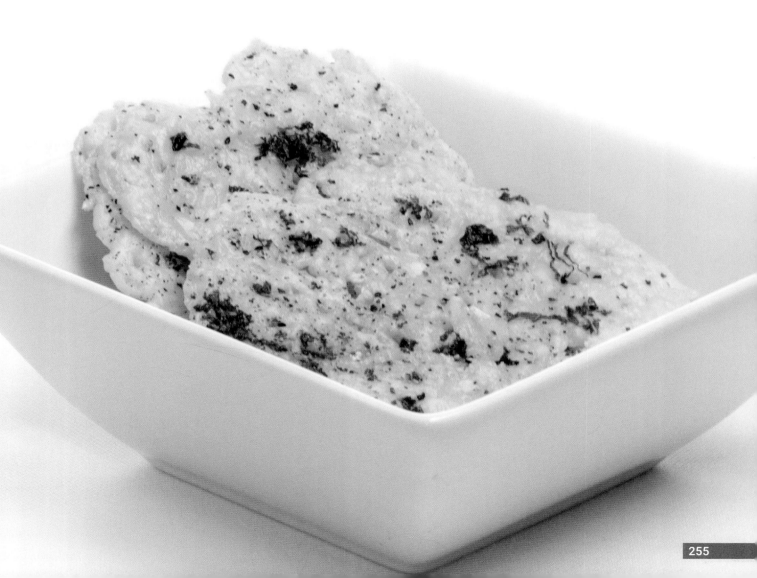

BREADED MOZZARELLA STICKS

Macronutrients per serving: **Calories 312** | **Fat 23g** | **Carbohydrate 7.5g** | **Fiber 5.1g** | **Protein 18.7g**

Makes: **12 sticks (3 sticks per serving)** | Prep time: **10 minutes, plus 2 hours to freeze** | Cook time: **About 12 minutes**

Some oils are better than others for deep-frying; reference the oils and smoke points information on page 199 for details. For this recipe, use an oil such as sunflower, safflower, or peanut oil that can withstand high temperatures.

FOR THE BREADING:

⅓ cup blanched almond flour

⅓ cup high-fiber coconut flour

¼ teaspoon garlic powder

¼ teaspoon onion powder

¼ teaspoon xanthan gum

¼ teaspoon kosher salt

Pinch of ground black pepper

FOR THE EGG WASH:

2 eggs

2 tablespoons heavy cream

6 mozzarella cheese sticks, halved lengthwise

1 cup vegetable oil, for frying

½ cup low-sugar tomato sauce, warmed, for serving

01 Line a sheet pan with parchment paper. (If a typical sheet pan, about 18 by 13 inches, won't fit in your freezer, line two smaller rimmed trays instead.)

02 Make the breading: Sift the almond flour, coconut flour, garlic powder, onion powder, xanthan gum, salt, and pepper into a mixing bowl.

03 Make the egg wash: In a small bowl, whisk together the eggs and heavy cream.

04 Take a mozzarella stick and, using one hand, bread it following this sequence: dip it into the egg wash, then into the breading, then into the egg wash again, and then back into the breading. Place the breaded cheese stick on the lined sheet pan and repeat with the rest of the cheese sticks. When all the sticks are breaded, place the pan in the freezer for a minimum of 2 hours.

05 When ready to fry the cheese sticks, heat the oil to 400°F in a 1-quart saucepan or a deep-fryer. Fry the cheese sticks 2 or 3 at a time for 1 to 2 minutes, until golden brown.

06 Transfer the fried cheese sticks to a paper towel–lined plate. Serve hot with tomato sauce for dipping.

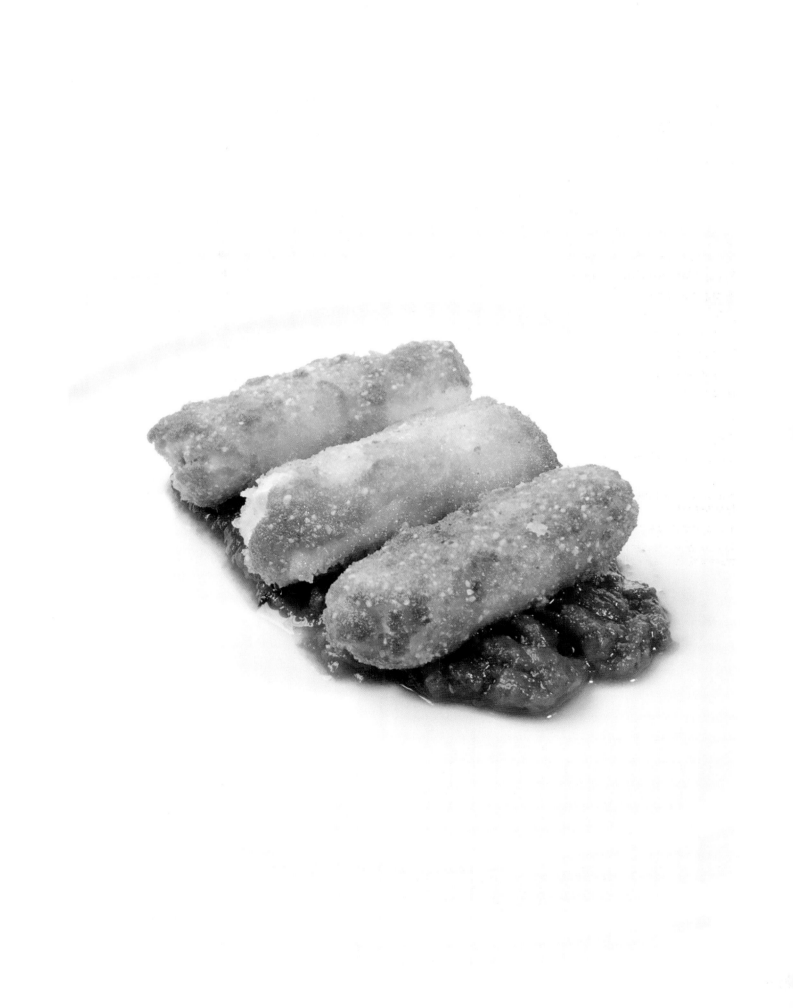

CHIPS AND SMOKY QUESO DIP

Macronutrients per serving: **Calories 354** | **Fat 32.3g** | **Carbohydrate 4.7g** | **Fiber 2.8g** | **Protein 11.1g**

Makes: **4 servings** | Prep time: **20 minutes, plus 1 hour to chill dough** | Cook time: **5 minutes**

FOR THE DIP:

1 tablespoon olive oil

2 tablespoons chopped onions

2 tablespoons chopped canned green chilies

1 tablespoon chopped canned chipotle peppers (packed in adobo sauce)

2 cloves garlic, chopped

½ cup chicken stock (page 345)

4 ounces cream cheese (½ cup), cubed, softened

½ cup cubed queso fresco (about 2 ounces)

½ cup shredded cheddar cheese (about 2 ounces)

2 tablespoons sour cream

1 tablespoon chopped fresh cilantro

1 teaspoon ground cumin

1 teaspoon smoked paprika

¼ teaspoon cayenne pepper (optional)

FOR THE CHIPS:

2 cups fresh spinach

¼ cup blanched almond flour

3 tablespoons high-fiber coconut flour

¼ ounce serving pork rinds (about ½ cup)

1½ teaspoons chia seeds

1 teaspoon psyllium husk powder

½ teaspoon kosher salt

½ teaspoon garlic powder

½ teaspoon onion powder

⅛ teaspoon xanthan gum

Pinch of cayenne pepper

½ cup water, warmed

2 tablespoons coconut oil or MCT oil, divided, for the pan

FOR GARNISH (OPTIONAL):

1 tablespoon chopped fresh cilantro

1 batch Pico de Gallo (page 224)

Lime wedges

01 Make the dip: Heat the olive oil in a 5-quart saucepan over medium heat. Add the onions, chilies, and chipotle peppers and sauté for 2 minutes, then add the garlic and sauté for 1 minute.

02 Add the chicken stock and simmer for 2 minutes. Whisk in the cheeses until the mixture is smooth and free of lumps.

03 Whisk in the sour cream, cilantro, cumin, paprika, and cayenne pepper, if using, until the spices are fully incorporated; set aside.

04 Make the dough for the chips: Combine the spinach, almond flour, coconut flour, pork rinds, chia seeds, psyllium husk powder, salt, garlic powder, onion powder, xanthan gum, and cayenne pepper in a food processor, then, while pulsing, slowly add the water until a dough comes together. Remove the dough from the food processor and knead on a greased flat surface for 1 to 2 minutes, until a smooth dough ball forms. Coat the inside of a mixing bowl with cooking spray, then place the dough in the bowl, cover with plastic wrap, and place in the refrigerator for 1 hour to chill.

05 After the dough has chilled, take it out of the bowl and place on a flat surface. Cover with parchment paper and use a rolling pin to roll it out to a thickness of ⅛ to ¼ inch. Remove the parchment and cut the dough into 9-inch circles using a 9-inch sauté pan or cake pan as a guide. Repeat the process until all the dough is used, gathering up the scraps and re-rolling the dough as needed.

06 Heat 1 tablespoon of the coconut oil in a 10-inch or larger skillet over medium-high heat. Add a circle of dough and cook for 3 to 4 minutes, until browned, then flip and cook on the other side until crisp. Repeat with the remaining dough circles, adding 1 teaspoon of coconut oil to the pan for each new tortilla. Set the cooked tortillas on a cutting board and cut each tortilla into 8 triangular chips.

07 Transfer the queso dip from the saucepan to a serving container and serve with the chips, garnished with cilantro, pico de gallo, and lime wedges, if desired. Store the queso in an airtight container in the refrigerator for up to 4 days, and store the chips in an airtight container at room temperature for up to 3 days.

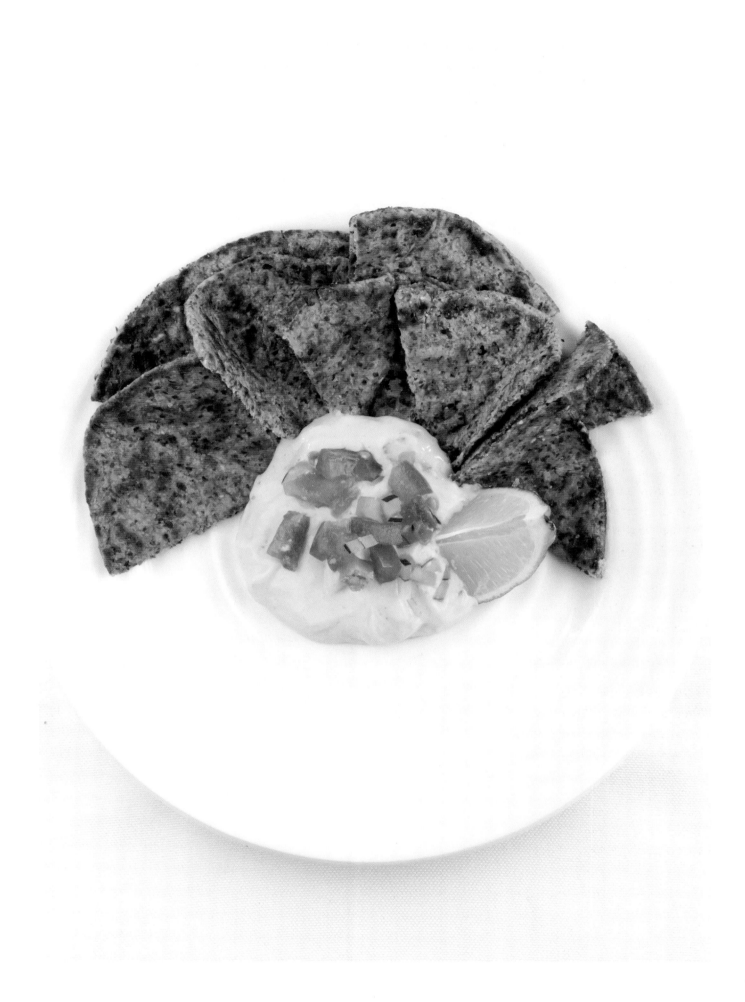

BACON-WRAPPED FETA

Macronutrients per serving: Calories **414** | Fat **33.3g** | Carbohydrate **7.5g** | Fiber **1.2g** | Protein **25g**
Makes: **4 servings** | Prep time: **10 minutes** | Cook time: **About 5 minutes**

12 ounces feta cheese

12 slices thick-cut bacon (about ⅛ inch thick)

12 cherry tomatoes, halved

SPECIAL EQUIPMENT:

Toothpicks

01   Portion the feta into twelve 1-ounce balls.

02   Lay a slice of bacon on a flat surface with a short end facing you. Place a feta ball on the bacon slice, at the short end nearest you. Begin to roll the bacon over the feta and keep rolling until you get to the middle of the strip. Once at the midway point, gently turn the feta ball 90 degrees, until the exposed side is facing the remaining portion of the bacon strip, and continue to roll until the feta is completely wrapped on all sides. Spear with a toothpick to hold the bacon in place. Repeat with the remaining slices of bacon and feta.

03   In a large sauté pan over medium heat, sear the bacon-wrapped feta balls for 2 to 3 minutes on each side, until the bacon is crisp. Remove from the pan and serve with cherry tomatoes. Store in an airtight container in the refrigerator for up to 1 week.

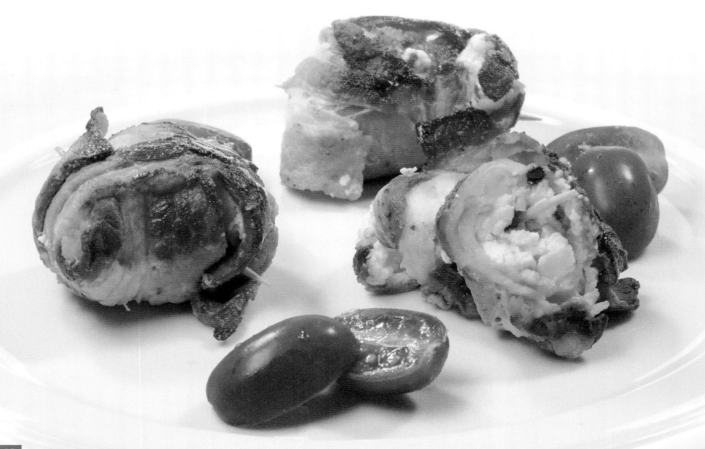

CHIPOTLE BLTS

Macronutrients per serving: **Calories 295** | **Fat 28.7g** | **Carbohydrate 2.7g** | **Fiber 1.8g** | **Protein 7g**

Makes: **12 BLTs (3 per serving)** | Prep time: **10 minutes** | Cook time: **5 minutes**

6 slices thick-cut bacon, cut in half crosswise

¼ cup mayonnaise

1 tablespoon canned chipotle peppers (packed in adobo sauce), finely chopped

1 teaspoon Sriracha sauce

2 large tomatoes, thinly sliced into 18 half-moons

12 leaves romaine lettuce

01 Preheat a sauté pan over medium-high heat, then cook the bacon in the pan for 4 to 5 minutes, until crispy. Remove from the pan and set aside.

02 In a small bowl, whisk together the mayonnaise, chipotle peppers, and Sriracha until smooth.

03 To assemble the BLTs, place 3 tomato slices and 1 half-slice of bacon on each lettuce leaf, then top with 1 teaspoon of the Sriracha mayo. Repeat with the remaining ingredients to make a total of 12 BLTs. Serve immediately. Store leftovers in an airtight container in the refrigerator for up to 2 days.

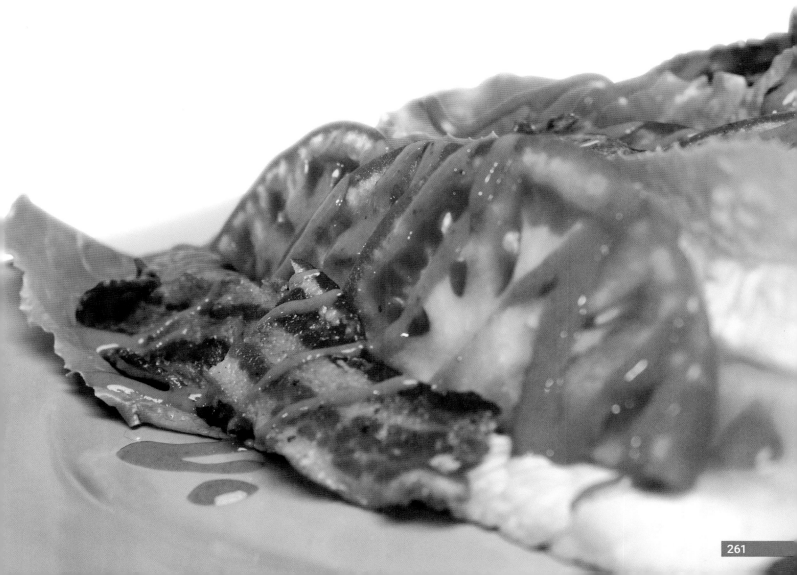

BUFFALO CHICKEN DIP

Macronutrients per serving (dip only): **Calories 185** | **Fat 14.3g** | **Carbohydrate 2.7g** | **Fiber 0g** | **Protein 9.9g**

Makes: **10 servings** | Prep time: **10 minutes** | Cook time: **About 25 minutes**

2 slices thick-cut bacon, roughly chopped

1 tablespoon olive oil

2 tablespoons chopped onions

1 clove garlic, chopped

8 ounces boneless, skinless chicken thighs

½ teaspoon kosher salt

6 ounces chicken stock (page 345)

1 (8-ounce) package cream cheese, cubed, softened

½ cup shredded mild or medium-sharp cheddar cheese (about 2 ounces)

¼ cup shredded sharp cheddar cheese (about 1 ounce)

2 tablespoons freshly grated Parmesan cheese

⅓ cup Buffalo wing sauce

1 tablespoon medium-hot hot sauce, such as Frank's RedHot

FOR GARNISH:

2 tablespoons bacon bits

1 tablespoon chopped onions

FOR SERVING:

Assorted crudités and/or pork rinds

01 In a sauté pan over medium heat, cook the bacon for about 4 minutes, until the fat begins to render and the bacon becomes crispy.

02 Add the olive oil, onions, and garlic to the pan and sauté for 1 to 2 minutes, until the onions are translucent. Remove from the pan and set aside.

03 Season the chicken with the salt, place in the pan, and sauté for 2 to 3 minutes on each side. Add the chicken stock and simmer until the chicken is fully cooked, 8 to 10 minutes. Remove the chicken from the pan, then roughly chop or shred the meat.

04 Return the bacon and onions to the sauté pan over medium heat. Add the cheeses and whisk until the mixture is smooth and warmed through, 5 to 7 minutes.

05 Add the Buffalo wing sauce and hot sauce to the cheese mixture and whisk until the sauces are fully incorporated.

06 Fold in the chicken, then transfer the dip to a serving dish. Garnish with the bacon bits and chopped onions. Serve with crudités and/or pork rinds. Store in an airtight container in the refrigerator for up to 4 days.

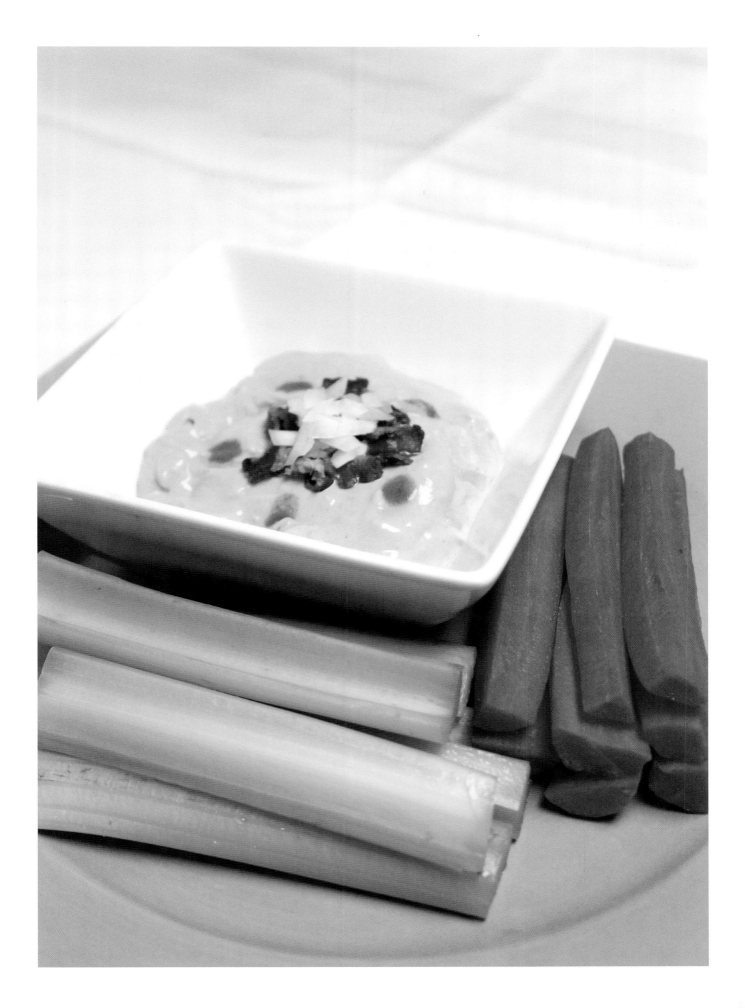

MAIN DISHES
& SIDES

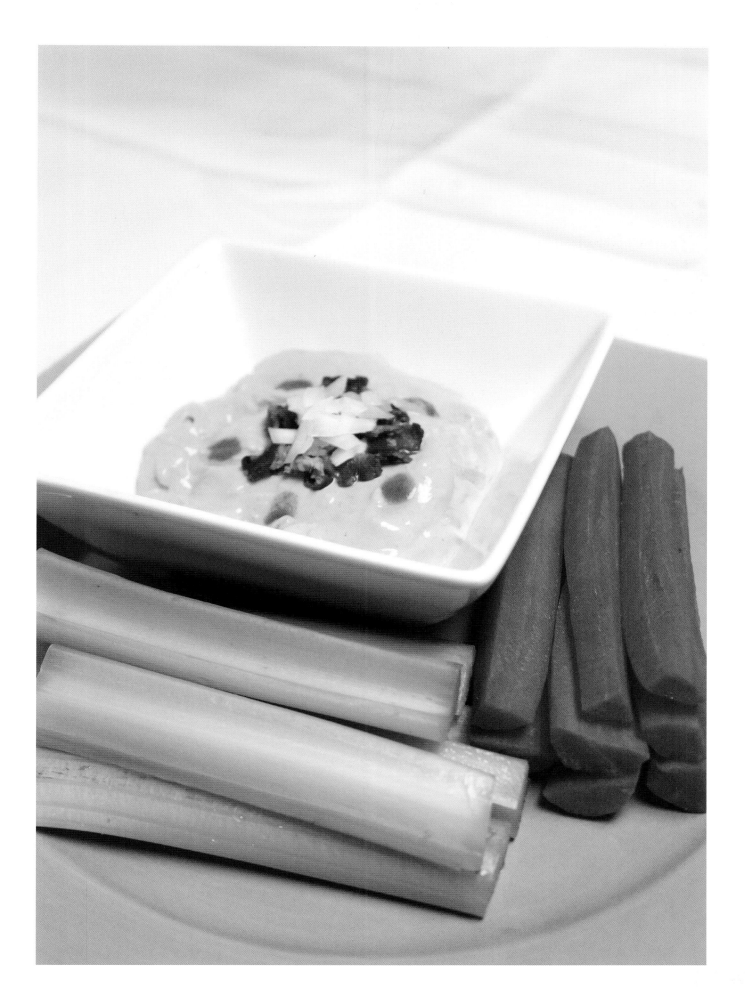

MAIN DISHES
& SIDES

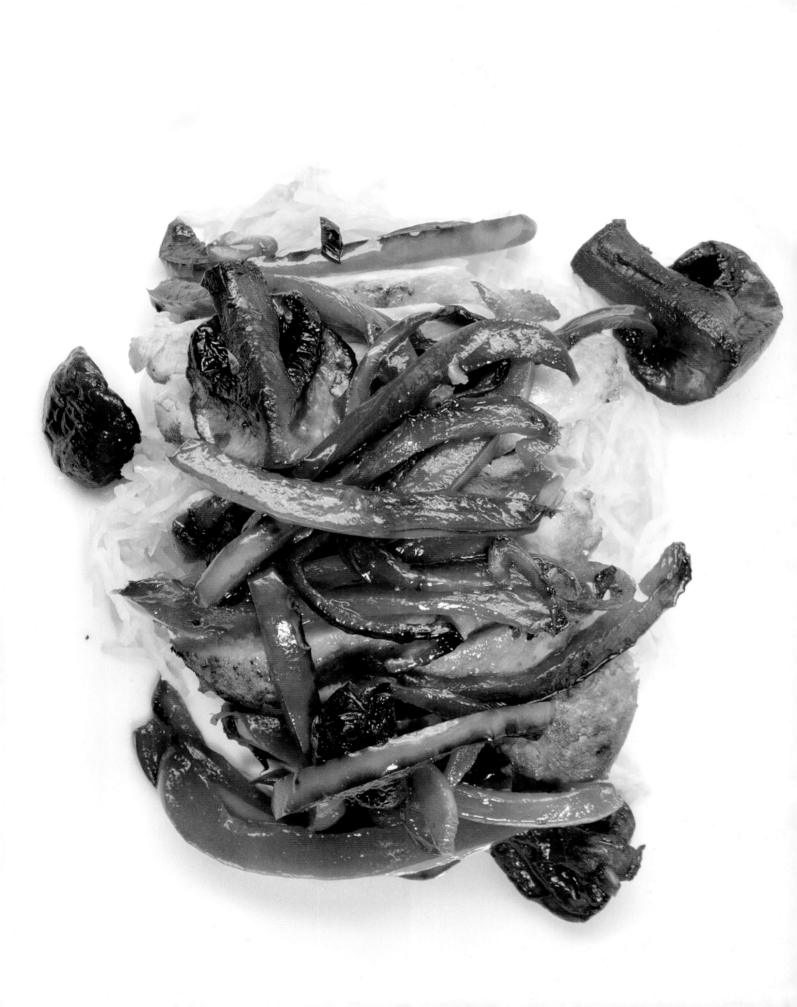

DRY-AGED STEAKS WITH DUCHESS "POTATOES" AND PAN-FRIED OKRA

Macronutrients per serving: **Calories 563** | **Fat 45.4g** | **Carbohydrate 8.3g** | **Fiber 2.5g** | **Protein 31.7g**

Makes: **4 servings** | Prep time: **15 minutes, plus 10 minutes to marinate** | Cook time: **About 25 minutes**

Grass-fed beef and butter are superior to their conventionally produced counterparts because they contain high amounts of antioxidants, omega-3 fatty acids, and conjugated linoleic acid, which may be beneficial for cardiovascular health.

FOR THE STEAKS:

4 (4-ounce) dry-aged boneless sirloin steaks, about 1¼ inches thick

¼ cup (½ stick) unsalted butter

½ teaspoon kosher salt

½ teaspoon fresh cracked peppercorn medley

1 tablespoon safflower oil

FOR THE OKRA:

2 tablespoons unsalted butter

12 okra spears

¼ teaspoon kosher salt

¼ teaspoon fresh cracked peppercorn medley

FOR THE DUCHESS "POTATOES":

1 small head cauliflower (4 to 5 inches in diameter), cored and florets grated

¼ cup shredded Gouda cheese (about 1 ounce)

3 tablespoons unsalted butter

2 tablespoons freshly grated Parmesan cheese

2 tablespoons heavy cream

1 egg

½ teaspoon kosher salt

¼ teaspoon ground nutmeg

¼ teaspoon ground white pepper

FOR GARNISH:

2 tablespoons freshly grated Parmesan cheese

01 Preheat the oven to 425°F. Line a sheet pan with parchment paper.

02 Remove the steaks from the refrigerator and allow them to come to room temperature for 10 minutes.

03 Marinate the steaks: Put the ¼ cup of butter in a microwave-safe bowl and microwave just until melted. Pour the butter into a sheet pan. Season the steaks with the salt and cracked pepper, then place the steaks in the melted butter to marinate for 10 minutes, flipping them over after 5 minutes.

04 Marinate the okra: In a microwave-safe bowl, melt the 2 tablespoons of butter, then add the okra, salt, and cracked pepper to the bowl. Marinate for 10 minutes, stirring occasionally.

05 Make the duchess "potatoes": Fill a 1-quart saucepan with water and bring to a boil. Blanch the grated cauliflower in the boiling water for 30 to 45 seconds. Drain the cauliflower in a fine-mesh sieve, then transfer to a food processor. Let the cauliflower cool for 3 to 4 minutes, then add the rest of the ingredients for the duchess "potatoes" to the food processor; process the mixture until it is smooth and free of lumps. Transfer the mixture to a pastry bag fitted with a piping tip (or to a plastic bag with a corner snipped off) and pipe twelve 2-inch rounds onto the lined sheet pan. Bake for 8 to 10 minutes, until the tops begin to brown.

06 Meanwhile, preheat a large oven-safe sauté pan over medium-high heat. Pour the butter used to marinate the steaks into the hot pan, along with the safflower oil; allow to heat for 1 to 2 minutes. Add the steaks to the pan and sear for 3 to 4 minutes, then flip and sear for 2 to 3 minutes on the other side. Place the steaks in the oven to finish cooking to your desired doneness (3 to 5 minutes for medium-rare). Allow the steaks to rest for 5 minutes before serving.

07 In another sauté pan over medium heat, heat the butter used to marinate the okra for 1 to 2 minutes. Add the okra to the pan and sear for 2 to 3 minutes, then flip and sear for an additional 2 to 3 minutes.

08 Plate each steak with 3 okra spears and 3 duchess "potato" rounds and serve immediately. Store leftovers in an airtight container in the refrigerator for up to 3 days.

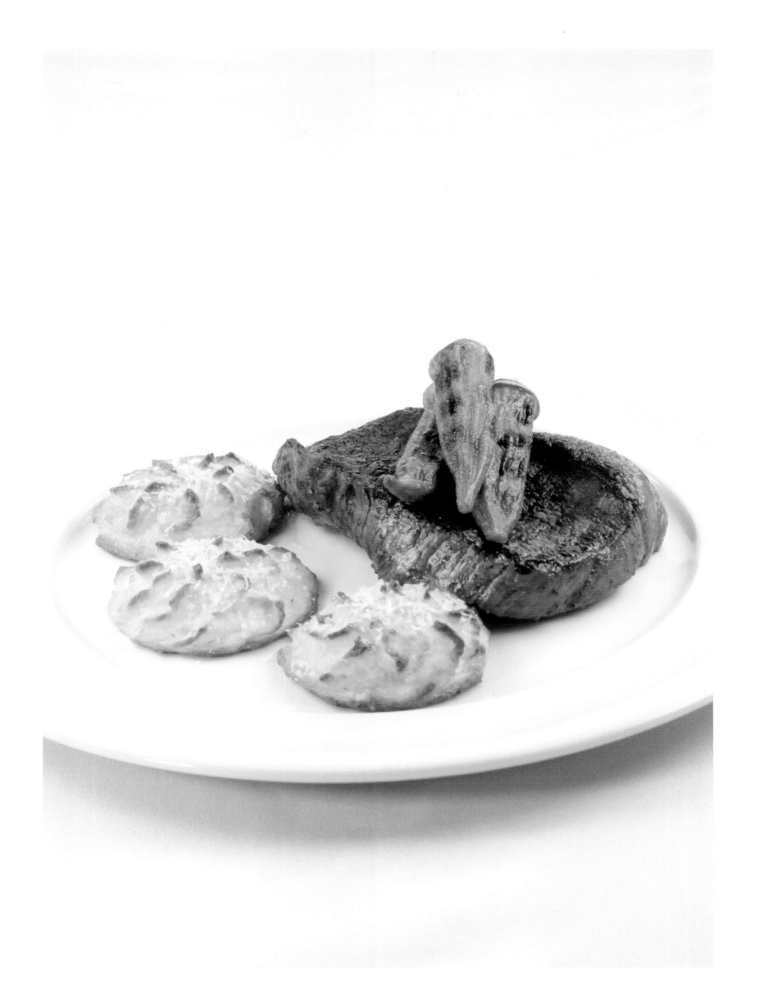

NEW YORK STYLE PIZZA

Macronutrients per serving: **Calories 136** | **Fat 10.6g** | **Carbohydrate 2.2g** | **Fiber 0.6g** | **Protein 8.8g**

Makes: **8 slices (1 per serving)** | Prep time: **15 minutes** | Cook time: **About 15 minutes**

FOR THE CRUST:

1 cup freshly grated mozzarella cheese (about 4 ounces)

¼ cup blanched almond flour

2 tablespoons cream cheese, softened

1 egg

½ teaspoon garlic salt

½ teaspoon onion powder

¼ cup chopped fresh basil

FOR THE TOPPINGS:

1 cup chopped spinach

¼ cup freshly grated mozzarella cheese (about 1 ounce)

¼ cup halved cherry tomatoes

10 slices pepperoni (about ½ ounce)

1 ounce thinly sliced prosciutto (optional)

01 Preheat the oven to 425°F. Place a pizza stone or round baking sheet in the oven to preheat.

02 To make the crust: Place the grated mozzarella and almond flour in a microwave-safe bowl. Microwave on high for 30 to 60 seconds, stir with a wooden spoon until homogenous, and then return to the microwave and cook on high for another 30 seconds.

03 Add the cream cheese and stir until well combined. Then add the egg, garlic salt, onion powder, and basil and stir until homogenous. With your hands, knead the dough until it becomes stiff.

04 Place a sheet of parchment paper on a flat surface. Dump the dough onto the parchment and cover with another piece of parchment paper. With a rolling pin, roll out the dough into a flat circle. Note: If the dough becomes too hard, place it back in the microwave for 20 to 30 seconds in 10-second increments to soften, but be careful not to cook the egg.

05 Remove the preheated pizza stone from the oven. Gently transfer the crust to the stone, then dock the dough with a fork. Bake for 6 to 8 minutes, until the dough begins to crisp around the edges.

06 Remove from the oven and top with the spinach, mozzarella, cherry tomatoes, and pepperoni, then place back in the oven for another 4 to 5 minutes to melt the cheese and warm the toppings. Remove from the oven and top with prosciutto if desired. Allow to rest for 2 minutes.

07 Cut the pizza into 8 equal slices and serve hot. Store leftovers in an airtight container in the refrigerator for up to 4 days.

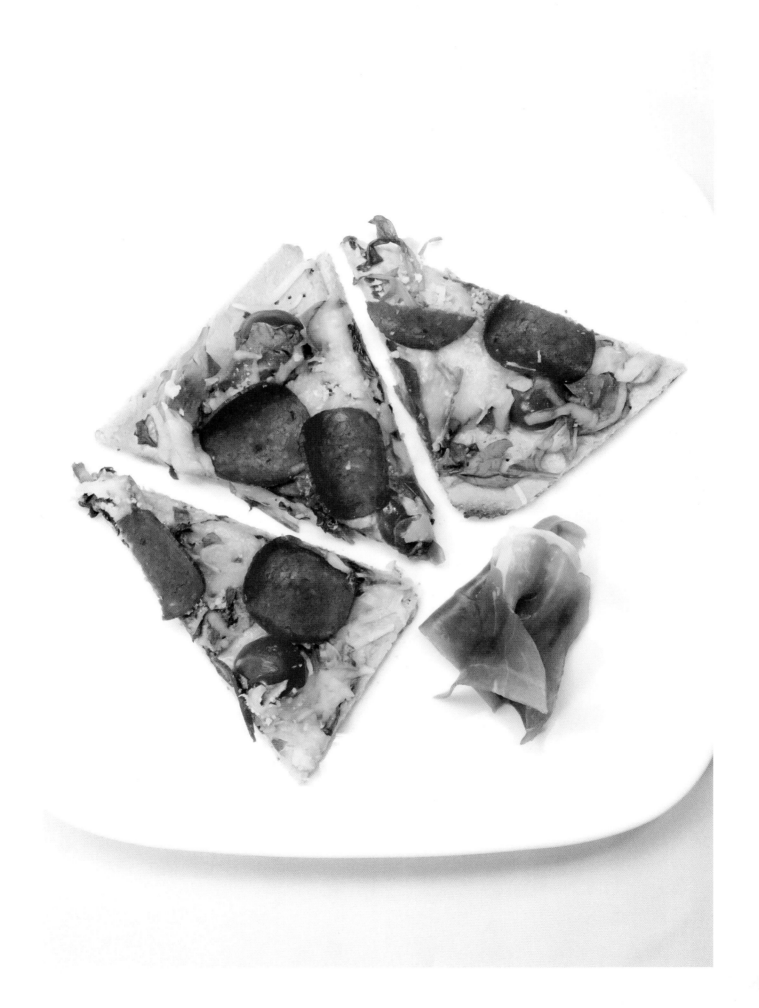

CHICKEN AVOCADO ROULADE

Macronutrients per serving: **Calories 653** | **Fat 50g** | **Carbohydrate 12.8g** | **Fiber 10g** | **Protein 41g**

Makes: **2 servings** | Prep time: **30 minutes** | Cook time: **About 25 minutes**

A *roulade* is a dish that is traditionally served in the form of a roll. Some kind of meat is flattened, filled, rolled, and then cooked.

6 slices thick-cut bacon, 2 slices cut in half lengthwise

2 (4-ounce) boneless, skinless chicken breast halves

2 medium avocados

¼ cup heavy cream

1 teaspoon onion powder

½ teaspoon garlic powder

½ teaspoon kosher salt

¼ teaspoon ground black pepper

01 Preheat the oven to 325°F. Set a cooling rack inside a sheet pan.

02 Lay 3 slices of bacon on a flat surface. Lay one of the chicken breasts on top of the bacon and roll the bacon around the breast. Repeat with the remaining bacon and chicken breast.

03 Preheat a large sauté pan over medium-high heat. Sear each of the four sides of the roulades for about 2 minutes, then remove the roulades from the pan and place on a sheet pan. Bake for 15 to 18 minutes, until the internal temperature reaches 165°F.

04 While the roulades are baking, prepare the avocado mash: Cut the avocados in half, remove the pits, and scoop the flesh into a medium-sized bowl. Add the heavy cream, onion powder, garlic powder, salt, and pepper, then mash until smooth.

05 Remove the roulades from the oven, place on a cutting board, and cut into 4 or 5 equal slices with a carving knife. Serve immediately with the avocado mash. Store leftovers in the refrigerator for up to 3 days.

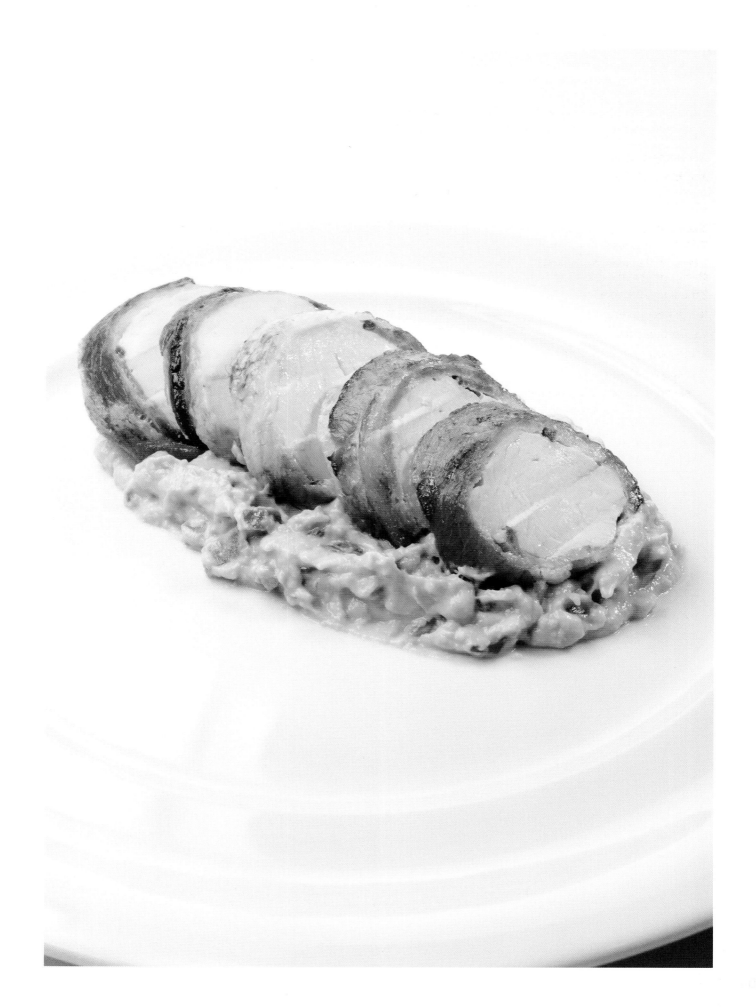

PUMPKIN CHILI

Macronutrients per serving: **Calories 318** | **Fat 23.4g** | **Carbohydrate 8.3g** | **Fiber 1.9g** | **Protein 14.5g**
Makes: **6 servings** | Prep time: **15 minutes** | Cook time: **About 40 minutes**

4 slices thick-cut bacon, cut cross-wise into lardons

8 ounces 85/15 ground sirloin

2 cups diced yellow squash

2 cups diced zucchini

1 cup diced carrots

¼ cup chopped onions

3 cloves garlic, chopped

2 cups chicken stock (page 345)

1 (15-ounce) can pumpkin puree

½ cup heavy cream

½ teaspoon ground cinnamon

¼ teaspoon ground cloves

¼ teaspoon ground nutmeg

¼ teaspoon red pepper flakes

1 teaspoon hot sauce, such as Tabasco

Kosher salt

½ cup raw pecans, finely chopped

FOR GARNISH:

1½ teaspoons coconut oil

¼ cup chopped onions

2 ounces ham, finely diced

01 Preheat the oven to 350°F.

02 In a 5-quart saucepan over medium-low heat, slowly cook the bacon to render the fat, about 10 minutes.

03 Add the ground sirloin, increase the heat to medium, and sauté for 1 to 2 minutes.

04 Add the yellow squash, zucchini, carrots, and onions and sauté, stirring constantly, until the onions are translucent. Add the garlic and cook for 2 to 3 minutes.

05 Deglaze the pan with the chicken stock, then add the pumpkin puree and simmer over low heat for about 20 minutes, until slightly reduced and thickened to the consistency of gravy. Stir in the heavy cream, spices, and hot sauce until well incorporated, then bring back up to a simmer for 1 to 2 minutes. Taste and season with salt, if needed.

06 Toast the pecans in the oven until fragrant and lightly browned, about 3 minutes, then stir them into the soup.

07 Prepare the garnish: Melt the coconut oil in a small skillet over medium-high heat, then add the onions and sauté for 2 to 3 minutes.

08 Serve the chili garnished with the sautéed onions and finely diced ham.

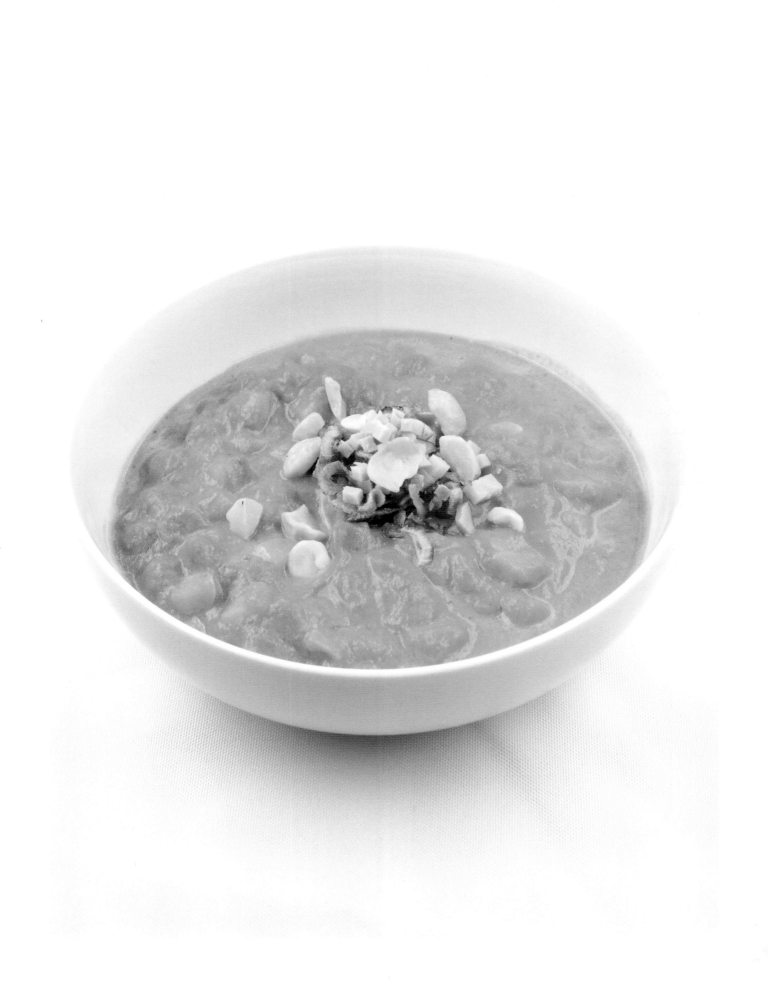

THAI COCONUT CURRY

Macronutrients per serving: **Calories 333** | **Fat 21.5g** | **Carbohydrate 8.9g** | **Fiber 1.8g** | **Protein 26.4g**

Makes: **4 servings** | Prep time: **15 minutes** | Cook time: **About 18 minutes**

FOR THE CHICKEN CURRY:

1 (13½-ounce) can full-fat coconut milk, divided

1 teaspoon red curry paste

2 cloves garlic, minced

1 lime, juiced

2 fresh Thai chilies, chopped (remove seeds for less heat)

1 pound boneless, skinless chicken thighs, flattened

1 tablespoon coconut oil

½ red bell pepper, cut into strips

½ yellow or green bell pepper, cut into strips

½ cup chicken stock (page 345)

Leaves from 1 bunch fresh Thai basil, chopped, divided

2 tablespoons unsweetened coconut flakes

FOR THE CAULIFLOWER RICE:

1 tablespoon coconut oil

¼ red onion, chopped

1 cup grated cauliflower florets

Chopped Thai basil leaves (reserved from above)

¼ teaspoon kosher salt

FOR GARNISH:

1 jalapeño pepper, sliced

1 lime, quartered

01 Marinate the chicken: Shake the can of coconut milk vigorously. In a mixing bowl, whisk together ¼ cup of the coconut milk, the red curry paste, garlic, lime juice, and Thai chilies. Add the chicken and toss to coat. Allow to marinate for 5 minutes.

02 Make the curry: In a large sauté pan, heat 1 tablespoon of coconut oil over medium-high heat, then add the bell peppers and sauté for 2 to 3 minutes. Put the marinated chicken and any remaining marinade in the pan and sauté for 3 to 4 minutes, then pour in the chicken stock and simmer for 5 minutes.

03 Whisk the remaining coconut milk, half of the Thai basil, and the coconut flakes into the pan and allow to simmer for about 3 minutes, until the chicken is no longer pink in the center and the internal temperature reaches 165°F.

04 While the chicken curry is simmering, make the rice: In another sauté pan, heat 1 tablespoon of coconut oil over medium-high heat, then add the red onion and cook for 2 to 3 minutes. Add the grated cauliflower and remaining Thai basil and cook for an additional 2 to 3 minutes, until the rice has begun to brown. Season with the salt and divide among 4 serving plates.

05 Serve the curry over the cauliflower rice, garnished with sliced jalapeño and lime quarters. Store leftovers in an airtight container in the refrigerator for up to 4 days.

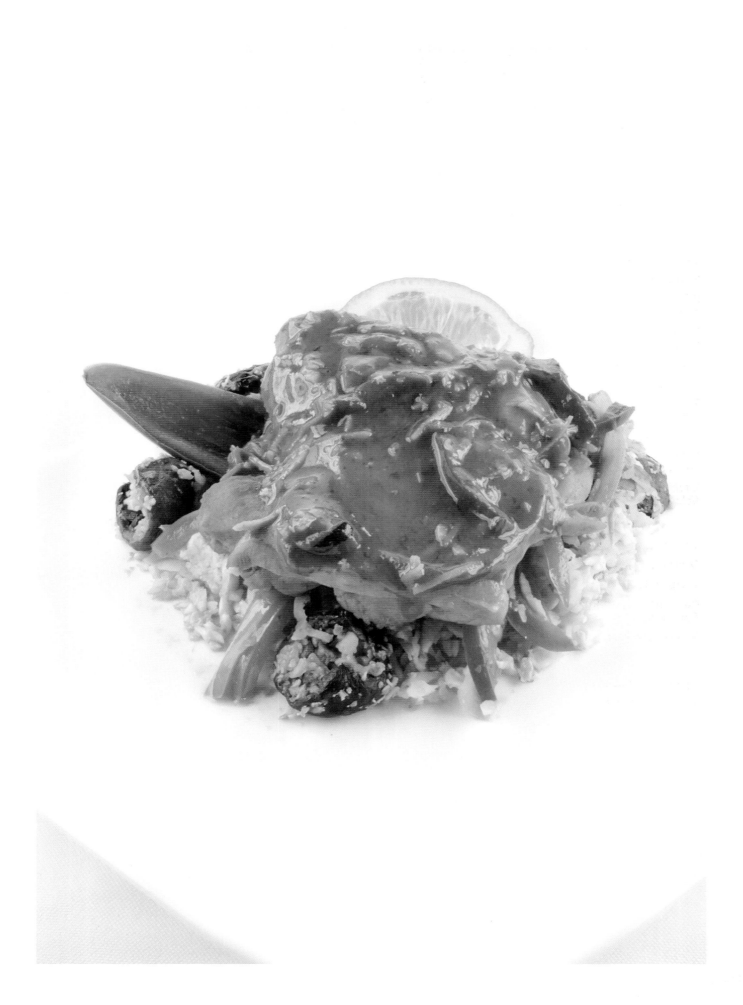

CHICKEN STIR-FRY

Macronutrients per serving: **Calories 469** | **Fat 33.2g** | **Carbohydrate 19g** | **Fiber 11g** | **Protein 23.6g**
Makes: **4 servings** | Prep time: **10 minutes** | Cook time: **About 30 minutes**

FOR THE "NOODLES":

1 medium spaghetti squash, halved lengthwise

2 tablespoons coconut oil

½ teaspoon kosher salt

½ teaspoon black pepper

FOR THE EGG WASH:

2 eggs

2 tablespoons heavy cream

FOR THE FLOUR COATING:

½ cup high-fiber coconut flour

1 teaspoon Chinese five-spice powder

4 tablespoons coconut oil, divided

12 ounces boneless, skinless chicken thighs, pounded to an even flatness

2 bell peppers (red, green, yellow, or a combination), cut into strips

½ small onion, sliced

2 cups mushrooms, halved or quartered depending on size

2 tablespoons soy sauce

01 Preheat the oven to 450°F.

02 Scoop out the seeds from the spaghetti squash. Rub the inside with the 2 tablespoons of coconut oil and season with the salt and pepper. Place on a sheet pan, cut side up, and roast for 15 to 17 minutes, until softened. Remove from the oven and, when cool enough to handle, remove the "noodle" strands with a fork; set aside.

03 Preheat a sauté pan over medium-high heat. While the pan is heating, prepare the egg wash and flour coating: In one bowl, whisk together the eggs and heavy cream; in another bowl, sift together the coconut flour and five-spice powder.

04 Heat 3 tablespoons of the coconut oil in the sauté pan over medium heat. Dip the chicken thighs in the egg wash, then toss in the flour coating. When the oil is hot, sear the chicken in batches for 2 to 3 minutes, then flip it over and sear for 2 to 3 minutes on the other side, until the outsides are browned and the internal temperature reaches 165°F; finish cooking the chicken in the oven if it starts to brown too much. Remove from the pan and set aside; repeat with the remaining chicken.

05 Wipe out the pan and place it over high heat. Heat the remaining tablespoon of coconut oil in the pan, then add the bell peppers, onion, and mushrooms and stir-fry for 3 to 4 minutes. Add the soy sauce and cook for 1 to 2 minutes, until the vegetables are tender and the sauce is completely cooked into the vegetables. While the vegetables are cooking, slice the cooked chicken into 1-inch-wide strips.

06 Divide the "noodles" among 4 plates. Top with the stir-fried vegetables and chicken and serve. Store leftovers in an airtight container in the refrigerator for up to 5 days.

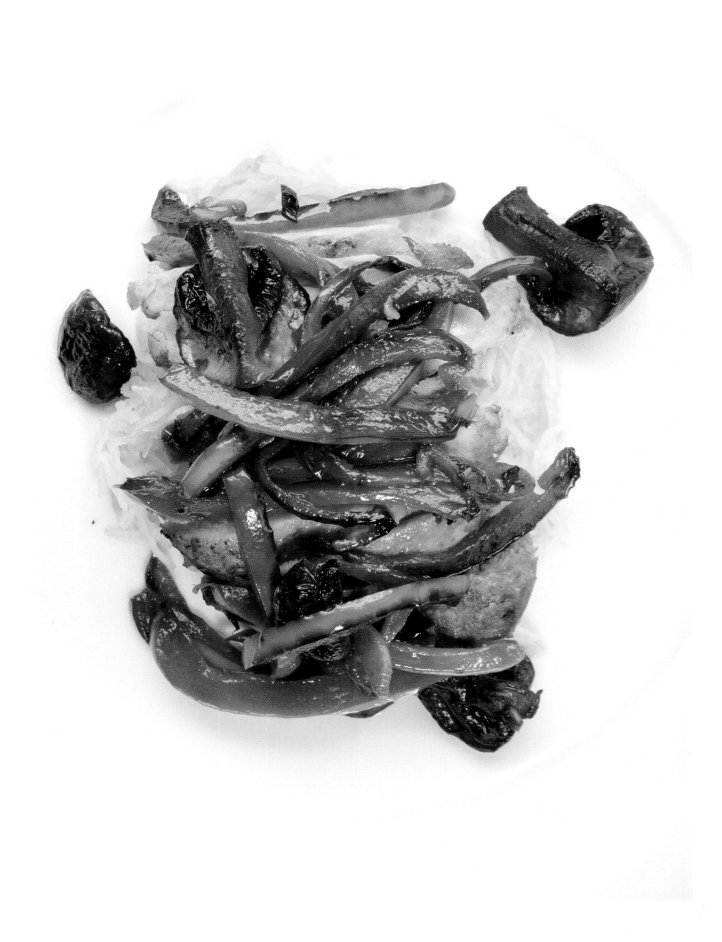

BRIE SIRLOIN SLIDERS

Macronutrients per serving: **Calories 693** | **Fat 52.5g** | **Carbohydrate 10.6** | **Fiber 3.2** | **Protein 45.6g**

Makes: **12 sliders (3 per serving)** | Prep time: **20 minutes** | Cook time: **About 10 minutes**

FOR THE BUNS:

7 eggs, room temperature

½ teaspoon baking soda

½ teaspoon kosher salt

¼ teaspoon cream of tartar

7 ounces cream cheese, softened

2 tablespoons grated Parmesan cheese

FOR THE BURGERS:

12 ounces 80/20 ground sirloin

1 tablespoon garlic powder

2 teaspoons onion powder

1 teaspoon kosher salt

½ teaspoon black pepper

2 teaspoons hot sauce

1 egg

2 tablespoons ricotta cheese

½ small bunch fresh basil, chopped

FOR THE AVOCADO SPREAD:

1 avocado, halved, peeled, and pitted

1 teaspoon lemon juice

¼ teaspoon kosher salt

ADDITIONAL TOPPINGS:

6 ounces Brie

2 Roma tomatoes, sliced

¼ small red onion, sliced

SPECIAL EQUIPMENT:

Toothpicks

01　Preheat the oven to 400°F, preheat a grill to medium-high heat, and coat two 12-well muffin tins with coconut oil or cooking spray.

02　Make the buns: Separate the eggs, placing the yolks in a mixing bowl and the whites in a separate, larger mixing bowl. Whisk the whites until frothy, then add the baking soda, salt, and cream of tartar. Whip until stiff peaks form, about 3 minutes. To the bowl with the yolks, add the cream cheese and Parmesan and beat until smooth. Using a rubber spatula, gently fold the yolk mixture into the whipped whites until fully incorporated. Pour the combined mixture into the prepared muffin tin, filling the cups half full. Bake for 7 to 9 minutes, until the tops are just starting to brown. Remove the buns to a cooling rack and let cool.

03　While the buns are baking, make the burgers: Mix together the ground sirloin, garlic powder, onion powder, salt, pepper, hot sauce, egg, ricotta, and basil. Divide into 12 patties, about 1 ounce each. Set aside.

04　Puree the avocado, lemon juice, and salt in a food processor, then transfer the puree to a pastry bag or a plastic bag with a corner snipped off. Pipe about 1½ teaspoons onto each of the 12 slider buns. (You can also simply spread the puree on the buns.)

05　Grill the burgers to the desired doneness (1½ to 2 minutes per side for medium). Assemble the sliders with 2 buns, 1 burger patty, and your choice of toppings. Pin each slider with a toothpick and serve.

06　Store leftovers in an airtight container in the refrigerator for up to 2 days.

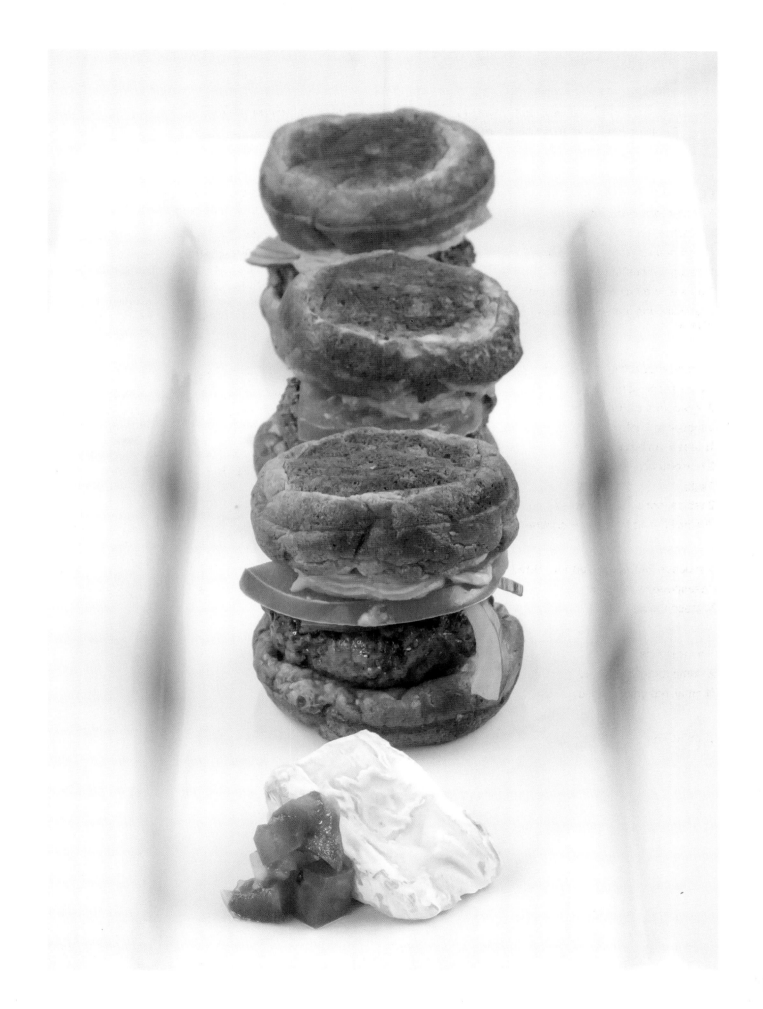

CALIFORNIA-STYLE SPAGHETTI AND MEATBALLS

Macronutrients per serving: **Calories 415** | **Fat 32.7g** | **Carbohydrate 9.8** | **Fiber 2.8g** | **Protein 23g**

Makes: **4 servings** | Prep time: **20 minutes** | Cook time: **About 20 minutes**

FOR THE MEATBALLS:

8 ounces 80/20 ground sirloin

4 ounces Italian sausage, casings removed

¼ small yellow onion, chopped

1 teaspoon garlic powder

1 teaspoon kosher salt

2 tablespoons unsalted butter, for the pan

FOR THE "SPAGHETTI":

2 tablespoons unsalted butter

2 small zucchini, spiral-sliced into noodles (about 2 cups)

2 small yellow squash, spiral-sliced into noodles (about 2 cups)

1 orange bell pepper, cut into strips

1 small tomato, diced

Kosher salt and ground black pepper

FOR THE SAUCE:

¼ cup half-and-half

1 medium avocado, mashed

Kosher salt and ground black pepper

¼ cup freshly grated Parmesan cheese (about ¾ ounce), for garnish

01 Preheat the oven to 300°F.

02 Make the meatballs: In a large bowl, mix together the ground sirloin, sausage, onion, garlic powder, and salt until well combined. Divide the mixture into twelve 1-ounce meatballs. In a large sauté pan over medium heat, heat 2 tablespoons of butter for 1 to 2 minutes. Add the meatballs and sear for 1 to 2 minutes on each side, then remove them to a sheet pan. Place in the oven to finish cooking, 4 to 7 minutes.

03 Make the "spaghetti": In the same sauté pan you used to cook the meatballs, heat 2 tablespoons of butter over medium heat. Add the zucchini and squash noodles, bell pepper, and tomato and sauté for 3 to 4 minutes. Reduce the heat to low and simmer until the noodles and bell pepper are tender, about 5 minutes. Season to taste with salt and pepper.

04 While the meatballs are cooking and the noodles are simmering, make the sauce: Place the half-and-half in a microwave-safe bowl and microwave for 1 to 2 minutes. Add the mashed avocado to the heated half-and-half and whisk until smooth. Season to taste with salt and pepper.

05 Divide the noodles and vegetables among 4 plates, then top each plate with 3 meatballs. Spoon the avocado sauce over the meatballs and garnish with Parmesan; serve immediately. Store leftovers in an airtight container in the refrigerator for up to 6 days.

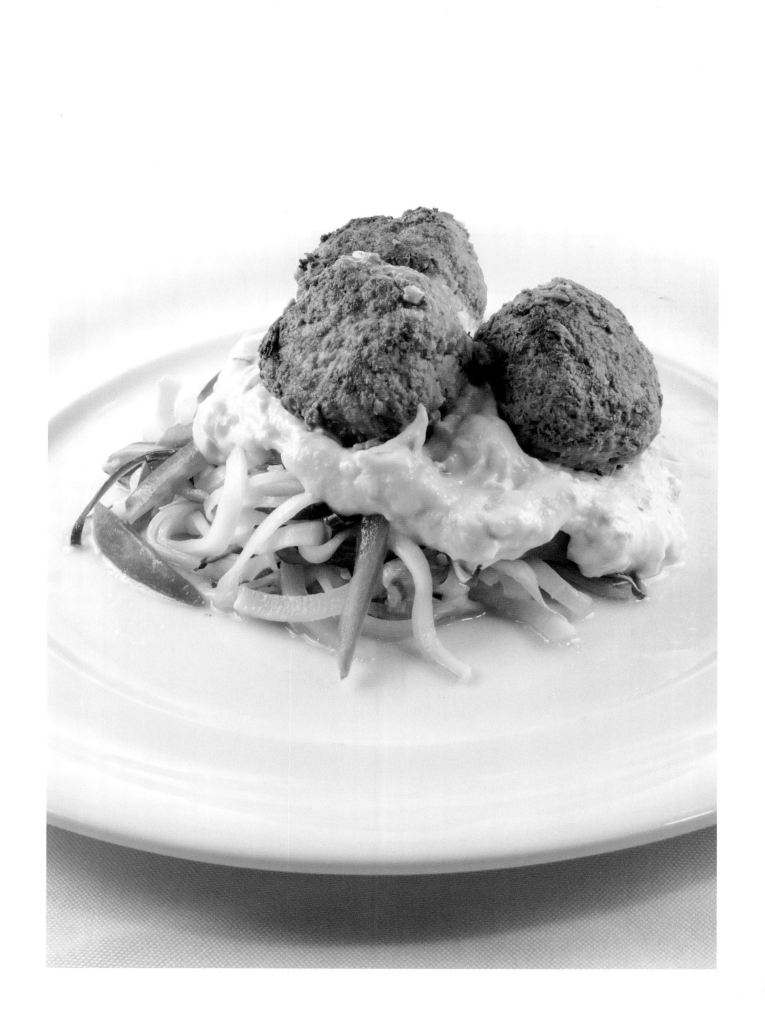

SHEPHERD'S PIE

Macronutrients per serving: **Calories 517** | **Fat 43.5g** | **Carbohydrate 8.5** | **Fiber 3.8** | **Protein 23g**

Makes: **6 servings** | Prep time: **20 minutes** | Cook time: **About 15 minutes**

¼ cup (½ stick) unsalted butter

2 eggs

½ small head cauliflower (4 to 5 inches in diameter), cored and florets grated

2 tablespoons blanched almond flour

1 tablespoon psyllium husk powder

1 teaspoon kosher salt

½ teaspoon ground black pepper

¼ teaspoon cream of tartar

½ cup shredded smoked Gouda (about 2 ounces)

4 fresh basil leaves, chopped

3 medium zucchini (about 6 ounces each), 1 diced, 2 sliced lengthwise into ¼-inch planks

1 medium carrot, diced

½ small onion, sliced

¼ cup raw almonds, chopped

1 pound ground lamb

4 ounces British-style pork sausages (bangers), casings removed

2 tablespoons olive oil

2 tablespoons chopped fresh basil, for garnish (optional)

01 Preheat the oven to 425°F.

02 Melt the butter in a 12-inch square or 14-inch round cast-iron pan over low heat.

03 Meanwhile, separate the eggs into two mixing bowls. To the yolks, add the cauliflower, almond flour, psyllium husk powder, salt, and pepper and mix until the ingredients are incorporated. Whisk the whites until frothy, then add the cream of tartar and continue to whisk until stiff peaks form, about 3 minutes. Fold the cauliflower mixture, Gouda, and basil into the whipped whites; set aside.

04 Increase the heat under the cast-iron pan to medium, then add the diced zucchini, carrot, onion, and almonds and sauté for 2 to 3 minutes, stirring constantly. Add the ground lamb and sausages and mix to combine with the vegetables. Press the mixture flat across the bottom of the pan; turn off the heat.

05 Pour the cauliflower/egg white mixture over the lamb mixture, then, using a spatula, press down until it is evenly distributed across the pan. Drizzle with the olive oil, then put the pan in the oven for 12 to 14 minutes, until the top is browned.

06 Meanwhile, blanch the zucchini planks: Fill a 2½-quart saucepan three-quarters full of water and bring to a boil. Blanch the zucchini until tender, 2 to 3 minutes, then drain.

07 Remove the shepherd's pie from the oven and serve hot over the blanched zucchini planks, garnished with fresh basil, if desired. Store leftovers in an airtight container in the refrigerator for up to 4 days.

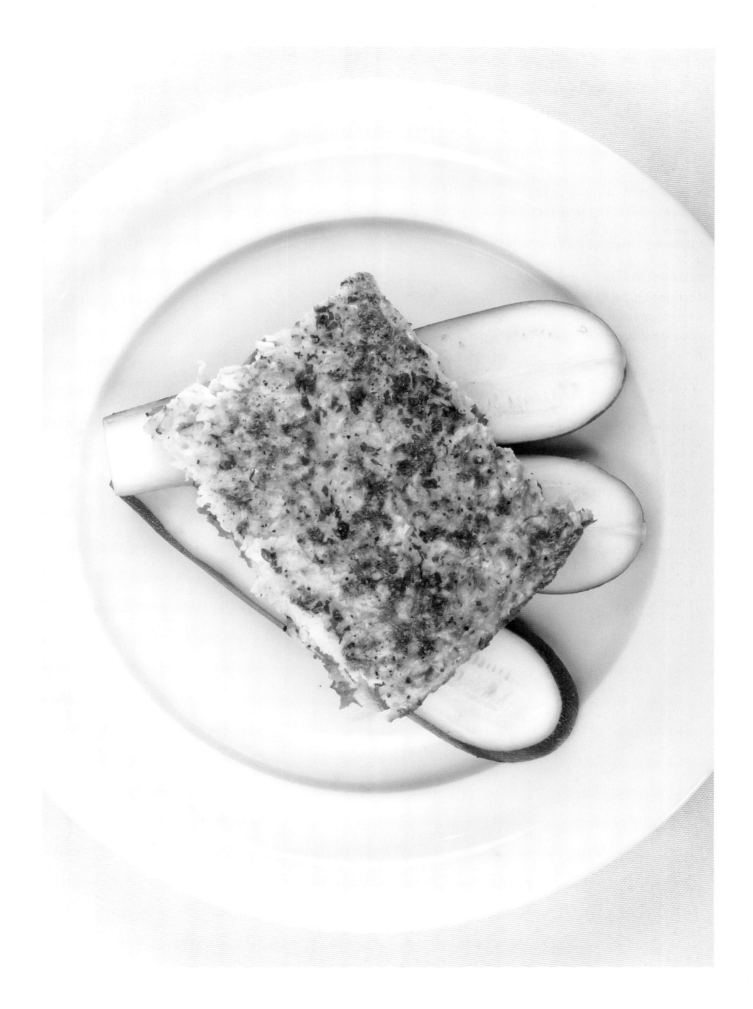

BACON-WRAPPED CAJUN CASSEROLE

Macronutrients per serving: **Calories 487** | **Fat 38.9g** | **Carbohydrate 4.5g** | **Fiber 0.7g** | **Protein 26.4g**

Makes: **6 servings** | Prep time: **15 minutes** | Cook time: **About 20 minutes**

14 slices thick-cut bacon

8 ounces andouille sausage, chopped

1 medium zucchini (about 6 ounces), sliced lengthwise into 3 planks

4 ounces cream cheese (½ cup), softened

½ head radicchio, thinly sliced

¼ small red onion, thinly sliced

¼ cup shredded cheddar cheese (about 1 ounce)

01 Preheat the oven to 375°F. Lay a large sheet of parchment paper on a flat surface. Lay the bacon slices on top of the parchment, cover with plastic wrap, and roll out the bacon with a rolling pin until it is ⅛ inch thick.

02 Line a 9 by 5-inch loaf pan with the bacon so that the inside of the pan is completely covered with bacon and the ends of the bacon slices hang over the edge.

03 Press the sausage into the bottom of the pan on top of the bacon, followed by layers of the zucchini, cream cheese, radicchio, red onion, and cheddar cheese.

04 Fold the bacon strips over the top so that all of the ingredients are completely covered by the bacon. Bake for 18 to 20 minutes, until the internal temperature reaches 155°F.

05 Remove from the oven, pour off any excess grease, then flip the casserole out onto a flat surface. Turn the oven to broil, then place the casserole back in the loaf pan with bottom side facing up. Return the pan to the oven for 3 to 5 minutes to crisp the top of the casserole.

06 Transfer the casserole to a cutting board, slice into 6 equal portions, and serve immediately. Store leftovers in an airtight container in the refrigerator for up to 4 days.

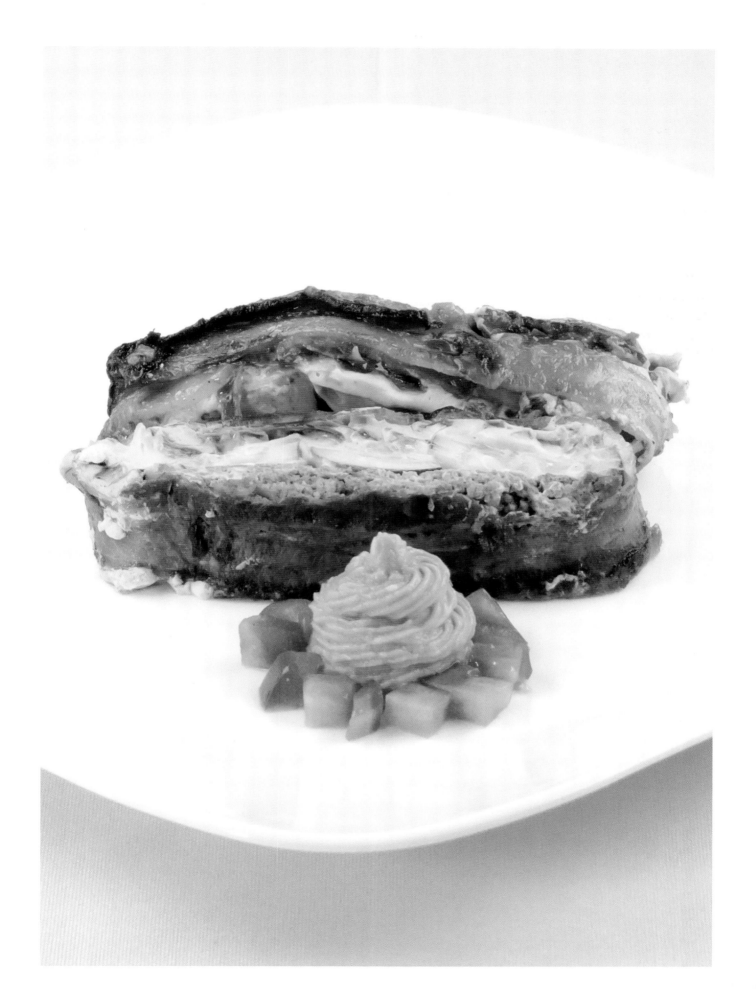

SALMON OVER SPINACH RISOTTO

Macronutrients per serving: **Calories 441** | **Fat 31.7g** | **Carbohydrate 6.6g** | **Fiber 3g** | **Protein 29.7g**

Makes: **4 servings** | Prep time: **15 minutes** | Cook time: **About 20 minutes**

4 (4-ounce) Atlantic salmon fillets

Kosher salt and ground black pepper

2 tablespoons chopped fresh dill, divided

4 tablespoons (½ stick) unsalted butter, divided

8 ounces spinach, chopped

½ small yellow onion, chopped

1 small stalk celery, chopped

½ medium head cauliflower (5 to 6 inches in diameter), cored and florets grated

2 cloves garlic, chopped

½ cup fish stock (page 346)

¼ cup heavy cream

¼ cup grated Parmesan cheese (about ¾ ounce)

01 Preheat the oven to 300°F. Season the salmon generously with salt, pepper, and 1 tablespoon of the dill.

02 Preheat a cast-iron skillet or other oven-safe skillet over medium heat. Heat 2 tablespoons of the butter in the skillet, then place the salmon in the pan, skin side down, and sear for 3 to 4 minutes. While searing, use a spoon to continuously baste the salmon with butter. Flip the salmon over, then transfer the skillet to the oven and bake for 5 to 7 minutes, until the fish flakes and a thermometer reads 145°F when inserted in the thickest part of the fillet.

03 While the salmon is baking, melt the remaining 2 tablespoons of butter in a sauté pan over medium heat. Add the spinach, onion, and celery and cook for 2 minutes, then add the cauliflower and sauté for 3 minutes. Add the garlic, remaining tablespoon of dill, and fish stock and simmer until the stock has evaporated and the cauliflower resembles rice, about 5 minutes.

04 Add the heavy cream and Parmesan to the risotto and stir until the cream has reduced by about three-quarters, about 2 minutes. Season to taste with salt and pepper. Divide the risotto among 4 plates and top each plate with a piece of salmon. Store leftovers in an airtight container in the refrigerator for up to 4 days.

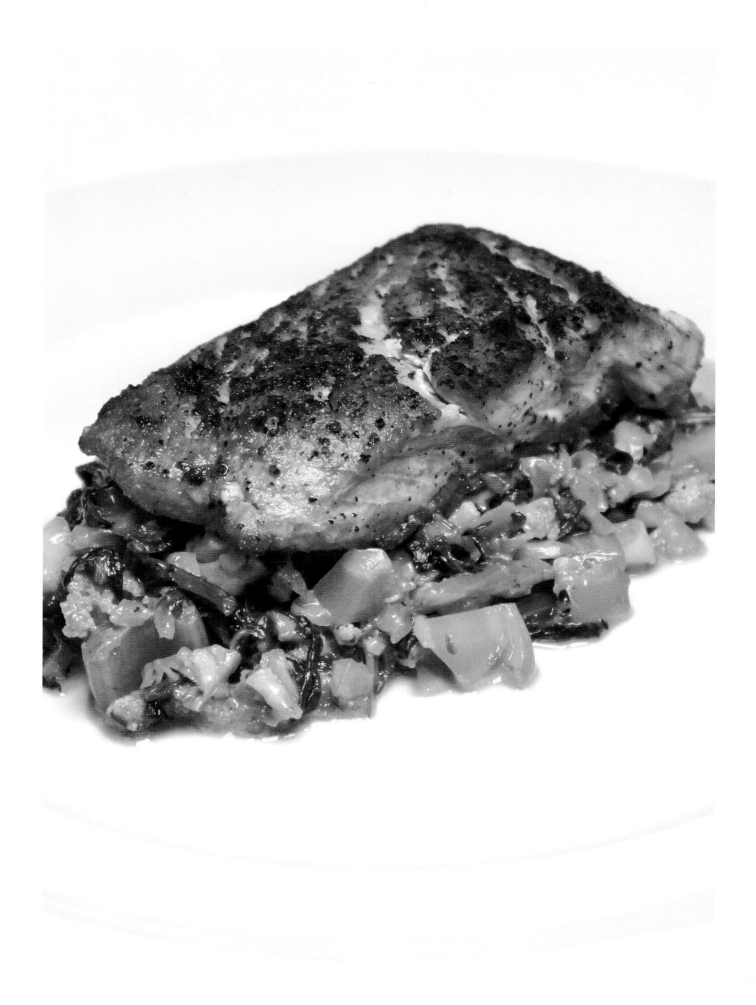

BRAISED PORK BELLY TACOS WITH CHIPOTLE RED PEPPER CHUTNEY AND PICKLED JALAPEÑOS

Macronutrients per serving: **Calories 767** | **Fat 66.6g** | **Carbohydrate 13.2g** | **Fiber 3.5g** | **Protein 28.6g**

Makes: **12 tacos (3 tacos per serving)** | Prep time: **20 minutes** | Cook time: **About 2 hours 15 minutes**

FOR THE PORK BELLY AND CHUTNEY:

2 tablespoons coconut oil, divided

1 medium tomato, chopped

1 small red onion, sliced, divided

1 medium carrot, chopped

3 canned chipotle peppers packed in adobo sauce, chopped

1 cup brown beef stock (page 343)

1 teaspoon lime juice

2 cloves garlic, minced

8 ounces pork belly

1 teaspoon kosher salt

1 teaspoon ground black pepper

FOR THE PICKLED JALAPEÑOS:

1 cup water

¼ cup white vinegar

1 tablespoon kosher salt

1 tablespoon pickling spice

2 jalapeño peppers, sliced

FOR THE SHELLS:

12 ounces shredded cheddar cheese (about 3 cups), divided into 1-ounce portions

FOR THE TOPPINGS:

6 cherry tomatoes, quartered

1 avocado, diced

Sliced red onion (reserved from above)

2 limes, quartered

01 Preheat the oven to 250°F.

02 Heat 1 tablespoon of the coconut oil in an oven-safe 5-quart saucepan over medium heat. Add the tomato, three-quarters of the sliced onion (reserve the remainder for topping), and the carrot and sauté for 3 to 4 minutes, until the vegetables have begun to brown. Add the chipotles and sauté for an additional 2 minutes. Add the stock, lime juice, and garlic, bring to a boil, then lower the heat to a simmer and simmer until the mixture is reduced by half. Remove from the heat.

03 Heat a sauté pan over high heat. Meanwhile, coat the pork belly with the remaining tablespoon of coconut oil and season liberally with the salt and pepper. Place the pork belly fat side down in the pan and sear for 1 to 2 minutes, until a thick browning has formed, then flip and sear on the other side for 1 to 2 minutes. Place the pork belly in the saucepan with the vegetable mixture, cover tightly with aluminum foil, and place in the oven to braise for 2 hours.

04 Make the pickled jalapeños: Bring the water, vinegar, salt, and pickling spice to a boil, then add the sliced jalapeños and boil for 1 minute. Remove from the heat, let cool, then transfer the brine and jalapeños to a jar and place in the refrigerator until needed.

05 After the pork belly has braised for 2 hours, remove it from the saucepan (leaving the braising liquid in the pan) and set it on a cutting board. Cut the pork belly into 12 slices (about 1 ounce each).

06 Make the chutney: Place the saucepan with the braising liquid over high heat. Once at a boil, lower the heat to a simmer and allow to simmer until the liquid is reduced by one-third to one-half and a thick sauce (chutney) has developed. For a smoother chutney, strain through cheesecloth or a fine-mesh sieve and/or puree in a food processor.

07 Make the taco shells: Place a wooden spoon over a large bowl and heat a large sauté pan over medium heat. Place 1 ounce of the cheese in the sauté pan and spread it out into a circle, 2 to 3 inches in diameter. Cook for 1 to 2 minutes, until the cheese has melted and begun to brown, then flip with a heatproof plastic spatula and cook on the other side for 30 to 60 seconds. Lay the cheese over the wooden spoon to mold it into a taco shell shape. When the draped shell has hardened, about 1 minute, remove it from the spoon. Repeat with the remaining cheese, making a total of 12 taco shells.

08 To assemble the tacos, fill each shell with a slice of pork belly, toppings, pickled jalapeños, and chutney. Serve with lime quarters. Store leftovers in an airtight container in the refrigerator for up to 2 days.

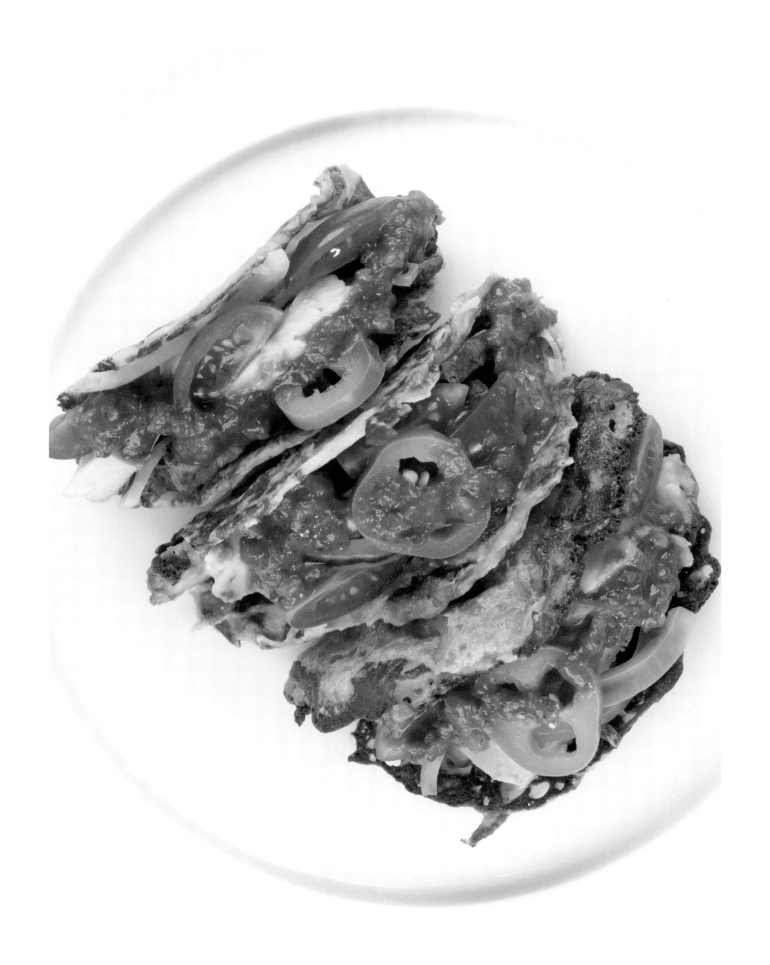

PAN-SEARED SCALLOPS WITH
PINK PEPPERCORN CREAM SAUCE AND ASPARAGUS

Macronutrients per serving: **Calories 520** | **Fat 41.2g** | **Carbohydrate 10.4g** | **Fiber 3g** | **Protein 27.1g**

Makes: **2 servings** | Prep time: **20 minutes** | Cook time: **About 15 minutes**

FOR THE ASPARAGUS:

1 tablespoon kosher salt

20 medium-thick asparagus spears (about 7 inches long), tough ends removed, peeled

FOR THE SCALLOPS:

⅓ cup unsalted butter

12 large sea scallops (about 1¼ pounds), rinsed and muscle removed

1 teaspoon kosher salt

¼ teaspoon fresh cracked black pepper

2 cloves garlic, peeled

1 tablespoon pink peppercorns

4 tablespoons heavy cream

Ground Himalayan salt, for garnish

01 Blanch the asparagus: Fill a 5-quart saucepan three-quarters full of water. Add the tablespoon of salt and bring to a boil, covered, over high heat. Blanch the asparagus in the boiling water for 1 to 2 minutes, then remove from the water and set aside.

02 Heat a large sauté pan over medium heat, then put the butter in the pan and allow it to heat up for 1 to 2 minutes.

03 Season the scallops with the salt and cracked pepper. Add the garlic and pink peppercorns to the pan and cook for 3 to 4 minutes. Add the scallops and sear for 2 to 3 minutes, then flip them over and sear for an additional 1 to 2 minutes for medium-cooked scallops. Remove the scallops from the pan and set aside.

04 Place the asparagus in the same pan you used to cook the scallops and sauté over medium heat for 2 to 3 minutes. Remove the asparagus from the pan and set aside.

05 Add the cream to the pan and whisk until the butter and cream have combined evenly.

06 To serve, divide the asparagus evenly among 4 plates, then place the scallops on top of the asparagus. Drizzle the cream sauce over the top and garnish with Himalayan salt. Store leftovers in an airtight container in the refrigerator for up to 2 days.

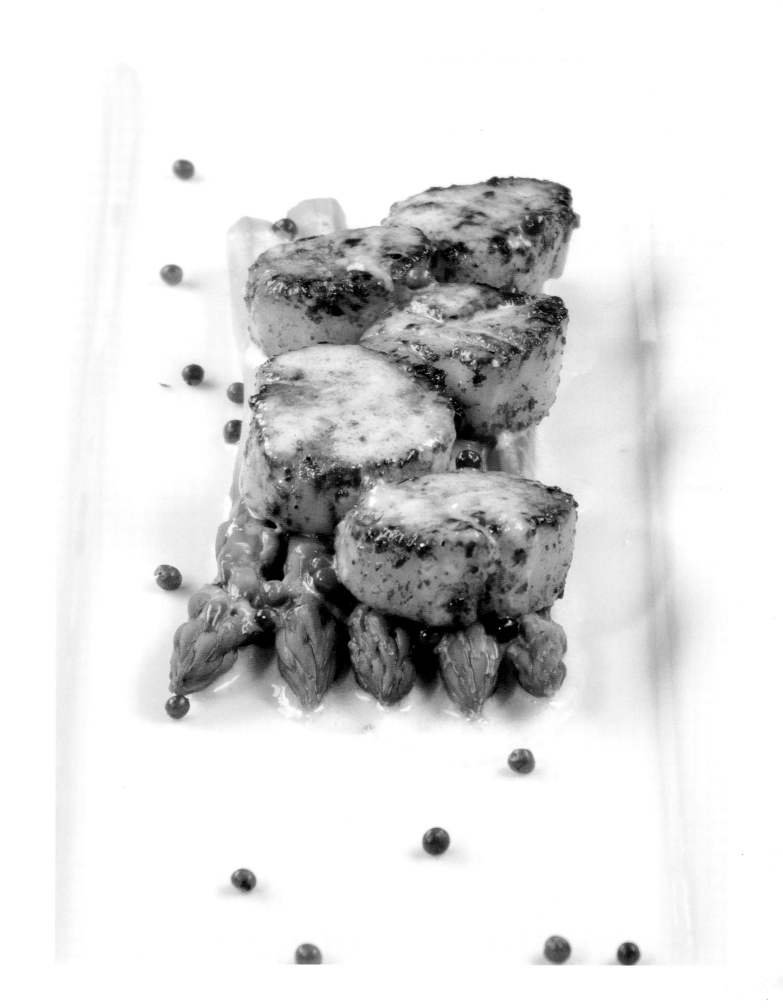

BRAISED PORK SHOULDER WITH DEMI-GLACE OVER PURPLE CABBAGE

Macronutrients per serving: **Calories 475** | **Fat 30.7g** | **Carbohydrate 11.5g** | **Fiber 3.2g** | **Protein 30.3g**

Makes: **4 servings** | Prep time: **20 minutes** | Cook time: **2½ to 3½ hours**

FOR THE PORK SHOULDER AND DEMI-GLACE:

2 tablespoons tomato paste, divided

1 tablespoon coconut oil or MCT oil

1 tablespoon smoked paprika

1 teaspoon kosher salt

1 pound boneless pork shoulder

2 tablespoons unsalted butter

1 small onion, chopped

1 medium carrot, chopped

2 medium stalks celery, chopped

¼ cup dry red wine, such as zinfandel or grenache

1 cup brown beef stock (page 343)

1 bay leaf

5 peppercorns

2 cloves garlic, peeled

5 sprigs fresh parsley

3 sprigs fresh thyme

2 sprigs fresh tarragon

⅛ to ¼ teaspoon xanthan gum (optional)

FOR THE CABBAGE:

1 tablespoon kosher salt

1 teaspoon white vinegar

½ head purple cabbage, sliced

2 tablespoons unsalted butter

¼ cup dry red wine, such as zinfandel or grenache

Kosher salt and ground black pepper

Very finely diced apple, for garnish (optional)

01 Preheat the oven to 250°F.

02 In a small dish, combine 1 tablespoon of the tomato paste, the coconut oil, smoked paprika, and 1 teaspoon of salt. Rub the mixture into the pork shoulder and set aside.

03 In a 4-quart oven-safe saucepan or Dutch oven, heat the butter over medium heat for 1 minute, then add the remaining tablespoon of tomato paste and the onion, carrot, and celery. Sauté for 2 to 3 minutes, until the vegetables begin to brown. Add the red wine and stock, bring to a boil, then reduce to a simmer.

04 Heat a sauté pan over high heat, then sear the pork shoulder on all sides in the hot pan (about 1 minute on each side). Place the seared pork in the saucepan with the vegetables.

05 Make a sachet: Wrap the bay leaf, peppercorns, garlic, parsley, thyme, and tarragon in a piece of cheesecloth, tying it closed with butcher twine. Place the sachet in the saucepan, cover the pan with a tight-fitting lid (or foil), and braise in the oven for 2 to 3 hours, until the meat can easily be cut with a knife.

06 About 20 minutes before the pork is done, blanch the cabbage: Bring a 5-quart saucepan of water to a boil, then add the tablespoon of salt and the vinegar. Blanch the cabbage in the boiling water for 30 to 45 seconds, then drain the cabbage and place it in a large bowl of ice water to stop the cooking and cool it. Once chilled, drain in a colander and set aside.

07 When the pork is done, remove it from the pan (reserving the braising liquid) and place it on a cutting board. Tent with foil and allow to rest.

08 Place a fine-mesh sieve or cheesecloth-lined colander over a clean saucepan. Pour the braising liquid through the sieve and discard the vegetables. Bring the strained liquid to a boil, then reduce to a simmer. After it simmers for 5 minutes, remove the fat (depouillage) from the top of the liquid. Then either simmer until the sauce is thick enough to coat the back of a spoon, about 10 minutes, or whisk in the optional xanthan gum to thicken.

09 Finish preparing the cabbage: In a large sauté pan over medium-high heat, melt 2 tablespoons of butter, then add the cabbage and sauté for 3 to 4 minutes, until the color begins to turn from purple to brown. Add the red wine, reduce the heat to low, cover, and simmer for 5 minutes. Remove the lid and simmer until all of the liquid has evaporated. Season with salt and pepper to taste.

10 Slice the pork into 4 equal portions and plate each portion with about ½ cup of cabbage and 2 tablespoons of demi-glace. Garnish with finely diced apple, if desired. Store leftovers in an airtight container in the refrigerator for up to 2 days.

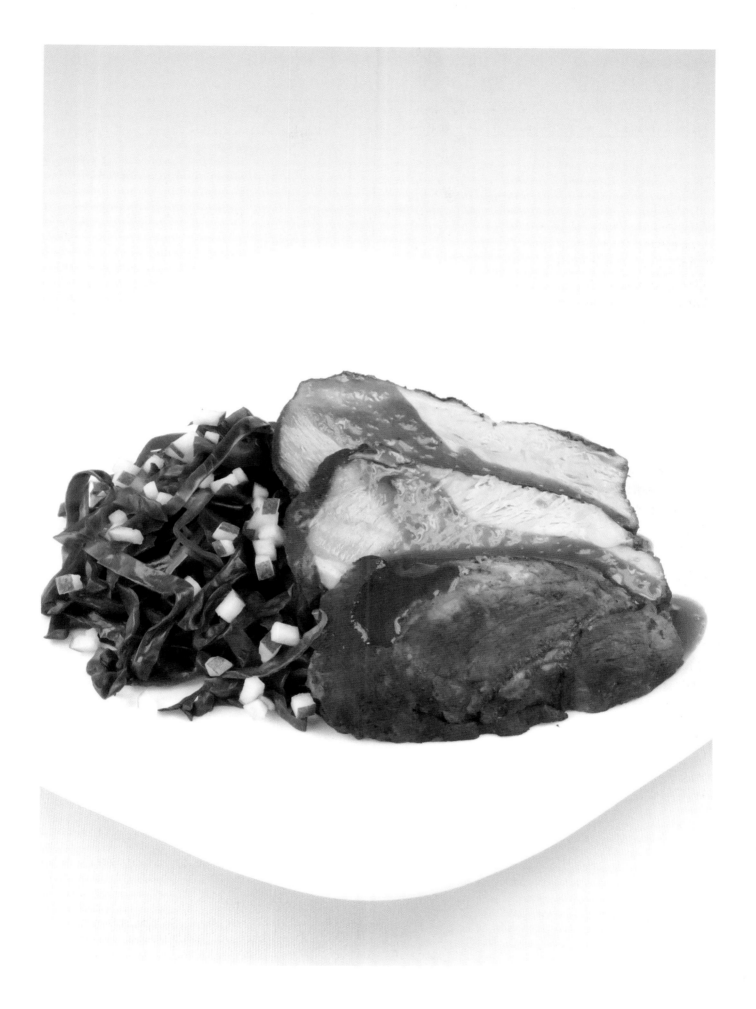

ITALIAN SAUSAGE–STUFFED BELL PEPPERS WITH TOMATO-MUSHROOM MARINARA

Macronutrients per serving: **Calories 659** | **Fat 47.4g** | **Carbohydrate 17.6g** | **Fiber 5.7g** | **Protein 37.7g**

Makes: **4 servings** | Prep time: **15 minutes** | Cook time: **About 45 minutes**

FOR THE MARINARA:

1 tablespoon olive oil

¼ small red onion, chopped

1 cup chopped mushrooms

1 large heirloom tomato, chopped

½ cup brown beef stock (page 343)

¼ bunch fresh basil, chopped

1 teaspoon garlic powder

¼ cup heavy cream

¾ cup grated Parmesan cheese (about 2 ounces)

FOR THE FILLING:

1 tablespoon coconut oil or MCT oil

¼ small white onion, chopped

3 green onions, chopped

2 cloves garlic, chopped

4 ounces spinach, chopped

8 ounces 80/20 ground sirloin

8 ounces Italian sausage, casings removed, crumbled

2 ounces cream cheese (¼ cup)

2 ounces feta cheese

2 teaspoons Italian seasoning

½ teaspoon kosher salt

¼ teaspoon ground black pepper

2 tablespoons high-fiber coconut flour

3 tablespoons hazelnut flour, divided

4 small bell peppers, any color, seeded and cored

1 tablespoon ground flax seeds

¾ cup grated Parmesan cheese (about 2 ounces)

01 Preheat the oven to 425°F. Line a sheet pan with parchment paper and set a cooling rack in it.

02 Make the marinara: Heat the olive oil in a small saucepan over medium heat for 1 to 2 minutes. When the oil is hot, add the red onion and mushrooms to the pan and sauté for 3 to 4 minutes, until the vegetables have begun to brown, stirring occasionally.

03 Add the tomato to the saucepan and cook for 3 to 4 minutes, then add the stock, basil, and garlic powder. Bring to a boil, then lower the heat and simmer for 15 to 20 minutes, until reduced by one-quarter. Stir in the heavy cream and Parmesan cheese.

04 While the marinara is simmering, make the filling for the peppers: In a large sauté pan over medium heat, heat the coconut oil for 1 to 2 minutes, then add the onions, garlic, and spinach and sauté, stirring occasionally, for 2 to 3 minutes. Transfer to a small mixing bowl and set aside to cool slightly.

05 In a large bowl, combine the ground sirloin, sausage, cream cheese, feta cheese, Italian seasoning, salt, and pepper with the spinach mixture and ¼ cup of the marinara; mix to incorporate all the ingredients.

06 Mix together the coconut flour and 1 tablespoon of the hazelnut flour, then evenly dust the inside of each bell pepper with the flour mixture. Stuff each pepper evenly with about 5 ounces of the filling and set on the cooling rack in the prepared sheet pan.

07 Combine the remaining 2 tablespoons of hazelnut flour, ground flax seeds, and Parmesan cheese in a small bowl, then evenly dust the tops of the stuffed bell peppers.

08 Bake for 18 to 20 minutes, until the internal temperature of the filling reaches 155°F. Remove from the oven, plate with the remaining marinara, and serve immediately. Store leftovers in an airtight container in the refrigerator for up to 4 days.

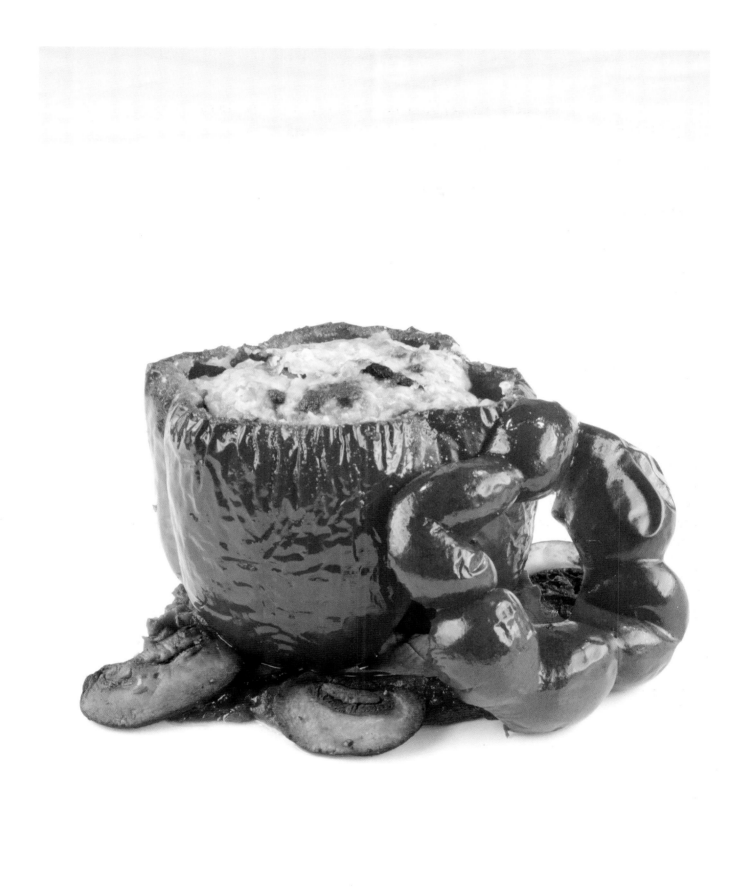

MEMPHIS-STYLE BARBECUED CHICKEN WITH GREEN BEANS AMANDINE

Macronutrients per serving: **Calories 440** | **Fat 28.8g** | **Carbohydrate 7.1g** | **Fiber 2.1g** | **Protein 38.2g**

Makes: **6 servings** | Prep time: **10 minutes, plus 20 minutes to marinate chicken** | Cook time: **20 minutes**

FOR THE MARINADE:

1 cup chicken stock (page 345)

¼ cup tomato paste

2 tablespoons Worcestershire sauce

2 tablespoons soy sauce

1 tablespoon apple cider vinegar

1 tablespoon prepared yellow mustard

1 teaspoon smoked paprika

1 teaspoon onion powder

1 teaspoon garlic powder

½ teaspoon ground cumin

⅛ teaspoon ground cinnamon

⅛ teaspoon ground cloves

⅛ teaspoon ground nutmeg

12 chicken legs

FOR THE GREEN BEANS:

1 tablespoon kosher salt

8 ounces green beans, cleaned and ends trimmed

2 tablespoons unsalted butter

¼ cup sliced almonds

1 ounce amaretto (optional)

FOR THE BARBECUE SAUCE:

Reserved marinade (from above)

1 bay leaf

01 Make the marinade: In a large bowl, whisk together the stock, tomato paste, Worcestershire sauce, soy sauce, vinegar, mustard, and spices.

02 Put the chicken legs in the marinade and allow to marinate for 20 minutes.

03 Preheat a grill to high heat.

04 Blanch the green beans: Fill a 5-quart saucepan three-quarters full of water, add the salt, and bring to a boil. Add the green beans and blanch for 2 to 3 minutes, then drain and set aside.

05 Remove the chicken legs from the marinade and grill for 2 to 3 minutes on each side, until the internal temperature reaches 185°F. If the outside begins to become too charred, reduce the grilling time to 1 to 2 minutes per side and finish cooking the chicken in a 350°F oven.

06 Transfer the marinade to a small saucepan, bring to a boil, and add the bay leaf, then simmer until reduced by one-quarter or until it has developed the consistency of barbecue sauce, about 10 minutes. Remove and discard the bay leaf.

07 While the marinade is reducing, finish the green beans: In a large sauté pan over medium heat, melt the butter. Add the green beans and sauté for 3 to 4 minutes, until crisp-tender. Stir in the almonds and amaretto, if using, then cook until all the liquid has evaporated.

08 Plate the green beans with the chicken legs and barbecue sauce. Store in an airtight container in the refrigerator for up to 4 days.

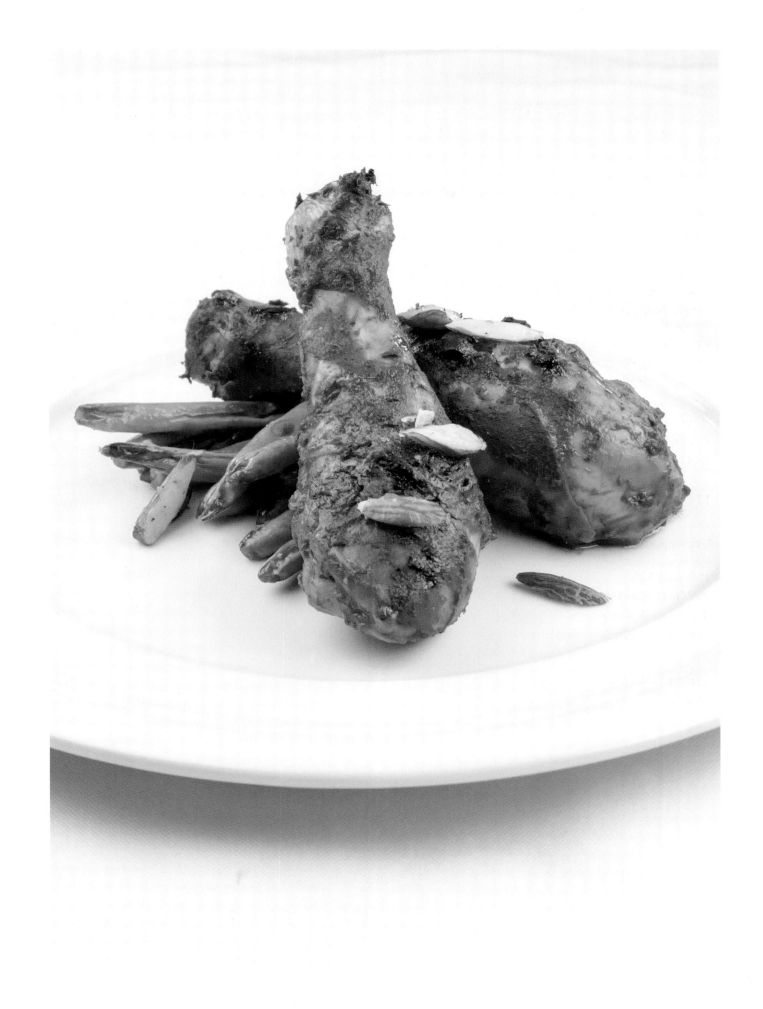

ALASKA ROLLS
WITH SRIRACHA AIOLI

Macronutrients per serving (rolls only): **Calories 304** | **Fat 23.1g** | **Carbohydrate 3.9g** | **Fiber 0.1g** | **Protein 20g**

Makes: **4 servings** | Prep time: **15 minutes** | Cook time: —

FOR THE ROLLS:

1 (8-ounce) package cream cheese, softened

½ teaspoon onion powder

½ teaspoon kosher salt

4 sheets nori

½ cucumber, shaved thin

12 ounces lox, divided

FOR THE SRIRACHA AIOLI:

3 tablespoons Classic Aioli (page 349)

2 teaspoons Sriracha sauce

01 In a small bowl, use a hand mixer to blend together the cream cheese, onion powder, and salt.

02 Lay a sheet of nori on a sushi mat or piece of parchment paper. Line it horizontally, 1 inch from the edge closest to you, with 2 ounces of the cream cheese mixture, 2 pieces of shaved cucumber, and 3 ounces of lox. Roll up the sushi, using the mat or parchment paper to guide you, ensuring that the mat or parchment does not roll up inside of the sushi roll. Repeat with the remaining ingredients, making a total of 4 rolls. Set the sushi rolls aside.

03 In a small bowl, whisk together the aioli and Sriracha.

04 Cut each sushi roll into 8 pieces and serve with the Sriracha aioli. Store the rolls and aioli in separate airtight containers in the refrigerator for up to 4 days.

ROASTED ASPARAGUS
WITH PARMESAN AND HIMALAYAN SALT

Macronutrients per serving: **Calories 137** | **Fat 10.7g** | **Carbohydrate 4.4g** | **Fiber 1.6g** | **Protein 7.4g**

Makes: **4 servings** | Prep time: **5 minutes** | Cook time: **About 15 minutes**

1½ teaspoons kosher salt

20 medium-thick asparagus spears, tough ends trimmed

1 tablespoon coconut oil or MCT oil

¼ small red onion, sliced

¾ cup freshly grated Parmesan cheese (about 2 ounces)

1 tablespoon extra-virgin olive oil, for drizzling

Coarsely ground Himalayan salt

01 Preheat the oven to 400°F and line a sheet pan with parchment paper.

02 Fill a wide pan (wide enough for the asparagus to lie flat) about one-third full with water. Add the salt and bring to a boil, then add the asparagus and blanch for 2 minutes or until tender. Remove from the heat, drain, and set aside.

03 Heat the coconut oil in a sauté pan over medium-high heat for 1 to 2 minutes. Add the onion and sauté until browned, 2 to 3 minutes, then remove from the pan and set aside.

04 Place the asparagus on the lined sheet pan, sprinkle with the Parmesan cheese, and bake for 5 to 6 minutes, until the cheese has melted and is beginning to brown. Remove from the oven, drizzle with the olive oil, and sprinkle with Himalayan salt.

05 Plate the asparagus with the sautéed onion and serve immediately. Store in an airtight container in the refrigerator for up to 5 days.

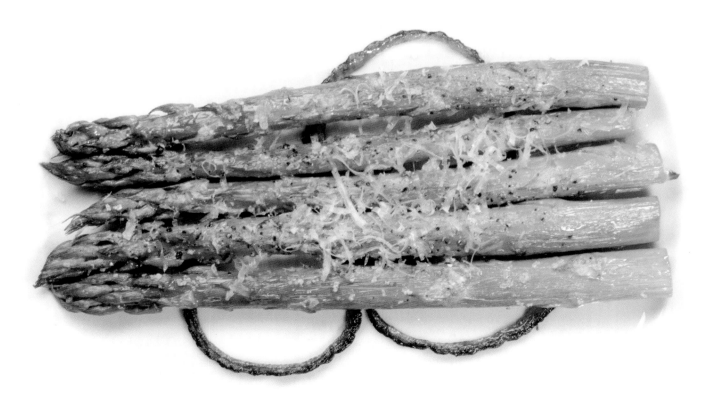

ROASTED RED PEPPER
BROWN BUTTER GREEN BEANS

Macronutrients per serving: **Calories 151** | **Fat 12.3g** | **Carbohydrate 10.2g** | **Fiber 3.9g** | **Protein 2.6g**

Makes: **4 servings** | Prep time: **10 minutes** | Cook time: **About 15 minutes**

1 red bell pepper

1 tablespoon olive oil

3 tablespoons unsalted butter

1 pound green beans, cleaned, ends trimmed

½ cup vegetable stock (page 342)

Kosher salt and ground black pepper

Tip: *If you do not have a gas cooktop to roast the bell pepper, you can use your oven's broiler setting. Place the olive oil–coated bell pepper on a sheet pan, set your broiler to high, and roast for 4 to 5 minutes, flipping halfway through. Or you can achieve the same result with a grill.*

01 Coat the bell pepper in the olive oil and roast over an open flame until charred. Place the pepper in a heatproof bowl, cover with plastic wrap, and set aside.

02 Heat the butter in a large sauté pan over medium heat, allowing it to come up to temperature and brown for 2 to 3 minutes. Add the green beans and sauté for 5 to 6 minutes, stirring frequently, until they begin to caramelize. Reduce the heat to low, add the stock, and simmer on low for 4 to 5 minutes, until tender.

03 While the green beans are simmering, remove the charred skin, core, and seeds from the bell pepper, dice the pepper, and add it to the green beans. Season with salt and pepper to taste and divide among 4 plates.

04 Serve hot or cool. Store in an airtight container in the refrigerator for up to 4 days.

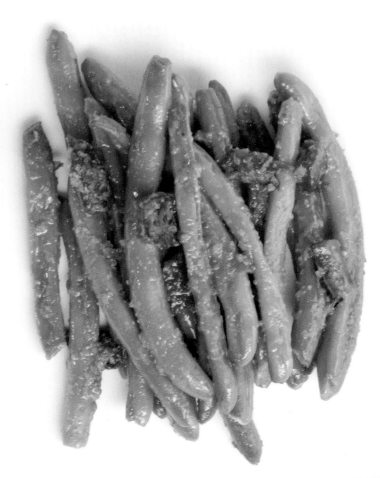

BRAISED BACON-Y BRUSSELS

Macronutrients per serving: **Calories 189** | **Fat 14g** | **Carbohydrate 11.4g** | **Fiber 4.3g** | **Protein 8g**

Makes: **4 servings** | Prep time: **5 minutes** | Cook time: **15 minutes**

4 slices thick-cut bacon, chopped

1 pound Brussels sprouts, halved

3 tablespoons unsalted butter

½ cup brown beef stock (page 343)

Kosher salt and ground black pepper

10 canned or jarred pearl onions, halved

01 In a large sauté pan, cook the bacon over medium-low heat for 5 to 6 minutes to render the fat.

02 Increase the heat to medium and add the butter to the pan. Allow to come up to temperature for 1 to 2 minutes before adding the Brussels sprouts. Sauté for 3 to 4 minutes, stirring frequently, until the outsides begin to crisp. Add the stock and simmer over low heat for 4 to 5 minutes, until the Brussels are tender, then season to taste with salt and pepper.

03 Serve the Brussels sprouts hot with the pearl onions sprinkled around them. Store in an airtight container in the refrigerator for up to 4 days.

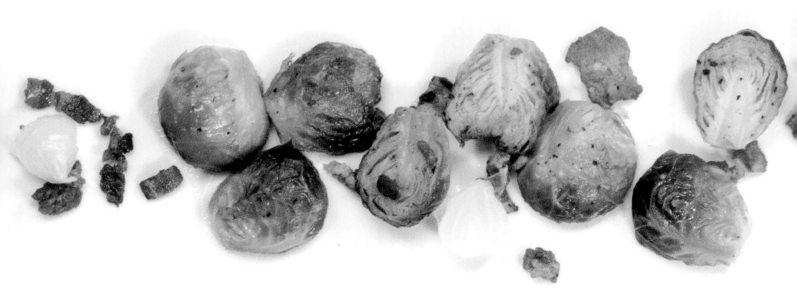

EGGPLANT PARMESAN
WITH MARINARA

Macronutrients per serving: **Calories 323** | **Fat 27.3g** | **Carbohydrate 8.6g** | **Fiber 3.4g** | **Protein 10.7g**

Makes: **4 servings** | Prep time: **25 minutes** | Cook time: **20 minutes**

1 eggplant (about 10 ounces), sliced into ¼-inch-thick rounds

1 quart water

2 tablespoons kosher salt

3 tablespoons olive oil, for pan-frying

FOR THE MARINARA:

1 tablespoon olive oil

2 Roma tomatoes, chopped

¼ small red onion, chopped

2 cloves garlic, chopped

½ cup vegetable stock (page 342)

½ bunch fresh basil, chopped

FOR THE BREADING:

¼ cup blanched almond flour

¾ cup freshly grated Parmesan cheese (about 2 ounces)

1 teaspoon kosher salt

1 tablespoon extra-virgin olive oil, for drizzling

O1 Place the sliced eggplant in a large bowl with the water and salt and let sit for 15 to 20 minutes. Remove the eggplant from the water, place in a colander set over a bowl, and allow to drain for 5 minutes, then pat dry.

O2 To make the marinara, heat 1 tablespoon of olive oil in a 2½-quart saucepan over medium heat. Add the tomatoes, onion, and garlic and sauté for 4 to 5 minutes, until the onion is translucent. Add the stock and basil and simmer for 15 minutes.

O3 While the marinara is simmering, combine the almond flour, Parmesan, and salt in a small bowl. Heat 1 tablespoon of the olive oil in a large skillet over medium heat for 1 to 2 minutes. Lightly dredge both sides of the eggplant slices in the almond flour mixture. Sauté the eggplant in three batches in the skillet for 2 to 3 minutes on each side, then remove from the pan. Repeat two more times with the remaining olive oil and eggplant.

O4 Remove the marinara from the heat. If desired, blend the marinara with an immersion blender for a smoother sauce, or leave it chunky. To serve, spoon some of the sauce onto a plate and top with 4 or 5 eggplant slices, then drizzle with extra-virgin olive oil. Store the eggplant and marinara in separate airtight containers in the refrigerator for up to 5 days.

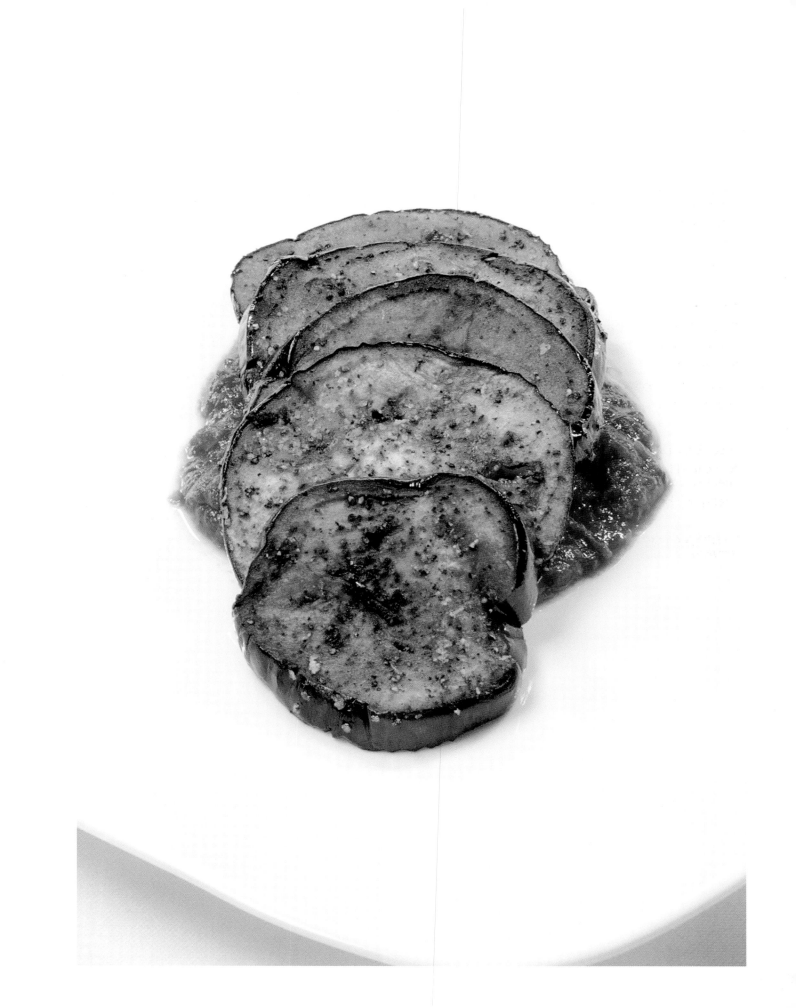

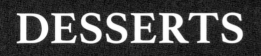

DESSERTS

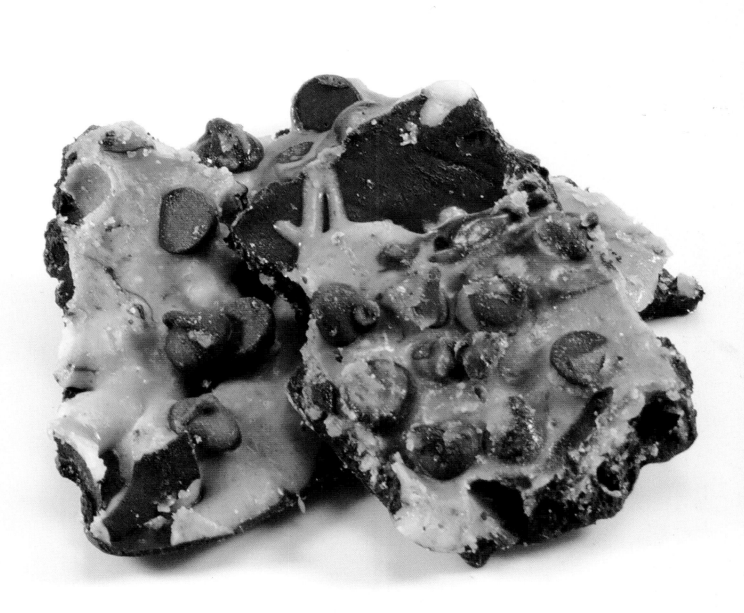

CLASSIC
CHOCOLATE CHIP COOKIES

Macronutrients per cookie: Calories 111 | Fat 9.9g | Carbohydrate 2.4g | Fiber 1.5g | Protein 3.5g

Makes: 10 to 12 cookies | Prep time: 10 minutes | Cook time: 15 to 18 minutes

½ cup blanched almond flour

¼ cup high-fiber coconut flour

¼ cup Quest Protein Powder Multi-Purpose Mix

1 teaspoon baking powder

¼ teaspoon kosher salt

½ cup (4 ounces) unsalted butter, softened

½ cup granulated erythritol

2 tablespoons sugar-free maple syrup

1 egg

1 teaspoon vanilla extract

⅓ cup Lily's Dark Chocolate Baking Chips

01 Preheat the oven to 350°F and line a cookie sheet with a silicone baking mat or parchment paper.

02 Sift the almond flour, coconut flour, protein powder, and baking powder into a large bowl, then add the salt and whisk until homogenous; set aside.

03 With a mixer fitted with the paddle attachment, cream the butter on low. Slowly add the erythritol and continue to mix for about 30 seconds, until combined; set aside.

04 In a small bowl, whisk together the maple syrup, egg, and vanilla extract until combined. With the mixer running on low, slowly pour the maple syrup mixture into the butter mixture and continue to cream for 45 to 60 seconds, until well combined.

05 With the mixer on low, slowly dust the flour mixture into the butter mixture until fully incorporated. You may need to finish mixing by hand. Once combined, fold in the chocolate chips.

06 Using two 1-tablespoon measures, portion the dough, roll into balls between your palms, then press flat on the cookie sheet. Space the cookies about 1 inch apart.

07 Bake for 15 to 18 minutes, until the corners begin to brown. Using a spatula, gently transfer the cookies to a cooling rack and allow to cool for 5 to 10 minutes.

08 Store in an airtight container for up to 5 days.

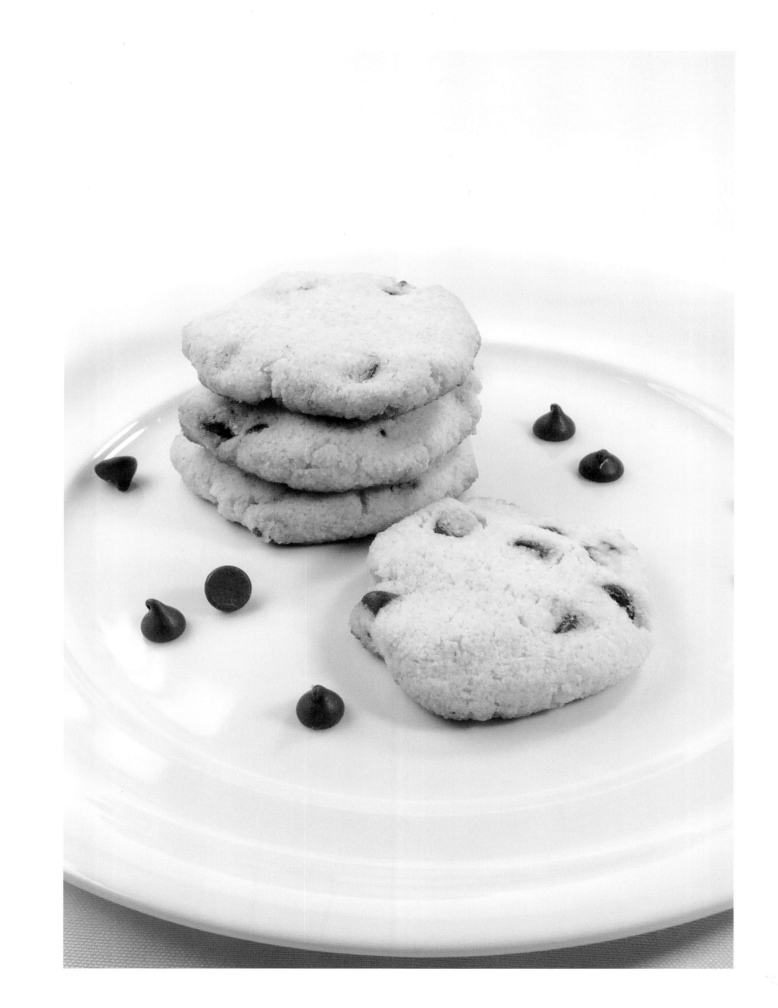

DOUBLE CHOCOLATE CHIP COOKIES

Macronutrients per cookie: Calories 110 | Fat 9.9g | Carbohydrate 2.7g | Fiber 1.5g | Protein 3.4g

Makes: 10 to 12 cookies | Prep time: 10 minutes | Cook time: 15 to 18 minutes

½ cup blanched almond flour

¼ cup Quest Protein Powder Chocolate Milkshake

3 tablespoons high-fiber coconut flour

1 tablespoon dark cocoa powder

1 teaspoon baking powder

¼ teaspoon kosher salt

½ cup (4 ounces) unsalted butter, softened

½ cup granulated erythritol

2 tablespoons sugar-free maple syrup

1 egg

1 teaspoon vanilla extract

⅓ cup Lily's Dark Chocolate Baking Chips

01 Preheat the oven to 350°F and line a cookie sheet with a silicone baking mat or parchment paper.

02 Sift the almond flour, protein powder, coconut flour, cocoa powder, and baking powder into a large bowl, then add the salt and whisk until homogenous; set aside.

03 With a mixer fitted with the paddle attachment, cream the butter on low. Slowly add the erythritol and continue mixing for about 30 seconds, until combined; set aside.

04 In a small bowl, whisk together the maple syrup, egg, and vanilla extract until combined. With the mixer running on low, slowly pour the maple syrup mixture into the butter mixture and continue to cream for 45 to 60 seconds, until well combined.

05 With the mixer on low, slowly dust the flour mixture into the butter mixture until fully incorporated. You may need to finish mixing by hand. Once combined, fold in the chocolate chips.

06 Using two 1-tablespoon measures, portion the dough, roll into balls between your palms, then press flat on the cookie sheet. Space the cookies about 1 inch apart.

07 Bake for 15 to 18 minutes, until the edges begin to brown. Using a spatula, gently transfer the cookies to a cooling rack and allow to cool for 5 to 10 minutes.

08 Store in an airtight container for up to 5 days.

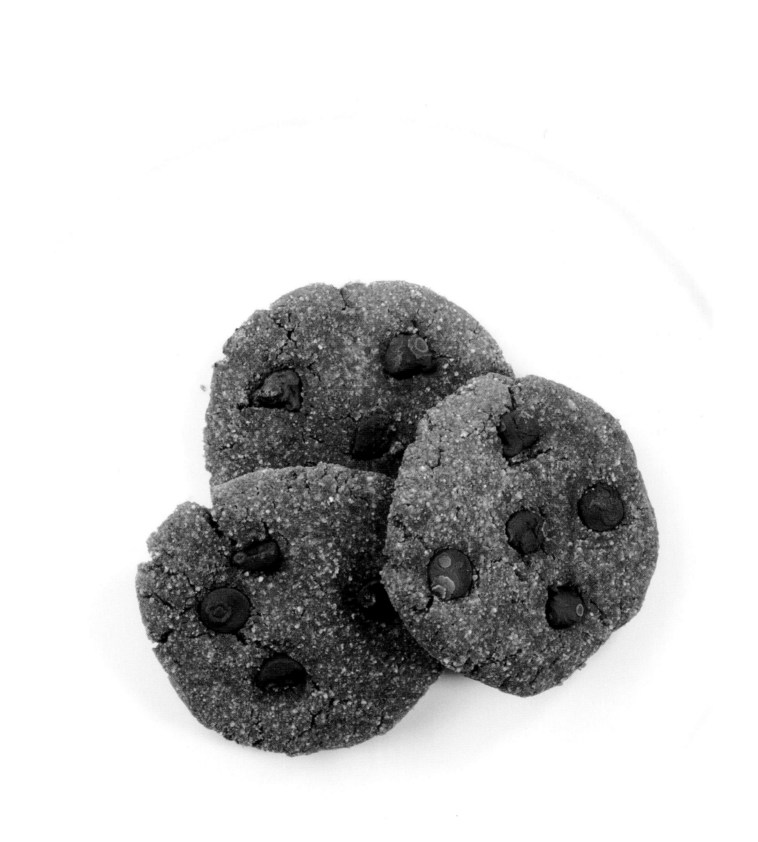

CARDAMOM SNICKERDOODLES
WITH MAPLE BOURBON CARAMEL

Macronutrients per cookie: Calories 144 | Fat 13.5g | Carbohydrate 3.6g | Fiber 2.5g | Protein 2.1g

Makes: 8 to 10 cookies (1 per serving) | Prep time: 15 minutes | Cook time: 8 to 11 minutes

When presenting these cookies, a garnish of halved grapes offers a nice contrast in texture and flavor, but the grapes are not necessary.

FOR THE COOKIES:

½ cup high-fiber coconut flour

2 tablespoons blanched almond flour

2 tablespoons hazelnut flour

1 tablespoon psyllium husk powder

½ teaspoon kosher salt

½ teaspoon ground cinnamon

¼ teaspoon ground cardamom

⅛ teaspoon ground nutmeg

⅛ teaspoon xanthan gum

⅛ teaspoon raw sucralose

⅛ teaspoon baking soda

½ cup unsweetened almond milk

1 tablespoon heavy cream

1 egg

2 tablespoons unsalted butter, softened

1 tablespoon coconut oil

1 tablespoon Splenda Brown Sugar Blend

1½ teaspoons vanilla extract

½ teaspoon maple extract

FOR THE TOPPING:

1 teaspoon powdered erythritol

1 teaspoon ground cinnamon

¼ teaspoon ground cardamom

FOR THE CARAMEL:

3 tablespoons clarified butter (page 348)

1 tablespoon granulated erythritol

1 tablespoon bourbon (optional)

½ teaspoon maple extract

¼ cup heavy cream

01 Preheat the oven to 350°F and line a baking sheet with a silicone baking mat or coat with cooking spray.

02 In a large bowl, sift together the coconut flour, almond flour, hazelnut flour, psyllium husk powder, salt, spices, xanthan gum, sucralose, and baking soda; set aside.

03 In a medium-sized bowl, whisk together the remaining cookie ingredients until thoroughly combined.

04 Pour the wet ingredients into the dry ingredients and combine with a rubber spatula until a dough forms.

05 Scoop up 2 tablespoons of the dough, roll it into a ball between your palms, place it on the baking sheet, and press down with your palm to flatten slightly. Repeat with the rest of the dough, leaving 1 inch of space between cookies. Bake for 8 to 11 minutes, until the edges of the cookies begin to brown.

06 While the cookies are baking, whisk together the ingredients for the topping and set aside.

07 To make the caramel, heat the clarified butter in a sauté pan over high heat for 2 to 3 minutes, until it gives off a nutty flavor. Whisk in the erythritol, bourbon (if using), and maple extract until the erythritol dissolves. Whisk in the cream until the mixture is fully combined. Remove from the heat.

08 Remove the cookies from the oven, coat with cooking spray, and dust with the topping. Using a flat surface (like a drinking glass), press the topping into the cookies. You can also place the topped cookies under the broiler for 1 minute to toast the topping.

09 Transfer the cookies to a cooling rack and allow to cool for 10 to 15 minutes. Serve each cookie with 1 tablespoon of the caramel.

10 Store leftover cookies in an airtight container at room temperature for up to 5 days. Store leftover caramel in an airtight container in the refrigerator for up to 1 week. To reheat the caramel, microwave in 20-second increments for 1 to 2 minutes, until it is less viscous.

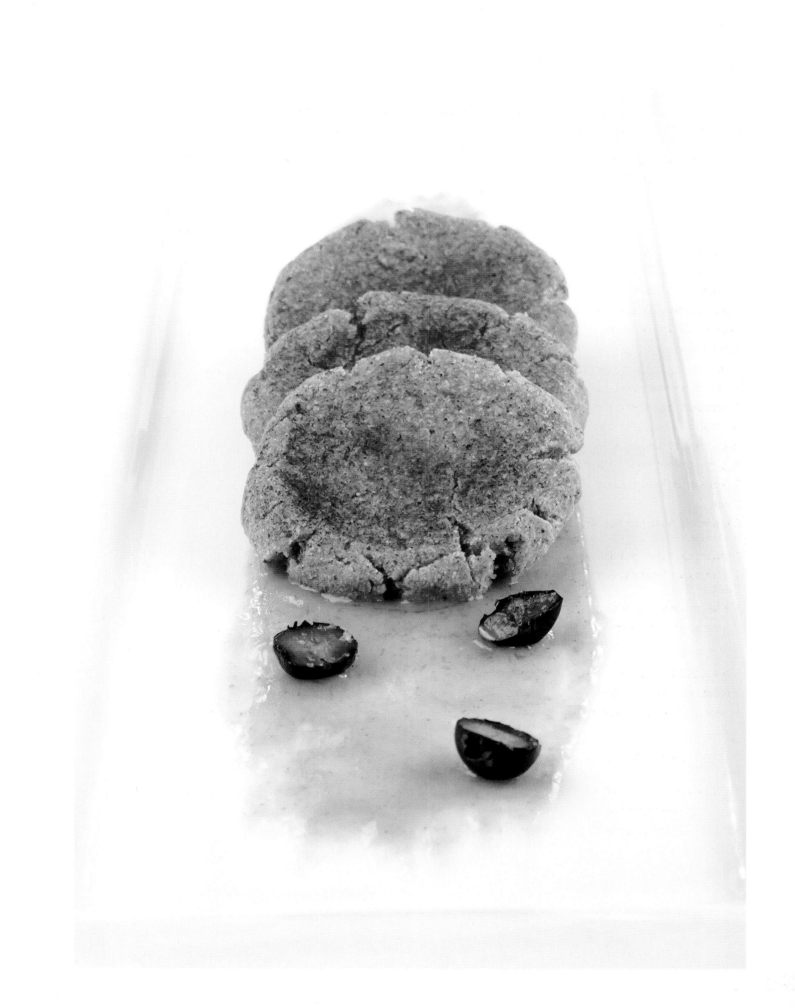

CHOCOLATE BARK

Macronutrients per serving: Calories 170 | Fat 16.5g | Carbohydrate 3.3g | Fiber 1.7g | Protein 2g

Makes: 16 servings | Prep time: 10 minutes | Cook time: —

2 ounces unsweetened chocolate, chopped

2 ounces cocoa butter

Raw stevia powder

Kosher salt

4 ounces macadamia nuts, crushed

¼ cup (½ stick) unsalted butter, melted

Pinch of raw sucralose

¼ cup coconut butter, softened

¼ cup unsweetened peanut butter, at room temperature

¼ cup Lily's Dark Chocolate Chips

01 In a microwave-safe bowl, melt the chocolate and cocoa butter on high in 30-second increments for 2 to 3 minutes, stirring often. Add stevia and salt to taste and stir until thoroughly combined. Coat a 12-inch dinner plate with cooking spray, then pour the chocolate mixture onto the plate to cover the plate.

02 Stir the macadamia nuts into the melted butter, season with the sucralose and salt to taste, and spread evenly over the chocolate on the plate.

03 Place the coconut butter and peanut butter in a small bowl, season with salt to taste, and stir until well combined. Pour the mixture evenly over the macadamia nuts, top with the chocolate chips, and place in the refrigerator to set for 3 to 4 minutes.

04 Divide the bark into 16 equal portions and serve. Store in the refrigerator for up to 1 week.

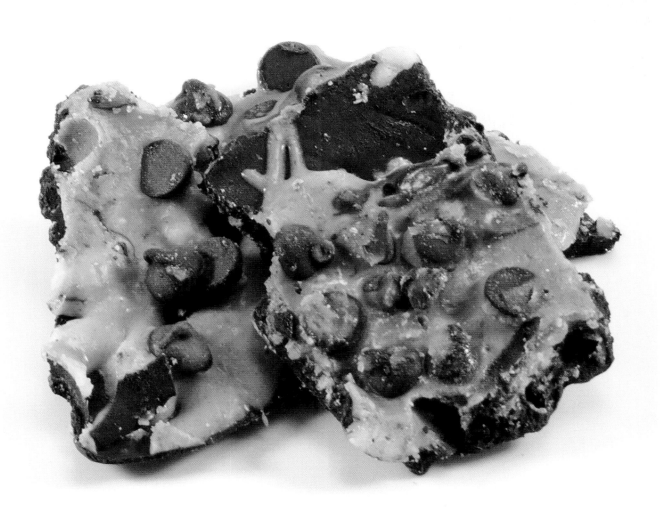

CHOCOLATE MOUSSE

Macronutrients per serving (without toppings): Calories 323 | Fat 27.6g | Carbohydrate 7g | Fiber 2.9g | Protein 10.4g

Makes: 4 servings | Prep time: 10 minutes, plus 2 hours to chill | Cook time: 2 to 4 minutes

2 ounces unsweetened chocolate (100% cacao)

½ cup heavy whipping cream

2 tablespoons powdered erythritol

4 ounces (½ cup) cream cheese, softened

¼ cup Quest Protein Powder Chocolate Milkshake

½ teaspoon almond extract

Cocoa powder, for dusting the rims (optional)

TOPPING SUGGESTIONS (OPTIONAL):

Chopped raw hazelnuts

Whipped cream

Blueberries

Shaved dark chocolate (80% to 100% cacao)

01 Chop the chocolate into ¼-inch pieces. Place in a medium-sized microwave-safe bowl and microwave on high in 15-second increments for 2 to 4 minutes, stirring after each increment, until the chocolate is melted.

02 Whip the heavy cream and erythritol until medium peaks form, 3 to 4 minutes.

03 Mix together the cream cheese, protein powder, almond extract, and melted chocolate until homogenous, then gently fold into the sweetened whipped cream.

04 Portion the mousse into four 6-ounce ramekins, jars, or cocktail glasses. For an elegant presentation, before filling the glasses with the mousse, dampen the rims with water, then dust them with cocoa powder. Chill for at least 2 hours.

05 Serve with your favorite keto toppings.

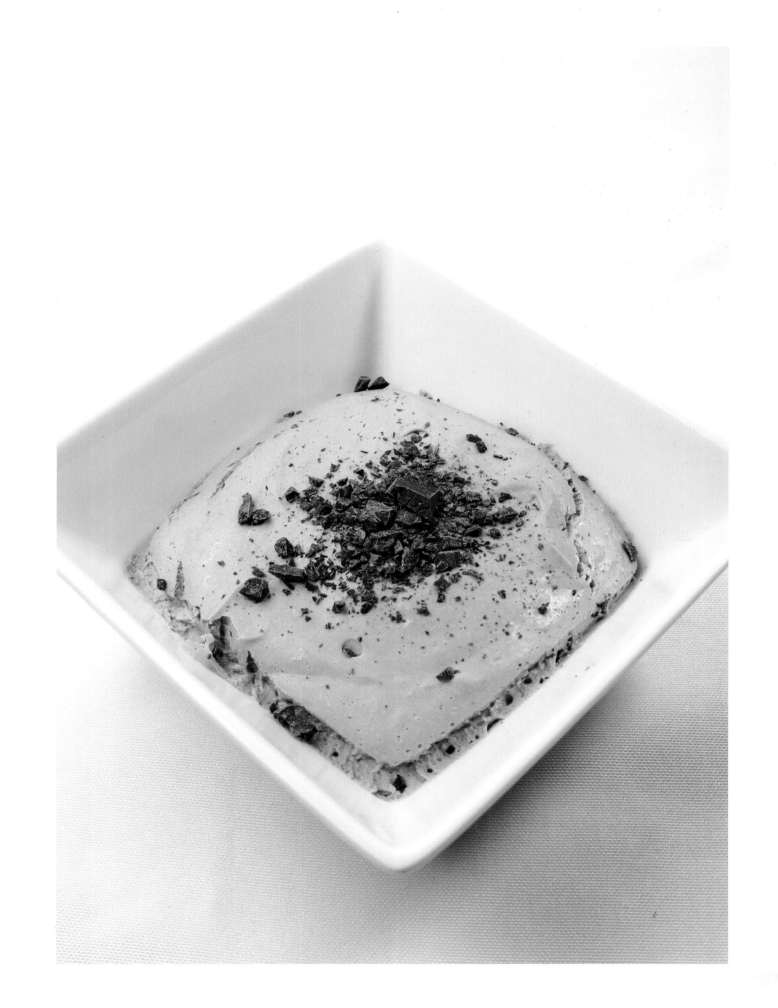

SINGLE-SERVING BROWNIE MUG CAKE

Macronutrients per serving: Calories 466 | Fat 35.2g | Carbohydrate 12g | Fiber 6.3g | Protein 31.7 g

Makes: 1 serving | **Prep time:** 5 minutes | **Cook time:** About 2 minutes

2 tablespoons heavy cream

2 teaspoons granulated erythritol

¼ cup Quest Protein Powder Chocolate Milkshake

2 tablespoons MCT oil powder

¼ teaspoon baking soda

Pinch of kosher salt

½ cup unsweetened almond milk

1 teaspoon vanilla extract

1 egg

1 tablespoon cocoa powder

1 tablespoon chopped raw macadamia nuts, for topping (optional)

01 In a large bowl, whip the heavy cream with a whisk until stiff peaks form, 2 to 3 minutes. Gently fold in the erythritol. Set aside in the refrigerator until needed.

02 Sift the protein powder, MCT oil powder, baking soda, and salt into a mixing bowl.

03 In a blender, pulse the almond milk, vanilla extract, egg, and cocoa powder until smooth. While whisking, pour the almond milk mixture into the dry ingredients and continue to whisk until smooth. Gently fold this mixture into the sweetened whipped cream.

04 Pour the batter into a 16-ounce or larger mug, leaving at least 2 inches of space at the top. Cover with plastic wrap and microwave on high for 1 minute. Remove from the microwave and carefully lift off the plastic wrap (it will be hot, so be careful not to get a steam burn).

05 Place the mug back in the microwave, uncovered, and microwave on high for 30 to 45 seconds, until a toothpick inserted in the middle of the cake comes out clean.

06 Top the cake with chopped nuts, if desired, and serve hot.

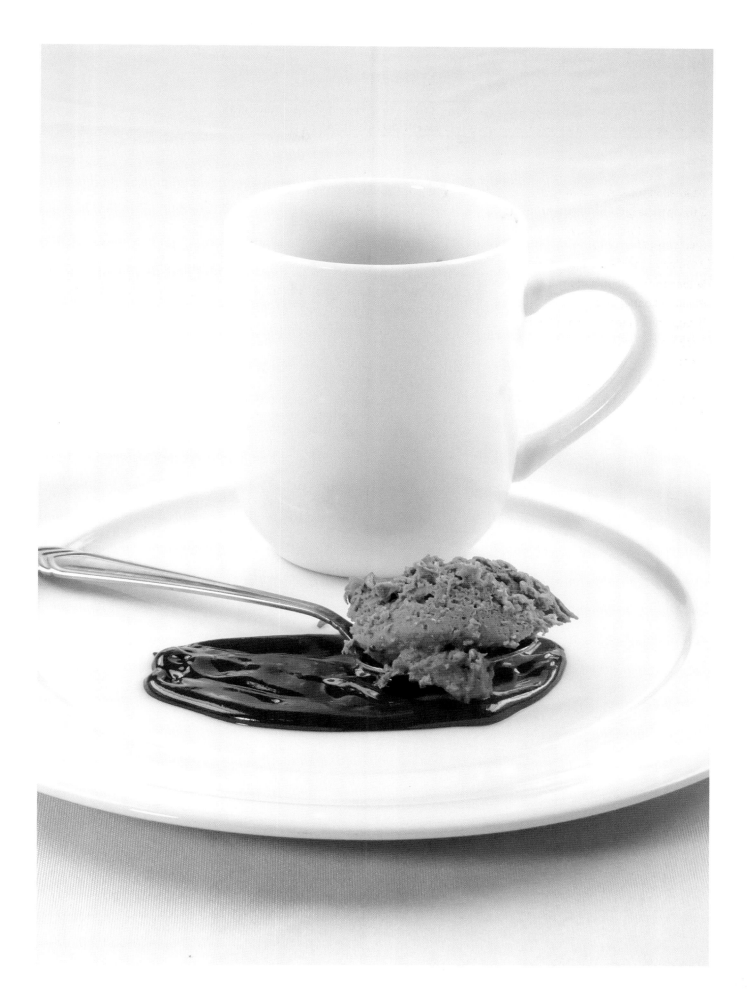

CLASSIC CHEESECAKE

Macronutrients per serving: Calories 258 | Fat 22.1g | Carbohydrate 4g | Fiber 1.2g | Protein 7.8g

Makes: One 12-inch cake (16 servings) | Prep time: 10 minutes, plus time to chill | Cook time: About 40 minutes

FOR THE FILLING:

3 (8-ounce) packages cream cheese, softened

5 egg yolks

2 whole eggs

¼ cup Quest Protein Powder Vanilla Milkshake

3 tablespoons granulated erythritol

1 teaspoon vanilla extract

½ teaspoon kosher salt

FOR THE CRUST:

½ cup (1 stick) unsalted butter, softened

¼ cup Quest Protein Powder Vanilla Milkshake

¼ cup high-fiber coconut flour

FOR GARNISH (OPTIONAL):

Fresh berries

01 Preheat the oven to 350°F and coat a 12-inch springform pan with cooking spray.

02 Using a stand mixer fitted with the whisk attachment or a large mixing bowl with a hand mixer, blend the filling ingredients until smooth.

03 Place the ingredients for the crust in another mixing bowl and mix together with a fork until a rough dough forms.

04 Press the crust into the bottom of the greased springform pan and par-bake for 4 to 5 minutes.

05 Remove the par-baked crust from the oven. Lower the oven temperature to 300°F.

06 Place a sheet pan in the oven and fill it ⅓ full of water to make a water bath for the springform pan. Pour the filling over the par-baked crust and place the springform pan in the water bath. Bake for 32 to 35 minutes, until the cheesecake is firm but not browned.

07 Remove the cheesecake from the oven and allow to cool to room temperature in the pan, then remove the outer ring from the pan and place the cake in the refrigerator to chill.

08 To serve, cut the cake into 16 equal slices and garnish with berries, if desired. Store in an airtight container in the refrigerator for up to 1 week.

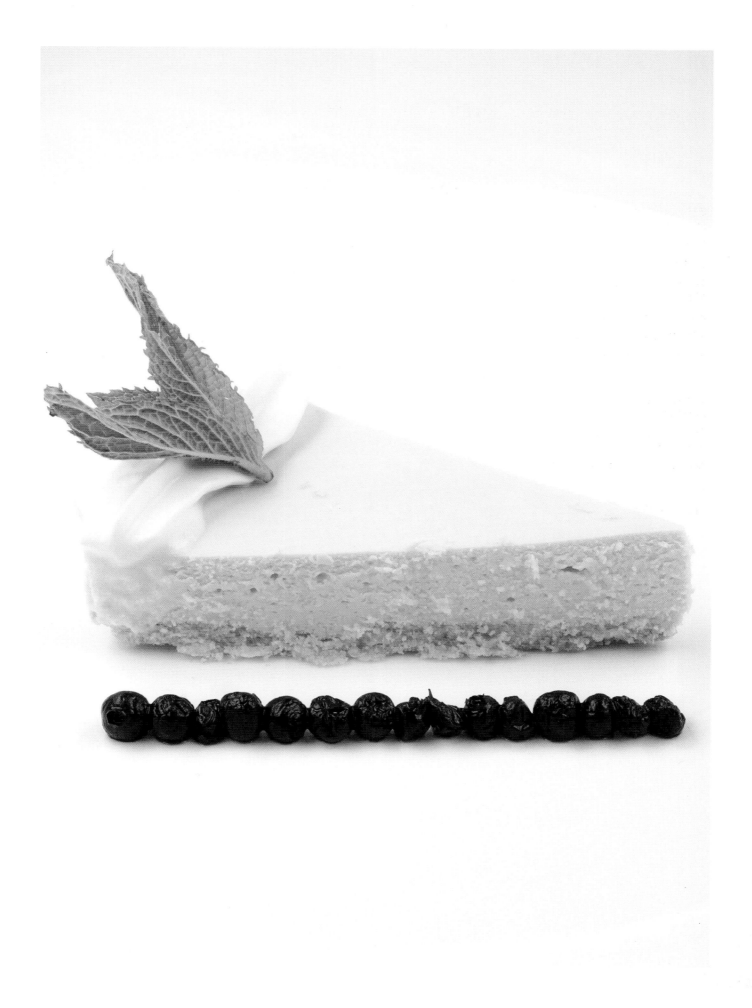

SUGAR COOKIES

Macronutrients per cookie: Calories 92 | Fat 7.8g | Carbohydrate 2.9g | Fiber 1.3g | Protein 3g

Makes: 10 to 12 cookies | Prep time: 20 minutes, plus 1 hour to chill dough | Cook time: 7 to 10 minutes

⅓ cup plus 2 tablespoons high-fiber coconut flour

⅓ cup blanched almond flour

⅓ cup Quest Protein Powder Vanilla Milkshake

½ teaspoon baking powder

¼ teaspoon salt

1 egg

2 tablespoons almond milk

1 teaspoon vanilla extract

⅛ teaspoon raw sucralose

½ cup (1 stick) unsalted butter, softened

2 tablespoons powdered erythritol

⅓ cup granulated erythritol

01 Sift the coconut flour, almond flour, protein powder, baking powder, and salt into a mixing bowl.

02 In another bowl, whisk the egg, almond milk, vanilla extract, and sucralose until smooth, then set aside.

03 In another bowl, using a hand mixer fitted with the paddle attachment, cream the butter and powdered erythritol until smooth. Slowly add the egg mixture until fully incorporated.

04 Fold the flour mixture into the butter mixture until a homogenous cookie dough develops. Cover the dough with plastic wrap and place in the refrigerator to chill for 1 hour.

05 Preheat the oven to 350°F. Line a baking sheet with parchment paper.

06 Using two 1-tablespoon measures, portion the dough, rolling into balls, and press flat onto the cookie sheet. Space the cookies about 1 inch apart.

07 Bake the cookies for 7 to 10 minutes, until the edges have begun to crisp (do not allow them to brown). Transfer the cookies to a cooling rack to cool for 5 minutes.

08 Place the granulated erythritol in a large bowl and toss each cooled cookie in the sweetener until coated.

09 Store in an airtight container at room temperature for up to 3 days.

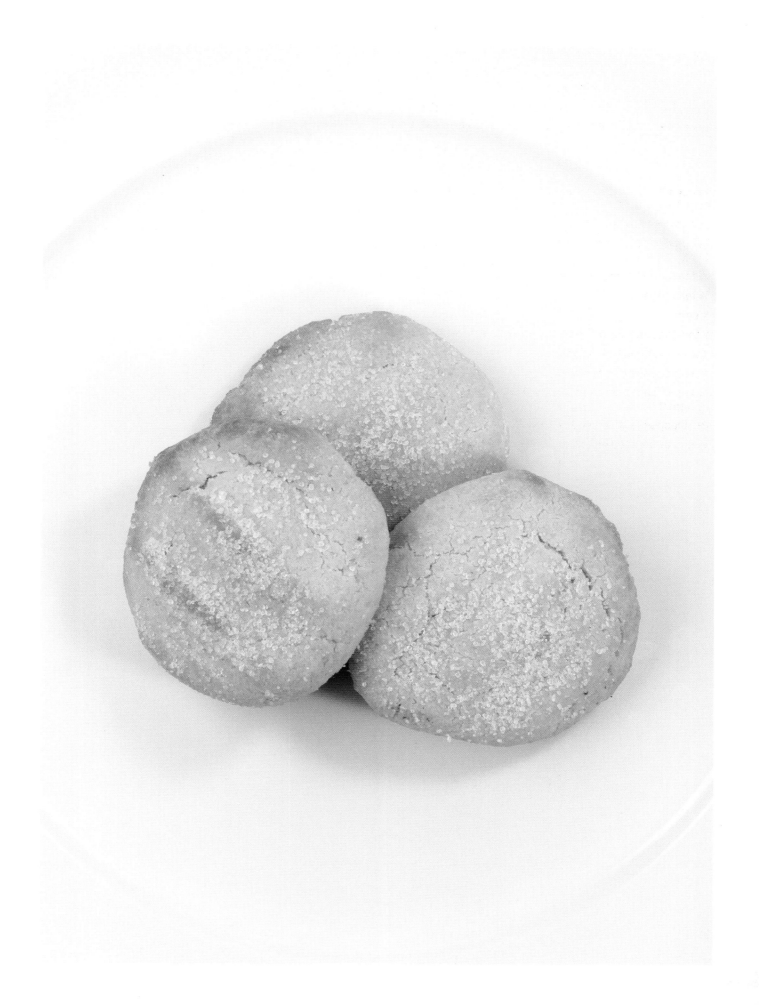

CHOCOLATE-COVERED BACON

Macronutrients per serving: Calories 276 | Fat 24.5g | Carbohydrate 8.2g | Fiber 4.8g | Protein 6.2g
Makes: 6 slices (3 per serving) | Prep time: 5 minutes | Cook time: About 10 minutes

6 slices thick-cut bacon

2 ounces unsweetened chocolate (100% cacao), roughly chopped

1 ounce cacao butter (sometimes called cocoa butter)

½ teaspoon vanilla extract

¼ teaspoon raw sucralose

⅛ teaspoon kosher salt

01 Place a piece of parchment paper (about 10 inches long) on a work surface.

02 Heat a large sauté pan over medium heat for 1 to 2 minutes. Put the bacon in the pan and cook until more or less crispy, depending on your desired doneness—about 6 minutes for less-crisp bacon, 10 minutes for crisper bacon. Remove the bacon from the pan, pat with paper towels to remove the excess grease, and set aside.

03 Place the chocolate and cacao butter in a microwave-safe bowl. Microwave on high in 15-second increments for 2 to 4 minutes, stirring often, until melted. Add the vanilla extract, sucralose, and salt and stir to combine; allow to cool for 2 to 3 minutes.

04 Take a bacon slice and dip half of it into the melted chocolate mixture. Place the chocolate-coated bacon on the parchment paper. Repeat with the rest of the bacon. Allow the chocolate to set for 5 minutes before serving.

05 Store in an airtight container in the refrigerator for up to 3 days.

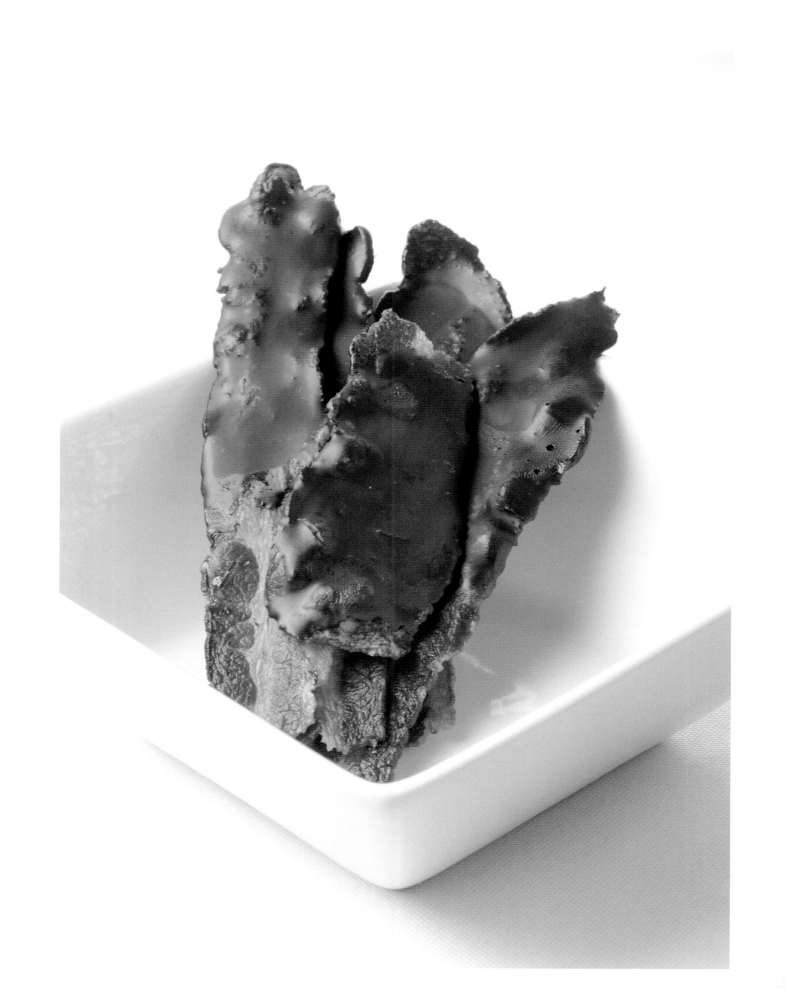

RICH CHOCOLATE CUPCAKES WITH SWISS BUTTERCREAM

Macronutrients per cupcake: Calories 300 | Fat 27.8g | Carbohydrate 6g | Fiber 4.4g | Protein 7.3g

Makes: 12 cupcakes (1 per serving) | Prep time: 15 minutes | Cook time: 12 to 15 minutes

FOR THE CUPCAKES:

½ cup blanched almond flour

½ cup high-fiber coconut flour

¼ cup Quest Protein Powder Chocolate Milkshake

¼ cup cocoa powder

½ teaspoon baking powder

½ teaspoon baking soda

¼ teaspoon kosher salt

⅛ teaspoon xanthan gum

2 eggs

½ cup unsweetened almond milk

⅓ cup heavy cream

6 tablespoons (¾ stick) unsalted butter, melted but not hot

2 ounces unsweetened chocolate, melted but not hot

FOR THE BUTTERCREAM:

½ cup water

3 egg whites, at room temperature

¼ cup granulated erythritol

¾ cup (1½ sticks) unsalted butter, softened

1 teaspoon vanilla extract

Pinch of kosher salt

Raw stevia powder

FOR GARNISH:

1 ounce unsweetened chocolate, shaved

1 tablespoon cocoa powder

01 Preheat the oven to 350°F and line a 12-well muffin tin with cupcake liners.

02 Sift the almond flour, coconut flour, protein powder, cocoa powder, baking powder, baking soda, salt, and xanthan gum into a large bowl; set aside.

03 In another bowl, whisk together the eggs, almond milk, heavy cream, butter, and chocolate.

04 Fold the wet ingredients into the dry ingredients until the mixture is homogenous. Pour the batter into the lined muffin tin, filling each well about two-thirds full. Bake for 12 to 15 minutes, until a toothpick inserted into a cupcake comes out clean.

05 While the cupcakes are baking, make the buttercream. Pour the water into a 2½-quart saucepan and bring to a simmer over medium heat.

06 Place the egg whites and erythritol in a medium-sized heatproof bowl, set over the water bath, and whisk until the erythritol has dissolved. Heat the egg white mixture, stirring with the whisk, until the temperature reaches 160°F; do not allow the temperature to exceed 160°F. Remove from the heat and whip the egg whites with a hand mixer on high until glossy, stiff peaks form, about 3 minutes.

07 Continue to whip while adding the butter 1 tablespoon at a time; each addition of butter should be thoroughly mixed into the egg whites until it disappears. After all the butter has been added, mix in the vanilla extract, salt, and stevia to taste. If the frosting looks lumpy, continue to whip until it becomes smooth. Transfer to a pastry bag fitted with the desired tip; set aside.

08 Transfer the cupcakes to a cooling rack and allow to cool for 5 to 10 minutes. Top each cupcake with buttercream, some shaved chocolate, and a dusting of cocoa powder. Store the frosted cupcakes in an airtight container on the counter for up to 3 days or in the refrigerator for up to 1 week.

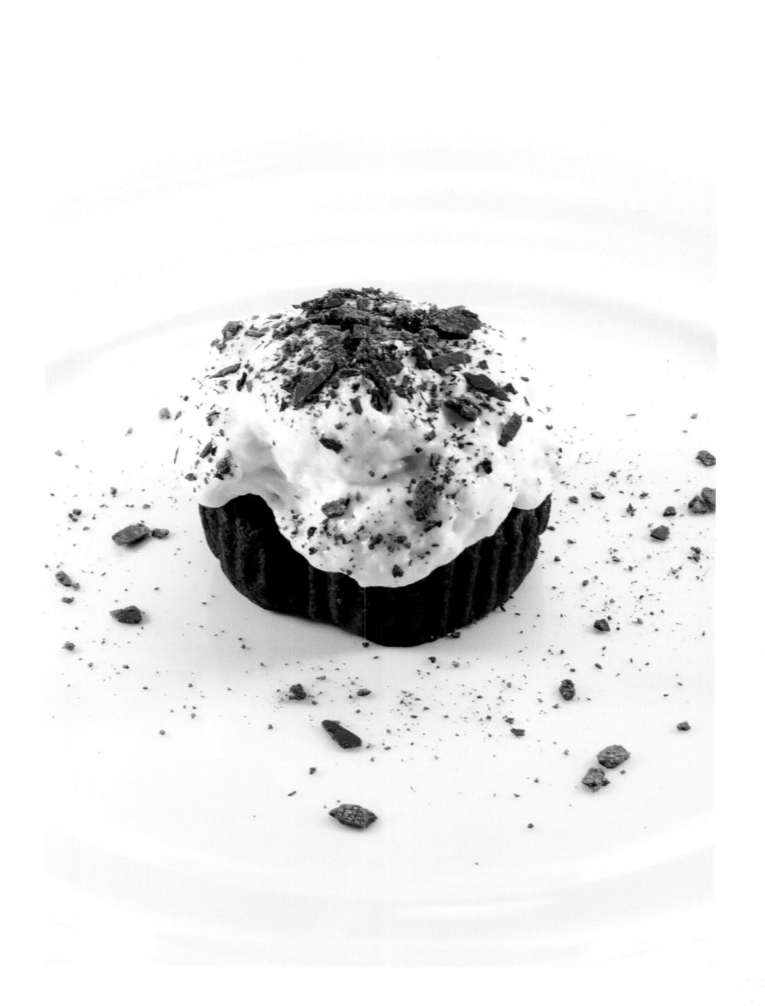

CHOCOLATE PEANUT BUTTER FUDGE

Macronutrients per serving: Calories 110 | Fat 10.3g | Carbohydrate 1.5g | Fiber 0.6g | Protein 3.9g

Makes: 16 servings | Prep time: 5 minutes, plus 1 to 2 hours to chill | Cook time: Less than 1 minute

¾ cup heavy cream

3 tablespoons cocoa butter (1½ ounces), melted

3 tablespoons coconut oil, melted

2 tablespoons unsweetened crunchy peanut butter, at room temperature

½ teaspoon kosher salt

⅛ teaspoon raw sucralose

3 tablespoons cocoa powder

2 scoops Quest Protein Powder Multi-Purpose Mix (about ½ cup)

FOR THE TOPPING:

1 teaspoon coarse sea salt

01 Place the heavy cream in a microwave-safe bowl and microwave on high for 30 to 45 seconds, until warm to the touch but not scalding. Add the cocoa butter, coconut oil, peanut butter, salt, and sucralose and whisk until thoroughly combined.

02 Sift the cocoa powder and protein powder into the cream mixture and stir until a thick batter forms. Pour the mixture into an 8-inch square baking pan, then refrigerate for 1 to 2 hours, until firm.

03 Remove the fudge from the refrigerator and sprinkle with the sea salt. Cut into 16 squares and serve. Store in the refrigerator for up to 1 week.

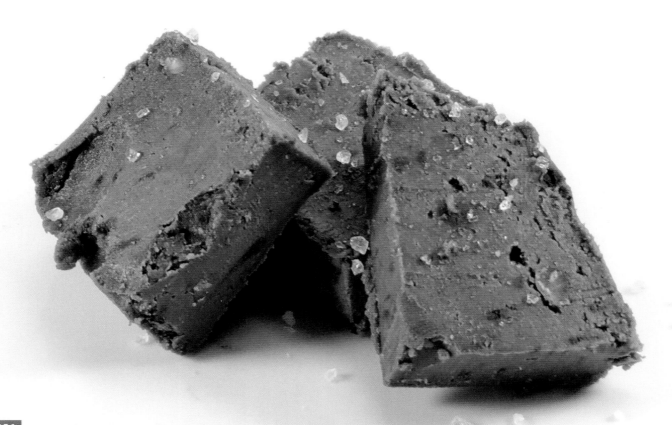

FUDGE BROWNIES

Macronutrients per brownie: Calories 148 | Fat 13.9g | Carbohydrate 2.9g | Fiber 1.6g | Protein 2.7g

Makes: 16 brownies (1 per serving) | Prep time: 10 minutes | Cook time: 13 to 16 minutes

½ cup plus 1 tablespoon blanched almond flour

2 tablespoons cocoa powder

1 teaspoon baking powder

½ cup macadamia nuts, crushed

2 ounces unsweetened chocolate

¼ cup coconut oil

¼ cup unsalted butter

⅓ cup granulated erythritol

2 eggs

01 Preheat the oven to 350°F and coat an 8-inch square baking pan with cooking spray.

02 Sift the almond flour, cocoa powder, and baking powder into a small bowl, then add the macadamia nuts.

03 Melt the chocolate and coconut oil in the microwave for 2 to 3 minutes, then stir in the butter.

04 Whisk together the erythritol and eggs until homogenous.

05 Fold the chocolate mixture into the dry ingredients and stir until combined. Then fold in the egg mixture and stir until a homogenous batter forms.

06 Pour the batter into the prepared pan and bake until a toothpick inserted into the center comes out clean, 13 to 16 minutes. Let cool in the pan for 5 to 10 minutes.

07 Cut into 16 squares and enjoy. Store in an airtight container at room temperature for up to 4 days.

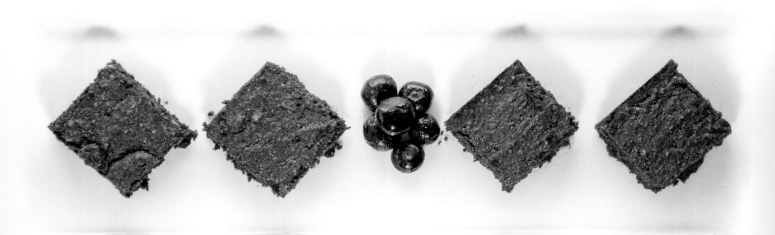

SINGLE-SERVING LEMON BLUEBERRY CAKE

Macronutrients per serving: Calories 427 | Fat 37g | Carbohydrate 12.3g | Fiber 6.7g | Protein 11.3g

Makes: 1 serving | Prep time: 5 minutes | Cook time: 1 minute

2 tablespoons blanched almond flour

2 tablespoons high-fiber coconut flour

½ teaspoon baking soda

⅛ teaspoon xanthan gum

2 tablespoons unsalted butter, melted but not hot

1 egg

1 teaspoon Splenda Brown Sugar Blend

2 tablespoons blueberries

1 teaspoon grated lemon zest

1 teaspoon grated lemon juice

FOR GARNISH:

1 blueberry

1 mint leaf

1 teaspoon powdered erythritol

01 In a small bowl, sift together the almond flour, coconut flour, baking soda, and xanthan gum.

02 In another small bowl, mix together the butter, egg, and Splenda Brown Sugar Blend until thoroughly combined.

03 Pour the wet ingredients into the dry ingredients and mix until homogenous. Fold in the blueberries, lemon zest, and lemon juice, then transfer the batter to a 10- to 12-ounce microwave-safe serving dish. Cover with plastic wrap and microwave on high for 1 minute.

04 Remove from the microwave, then garnish with a blueberry, a mint leaf, and a dusting of erythritol. Serve immediately or let cool, cover, and refrigerate for up to 1 week.

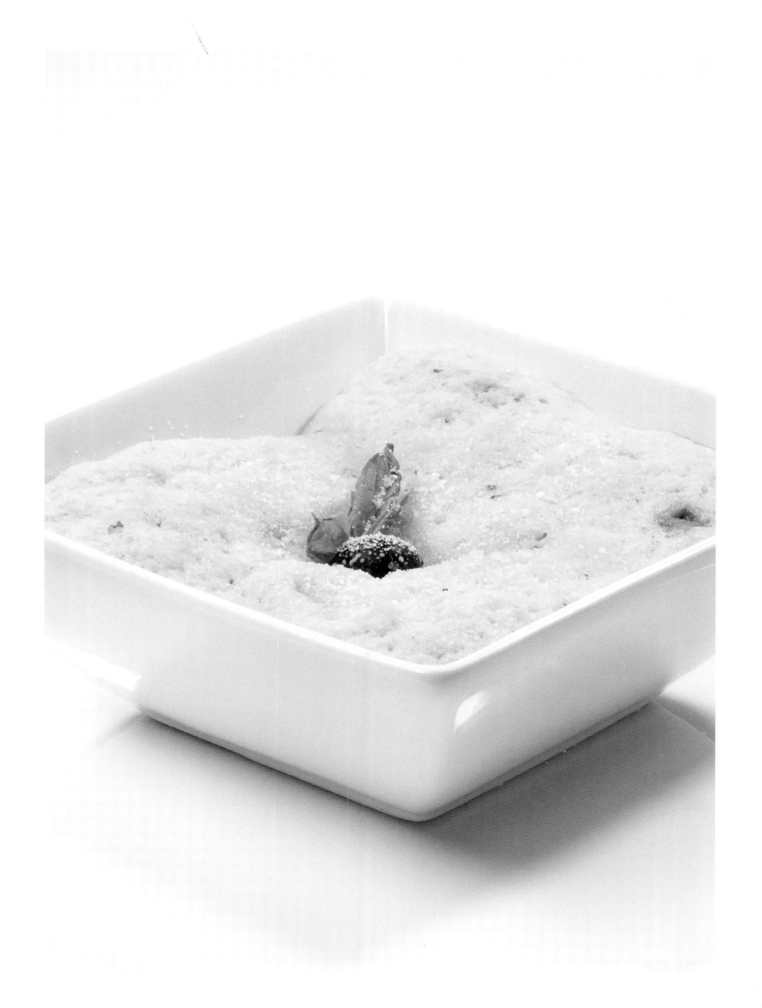

RICH CHOCOLATE AVOCADO ICE CREAM

Macronutrients per serving (based on 4 servings): Calories 353 | Fat 29.8g | Carbohydrate 11.3g | Fiber 6.7g | Protein 12g

Makes: 4 to 6 servings | Prep time: 5 minutes, time to chill ice cream base, churn, and set up in freezer | Cook time: 5 minutes

1 cup full-fat coconut milk

½ cup unsweetened almond milk

½ teaspoon kosher salt

1 tablespoon granulated erythritol

⅛ teaspoon raw sucralose

2 eggs

2 avocados (about 8 ounces each), halved and pitted

¼ cup Quest Protein Powder Chocolate Milkshake

3 tablespoons cocoa powder

SPECIAL EQUIPMENT:

Ice cream maker

01 Twenty-four hours before you plan to make ice cream, place the freezer bowl for your ice cream maker in the freezer.

02 In a 5-quart saucepan over medium heat, heat the coconut milk, almond milk, salt, erythritol, and sucralose until simmering, then pour into a blender and pulse until smooth.

03 Whisk the eggs in a medium-sized heatproof bowl. Temper the eggs by slowly pouring about a quarter of the hot coconut milk mixture into the eggs, 2 tablespoons at a time, whisking continuously, until the mixture is homogenous. Place the lid back on the blender but remove the fill cap. Turn the blender on to low, then slowly pour the egg and coconut milk mixture into the blender.

04 Remove the lid and scoop the flesh of the avocados into the blender. Place the lid back on, with the fill cap removed, and turn the blender on to low. While the blender is running, add the protein powder and cocoa powder and continue blending until the mixture is homogenous.

05 Place the blender jar in the refrigerator until the mixture is thoroughly chilled, at least 4 hours.

06 Insert the freezer bowl into the ice cream maker and churn the chilled ice cream base according to the manufacturer's directions.

07 Transfer the ice cream to an airtight container and place in the freezer until a thicker consistency develops, about 20 minutes. Store in the freezer for up to 1 month.

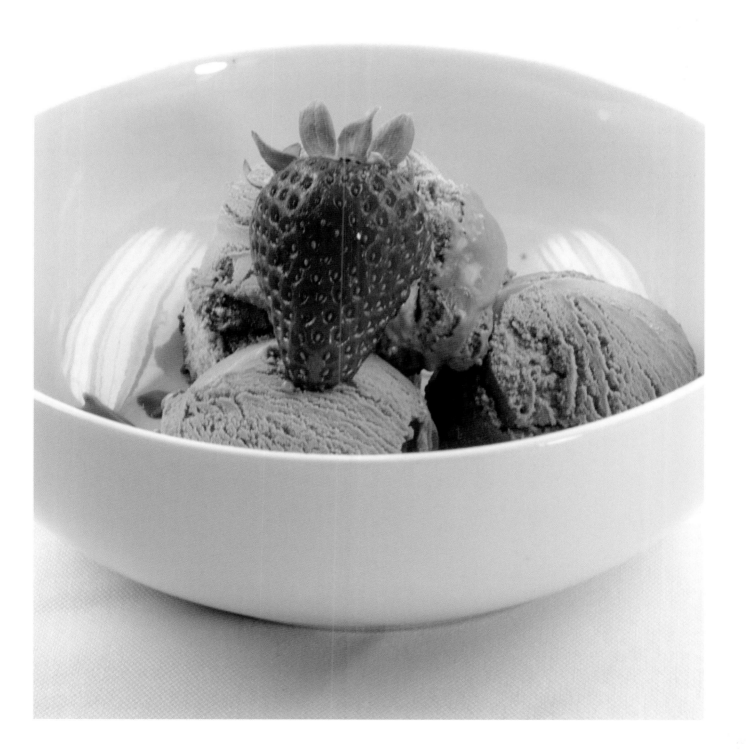

MAPLE BOURBON PECAN AVOCADO ICE CREAM

Macronutrients per serving (based on 4 servings): Calories 285 | Fat 29.7g | Carbohydrate 8.7g | Fiber 4.3g | Protein 11.6g

Makes: 4 to 6 servings | Prep time: 5 minutes, plus time to chill ice cream base, churn, and set up in freezer | Cook time: 5 minutes

1 cup full-fat coconut milk

½ cup unsweetened almond milk

½ teaspoon kosher salt

1 tablespoon granulated erythritol

⅛ teaspoon raw sucralose

2 eggs

2 avocados (about 8 ounces), halved and pitted

¼ cup Quest Protein Powder Vanilla Milkshake

½ teaspoon vanilla extract

½ teaspoon maple extract

½ ounce bourbon (optional)

¼ cup chopped pecans

FOR THE TOPPING:

Chopped pecans

SPECIAL EQUIPMENT:

Ice cream maker

01 Twenty-four hours before you plan to make ice cream, place the freezer bowl for your ice cream maker in the freezer.

02 In a 5-quart saucepan over medium heat, heat the coconut milk, almond milk, salt, erythritol, and sucralose until simmering, then pour into a blender and pulse until smooth.

03 Whisk the eggs in a medium-sized heatproof bowl. Temper the eggs by slowly pouring about a quarter of the hot coconut milk mixture into the eggs, 2 tablespoons at a time, whisking continuously, until the mixture is homogenous. Place the lid back on the blender but remove the fill cap. Turn the blender on to low, then slowly pour the egg and coconut milk mixture into the blender.

04 Remove the lid and scoop the flesh of the avocados into the blender. Place the lid back on, with the fill cap removed, and turn the blender on to low. While the blender is running, add the protein powder, vanilla extract, maple extract, and bourbon, if using, and continue to blend until the mixture is homogenous.

05 Place the blender jar in the refrigerator until the mixture is thoroughly chilled, at least 4 hours.

06 Insert the freezer bowl into the ice cream maker and churn the chilled ice cream base according to the manufacturer's directions. Add the pecans during the last 2 minutes of churning.

07 Transfer the ice cream to an airtight container and place in the freezer until a thicker consistency develops, about 20 minutes. Serve topped with chopped pecans. Store in the freezer for up to 1 month.

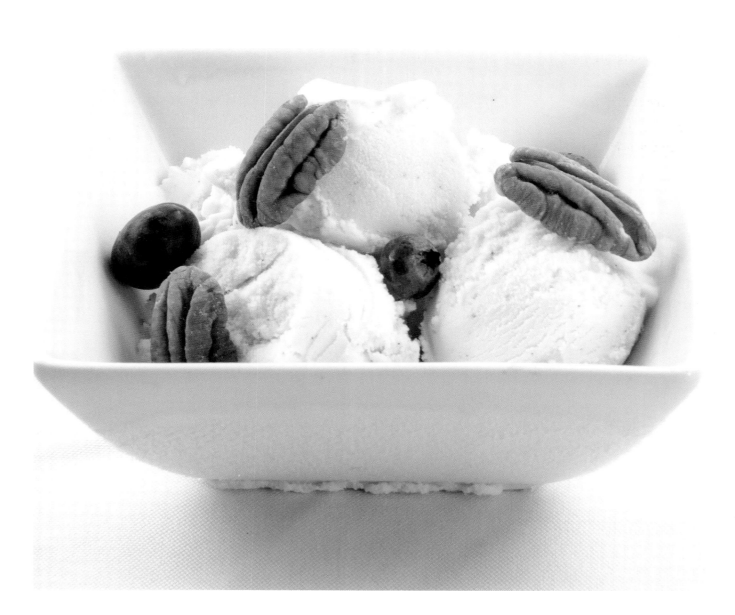

CARROT CAKE
WITH SALTED CARAMEL FROSTING

Macronutrients per serving: Calories 464 | Fat 40.1g | Carbohydrate 7.6g | Fiber 3.9g | Protein 14.2g

Makes: One 3-layer, 9-inch cake (8 servings) | Prep time: 30 minutes | Cook time: 15 minutes

FOR THE CAKE:

¾ cup blanched almond flour

½ cup high-fiber coconut flour

¼ cup Quest Protein Powder Multi-Purpose Mix

1 tablespoon ground flax seeds

1 teaspoon baking powder

½ teaspoon xanthan gum, divided

2 teaspoons ground cinnamon

¼ teaspoon ground allspice

¼ teaspoon ground cloves

¼ teaspoon ground nutmeg

½ teaspoon kosher salt

5 eggs

½ cup (1 stick) unsalted butter, melted

3 tablespoons coconut oil or MCT oil

2 tablespoons heavy cream

2 teaspoons vanilla extract

1 teaspoon Splenda Brown Sugar Blend

¼ teaspoon raw sucralose (optional)

¾ cup unsweetened almond milk

1 carrot (about 8 ounces), shredded, plus extra for garnish

¼ cup pecans, chopped

FOR THE FROSTING:

2 (8-ounce) packages cream cheese, softened

¼ cup Quest Protein Powder Salted Caramel

2 tablespoons unsalted butter, softened

1½ teaspoons ground cinnamon

¼ teaspoon kosher salt

FOR GARNISH:

¼ cup whole pecans

01 Preheat the oven to 325°F and coat three 9-inch round cake pans with cooking spray.

02 To make the cake, sift together the almond flour, coconut flour, protein powder, flax seeds, baking powder, ¼ teaspoon of the xanthan gum, spices, and salt; set aside.

03 Separate the eggs into two large bowls. To the bowl with the yolks, add the butter, coconut oil, heavy cream, vanilla extract, Splenda Brown Sugar Blend, and sucralose, if using. Using a hand mixer fitted with the paddle attachment, blend until the mixture is fully combined.

04 Whisk the egg whites until frothy, then add the remaining ¼ teaspoon of xanthan gum. Using a hand mixer fitted with the whisk attachment, whip until stiff peaks form, 2 to 3 minutes.

05 Fold the dry ingredients into the egg yolk mixture until homogenous, then gently fold the mixture into the egg whites. Fold in the almond milk, shredded carrot, and pecans, then portion the batter equally among the prepared pans. Bake for 11 to 15 minutes, until the sides of the cakes start to brown and pull away from the pans.

06 While the cakes are baking, make the frosting: Using a hand mixer fitted with the paddle attachment, blend together the cream cheese, protein powder, butter, cinnamon, and salt until smooth; set aside.

07 Remove the cakes from the pans and place on a cooling rack for 10 to 15 minutes, until cool and firm.

08 To assemble, place one cake on a plate and spread a thin layer of frosting on top. Repeat with the second cake on top of the first. Place the third cake as the final layer and evenly cover the top and sides of the cake with the remaining frosting.

09 Once the cake is frosted, cut into 8 equal slices and plate with whole pecans and shredded carrot. Store in an airtight container in the refrigerator for up to 1 week.

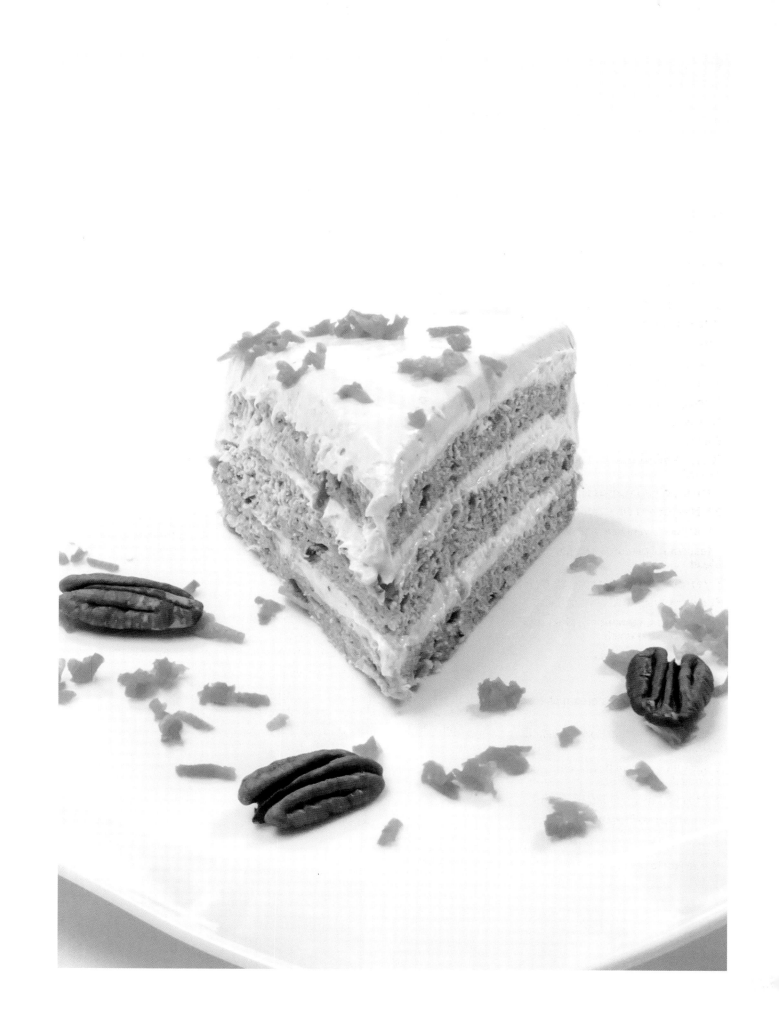

CHOCOLATE PEANUT BUTTER BANANA TRUFFLES

Macronutrients per truffle: Calories 212 | Fat 18.5g | Carbohydrate 5.5g | Fiber 2.6g | Protein 6.9g

Makes: 6 truffles (1 per serving) | Prep time: 10 minutes, plus 10 minutes to freeze | Cook time: 5 minutes

FOR THE PEANUT BUTTER FILLING:

¼ cup Quest Protein Powder Chocolate Milkshake

1 ounce cream cheese (2 tablespoons), softened

2 tablespoons unsweetened peanut butter

2 tablespoons unsweetened almond milk

1 tablespoon unsalted butter

1 tablespoon granulated erythritol

1 tablespoon cocoa powder

¼ teaspoon kosher salt

FOR THE CHOCOLATE SHELL:

3 ounces unsweetened chocolate

1½ ounces cocoa butter

⅛ teaspoon raw sucralose

Pinch of kosher salt

FOR THE DRIZZLE:

1 ounce cocoa butter

¼ teaspoon banana extract

1 drop yellow food coloring (optional)

01 In a bowl, mix all of the ingredients for the filling until homogenous. Form the mixture into six balls about the size of golf balls and place on a sheet pan. Insert a toothpick into each ball and freeze for 10 minutes.

02 Meanwhile, place the ingredients for the shell in a microwave-safe bowl and microwave on high in 30-second increments for 2 to 3 minutes, stirring often, until melted and homogenous and the temperature is about 118°F. Allow to cool to between 82°F and 85°F, then reheat in the microwave for 5 to 8 seconds, until the temperature is between 87°F and 91°F. The chocolate has to stay in this range so that it tempers correctly; if it drops below 82°F or rises above 91°F, you will need to repeat the process.

03 Remove the peanut butter balls from the freezer and submerge them in the chocolate mixture to coat evenly. (You may need to reheat the chocolate to keep it within the optimal temperature range.) Return the coated balls to the sheet pan and remove the toothpicks; set aside.

04 To make the drizzle, microwave the cocoa butter on high in 15-second increments for 2 to 3 minutes. Add the banana extract and yellow food coloring, if desired, stir until homogenous, and transfer to a plastic bag or pastry bag fitted with a piping tip. If using a plastic bag, cut off the tip of one corner. Drizzle the mixture over each ball and allow to set at room temperature for 3 to 5 minutes, until the drizzle is firm.

05 Serve immediately or transfer to an airtight container and store in the refrigerator for up to 1 week.

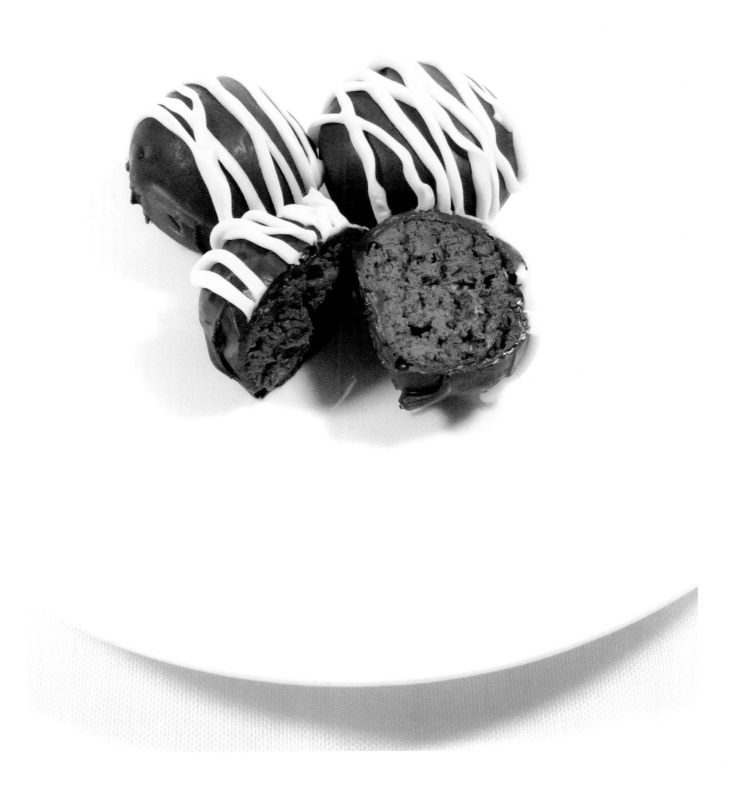

IRISH CREAM PISTACHIO CAKE SQUARES

Macronutrients per serving: Calories 392 | Fat 26.9g | Carbohydrate 9.5g | Fiber 4.6g | Protein 11.2g

Makes: 12 servings | Prep time: 10 minutes | Cook time: 35 to 40 minutes

FOR THE CRUST:

½ cup high-fiber coconut flour

2 tablespoons Quest Protein Powder Vanilla Milkshake

Pinch of kosher salt

¼ cup (½ stick) unsalted butter, melted

1 tablespoon coconut manna

½ teaspoon ground cinnamon

1 teaspoon heavy cream

FOR THE CAKE:

¼ cup blanched almond flour

2 tablespoons high-fiber coconut flour

2 tablespoons Quest Protein Powder Vanilla Milkshake

1 (8-ounce) package cream cheese, softened

¼ cup (½ stick) unsalted butter, melted

3 eggs, at room temperature

2 tablespoons Baileys Irish Cream (optional)

½ teaspoon vanilla extract

2 tablespoons granulated erythritol

½ teaspoon ground cinnamon

¼ teaspoon raw stevia powder

¼ teaspoon kosher salt

Pinch of ground nutmeg

8 ounces pistachios, divided

01 Preheat the oven to 400°F and coat an 8-inch square baking dish with cooking spray.

02 To make the crust, mix together all of the crust ingredients in a medium-sized bowl until a crumbly dough forms. Press the dough into the bottom of the baking dish and par-bake for 7 to 9 minutes, until the corners begin to brown. Set aside.

03 To make the cake, sift the almond flour, coconut flour, and protein powder into a large bowl.

04 In another bowl, using a hand mixer, cream the cream cheese, butter, eggs, Baileys (if using), vanilla extract, erythritol, cinnamon, stevia, salt, and nutmeg. Pour the wet ingredients into the dry ingredients and whisk until homogenous, then fold 5 ounces of the pistachios into the batter. Pour the batter over the par-baked crust and bake for 35 to 40 minutes, until the edges begin to brown and pull from the sides of the pan.

05 Let cool in the pan, then cut into 12 squares and serve. Store in an airtight container in the refrigerator for up to 5 days.

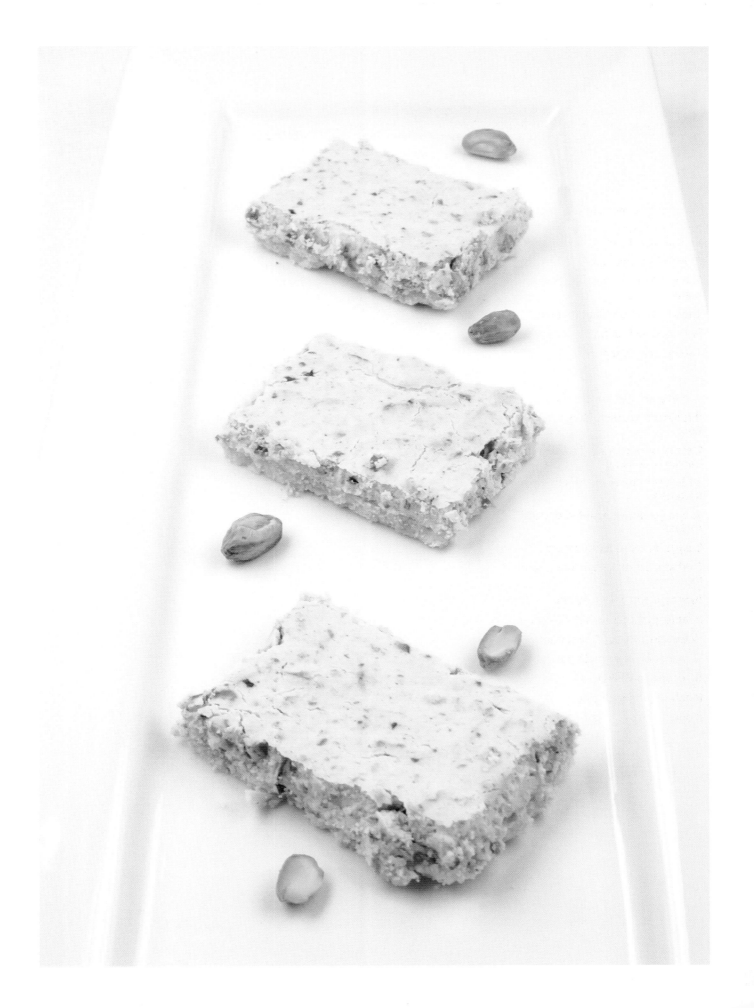

BASICS

VEGETABLE STOCK

Macronutrients per serving: **Calories 8** | **Fat 0.5g** | **Carbohydrate 0.3g** | **Fiber 0.1g** | **Protein 0.1g**

Makes: **2 quarts (64 ounces) (1 cup per serving)** | Prep time: **10 minutes** | Cook time: **30 to 35 minutes**

Vegetable stock is a great substitute for water when making a soup or sauce. It does not have the same strong flavor that a beef, chicken, or fish stock would have. It can be used as a braising liquid for vegetables, as the liquid base in a soup, or as a deglazing liquid when sautéing meats or vegetables.

2 tablespoons unsalted butter

1 red onion (about 8 ounces), roughly chopped into 1-inch pieces

2 stalks celery (about 4 ounces each), roughly chopped into 1-inch pieces

2 carrots (about 4 ounces each), peeled and roughly chopped into 1-inch pieces

6 cloves garlic, chopped

2 quarts water

6 sprigs fresh parsley

6 sprigs fresh thyme

2 bay leaves

1 teaspoon kosher salt

01 In a stockpot, heat the butter over medium heat for 1 to 2 minutes. Add the onion, celery, carrots, and garlic and sauté for 2 to 3 minutes, stirring frequently.

02 Pour in the water and stir. Add the parsley, thyme, bay leaves, and salt and stir once more. Bring to a boil, then reduce the heat to a simmer and continue to simmer for 30 to 35 minutes.

03 Line a colander with cheesecloth and set over a heatproof container. Pour the stock through the colander into the container; discard the vegetables.

04 Store in an airtight container in the refrigerator for up to 1 week, or freeze for up to 2 months.

BROWN BEEF STOCK

Macronutrients per serving: Calories 14 | Fat 0.5g | Carbohydrate 0.3g | Fiber 0.1g | Protein 2g
Makes: 2 quarts (64 ounces) (1 cup per serving) | Prep time: 15 minutes | Cook time: 5 to 6 hours

2 pounds beef bones, sawed into 2-inch pieces

2 tablespoons unsalted butter

1 red onion (about 8 ounces), roughly chopped into 1-inch pieces

2 stalks celery (about 4 ounces each), roughly chopped into 1-inch pieces

2 carrots (about 4 ounces each), peeled and roughly chopped into 1-inch pieces

6 cloves garlic, chopped

½ cup dry red wine (optional)

2 quarts water

6 sprigs fresh parsley

6 sprigs fresh thyme

2 bay leaves

1 teaspoon kosher salt

Tip: *When the stock is thoroughly chilled, its fat content rises to the top to form a solid white layer. It then can easily be removed with a spoon.*

01 Preheat the oven to 400°F.

02 Rinse the bones under cold water, then place on a sheet pan. Roast the bones for 45 to 60 minutes, until browned but not charred; if they become charred, the stock will taste burnt.

03 When the bones are done roasting, heat the butter in a stockpot over medium heat for 1 to 2 minutes. Add the onion, celery, carrots, and garlic and sauté for 2 to 3 minutes, stirring frequently. Add the red wine, if using, and allow to simmer for 1 to 2 minutes.

04 Pour in the water and stir. Add the bones and any juices that have accumulated in the roasting pan, parsley, thyme, bay leaves, and salt and stir once more. Bring to a boil, then reduce the heat to a simmer and continue to simmer for 4 to 5 hours, until the stock has a rich brown color and a layer of white fat has developed on the surface. Use a spoon to remove the layer of fat from the top (depouillage) by moving the pan so that only half of it is over the heat. This will cause the fat to float to one side, making it easier to remove.

05 Line a colander with cheesecloth and set over a heatproof container. Pour the stock through the colander into the container; discard the vegetables and bones. Return the stock to the heat in a clean stockpot, bring to a boil, and remove any remaining white fat that rises to the surface.

06 Store in an airtight container in the refrigerator for up to a week, or freeze for up to 2 months.

WHITE BEEF STOCK

Macronutrients per serving: Calories 14 | Fat 0.5g | Carbohydrate 0.3g | Fiber 0.1g | Protein 2g

Makes: 2 quarts (64 ounces) (1 cup per serving) | Prep time: 15 minutes | Cook time: 2½ to 3½ hours

2 pounds beef bones, sawed into 2-inch pieces

4 quarts water, divided

2 tablespoons unsalted butter

1 red onion (about 8 ounces), roughly chopped into 1-inch pieces

2 stalks celery (about 4 ounces each), roughly chopped into 1-inch pieces

2 carrots (about 4 ounces each), peeled and roughly chopped into 1-inch pieces

6 cloves garlic, chopped

6 sprigs fresh parsley

6 sprigs fresh thyme

2 bay leaves

1 teaspoon kosher salt

01 Rinse the bones under cold water, then place them in a stockpot. Add 2 quarts of the water and bring to a boil. Boil for 3 to 4 minutes, then remove the bones and rinse again; set aside. Discard the boiling water.

02 Heat the butter in a stockpot over medium heat for 1 to 2 minutes. Add the onion, celery, carrots, and garlic and sauté for 2 to 3 minutes, stirring frequently.

03 Pour in the remaining 2 quarts of water and stir. Add the boiled and rinsed bones, parsley, thyme, bay leaves, and salt and stir once more. Bring to a boil, then reduce the heat to a simmer and continue to simmer for 2 to 3 hours, until a white layer of fat has developed on the surface of the stock. Use a spoon to remove the layer of fat from the top (depouillage) by moving the pan so that only half of it is over the heat. This will cause the fat to float to one side, making it easier to remove.

04 Line a colander with cheesecloth and set over a heatproof container. Pour the stock through the colander into the container; discard the vegetables and bones. Return the stock to the heat in a clean stockpot, bring to a boil, and remove any remaining white fat that rises the surface.

05 Store in an airtight container in the refrigerator for up to 1 week, or freeze for up to 2 months.

CHICKEN STOCK

Macronutrients per serving: Calories 6 | Fat 0.4g | Carbohydrate 0.3g | Fiber 0.1g | Protein 0.3g
Makes: 2 quarts (64 ounces) (1 cup per serving) | Prep time: 15 minutes | Cook time: 2 to 2½ hours

2 pounds chicken bones (backs, necks, feet, and/or wings), cut into 2-inch pieces

4 quarts water, divided

2 tablespoons unsalted butter

1 red onion (about 8 ounces), roughly chopped into 1-inch pieces

2 stalks celery (about 4 ounces each), roughly chopped into 1-inch pieces

2 carrots (about 4 ounces each), peeled and roughly chopped into 1-inch pieces

6 cloves garlic, chopped

6 sprigs fresh parsley

6 sprigs fresh thyme

2 bay leaves

1 teaspoon kosher salt

01 Rinse the bones under cold water, then place them in a stockpot. Add 2 quarts of the water and bring to a boil. Boil for 3 to 4 minutes, then remove the bones and rinse again; set aside. Discard the boiling water.

02 Heat the butter in a stockpot over medium heat for 1 to 2 minutes. Add the onion, celery, carrots, and garlic and sauté for 2 to 3 minutes, stirring frequently.

03 Pour in the remaining 2 quarts of water and stir. Add the boiled and rinsed bones, parsley, thyme, bay leaves, and salt and stir once more. Bring to a boil, then reduce the heat to a simmer and continue to simmer for 1½ to 2 hours, until a thin white layer of fat has developed on the surface of the stock. Use a spoon to remove the layer of fat from the top (depouillage) by moving the pan so that only half of it is over the heat. This will cause the fat to float to one side, making it easier to remove.

04 Line a colander with cheesecloth and set over a heatproof container. Pour the stock through the colander into the container; discard the vegetables and bones. Return the stock to the heat in a clean stockpot, bring to a boil, and remove any remaining white fat that rises to the surface.

05 Store the stock in an airtight container in the refrigerator for up to 5 days, or freeze for up to 2 months.

FISH STOCK

Macronutrients per serving: Calories 3 | Fat 0.2g | Carbohydrate 0.3g | Fiber 0.1g | Protein 0.1g

Makes: 2 quarts (64 ounces) (1 cup per serving) | Prep time: 15 minutes | Cook time: 1 to 1½ hours

2 tablespoons unsalted butter

1 red onion (about 8 ounces), roughly chopped into 1-inch pieces

2 stalks celery (about 4 ounces each), roughly chopped into 1-inch pieces

2 carrots (about 4 ounces each), peeled and roughly chopped into 1-inch pieces

6 cloves garlic, chopped

½ cup dry white wine (optional)

2 quarts water

2 pounds whitefish bones, such as snapper, bass, and/or halibut, cut into 2-inch pieces

6 sprigs fresh parsley

6 sprigs fresh thyme

2 bay leaves

1 teaspoon kosher salt

01 Heat the butter in a stockpot over medium heat for 1 to 2 minutes. Add the onion, celery, carrots, and garlic and sauté for 2 to 3 minutes, stirring frequently. Stir in the white wine, if using.

02 Pour in the water and stir. Add the fish bones, parsley, thyme, bay leaves, and salt and stir once more. Bring to a boil, reduce the heat to a simmer, and continue to simmer for 60 to 90 minutes, until a thin white layer of fat has developed on the surface of the stock. Use a spoon to remove the layer of fat from the top (depouillage) by moving the pan so that only half of it is over the heat. This will cause the fat to float to one side, making it easier to remove.

03 Line a colander with cheesecloth and set over a heatproof container. Pour the stock through the colander into the container; discard the vegetables and bones. Return the stock to the heat in a clean stockpot, bring to a boil, and remove any remaining white fat that rises to the surface.

04 Store in an airtight container in the refrigerator for up to 4 days, or freeze for up to 2 months.

HOLLANDAISE

Macronutrients per serving: **Calories 134 | Fat 14.2g | Carbohydrate 0g | Fiber 0g | Protein 1.6g**
Makes: **1 cup (2 tablespoons per serving)** | Prep time: **5 minutes** | Cook time: **10 minutes**

½ cup water

4 egg yolks, at room temperature

1 tablespoon lemon juice

4 ounces clarified butter (page 348)
or unsalted butter, melted

Hot sauce, such as Tabasco

Kosher salt and ground white pepper

01 In a small saucepan, heat the water until simmering.

02 Place the egg yolks in a medium-sized heatproof bowl and whisk until liquefied. Whisk in the lemon juice until the mixture has thickened and doubled in volume. Place the bowl over the simmering water and whisk the yolk mixture for 2 to 3 minutes, until air bubbles begin to develop and the mixture starts to thicken. It's important to keep whisking to prevent the yolks from cooking or traveling up the side of the bowl; do not allow the temperature of the mixture to exceed 160°F, or the egg yolks will start to cook.

03 Slowly whisk in the butter in 1-tablespoon increments; the butter should be fully blended in before you add more. Repeat until the mixture has doubled in volume again, has lightened in color, and is creamy; this is called the ribbon stage because when you pull a whisk through the mixture, it leaves trails that are visible for a short while.

04 Remove the hollandaise from the heat, season to taste with hot sauce, salt, and pepper, and keep warm over a water bath until needed or let cool, place in an airtight container, and refrigerate for up to 1 day. To rewarm the hollandaise, place it in a heatproof bowl over a pan of simmering water and whisk until the temperature reaches 140°F to 160°F. Once reheated, the sauce should be used within 10 minutes. If you hold it too long, it might separate.

CLARIFIED BUTTER
AND GHEE

Macronutrients per serving: **Calories 119** | **Fat 13.5g** | **Carbohydrate 0g** | **Fiber 0g** | **Protein 0g**

Makes: **12 ounces** | Prep time: **5 minutes** | Cook time: **about 15 minutes for clarified butter, 25 minutes for ghee**

The initial steps to make clarified butter and ghee are exactly the same. To make ghee, you simply take the process a bit further. When butter is heated, it separates into three layers, at which point it can be strained to make clarified butter. If you continue to heat the butter to allow more of the water content to evaporate and the milk solids to brown, you end up with ghee, a fat with a slightly nutty flavor, a high smoke point, and an extended shelf life.

16 ounces unsalted butter

01 Melt the butter in a small saucepan over low heat. Place a fine-mesh sieve lined with cheesecloth over a heatproof container.

02 Allow the butter to foam and slowly come to a boil over low heat; it will begin to separate into three layers. After 12 to 15 minutes, the top will be a thin layer of foam, the middle layer will be a transparent golden color, and the butter layer or milk solids will be on the bottom of the pan. The golden layer in the middle is the clarified butter, which has to be separated from the other two layers. Once the three layers have developed, you're ready to make clarified butter (see Step 3). To make ghee, skip ahead to Step 4.

03 To make clarified butter, remove the pan from the heat and allow to cool for about 5 minutes. With a large spoon, remove and discard the thin layer of foam from the top, then pour the butter through the cheesecloth into the heatproof container to remove any remaining foam from the top layer and the milk solids from the bottom layer. The clarified butter can be used warm or cooled and stored for later use (see Step 5).

04 To make ghee, after the three layers have developed, cook the butter for an additional 5 to 10 minutes, until it gives off a nutty aroma and the milk solids at the bottom of the pan have browned. (Be careful not to burn them!) Then, with a large spoon, remove and discard the thin layer of foam from the top and pour the butter through the cheesecloth into the heatproof container to remove any remaining foam from the top layer and the milk solids from the bottom layer. The ghee can be used warm or cooled and stored for later use.

05 Store the clarified butter or ghee in an airtight container in the refrigerator; clarified butter will keep for about 3 weeks, ghee for about 4 weeks.

CLASSIC AIOLI

Macronutrients per serving: **Calories 126** | **Fat 14.1g** | **Carbohydrate 0.3g** | **Fiber 0g** | **Protein 0g**

Makes: **About ½ cup (1 tablespoon per serving)** | Prep time: **10 minutes** | Cook time: —

1 egg yolk

1 teaspoon lemon juice

2 cloves garlic, smashed to a paste

½ teaspoon kosher salt

½ teaspoon Dijon mustard

½ cup extra-virgin olive oil, divided

½ cup grapeseed oil

Grond black pepper

01 In a medium-sized bowl, whisk together the egg yolk, lemon juice, garlic paste, salt, and mustard.

02 Add 1 tablespoon of the olive oil and stir until it begins to combine with the other ingredients. Then, in a steady stream, pour in the remaining olive oil and the grapeseed oil, whisking constantly to emulsify (combine) the oil and egg yolk. The egg yolk mixture should look like it is absorbing the oil.

03 Season to taste with pepper. Use immediately or store in an airtight container in the refrigerator for up to 10 days.

Variation: Bacon Aioli. Substitute warmed bacon fat for the ½ cup of grapeseed oil. The bacon fat should be liquid, but not so hot that it cooks the egg yolk. A safe temperature would be 100°F to 120°F.

Chapter 9:

FREQUENTLY ASKED QUESTIONS

General

How are ketones produced?

Ketones are produced during the breakdown of fat by the liver. Fat is primarily broken down for fuel when carbohydrate consumption (and therefore insulin) is low.

Can the brain use ketones?

Unlike most fatty acids, ketones can be taken in and used as an energy source for the brain. In fact, the brain might actually prefer ketones to glucose; studies have shown that ketone uptake by the brain increases as blood ketone levels rise (Cunnane et al., 2011). There is also a lot of research demonstrating that a ketogenic diet can have brain-protecting effects in various types of damaged neurons, possibly due to the neurons receiving greater fuel reserves through ketones, less oxidative stress, and less inflammation (Gasior, Rogawski, and Hartman, 2006). Even when glucose uptake by the brain is impaired, as it is in people with Alzheimer's, Parkinson's, and traumatic brain injury, ketones can be utilized.

Which tissues use ketones?

Ketones can be used by nearly all of the cells and tissues in the body, though not by the liver (where they are made). Some cells, like those in certain regions of the brain and red blood cells, can use only glucose for energy, but the body can produce plenty of glucose from gluconeogenesis (see page 18) to provide those cells with what they need when carbohydrate consumption is low.

Is a ketogenic diet safe?

Yes, the ketogenic diet is safe for most people when properly formulated (Kang et al., 2007; Suo et al., 2013; Freeman et al., 1998). However, if any of the conditions outlined in Figure 9.1 affect you, a ketogenic diet may not be right for you—talk to your doctor.

KETOSIS IS NOT RECOMMENDED FOR

- Carnitine deficiency
- CPT I/II deficiency
- Beta oxidation defects
- Mitochondrial 3-hydroxy-3-methylglutaryl-CoA synthase deficiency
- Medium-chain Acyl dehydrogenase deficiency
- Long-chain Acyl dehydrogenase
- Impaired gastrointestinal motility
- Pregnancy
- Kidney failure
- Pyruvate carboxylase deficiency
- Porphyria
- Pancreatitis
- Gallbladder disease
- Impaired liver function
- Impaired fat digestion
- Gastric bypass surgery
- Abdominal tumors

Figure 9.1. *Conditions and situations in which a ketogenic diet may not be advised or should be thoroughly monitored.*

What's the difference between a low-carb diet and a ketogenic diet?

There is no strict definition of "low-carb." Some studies suggest that a low-carb diet is any diet with less than 30 percent of calories coming from carbohydrates (Bueno et al., 2013). A ketogenic diet generally restricts carbohydrates even further, to as low as 5 percent of total calories (Freeman, Kossoff, and Hartman, 2007). So, while a ketogenic diet is certainly low-carb, not all low-carb diets are ketogenic. The ketogenic diet's greater restriction of carbohydrates results in the production of ketones (Young, 1971).

What is the difference between the Atkins diet and a ketogenic diet?

Although the Atkins diet and ketogenic diet have similar features, they differ in their carbohydrate, protein, and fat intake. The induction phase of the Atkins diet is very similar to the ketogenic diet; however, eventually the Atkins diet introduces higher carbohydrate and protein recommendations. In the beginning especially, the ketogenic diet consists of a moderate amount of protein and very low carbohydrate intake. Over time and as you learn your body, you will be able to play around with protein and carbohydrate levels while still filling in the rest of your calories with fat.

What is the difference between nutritional ketosis and ketoacidosis?

Nutritional ketosis is characterized by a *controlled* increase in ketones, along with reductions in blood glucose and normal blood pH. Ketoacidosis is characterized by an *uncontrolled* increase in ketone production (higher than 15 mmol/L) despite elevated blood glucose levels and results in dangerous decreases in blood pH (Cartwright et al., 2012); it is a concern mainly for type 1 diabetics. Ketogenic diets and ketone supplementation typically do not raise ketone levels above 5 to 7 mmol/L (Veech, 2004).

Will I be hungry?

If you follow a well-formulated ketogenic diet, then no; not only is the high amount of fat on a ketogenic diet satiating, but ketones also seem to reduce hunger signals (see page 69). Studies have allowed subjects on a ketogenic diet to eat as much as they want, yet they still tend to eat fewer calories, report less hunger, and lose more weight than those on a non-ketogenic diet (Johnstone et al., 2008). It is possible that this is because fat is more calorically dense; however, studies have also demonstrated that being in a state of ketosis can reduce hunger signals (Sumithran et al., 2011). Additional research has found that the consumption of fat reduces hormones responsible for appetite signaling (Sumithran et al., 2013), so long-term hunger shouldn't be a problem.

Do I need to count calories?

When you first start following a ketogenic diet, we recommend tracking macronutrients and calories just to get the hang of it and to make sure that you're getting the right amount of each. However, soon after adapting, you should simply be able to eat until you are full while monitoring your carbohydrate intake. Don't let those sneaky carbs creep up too high. In fact, people who are keto-adapted often reduce their calories unintentionally because they feel full faster. If possible, eat to satiety once you get the hang of it; your keto-adapted appetite should ensure that you consume enough calories without overeating (Volek et al., 2002). Those individuals using the ketogenic diet for therapeutic applications should incorporate some level of calorie control/restriction in order to achieve the best results.

Should I track net carbs or total carbs?

This is one of the most common questions we get, and we talk about it in depth on page 42 (where we urge you to be cautious of misleading "fiber" labels). Our general recommendation is to track total carbs when starting out on the ketogenic diet and then, once you get the hang of it, to transition to net carbs, which can help ensure that you're getting enough fiber (see page 42). Be your own scientist and see what works best for you!

Do I have to stick to certain macronutrient ratios (such as 75 percent fat, 20 percent protein, and 5 percent carbs)?

Target macronutrient ratios can be a good place to start, but keep in mind that the macro ratios that work best for you and your lifestyle may differ from what works best for someone else. The key is to keep carbohydrate intake low, protein intake moderate, and fat intake moderate to high. Have fun with it and tinker with your diet until you figure out what is optimal for you. Once you have individualized the ketogenic diet to suit your needs, and after you have been eating this way for a while, you will learn what you should and shouldn't consume to maintain your optimal ratios, and you may not need to count macronutrient content as strictly.

Do I need to exercise in order to lose weight and improve my health while on a ketogenic diet?

There are plenty of studies demonstrating improvements in body composition (i.e., reduced fat mass and maintained or increased lean muscle mass) and blood lipids (i.e., reduced triglyceride and total cholesterol levels and increased HDL cholesterol levels) on a ketogenic diet without exercise (Yancy et al., 2004; Volek et al., 2004). However, exercise is a key component of a healthy lifestyle, and it can dramatically improve your results on a ketogenic diet. For this reason, we highly recommend some type of physical activity or exercise, even if it is just walking 10,000 steps per day (about 5 miles). Our colleague Dr. Stephen Cunnane found that even moderate walking increased brain ketone uptake, so get out there and move!

Do I have to stay on a ketogenic diet every single day?

On page 74, we touch on the traditional cyclic approach to ketogenic dieting, where people tend to eat ketogenic on weekdays and then go back to consuming carbohydrates on weekends. While we don't believe that is the best approach, we do tend to eat "ketogenic" six days a week and have a low-carb, high-protein, moderate-fat day sometime during the week. For us, this isn't a "carb up" day but rather a "protein up" day, where we eat more protein yet still consume lower-carbohydrate foods. This approach may help people who are training or are hitting a plateau on the diet. Rather than going crazy with a carbohydrate refeed, changing it up with protein can help you continue to progress toward your goals.

Nutrients and Supplements

Do I need to consume carbohydrates to replenish glycogen?

Studies suggest that the body does not require carbohydrates to replenish glycogen (Pascoe et al., 1993), and research on keto-adapted athletes has found that they spare and replenish muscle glycogen at similar rates as carbohydrate-adapted athletes (Volek et al., 2016). At the beginning of a ketogenic diet, as your body is adapting to burning fat, your glycogen stores may be limited, but they will soon rebound once you're fully adapted. We discuss this more on page 138.

Should I increase my sodium intake?

Sodium levels do drop on a ketogenic diet, so it's a good idea to consume more sodium (Tiwari, Riazi, and Ecelbarger, 2007). (See page 48 for more on sodium and other electrolytes.) Himalayan sea salt can be a beneficial source because it contains many minerals, including sodium, calcium, potassium, iodine, and magnesium, with a sodium content similar to table salt but with larger crystals for more flavor.

Are there other electrolytes I should replenish?

Potassium, magnesium, and calcium also can become depleted on a ketogenic diet. See page 48 for more on electrolytes and supplements.

Should I worry about fiber?

It's common for fiber intake to drop when switching to a ketogenic diet, simply because fiber is most abundant in foods that are high in carbohydrates, particularly vegetables and grains. Fiber is an important nutrient that is essential for good health. Although it is technically a carbohydrate, it does not increase blood glucose or insulin levels, so we highly recommend making an effort to eat enough fiber. However, be aware that isomaltooligosaccharides (IMOs), the kind of fiber commonly found in "high-fiber" protein bars, produces a blood sugar and insulin response. A few brands of high-fiber protein bars contain soluble corn fiber instead, which does not raise blood sugar or insulin, so check ingredient labels. (See page 42 for more on fiber.)

Will eating too much protein kick me out of ketosis?

While some amino acids, such as leucine and lysine, can be converted to ketones, others can be converted to glucose and may therefore raise blood glucose and insulin levels if consumed in excessive amounts. For this reason, we suggest getting no more than 20 to 35 percent of your calories from protein. Keep in mind that the optimal level varies from individual to individual—for instance, someone using a ketogenic diet to help with epilepsy may need less protein than someone using it to try to gain muscle mass. Be your own scientist! (See page 47 for more on protein.)

Will carbs make me fat?

We do not intend to demonize carbohydrates as the sole culprit for the obesity epidemic our society is facing. Instead, we hope to change the paradigm of a "healthy" diet to help people look at carbohydrates as a useful tool rather than as a dietary necessity. Although it is true that chronic high carbohydrate consumption can lead to chronic high blood glucose and insulin levels, resulting in metabolic changes such as insulin resistance that increase the likelihood of obesity, it is possible for many people to consume carbohydrates and maintain a healthy profile.

Are there certain fats I should avoid?

While we love fat, it is important to note that not all fat is created equal. Omega-6 fatty acids are known for contributing to inflammation, which is associated with many chronic diseases. Make sure to balance your omega-3 fatty acids with your omega-6 fatty acids to ensure the best outcome. Similarly, trans fats are harmful to health and should be limited. (See pages 44 and 45 for more on the types of fat.) Finally, if you hit a plateau or obstacle while on a ketogenic diet, we have found that lowering dairy fat and saturated fat as a whole slightly while increasing unsaturated fats can help.

Is it possible to eat too much fat?

When you are keto-adapted, you become much more efficient at utilizing fat as fuel, and some studies show that slightly overfeeding on fat alone may not cause significant weight gain. However, keep in mind that fat is calorically dense, containing 9 calories per gram. Eating excessive amounts of fat can increase calorie intake to an extent that may prevent fat loss; too much dietary fat might keep your body from breaking down its own fat stores for energy. As with everything, keep the fat content of the diet in context—and don't binge on fat bombs or eat sticks of butter like candy bars!

Should all my fat come from saturated fat?

We discuss the different types of fat and their impact on the body on pages 44 and 45. As explained earlier, saturated fat should not be demonized, especially on a ketogenic diet. However, we have found that our bodies adapt best when saturated fat represents about 50 percent of our total fat intake and the rest comes from monounsaturated fats like coconut oil and avocados. This could, in part, explain why so many studies have differing findings in regard to cholesterol and triglyceride levels when following a ketogenic diet. If you are concerned about these factors, ensuring that you consume a balance of saturated and monounsaturated fats may be a smart approach. Regardless of what some health organizations and media outlets might claim, don't be afraid of coconut oil or saturated fats when taken in the context of a well-formulated diet.

What are exogenous ketones?

Exogenous ketones are supplemental ketones that are found in either powdered or liquid form. The powdered versions are typically bound to minerals such as calcium, sodium, and magnesium, while the liquid forms consist primarily of ketone esters. (See Chapter 4 for more on exogenous ketones.)

Will exogenous ketones make me lose weight?

Exogenous ketones likely do not directly cause fat loss. Keep in mind that they are an energy source and do have calories. However, elevated ketone levels have been shown to reduce hunger (Sumithran et al., 2011), increase the production of new mitochondria, and decrease the ratio of weight gained to amount of food consumed (Bough et al., 2006), which could allow for greater fat burning and incidentally reduce body weight indirectly. (See page 75 for more on exogenous ketones and weight loss.)

Are MCTs the same as exogenous ketones?

No. MCTs can be converted to ketones once they're broken down in the liver (Rebello et al., 2015). However, some research suggests that it takes extremely high amounts of MCT (more than 20 grams) to get the same effects that just a couple grams of exogenous ketones could achieve (Misell, Lagomarcino, Schuster, and Kern, 2001). (See page 55 for more on MCTs.)

Are MCT supplements safe?

Yes! No adverse effects were found in people taking 30 grams of MCTs a day (a much higher dose than is typically consumed) for thirty days (Courchesne-Loyer et al., 2013). Additionally, 1 gram of MCTs per kilogram of body weight has been established as safe (Traul, Driedger, Ingle, and Nakhasi, 2000). However, MCTs can have gastrointestinal side effects, such as nausea and diarrhea, so we highly recommend starting out slowly and building up your tolerance.

Are exogenous ketones safe?

Exogenous ketone esters have been found to be safe in humans and in animals (Clarke et al., 2012; Kesl et al., 2016; Evans, Cogan, and Egan, 2016). Additionally, ketone salts have been granted GRAS (generally recognized as safe) status. Several studies have used both ketone salts and ketone esters in both animals and humans with no adverse side effects. As with any supplement, look for exogenous ketones that are third party tested by a company like Informed Choice or NSF to ensure quality and clinical research behind their use.

Becoming Keto-Adapted

How long does it take to get into ketosis?
Ketosis is generally recognized to occur when ketone levels rise to 0.3 to 0.5 mmol/L. Two days of carbohydrate restriction can be enough to reach this level (Bilsborough and Crowe, 2003). However, achieving this level of ketosis does not mean that you are keto-adapted—that your body is primarily using fat as fuel. Becoming fully keto-adapted may take longer; exactly how long varies from person to person.

What does it mean to be keto-adapted?
When you're keto-adapted, your body has transitioned from primarily using glucose as fuel to primarily using fat and ketones. Once adapted, you will start to see changes in satiety, hunger, and even cognitive function/focus. (For more on keto adaptation, see page 16.)

How do I know if I'm in ketosis?
Ketone levels can be tested using urine strips, blood ketone meters, and breath ketone meters. Blood meters, which test for BHB, are considered the gold standard. Breath analysis has been shown to be effective at measuring acetone (Musa-Veloso, Likhodii, and Cunnane, 2002), while urine analysis measures acetoacetate. Urine test strips can provide good feedback at the beginning of the diet, but once you're keto-adapted and using ketones more efficiently, fewer ketones are expelled in the urine, so they are not a reliable indicator of your degree of ketosis.

If I take exogenous ketones, am I keto-adapted?
Taking ketone supplements without lowering carbohydrate intake will not likely make you fully keto-adapted. It is unknown whether taking these supplements long-term can lead to certain changes that typically occur with keto adaptation (such as an enhanced capacity to allow ketones to enter tissues to be used for fuel by increasing the number of ketone transporter proteins), but to be fully keto-adapted, some degree of carbohydrate restriction needs to occur.

What is the optimal ketone level on the diet?
This is difficult to say; it depends on the reason for ketosis. As long as ketone levels are greater than 0.3 mmol/L, you're in ketosis. Many people think that higher ketone levels are better, but this has not been established. Some individuals who have been keto-adapted for an extended period may become particularly efficient at using ketones and therefore don't have a lot of them circulating in the blood. For health concerns such as epilepsy and other neurological conditions, higher ketone levels may be beneficial—exogenous ketones or high-dose MCTs may be especially helpful for accomplishing those levels.

What is the keto flu?
The keto flu is a constellation of symptoms that can occur when you're adjusting to a ketogenic diet. Symptoms include a lack of mental clarity, nausea, headaches, and constipation. A well-formulated ketogenic diet that takes into account electrolytes, fiber, and hydration can help mitigate these symptoms. (For more on the keto flu and how to handle it, see page 191.)

I just started a ketogenic diet and I feel sick. What can I do?
The ill feeling that may occur in the first few days after initiating a ketogenic diet is commonly referred to as the keto flu. Fortunately, this feeling is temporary and can be completely or partially alleviated by taking a few precautionary measures. First, consider your electrolytes. A deficiency in sodium, potassium, or calcium could make you feel sick. (See page 48 for more on electrolytes.) Second, consider your hydration level. It's easy to get dehydrated at the beginning of a ketogenic diet. Third, consider your fiber intake. If you're not getting enough fiber, you could become constipated. (See page 42 for more on fiber.) The takeaway: replenish your electrolytes, drink a lot of water, and make sure you're getting enough fiber.

Can I speed up the transition phase to becoming keto-adapted?
Our lab has found that doing so is possible. Exercise, particularly high-intensity exercise, tends to speed up the transition phase because it helps deplete glycogen stores quickly, forcing the body to rely more on fat. Additionally, starting the transition with fasting or intermittent fasting (see page 49) can rapidly increase ketone production.

Foods to Eat and to Avoid

Can I drink alcohol on a ketogenic diet?

Certain alcohols, such as wine, whiskey, and vodka, may be safe to consume in moderation on a ketogenic diet. Some studies have found that consuming red wine does not seem to impair the state of ketosis (Pérez-Guisado, Muñoz-Serrano, and Alonso-Moraga, 2008). In fact, some winemakers, like Dry Farm Wines, are going so far as to remove sugar entirely in order to make their wines even more keto-friendly. Be careful of dark beers (such as lagers, stouts, porters, and ales) and mixed-liquor drinks that are known to be higher in carbohydrate content.

Can I have coffee?

Coffee intake is allowed on a ketogenic diet; just hold the sugar. It is worth pointing out that some studies have found that caffeine is ketogenic—it could actually increase ketone production (Johnston, Clifford, and Morgan, 2003; Vandenberghe et al., 2016). Therefore, some people enjoy a cup of coffee with heavy cream and MCT oil to start the day.

Can I have fruit?

Most fruit is filled with natural sugar, so it's important to carefully consider fruit intake on a ketogenic diet. There are lower-glycemic fruits, like berries, that may be tolerated in moderate amounts. While fruit does contain vitamins and other nutrients, it's easy to get these from other sources on a well-formulated ketogenic diet.

Can I have dairy?

Dairy that's low in lactose (the sugar found in milk), such as heavy cream, butter, and cheese, can be consumed in moderation on a ketogenic diet. Dairy products that are high in lactose, such as milk and yogurt, should be limited or, for some people, eliminated entirely. We often find that individuals who are struggling with the diet are consuming too much dairy, and pulling back even slightly can help significantly.

Which sweeteners are best on a ketogenic diet?

We recommend that you use natural sweeteners whenever possible. Stevia, erythritol, monk fruit (luo han guo), and a new natural sweetener called allulose are the preferred choices. Inulin is also common, but many people don't tolerate it well and experience gastrointestinal symptoms after consuming it. Among artificial sweeteners, the best choices are raw sucralose and aspartame. These are common ingredients in commercial artificial sweetener products, but those products also include ingredients such as maltodextrin and dextrose—which are sugars—so the raw versions of sucralose and aspartame are best.

Training and Athletic Performance

How does a ketogenic diet affect performance?

At the onset of the diet, performance may decline (Burke et al., 2000; Phinney et al., 1980). However, research has found that over time, these performance decrements disappear (Phinney et al., 1980; Paoli et al., 2012). Some studies, including those conducted in our lab, have even found that people following a ketogenic diet and doing resistance training can gain the same amount of strength compared to controls (Sharp et al., 2015; Gregory, 2016). (See Chapter 5, section 5 for more on exercise and performance.)

Will I lose muscle on a ketogenic diet?

Research suggests that keeping protein to around 1.2 to 1.6 grams per kilogram of body weight allows people to maintain or gain lean mass. Even among individuals in a calorie-restricted state, studies have found fat loss to be as high as 95 percent of total weight lost on a ketogenic diet (Young, Scanlan, Im, and Lutwak, 1971) and that consuming a ketogenic diet at maintenance calories leads to increases in muscle mass (Volek et al., 2002). The positive effects on muscle mass are due in part to the protein-sparing and anabolic effects of ketones. (See page 143 for more on muscle maintenance.)

Should I do targeted ketogenic dieting (TKD) for performance?

Targeted ketogenic dieting involves incorporating carbohydrates around a training session (before, during, and/or after training). By doing so, the adrenaline from the training session blunts the insulin response you would get from the carbohydrates (thereby preventing the negative, anti-ketogenic effects of eating carbs) but could potentially give you an acute cognitive effect (King et al., 1988). No studies have looked directly at TKD, but individuals who are training hard have reported great benefits with this type of approach. Keep in mind that your particular goal (fat loss, muscle gain, performance, etc.) will determine what is optimal for you.

Regardless, we do not recommend attempting TKD until you are thoroughly keto-adapted, and then we suggest that you start by experimenting with consuming a small amount of carbohydrates (i.e., less than 30 grams) before or during your workout.

What type of exercise is best on a ketogenic diet?

Any exercise is better than no exercise! However, we have found in our lab that training at a high intensity can increase the production of ketones. So train hard and try to incorporate resistance training with some type of cardio, even if that means just going for a walk after each meal.

Fasting

Can I fast on a ketogenic diet?

Not only can fasting be done on a ketogenic diet, but it may be beneficial for increasing ketone production (Reichard et al., 1974). However, research has found that fasting is not a requirement—you can produce ketones without fasting (Kim, Kang, Park, and Kim, 2004). We recommend that you give it a try at some point during your ketogenic journey to see if it's for you. (See page 49 for more on fasting.)

Is fasting safe?

We all go through periods of fasting—we fast while we're asleep, for example. Our hunter-gatherer ancestors went through periods of fasting throughout their lives. While there may be cases in which extended periods of fasting might not be beneficial, such as when cortisol levels are uncontrollable or possibly during pregnancy, studies have found that in general fasting can be safely implemented into an individual's lifestyle (Michalsen et al., 2005).

What fasting approaches can I use?

There are three main fasting protocols:

- **Intermittent eating:** fasting for a portion of the day followed by an eating window
- **Alternate-day eating:** fasting for an entire day followed by a day of normal eating
- **Total fasting:** complete restriction of food for days or even weeks

See page 49 for more on fasting.

Do I have to eat breakfast?

Contrary to what you have probably been told your whole life, breakfast isn't necessarily the most important meal of the day. If you choose to fast, you can certainly skip breakfast—or even have a "fat fast" breakfast (see the next question) of coffee with MCTs—and then eat your first meal in the afternoon.

What is fat fasting?

Fat fasting is exactly what it sounds like: consuming only fat during a fasting period. Research has shown that consuming fat alone does not increase insulin levels (Welle, Lilavivat, and Campbell, 1981), can improve insulin sensitivity (Boden, Chen, Rosner, and Barton, 1995), and mimics the body's reactions that occur during normal fasting. Therefore, having coffee with some MCT oil or heavy cream might mimic the response you would achieve with fasting.

Health Concerns

Can the ketogenic diet help me manage specific health problems?

Absolutely. Obesity and insulin resistance are at the root of many diseases, including type 2 diabetes and heart disease, and the fact that both can be improved on a ketogenic diet may suggest that the diet can help with those situations. Additionally, there is strong evidence that a ketogenic diet benefits conditions such as epilepsy and Glut1 deficiency (Veech, 2004). In section 6 of Chapter 5, we discuss how the diet may help with conditions such as type 2 diabetes, Alzheimer's, Parkinson's, ALS, multiple sclerosis, depression, PTSD, and cancer.

What is insulin resistance, and how do I know if I have it?

Insulin resistance is the inability to effectively utilize insulin, the hormone that moves glucose from the bloodstream into the cells. Insulin resistance means that insulin is not properly communicating with cells, and it can contribute to many metabolic diseases, particularly type 2 diabetes. If you often feel lethargic and easily gain weight from consuming carbohydrates, there is a high probability that you have some degree of insulin resistance. Ask your doctor to test your fasting blood glucose and insulin levels or, if possible, run an oral glucose tolerance test. (See page 19 for more on insulin resistance.)

To run an oral glucose tolerance test at home:

1) Do an overnight fast of twelve hours. Upon waking in the morning, measure your fasting blood glucose. This is your baseline (ideally between 80 and 120 mg/dL).

2) Drink 75 grams of a glucose/sugar-containing drink, such as orange juice or a sports drink.

3) Measure your blood glucose over a period of 120 minutes (at 0, 30, 60, 90, and 120 minutes after the initial measurement).

4) Record your numbers and see how they compare to your baseline.

My cholesterol has gone up since starting a ketogenic diet. What should I do?

Total cholesterol is not the best marker to look at because it does not take into consideration the composition of the cholesterol. The ketogenic diet has been shown to increase HDL (good) cholesterol (Yancy et al., 2004), which would lead to an increase in total cholesterol but would be beneficial overall. Be sure to have your doctor check the breakdown of your blood lipid tests and look for better markers, such as VLDL, LCL particle size, LDL-to-HDL ratio, triglycerides, and even high-sensitivity CRP (not traditionally part of a cholesterol panel). Also, see the question that discusses potential reasons why altering the fat composition of a ketogenic diet can help with cholesterol profiles. (For more on cholesterol and triglycerides, see page 88.)

I'm concerned about raising my triglyceride levels. Will a high-fat diet raise triglycerides?

No! It's a common myth that eating a lot of fat causes high triglyceride levels. Research has found that when a high-fat diet is paired with carbohydrate restriction, triglyceride levels actually drop (Sharman et al., 2002).

My doctor said that a ketogenic diet is bad. What should I do?

We hear this all the time, in spite of all the research showing the benefits of keto. The best thing you can do is to educate yourself and offer educational materials to your doctor. If that approach doesn't work, it may be time to consider a new physician who is supportive of your nutitional choices. A solid list of doctors who support the ketogenic diet can be found at http://ketogenic.com/tools/keto-clinicians-finder/.

Everyday Considerations

Can I eat out on a ketogenic diet?

Absolutely. In fact, we find that eating out on a ketogenic diet is much easier than eating out on a low-fat diet. You can never go wrong with a nice Cobb salad or a fatty cut of meat with a side of vegetables cooked in melted butter. Be careful of hidden carbs, such as those used in sauces and salad dressings. Don't be afraid to ask your server how a dish is prepared prior to ordering.

If you're traveling and want to take along a snack, pack some nuts, pork rinds (or pork skins), and/or Parmesan crisps.

What should I do if I hit a weight-loss plateau?

As with any eating plan, it is possible to hit a plateau on the ketogenic diet. If this happens to you, it is time to reassess your diet. Ask yourself the following questions:

- Are my carbs low enough?
- Have I tried increasing or decreasing my protein intake?
- What is my total calorie intake?
- Have I tried cutting out dairy?
- Am I consuming too many artificial sweeteners?
- Have I tried tracking my macros and measuring my food?

Keep in mind that the number on the scale doesn't always tell you what's really going on inside. If you lose 2 pounds of fat and gain 2 pounds of muscle, you may not have lost any weight, but you are losing fat and gaining muscle, which is exactly what you want.

What happens if I cheat one weekend?

While eating more carbs every weekend may not be ideal (see the question on carb refeeds on page 353), slip-ups do happen, and while they should be rare, they should not cause you to panic. If you get kicked out of ketosis, you may feel groggy or have a hard time focusing for a short time, but get back on track and you'll feel normal again soon. The longer you've been keto-adapted, the quicker you'll return to ketosis after a cheat day. Remember, this is a lifestyle and not a temporary fix. We are in this for the long game.

I want to help a family member or friend try keto. How can I get them on board?

Start by telling them about the ketogenic diet and offering them educational materials such as this book or pointing them to online resources, such as the website Ketogenic.com. Tell them about your own background with the ketogenic diet, too: hearing about others' experiences often helps people open their minds to something new.

References

American Heart Association. "How much sodium should I eat per day?" Accessed December 7, 2016. https://sodiumbreakup.heart.org/how_much_sodium_should_i_eat.

Bilsborough, S. A., and T. C. Crowe. "Low carbohydrate diets: what are the potential short and long term health implications?" *Asia Pacific Journal of Clinical Nutrition* 12, no. 4 (2003): 396–404.

Boden, G., X. Chen, J. Rosner, and M. Barton. "Effects of a 48-h fat infusion on insulin secretion and glucose utilization." *Diabetes* 44, no. 10 (1995): 1239–42.

Bough, K. J., J. Wetherington, B. Hassel, J. F. Pare, J. W. Gawryluk, J. G. Greene, R. Shaw, Y. Smith, J. D. Geiger, and R. J. Dingledine. "Mitochondrial biogenesis in the anticonvulsant mechanism of the ketogenic diet." *Annals of Neurology* 60, no. 2 (2006): 223–35. doi: 10.1002/ana.20899.

Bueno, N. B., I. S. de Melo, S. L. de Oliveira, and T. da Rocha Ataide. "Very-low-carbohydrate ketogenic diet v. low-fat diet for long-term weight loss: a meta-analysis of randomised controlled trials." *British Journal of Nutrition* 110, no. 07 (2013): 1178–87. doi: 10.1017/S0007114513000548.

Burke, L. M., D. J. Angus, G. R. Cox, N. K. Cummings, M. A. Febbraio, K. Gawthorn, J. A. Hawley, M. Minehan, D. T. Martin, and M. Hargreaves. "Effect of fat adaptation and carbohydrate restoration on metabolism and performance during prolonged cycling." *Journal of Applied Physiology* 89, no. 6 (2000): 2413–21.

Cartwright, M. M., W. Hajja, S. Al-Khatib, M. Hazeghazam, D. Sreedhar, R. N. Li, E. Wong-McKinstry, and R. W. Carlson. "Toxigenic and metabolic causes of ketosis and ketoacidotic syndromes." *Critical Care Clinics* 28, no. 4 (2012): 601–31. doi: 10.1016/j.ccc.2012.07.001.

Civitarese, A. E., M. K. Hesselink, A. P. Russell, E. Ravussin, and P. Schrauwen. "Glucose ingestion during exercise blunts exercise-induced gene expression of skeletal muscle fat oxidative genes." *American Journal of Physiology-Endocrinology and Metabolism* 289(6) (2005): E1023–29. doi: 10.1152/ajpendo.00193.2005.

Clarke, K., K. Tchabanenko, R. Pawlosky, E. Carter, M. T. King, K. Musa-Veloso, M. Ho, A. Roberts, J. Robertson, T. B. Vanitallie, and R. L. Veech. "Kinetics, safety and tolerability of (R)-3-hydroxybutyl (R)-3-hydroxybutyrate in healthy adult subjects." *Regulatory Toxicology and Pharmacology* 63, no. 3 (2012): 401–8. doi: 10.1016/j.yrtph.2012.04.008.

Courchesne-Loyer A., M. Fortier, J. Tremblay-Mercier, R. Chouinard-Watkins, M. Roy, S. Nugent, C. A. Castellano, and S. C. Cunnane. "Stimulation of mild, sustained ketonemia by medium-chain triacylglycerols in healthy humans: estimated potential contribution to brain energy metabolism." *Nutrition* 29, no. 4 (2013): 635–40. doi: 10.1016/j.nut.2012.09.009.

Cunnane S., S. Nugent, M. Roy, A. Courchesne-Loyer, E. Croteau, S. Tremblay, A. Castellano, F. Pifferi, C. Bocti, N. Paquet, H. Begdouri, M. Bentourkia, E. Turcotte, M. Allard, P. Barberger-Gateau, T. Fulop, and S. I. Rapoport. "Brain fuel metabolism, aging, and Alzheimer's disease." *Nutrition* 27, no. 1 (2011): 3–20. doi: 10.1016/j.nut.2010.07.021.

Evans, M., K. E. Cogan, and B. Egan. "Metabolism of ketone bodies during exercise and training: physiological basis for exogenous supplementation." *Journal of Physiology* 595, no. 9 (2016): 2857–71. doi: 10.1113/JP273185.

Freeman, J. M., E. H. Kossoff, and A. L. Hartman. "The ketogenic diet: one decade later." *Pediatrics* 119, no. 3 (2007): 535–43. doi: 10.1542/peds.2006-2447.

Freeman, J. M., E. P. Vining, D. J. Pillas, P. L. Pyzik, J. C. Casey, and L. M. Kelly. "The efficacy of the ketogenic diet–1998: a prospective evaluation of intervention in 150 children." *Pediatrics* 102(6) (1998): 1358–63.

García-Cáceres, C., E. Fuente-Martín, J. Argente, and J. A. Chowen. "Emerging role of glial cells in the control of body weight." *Molecular Metabolism* 1, nos. 1–2 (2012): 37–46. doi: 10.1016/j.molmet.2012.07.001.

Gasior, M., M. A. Rogawski, and A. L. Hartman. "Neuroprotective and disease-modifying effects of the ketogenic diet." *Behavioural Pharmacology* 17, nos. 5–6 (2006): 431–9.

Gregory, R. M. "A low-carbohydrate ketogenic diet combined with 6 weeks of CrossFit training improves body composition and performance." Dissertation/Thesis, James Madison University (2016).

Horowitz, J. F., R. Mora-Rodriguez, L. O. Byerley, and E. F. Coyle. "Lipolytic suppression following carbohydrate ingestion limits fat oxidation during exercise." *American Journal of Physiology-Endocrinology and Metabolism* 273, no. 4, Pt. 1 (1997): E768–75.

Johnston, K. L., M. N. Clifford, and L. M. Morgan. "Coffee acutely modifies gastrointestinal hormone secretion and glucose tolerance in humans: glycemic effects of chlorogenic acid and caffeine." *American Journal of Clinical Nutrition* 78, no. 4 (2003): 728–33.

Johnstone, A. M., G. W. Horgan, S. D. Murison, D. M. Bremner, and G. E. Lobley. "Effects of a high-protein ketogenic diet on hunger, appetite, and weight loss in obese men feeding ad libitum." *American Journal of Clinical Nutrition* 87, no. 1 (2008): 44–55.

Kang, H. C., Y. M. Lee, H. D. Kim, J. S. Lee, and A. Slama. "Safe and effective use of the ketogenic diet in children with epilepsy and mitochondrial respiratory chain complex defects." *Epilepsia* 48, no. 1 (2007): 82–88.

Kesl, S. L., A. M. Poff, N. P. Ward, T. N. Fiorelli, A. Csilla, A. J. Van Putten, J. W. Sherwood, P. Arnold, and D. P. D'Agostino. "Effects of exogenous ketone supplementation on blood ketone, glucose, triglyceride, and lipoprotein levels in Sprague–Dawley rats." *Nutrition & Metabolism* 13 (2016): 9. doi: 10.1186/s12986-016-0069-y.

Kim, D. W., H. C. Kang, J. C. Park, and H. D. Kim. "Benefits of the nonfasting ketogenic diet compared with the initial fasting ketogenic diet." *Pediatrics* 114, no. 6 (2004): 1627–30. doi: 10.1542/peds.2004-1001.

King, D. S., G. P. Dalsky, W. E. Clutter, D. A. Young, M. A. Staten, P. E. Cryer, and J. O. Holloszy. "Effects of lack of exercise on insulin secretion and action in trained subjects." *American Journal of Physiology-Endocrinology and Metabolism* 254, no. 5 (1988): E537–42.

Michalsen, A., B. Hoffmann, S. Moebus, M. Bäcker, J. Langhorst, and G. J. Dobos. "Incorporation of fasting therapy in an integrative medicine ward: evaluation of outcome, safety, and effects on lifestyle adherence in a large prospective cohort study." *Journal of Alternative & Complementary Medicine* 11, no. 4 (2005): 601–7.

Misell, L. M., N. D. Lagomarcino, V. Schuster, and M. Kern. "Chronic medium-chain triacylglycerol consumption and endurance performance in trained runners." *Journal of Sports Medicine and Physical Fitness* 41, no. 2 (2001): 210–5.

Musa-Veloso, K., S. S. Likhodii, and S. C. Cunnane. "Breath acetone is a reliable indicator of ketosis in adults consuming ketogenic meals." *American Journal of Clinical Nutrition* 76, no. 1 (2002): 65–70.

Nielsen, Jörgen V., and Eva A. Joensson. "Low-carbohydrate diet in type 2 diabetes: stable improvement of bodyweight and glycemic control during 44 months follow-up." *Nutrition & Metabolism* (London) 5 (2008): 14. doi: 10.1186/1743-7075-5-14.

Paoli, A., K. Grimaldi, D. D'Agostino, L. Cenci, T. Moro, A. Bianco, and A. Palma. "Ketogenic diet does not affect strength performance in elite artistic gymnasts." *Journal of the International Society of Sports Nutrition* 9, no. 1 (2012): 34. doi: 10.1186/1550-2783-9-34.

Paoli, A., A. Bianco, K. A. Grimaldi, A. Lodi, and G. Bosco. "Long term successful weight loss with a combination biphasic ketogenic Mediterranean diet and Mediterranean diet maintenance protocol." *Nutrients* 5, no. 12 (2013): 5205–17. doi: 10.3390/nu5125205.

Pascoe, D. D., D. L. Costill, W. J. Fink, R. A. Robergs, and J. J. Zachwieja. "Glycogen resynthesis in skeletal muscle following resistive exercise." *Medicine and Science in Sports and Exercise* 25, no. 3 (1993): 349–54.

Pérez-Guisado, J., A. Muñoz-Serrano, and Á. Alonso-Moraga. "Spanish ketogenic Mediterranean diet: a healthy cardiovascular diet for weight loss." *Nutrition Journal* 7, no. 1 (2008): 30. doi: 10.1186/1475-2891-7-30.

Phinney, S. D., E. S. Horton, E. A. Sims, J. S. Hanson, E. Danforth Jr., and B. M. Lagrange. "Capacity for moderate exercise in obese subjects after adaptation to a hypocaloric, ketogenic diet." *Journal of Clinical Investigation* 66, no. 5 (1980): 1152–61. doi: 10.1172/JCI109945.

Rebello, C. J., J. N. Keller, A. G. Liu, W. D. Johnson, and F. L. Greenway. "Pilot feasibility and safety study examining the effect of medium chain triglyceride supplementation in subjects with mild cognitive impairment: A randomized controlled trial." *BBA Clinical* 3 (2015): 123–5.

Reichard Jr., G. A., O. E. Owen, A. C. Haff, P. Paul, and W. M. Bortz. "Ketone-body production and oxidation in fasting obese humans." *Journal of Clinical Investigation* 53, no. 2 (1974): 508–15. doi: 10.1172/JCI107584.

Seaton T. B., S. L. Welle, M. K. Warenko, and R. G. Campbell. "Thermic effect of medium-chain and long-chain triglycerides in man." *American Journal of Clinical Nutrition* 44, no. 5 (1986): 630–4.

Sharman, M. J., W. J. Kraemer, D. M. Love, N. G. Avery, A. L. Gómez, T. P. Scheett, and J. S. Volek. "A ketogenic diet favorably affects serum biomarkers for cardiovascular disease in normal-weight men." *Journal of Nutrition* 132, no. 7 (2002): 1879–85.

Sharp, M. S., R. P. Lowery, K. A. Shields, C. A. Hollmer, J. R. Lane, J. M. Partl, ... and J. M. Wilson. "The 8 week effects of very low carbohydrate dieting vs very low carbohydrate dieting with refeed on body composition." NSCA National Conference, Orlando, FL. (2015).

Sumithran, P., L. A. Prendergast, E. Delbridge, K. Purcell, A. Shulkes, A. Kriketos, et al. "Long-term persistence of hormonal adaptations to weight loss." *New England Journal of Medicine* 365 (2011): 1597–604. doi: 10.1056/NEJMoa1105816.

Sumithran, P., L. A. Prendergast, E. Delbridge, K. Purcell, A. Shulkes, A. Kriketos, et al. "Ketosis and appetite-mediating nutrients and hormones after weight loss." *European Journal of Clinical Nutrition* 67 (2013): 759–64. doi: 10.1038/ejcn.2013.90.

Suo, C., J. Liao, X. Lu, K. Fang, Y. Hu, L. Chen, ... and C. Li. "Efficacy and safety of the ketogenic diet in Chinese children." *Seizure* 22, no. 3 (2013): 174–8.

Tiwari, S., S. Riazi, and C. A. Ecelbarger. "Insulin's impact on renal sodium transport and blood pressure in health, obesity, and diabetes." *American Journal of Physiology-Renal Physiology* 293, no. 4 (2007): F974–84.

Traul, K. A., A. Driedger, D. L. Ingle, and D. Nakhasi. "Review of the toxicologic properties of medium-chain triglycerides." *Food and Chemical Toxicology* 38, no. 1 (2000): 79–98.

Vandenberghe, C., V. St-Pierre, A. Courchesne-Loyer, M. Hennebelle, C. A. Castellano, and S. C. Cunnane. "Caffeine intake increases plasma ketones: an acute metabolic study in humans." *Canadian Journal of Physiology and Pharmacology* 95, no. 4 (2017): 455–8. doi: 10.1139/cjpp-2016-0338.

Veech, R. L. "The therapeutic implications of ketone bodies: the effects of ketone bodies in pathological conditions: ketosis, ketogenic diet, redox states, insulin resistance, and mitochondrial metabolism." *Prostaglandins, Leukotrienes and Essential Fatty Acids* 70, no. 3 (2004): 309–19.

Volek, J. S., D. J. Freidenreich, C. Saenz, L. J. Kunces, B. C. Creighton, J. M. Bartley, ... and E. C. Lee. "Metabolic characteristics of keto-adapted ultra-endurance runners." *Metabolism* 65, no. 3 (2016): 100–10.

Volek, J. S., M. J. Sharman, A. L. Gómez, D. A. Judelson, M. R. Rubin, G. Watson, ... and W. J. Kraemer. "Comparison of energy-restricted very low-carbohydrate and low-fat diets on weight loss and body composition in overweight men and women." *Nutrition & Metabolism* 1, no. 1 (2004): 13.

Volek, J. S., M. J. Sharman, D. M. Love, N. G. Avery, T. P. Scheett, and W. J. Kraemer. "Body composition and hormonal responses to a carbohydrate-restricted diet." *Metabolism* 51, no. 7 (2002): 864–70.

Wallace, T. M., N. M. Meston, S. G. Gardner, and D. R. Matthews. "The hospital and home use of a 30-second hand-held blood ketone meter: guidelines for clinical practice." *Diabetic Medicine* 18, no. 8 (2001): 640–5.

Welle, S., U. Lilavivat, and R. G. Campbell. "Thermic effect of feeding in man: increased plasma norepinephrine levels following glucose but not protein or fat consumption." *Metabolism* 30, no. 10 (1981): 953–8.

Westman, E. C., R. D. Feinman, J. C. Mavropoulos, M. C. Vernon, J. S. Volek, J. A. Wortman, ... and S. D. Phinney. "Low-carbohydrate nutrition and metabolism." *American Journal of Clinical Nutrition* 86, no. 2 (2007): 276–84.

Westman, E. C., W. S. Yancy, J. C. Mavropoulos, M. Marquart, and J. R. McDuffie. "The effect of a low-carbohydrate, ketogenic diet versus a low-glycemic index diet on glycemic control in type 2 diabetes mellitus." *Nutrition & Metabolism* 5, no. 1 (2008): 36.

Yancy, W. S., M. K. Olsen, J. R. Guyton, R. P. Bakst, and E. C. Westman. "A low-carbohydrate, ketogenic diet versus a low-fat diet to treat obesity and hyperlipidemia: A randomized, controlled trial." *Annals of Internal Medicine* 140, no. 10 (2004): 769–77.

Young, C. M., S. S. Scanlan, H. S. Im, and L. Lutwak. "Effect on body composition and other parameters in obese young men of carbohydrate level of reduction diet." *American Journal of Clinical Nutrition* 24, no. 3 (1971): 290–6.

RECOMMENDED
BRANDS AND PRODUCTS

There are more keto-friendly foods on the market today than ever before. In the lists here, you will find some of our favorite brands and products. If an item isn't listed, it doesn't mean that we don't recommend it or that we don't like it, but rather that there may be multiple other brands or products that you could find at your local grocer.

Sweeteners	
ERYTHRITOL	Swerve
MONK FRUIT (LUO HAN GUO)	Lakanto
STEVIA	NuNaturals

Bagels, Breads, and Buns	
BAGELS	Great Low Carb Bread Company
CRUMBS/COATING	Know Foods
BUNS	Know Foods
PIZZA CRUST	ThinSlim Foods
SLICED BREAD	Great Low Carb Bread Company
WRAPS	Flat Out Bread (Light)

Drinks	
COLD BREW COFFEE	Caveman Coffee Co.
DIET SODA (NO ARTIFICIAL SWEETENERS)	Zevia
FLAVORED WATER	Hint
MUSHROOM COFFEE	Four Sigmatic
NOOTROPIC COFFEE	Kimera Koffee
READY-TO-MIX KETO COFFEE	Coffee Blocks
WATER FLAVORING	Sweet Leaf Drops

Crackers and Crunchies	
CHEESE CRISPS	Cello Whisps
CHEESE	Moon Cheese
COCONUT CHIPS	Made in Nature
CRACKER THINS	Know Better
FLAXSEED CRACKERS	Food Alive
KALE CHIPS	Rhythm Superfoods
PORK RINDS	4505 Chicharrones

Flours	
ALMOND FLOUR	Bob's Red Mill
ALMOND MEAL	Honeyville
COCONUT FLOUR	Nutiva
GROUND FLAXSEED	Spectrum Essentials
MULTIPURPOSE BAKING MIX	Quest Nutrition

Guilty Pleasures	
BROWNIES	Good Dee's Brownie Mix
CAKE	Smart Baking Company
CANDY BAR	Quest Hero Bar
CANDY SOURS	XyloBurst
CHOCOLATE BARS	Lily's
CHOCOLATE SQUARES	ChocZero
COOKIES	Keto Kookie
FUDGE	Phat Fudge
GUMMIES	Smart Sweets
ICE CREAM	Enlightened
MUFFINS AND CUPCAKES	Know Foods
PEANUT BUTTER CUPS	Eating Evolved
PIZZA	Real Good Pizza
SPAGHETTI AND NOODLES	Miracle Noodle
SYRUPS (PANCAKE AND CARAMEL)	Walden Farms

Meats, Jerky, and Bars	
BEEF JERKY	Chomps
CANNED TUNA	Wild Planet Foods
HOME-DELIVERED CHICKEN	ButcherBox
HOME-DELIVERED PORK	US Wellness Meats
HOME-DELIVERED BEEF	Crowd Cow
HOME-DELIVERED BISON	The Honest Bison
HIGH FAT, LOW CARB BAR	Keto Bar
MEAT BAR	EPIC
PROTEIN BAR	Quest Nutrition
WILD SALMON	Vital Choice

Protein	
ALL-NATURAL PROTEIN BLEND	Biotrust Nutrition
BONE BROTH	Kettle & Fire
BONE BROTH PROTEIN	Ancient Nutrition
COLLAGEN PROTEIN	Vital Proteins
MICELLAR CASEIN	EAS
PROTEIN SPREAD	G Butter
WHEY-CASEIN PROTEIN BLEND	Quest Nutrition
WHEY PROTEIN	Dymatize Nutrition Iso 100

Nuts and Nut Butters	
FLAVORED ALMONDS	Legendary Foods
FLAVORED FAT SHOT	Adapt Your Life
MACADAMIA NUT BUTTER	F-Bomb
MACADAMIA NUTS	Mauna Loa
PEANUT AND ALMOND BUTTERS	Legendary Foods
POWDERED PEANUT BUTTER	PB Fit
PILI NUTS	Hunter Gatherer Foods Sprouted Pili Nuts
SUNFLOWER BUTTER	Wild Friends

Oils and Condiments	
BBQ SAUCE	Stubbs
COCONUT MANNA	Nutiva
DUCK FAT	Fatworks
EMULSIFIED MCT OIL	Natural Force
FLAVORED GHEE	Pure Indian Foods
GHEE OIL	Fourth & Heart
HIMALAYAN SALT	San Francisco Salt Co.
HONEY MUSTARD	Primal Kitchen
MCT AND COCONUT OIL POWDER	Quest Nutrition
OLIVES	Oloves
SEASONINGS	Oh My Spice
SEA SALT	Real Salt
TERIYAKI	LC Foods

KETOGENIC
RESOURCES

Herbert Spencer, one of the best-known and most well-respected philosophers of the nineteenth century, said, "The great aim of education is not knowledge, but action." In this day and age, with the internet and various other research platforms, we have access to just about anything we want to know. The problem is that research can often be misinterpreted or misunderstood. When we built the Applied Science and Performance Institute, we set out on a mission to help change people's lives through science and innovation. We wanted to break down complex scientific information and relay it to people in an easy-to-understand manner. We wanted to become a trusted resource so that everyone would know that for any given topic, we would research everything relating to exercise, nutrition, or supplementation. We stand here today with that same mission to help change as many lives as possible through science, innovation, and education.

We want to bring you the best resources possible in order to help you make decisions about living an optimal lifestyle. We want you to be equipped with the best information, not only so that you can incorporate what you have learned in this book into your lifestyle, but also so that you can share these resources with other people who may be searching for answers as well.

With that in mind, we have compiled a list of some of our favorite books, websites, podcasts, and organizations, which we often refer people to when they have questions about the ketogenic lifestyle. These sources are backed by research and have been recommended by other established professionals and experts within the realm of exercise and nutrition science. We've also provided a curated list of doctors who are experienced with and supportive of the ketogenic lifestyle.

Books

Personal growth takes time and persistence. In life, it's the small, incremental steps you take every day toward self-improvement that add up over time to incredible changes. For example, taking just 3 percent of your day—thirty minutes—to read a book and explore a new area can add up over the

course of several months, a year, and even a lifetime. If ketogenic dieting is something you are truly interested in or you know someone who may benefit from the diet, then it may be advantageous to seek out the opinions of others by reading their books.

We hope to provide a lot of information within *The Ketogenic Bible,* but by no means is this the be-all, end-all resource on the ketogenic diet and ketosis. Many others have done incredible jobs presenting information that we may have only touched upon, and reading about something from a different viewpoint could help you nail down the concept and allow you to implement a change in your lifestyle. Below is a list of some of our favorite books from experts across the globe who have been pioneers in exploring various aspects of the ketogenic diet.

Some Recommended Reading	
KETOGENIC DIET AND METABOLIC THERAPIES	Susan A. Masino
KETOGENICA PRINCIPIA	A. Simmonds
NEW ATKINS FOR A NEW YOU	Eric C. Westman and Stephen D. Phinney
THE BIG FAT SURPRISE	Nina Teicholz
THE ART AND SCIENCE OF LOW CARBOHYDRATE LIVING/PERFORMANCE	Jeff Volek and Stephen D. Phinney
LOW CARB, HIGH FAT FOOD REVOLUTION	Andreas Eenfeldt
KETO CLARITY	Jimmy Moore and Eric C. Westman
THE REAL MEAL REVOLUTION	Tim Noakes and Jonno Proudfoot
TRIPPING OVER THE TRUTH	Travis Christofferson
CANCER AS A METABOLIC DISEASE: ON THE ORIGIN, MANAGEMENT, AND PREVENTION OF CANCER	Thomas Seyfried
SUGAR FREE: 8 WEEKS TO FREEDOM FROM SUGAR AND CARB ADDICTION	Karen Thompson
THE KETOGENIC COOKBOOK: NUTRITIOUS LOW-CARB, HIGH-FAT PALEO MEALS TO HEAL YOUR BODY	Jimmy Moore and Maria Emmerich
THE KETO DIET	Leanne Vogel

Websites, Podcasts, and Organizations

Several websites and podcasts have popped up with really intelligent individuals interviewing scientists, practitioners, and researchers on the ketogenic lifestyle. In addition, several organizations not only seek to educate people on the potential applications of the ketogenic diet but also help fund research studies to further the field. Below we have listed a number of outlets that provide exceptional information about ketogenic dieting. The websites listed contain articles and other content that can help you along your ketogenic journey. The organizations listed are either actively holding events and conferences around the ketogenic diet or doing research to help drive new findings in the field. Lastly, if you have a long commute to work or prefer listening to reading, we have listed some of our favorite podcasts, which often feature well-known experts on nutrition and fitness.

Top Websites

KETOGENIC.COM

RULED.ME

DIETDOCTOR.COM

KETOGENIC-DIET-RESOURCE.COM

KETONUTRITION.ORG

Top Organizations

CHARLIE FOUNDATION

EPIGENIX FOUNDATION AND KETOPET SANCTUARY

MATTHEW'S FRIENDS

EPILEPSY AND GLUT1 DEFICIENCY FOUNDATION

LOW CARB USA/UNIVERSE, FITCON, KETOKADEMY, METABOLIC THERAPEUTICS (KETO CONFERENCES)

Top Podcasts

LIVIN' LA VIDA LOW CARB / KETO TALK

BEN GREENFIELD FITNESS

THE KETO DIET PODCAST

KETOVANGELIST / THE KETOGENIC ATHLETE

BULLETPROOF RADIO

THE TIM FERRIS SHOW

PRIMAL EDGE HEALTH

FAT BURNING MAN

FIT 2 FAT 2 FIT

2 KETO DUDES

Keto Physicians

Finding a good doctor is hard enough as it is; when you're looking for a doctor who understands ketosis and the ketogenic diet, it can seem impossible. Most medical doctors receive just one or two classes on nutrition throughout their years of schooling, which limits many individuals' understanding of the benefits of certain diets, such as the ketogenic diet.

Currently, many doctors and researchers are conducting trials and case studies to investigate the implementation of a ketogenic diet on numerous disease states, including cancers. Furthermore, many physicians across the county use a low-carb nutritional approach to aid their patients with losing weight and overall health profiles.

We have provided a list of physicians, nutritionists, and other health experts who advocate for the use of a ketogenic diet. Please keep in mind that these doctors aren't necessarily utilizing the ketogenic diet for every condition or patient, and they may not necessarily be in favor of using it for your specific need. However, they are all knowledgeable about the ketogenic diet and support its use in certain situations. All of the doctors listed here have been contacted by our team and are ready and willing to help you achieve your goals! (If you aren't having any luck with this list, Ketogenic.com has a tool called Keto Clinicians Finder, which is constantly being updated with new doctors who support the ketogenic diet.)

Keto Physicians

Name	City	Practice	Phone
ALABAMA			
DR. JESSICA DIETRICH-MARSH	Pelham	Health Inc.	(205) 664-7707
CALIFORNIA			
DR. DEBORAH PENNER	Chico	Chico Creek Wellness & Chiropractic	(530) 342-8464
DR. ALLAN SOSIN	Irvine	Institute for Progressive Medicine	(949) 600-5100
DR. POUYA SHAFIPOUR	Los Angeles	Wellesley Medical	(310) 400-5565
DR. TRUDI PRATT	Redding	Chiropractic and Nutrition	(530) 244-7873
DR. ALLEN PETERS	Redondo Beach	Nourishing Wellness	(310) 373-7830
DR. SCOTT SHERR	Redwood City	Integrative Hyperbaric Oxygen Therapy	(650) 367-5544
DR. CARL KNOPKE	Riverside	Inland Empire Weight Loss	(951) 231-1363
DR. KELLY AUSTIN	San Diego	California Natural Health	(858) 675-7072
DR. LESLYN KEITH	San Luis Obispo	Central Coast Lymphedema Therapy	(805) 748-6519
DR. JEREMY KASLOW	Santa Ana	DrKaslow.com	(714) 565-1032
DR. ROBERT KROCHMAL	Woodland Hills	MD Integrative Wellness	(818) 999-9960
CONNECTICUT			
DR. KARA FITZGERALD	Sandy Hook	Functional Medicine	(203) 304-9502
DR. FRANK AIETA	West Prospect	Dr. Frank Aieta	(860) 232-9662
FLORIDA			
DR. OLIVER R. DI PIETRO	Bay Harbor Islands	The K-E Diet	(855) 553-3438
DR. CARRIE J. GRAVES	Clearwater	The Wellness Tree	(727) 346-6247
DR. DIEGO RUTENBERG	Miami	Holistic Specialists	(954) 394-9952
DR. JAYSON CALTON	Sarasota	Calton Nutrition	(941) 882-4297
DR. CYNTHIA CLARK	Sarasota	Longevity Wellness Clinic	(941) 923-9355

IDAHO

| DR. JASON WATSON | Boise | Active Health & Wellness | (208) 344-5433 |

INDIANA

| DR. JEFFREY GLADD | Fort Wayne | GladdMD Integrative Medicine | (260) 449-9698 |

IOWA

| DR. ZACHARY WATKINS | Clive | Livewell Clinic, LLC | (515) 279-9900 |

KANSAS

| DR. IRVING COHEN | Topeka | Preventive Medicine Associates, LLC | (785) 783-7779 |

KENTUCKY

| DR. PETER SWANZ | Louisville | Vital Force Naturopathy | (812) 716-4325 |

LOUISIANA

| DR. EDWARD C. LAFLEUR | Youngsville | | (337) 451-5952 |

MARYLAND

| DR. GEORGE YU | Annapolis | Totally Yu | (410) 897-0540 |
| DR. MARTIN PASSEN | Owings Mills | The Center for Medical Weight Loss | (410) 356-8446 |

MASSACHUSETTS

| DR. JUDY TSAFRIR | Newton Centre | JudyTsafrirMD.com | (617) 965-3020 |

MICHIGAN

| DR. JOSEPH WARDIE | Gross Pointe Woods | TRIAD Health Solutions | (586) 585-1494 |

MINNESOTA

| DR. KRISTI HUGHES | Alexandria | The Institute for Functional Medicine | (320) 762-4295 |
| DR. THOMAS SULT | New London | 3rd Opinion | (320) 347-1212 |

MISSOURI

| DR. REBECCA GOULD | Clayton | The Healing Center | (314) 727-2120 |
| DR. TIPU SULTAN | Florissant | Environmental Health and Allergy Center--St. Louis | (314) 921-5600 |

NEW HAMPSHIRE

| DR. PAULA DIAMOND-BEIR | Portsmouth | Human Nature Natural Health | (603) 610-7778 |

NEW JERSEY

| DR. MICHAEL ROTHMAN | East Brunswick | MD Wellness & Spa | (732) 268-7663 |

NEW MEXICO

| DR. JUSTIN HOFFMAN | Santa Fe | LightandLove.info | (505) 955-9919 |

NEW YORK

DR. KEITH BERKOWITZ	New York City	Center for Balanced Health	(212) 459-1700
DR. DENNIS GAGE	New York City	Thinderella Lifestyle Change	(212) 772-7628

NORTH CAROLINA

DR. ERIC WESTMAN	Durham	Duke Lifestyle Medicine Clinic	(919) 620-4060
DR. MARK O'NEAL SPEIGHT	Matthews	The Center for Wellness, PA	(704) 847-2022

OHIO

DR. GARY HUBER	Cincinnati	Huber Personalized Medicine	(513) 924-5300
CHELSEA CAITO, RD	Cincinnati	Huber Personalized Medicine	(513) 366-2123
DR. JIM LAVALLE	Cincinnati	LaValle Metabolic Institute	(513) 924-5300

OKLAHOMA

DR. DOUGLAS KELLY	Tulsa	Cancer Treatment Centers of America & Hillcrest Medical Center	(855) 504-5889

OREGON

DR. ELIE COLE	Milwaukie	The Nourishing Medicine Clinic	(503) 860-8998

SOUTH CAROLINA

DR. SHERRI JACOBS	Charleston	Health-E Coaching	(843) 408-0894
DR. PAMELA LYON	Columbia	WaistLines	(803) 419-3300

SWITZERLAND

DR. JEAN PIERRE SPINOSA	Lausanne	Dr méd. Jean-Pierre Spinosa	+41 21 329-0980

TENNESSEE

DR. CHAD YARBROUGH	Nashville	Center for Proactive Medicine	(615) 331-1973

TEXAS

DR. MARLENE MERRITT	Austin	Merritt Wellness Center	(512) 495-9015
DR. WILL MITCHELL	Austin	Merritt Wellness Center	(512) 495-9015
DR. STEVEN HOTZE	Katy	Hotze Health & Wellness Center	(877) 698-8698

VIRGINIA

DR. CHARLES SHAFFER	Christiansburg	The Weigh Station	(540) 381-2670

WASHINGTON

DR. TIM GERSTMAR	Redmond	Aspire Natural Health	(425) 202-7849
DR. TED NAIMAN	Issaquah	Virginia Mason Issaquah Medical Center	(425) 557-8000
DR. PATRICIA SYLWESTER	Olympia	Vital Rejuvenation	(360) 870-8616
DR. ROBERT THOMPSON	Seattle	LowGlycemicLoad.com	(206) 682-0757

WYOMING

DR. JESSE MILLER	Casper	eatmedicine.com	(307) 215-5750

Recipe Index

BREAKFAST

208 Classic Powdered Cake Doughnuts

210 Cauliflower Overnight "Oats"

212 Coconut Chocolate Chip Muffins

214 Breakfast Lasagna

216 Meat Lover's Quiche

218 Eggs Benedict

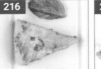
220 Maple Banana Pancakes

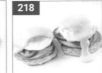
222 Bacon, Egg, and Cheese Sandwich

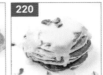
224 Breakfast Wraps with Pico de Gallo

226 Black Walnut Zucchini Bread with Maple Butter

228 Eggs in a Basket

229 Chorizo Hash Browns and Fried Eggs

230 Frittata Muffins

231 Green Goblin Breakfast Shake

APPETIZERS AND SMALL PLATES

234 Spinach Dip

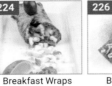
236 Stuffed Mushroom Caps

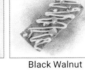
237 Bacon-Wrapped Asparagus

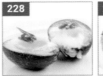
238 Jalapeño Poppers with Caramelized Onion Chutney

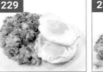
240 Stuffed Zucchini Boats with Spicy Ranch

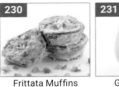
242 Broccoli Bites with Spicy Mustard

244 Barbecue Bacon-Wrapped Shrimp

246 Prosciutto-Wrapped Cocktail Sausages with Raspberry Maple Bacon Jam

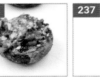
248 Bruschetta with Basil Oil

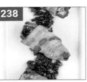
250 Jalapeño Pickled Deviled Eggs

252 Battered Buffalo Bites

254 Pistachio-Coated Goat Cheese with Raspberry Coulis

255 Basil–Cracked Pepper Parmesan Chips

256 Breaded Mozzarella Sticks

258 Chips and Smoky Queso Dip

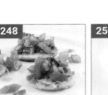
260 Bacon-Wrapped Feta

261 Chipotle BLTs

262 Buffalo Chicken Dip

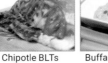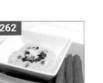

MAIN DISHES AND SIDES

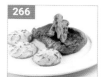
266
Dry-Aged Steaks with Duchess "Potatoes" and Pan-Fried Okra

268
New York Style Pizza

270
Chicken Avocado Roulade

272
Pumpkin Chili

274
Thai Coconut Curry

276
Chicken Stir-Fry

278
Brie Sirloin Sliders

280
California-Style Spaghetti and Meatballs

282
Shepherd's Pie

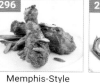
284
Bacon-Wrapped Cajun Casserole

286
Salmon over Spinach Risotto

288
Braised Pork Belly Tacos with Chipotle Red Pepper Chutney and Pickled Jalapeños

290
Pan-Seared Scallops with Pink Peppercorn Cream Sauce and Asparagus

292
Braised Pork Shoulder with Demi-Glace over Purple Cabbage

294
Italian Sausage–Stuffed Bell Peppers with Tomato-Mushroom Marinara

296
Memphis-Style Barbecued Chicken with Green Beans Amandine

298
Alaska Rolls with Sriracha Aioli

299
Roasted Asparagus with Parmesan and Himalayan Salt

300
Roasted Red Pepper Brown Butter Green Beans

301
Braised Bacon-y Brussels

302
Eggplant Parmesan with Marinara

DESSERTS

306
Classic Chocolate Chip Cookies

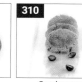
308
Double Chocolate Chip Cookies

310
Cardamom Snickerdoodles with Maple Bourbon Caramel

312
Chocolate Bark

314
Chocolate Mousse

316
Single-Serving Brownie Mug Cake

318
Classic Cheesecake

320
Sugar Cookies

322
Chocolate-Covered Bacon

324
Rich Chocolate Cupcakes with Swiss Buttercream

326
Chocolate Peanut Butter Fudge

327
Fudge Brownies

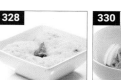
328
Single-Serving Lemon Blueberry Cake

330
Rich Chocolate Avocado Ice Cream

332
Maple Bourbon Pecan Avocado Ice Cream

334
Carrot Cake with Salted Caramel Frosting

336
Chocolate Peanut Butter Banana Truffles

338
Irish Cream Pistachio Cake Squares

Index